Heilmann / Paton

Atlas of Ophthalmic Surgery

Techniques – Complications

In Three Volumes · Volume II

Atlas of Ophthalmic Surgery

Edited by
Klaus Heilmann
David Paton

Techniques – Complications

In Three Volumes

Georg Thieme Verlag
Stuttgart · New York

Thieme Medical Publishers, Inc.
New York

Volume II

Cornea Glaucoma Lens

Editors
Douglas D. Koch
George L. Spaeth

With Contributions by

J. Draeger, Hamburg
J. M. Emery, Houston
C. S. Foster, Boston
J. C. Hays, Atlanta
K. Heilmann, Munich
S. H. Johnson, Newport Beach
H. E. Kaufman, New Orleans
D. D. Koch, Houston
R. P. Kratz, Newport Beach
D. B. Mark, Sunnyvale
M. B. McDonald, New Orleans
G. O. H. Naumann, Erlangen-Nürnberg
D. Paton, New York
I. P. Pollack, Baltimore
A. L. Robin, Baltimore
J. J. Rowsey, Oklahoma City
G. L. Spaeth, Philadelphia
R. Winter, Hamburg

561 Figures

Illustrated by Rudolf Brammer

Georg Thieme Verlag
Stuttgart · New York

Thieme Medical Publishers, Inc.
New York

1987

D-7000 Stuttgart 30, Germany
Thieme Medical Publishers, Inc.
381 Park Avenue South, New York, N.Y. 10016.
Typesetting: Kittelberger GmbH, Reutlingen
(System: 202 Linotype)
Printed in West-Germany by Grammlich, Pliezhausen

ISBN 3-13-656501-0 (Georg Thieme Verlag, Stuttgart)
ISBN 0-86577-180-4 (Thieme Medical Publishers, Inc., New York)

1 2 3 4 5 6

Library of Congress Cataloging-in-Publication Data
(Revised for vol. 2)

Atlas of ophthalmic surgery.

Vol. 2 – published in New York by Thieme Medical Publishers.
Includes bibliographies and index.
Contents: v. 1. Lids, orbits, extraocular muscles / editors, Charles K. Beyer-Machule, Gunter K. von Noorden – v. 2. Cornea, glaucoma, lens / editors, Douglas D. Koch, George L. Spaeth.
1. Eye–Surgery–Atlases. 2. Eyelids–Surgery–Atlases. 3. Eye-sockets – Surgery – Atlases. I. Heilmann, Klaus. II. Paton, David.
[RE80.A87 1985] 617.7'1 84-52205

Important Note: Medicine is an ever-changing science. Research and clinical experience are continually broadening our knowledge, in particular our knowledge of proper treatment and drug therapy. Insofar as this book mentions any dosage or application, readers may rest assured that the authors, editors and publishers have made every effort to ensure that such references are strictly in accordance with the state of knowledge at the time of production of the book. Nevertheless, every user is requested to examine carefully the manufacturer's leaflets accompanying each drug to check on his own responsibility whether the dosage schedules recommended therein or the contraindications stated by the manufacturers differ from the statements made in the present book. Such examination is particularly important with drugs that are either rarely used or have been newly released on the market.

Addresses

Jörg Draeger, M. D.
Augenklinik der Universität Hamburg
Martinistraße 52
D-2000 Hamburg 20
FRG

Jared M. Emery, M. D.
Cullen Eye Institute
Baylor College of Medicine
6501 Fannin
Houston, TX 77030
USA

C. Stephen Foster, M. D.
Massachusetts Eye and Ear Infirmary
243 Charles Street
Boston, MA 02114
USA

James C. Hays, M. D.
33 SW Upper Riverdale Rd., # 17
Riverdale, GA 30274
USA

Klaus Heilmann, M. D.
Beethovenplatz 2–3
D-8000 München 2
FRG

Stephen H. Johnson, M. D.
1441 Avocado Avenue, Suite 301
Newport Beach, CA 92660
USA

Herbert E. Kaufmann, M. D.
LSU Eye Center
136 South Roman Street
New Orleans, LA 70112
USA

Douglas D. Koch, M. D.
Cullen Eye Institute
Baylor College of Medicine
6501 Fannin
Houston, TX 77030
USA

Richard P. Kratz, M. D.
1441 Avocado Avenue, Suite 301
Newport Beach, CA 92660
USA

David B. Mark, M. D.
877 W. Freemont Ave.
Sunnyvale, CA 94087
USA

Marguerite B. McDonald, M. D.
LSU Eye Center
136 South Roman Street
New Orleans, LA 70112
USA

G. O. H. Naumann, M. D.
Augenklinik der Universität Erlangen-Nürnberg
Schwabachanlage 6
8520 Erlangen
FRG

David Paton, M. D.
120 East End Avenue
New York, NY 10028
USA

Irvin P. Pollack, M. D.
Wilmer Institute, Glaucoma Services
Johns Hopkins Hospital
Baltimore, MD
USA

Alan L. Robin, M. D.
Wilmer Institute, Glaucoma Services
Johns Hopkins Hospital
Baltimore, MD
USA

J. James Rowsey, M. D.
Dean A. McGee Eye Institute
University of Oklahoma
Oklahoma City, Oklahoma
USA

George L. Spaeth, M. D.
Wills Eye Hospital, Glaucoma Services
9th and Walnut Streets
Philadelphia, PA 19107
USA

Rolf Winter, M. D.
Augenklinik der Universität Hamburg
Martinistraße 52
D-2000 Hamburg 20
FRG

Preface

It is a source of great pleasure for the editors to present this second volume of the *Atlas of Ophthalmic Surgery,* covering microsurgical procedures on the cornea, the lens, and for treatment of glaucomas.

These topics make the breathtaking rate of progress in ophthalmic surgery in recent years particularly apparent: much that is possible in surgery today was considered impossible even a short time ago. We have tried to keep pace with developments, though without aspiring to furnish an overview of all recently publicized surgical procedures.

It was an honor and a pleasure for the editors to work with so many internationally renowned authors. We thank them for their unfailing cooperation and their patience in the protracted business of producing the book.

This volume also is written for physicians who, being conversant with the principles of general surgery and the fundamentals of ophthalmic diseases, wish to learn and/or practise special methods in ophthalmic surgery.

The tried and trusted didactic method used in Volume I has been retained: the descriptions of the procedures and the problems associated with them are built up entirely on the basis of the illustrations. Thus, the text serves as a link between series of illustrations. The texts and drawings are spatially related to one another; the result is a coherent, eminently "readable" sequence of illustrations and text.

All the illustrations were drawn by our medical artist, Rudolf Brammer, who was likewise responsible for the artwork in Volume I. He has wide knowledge of the subject and is an exceptionally talented artist. Thus it was that he was able to produce these illustrations, with their manifest scientific precision and outstanding artistic quality, on the basis of simple sketches made while the authors performed the various operations. The editors and authors admire his work with gratitude.

We owe a great debt of thanks to our colleagues George L. Spaeth of Philadelphia and Douglas D. Koch of Houston, for taking on the difficult task of specialist editors for this second volume. In our opinion they have accomplished it superbly.

The editors wish to extend thanks – also on behalf of the authors – to Nigel Rigby, for his valuable editorial work (and for translating several of the manuscripts into English), as well as Gert Krüger and Peter Helms, who were responsible for the layout.

Very special thanks are due to our publishers, Georg Thieme Verlag: were it not for their generosity and willingness to accommodate the authors' wishes, a work of this quality could never have been published.

The editors are proud of the fact that as a result of the unusually warm welcome accorded it by colleagues and critics, the *Atlas of Ophthalmic Surgery* is now also to be published simultaneously in German, Italian, and French. We hope that this second volume will be equally well received.

November 1986

Klaus Heilmann
David Paton

Volume Editors' Preface

This volume is designed to provide beginning and experienced ophthalmic surgeons with clear, concise descriptions of anterior segment surgical procedures. Ophthalmic microsurgery is evolving at an exhilaratingly rapid rate. This intensified the challenge that we as editors faced in selecting the techniques to be included. Our goal was to balance the new and the established, to incorporate innovation while emphasizing techniques that have withstood a reasonable amount of scrutiny and time.

By necessity, not all techniques or minor variations in techniques can be included. On the other hand, overlap in some of the procedures depicted is inevitable and intentional. We felt it important to include different authors' approaches in certain instances in order to illustrate better the nuances of these techniques.

We are grateful to our authors for the thought, concern, and time that they devoted to their contributions. We feel that one of the strengths of this volume is the diversity of views provided by our contributors from multiple centers in Germany and in the United States.

We wish to pay special thanks to Klaus Heilmann and David Paton, Nigel Rigby and Gert Krüger of Georg Thieme Verlag, our editor Adrienne Jacobson, and especially Rudolf Brammer, our medical illustrator. We are deeply appreciative of his astonishingly rapid grasp of our techniques, his tireless patience in dealing with us perfectionist authors, and his truly gifted ability to transform our microsurgical procedures into elegant, instructive illustrations.

November 1986

Douglas D. Koch
George L. Spaeth

Contents

4

Lens

Vol. I: Lids, Orbits, Extraocular Muscles
Edited by Charles K. Beyer-Machule
and Gunter K. von Noorden

Vol. III: Retina, Vitreous
Edited by Felipe I. Tolentino
and H. Mackenzie Freeman

1

Cornea

James C. Hays, Herbert E. Kaufman, Marguerite B. McDonald
David Paton, J. James Rowsey

Penetrating Keratoplasty

David Paton

Indications and Management Options

Penetrating keratoplasty has four main indications ranging from common to rare in the following order: optical, tectonic, therapeutic, and cosmetic.

Optical keratoplasty is usually the primary goal of keratoplasty, namely, to restore or enhance the visual role of the eye.

Tectonic keratoplasty is primarily for restoration of altered corneal structure and contour such as stromal thinning, descemetocele, and corneal perforation. Visual improvement may be a secondary goal, but is not the first priority.

Therapeutic keratoplasty is occasionally performed in situations where a portion of the cornea with active disease is replaced by a graft, as in progressive keratitis after failure of specific antimicrobial or anti-inflammatory therapy.

Cosmetic keratoplasty is rarely used, but is occasionally important, for example when a young adult is disfigured by an amblyopic eye with unilateral full-thickness corneal opacification, and the prognosis for successful corneal transplant is considered highly favorable.

It is obvious that measure of surgical success in each type of keratoplasty relates to the degree of accomplishment of the primary and secondary goals.

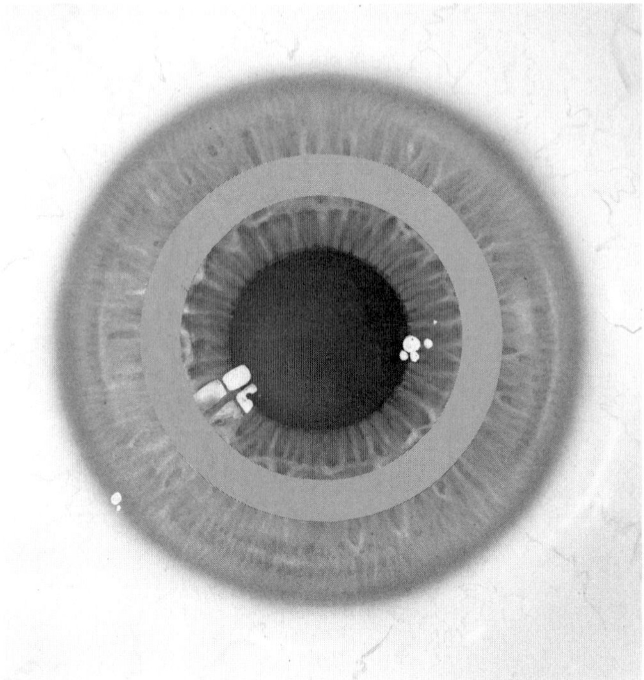

1.1 Every cornea of normal diameter has the same "optimal recipient zone," defined as that space located between the boundaries of hypothetical marks of a centered 6.5 mm trephine and a centered 8.0 mm trephine. If morphological characteristics of the individual diseased cornea are discounted, the ideal penetrating keratoplasty is a centered 7.5 mm graft. Smaller grafts produce more astigmatism depending upon the tissue status of the recipient, require precise centering, and are usually surrounded by a larger area of diseased recipient tissue (potentially an adverse factor in long-term graft success and in contact lens tolerance). Larger grafts have a higher incidence of allograft reaction, are more likely to be associated with iris adhesions (particularly if the anterior chamber is physiologically shallow), and lead to increased risk of regraft failure should the first graft opacify.

2

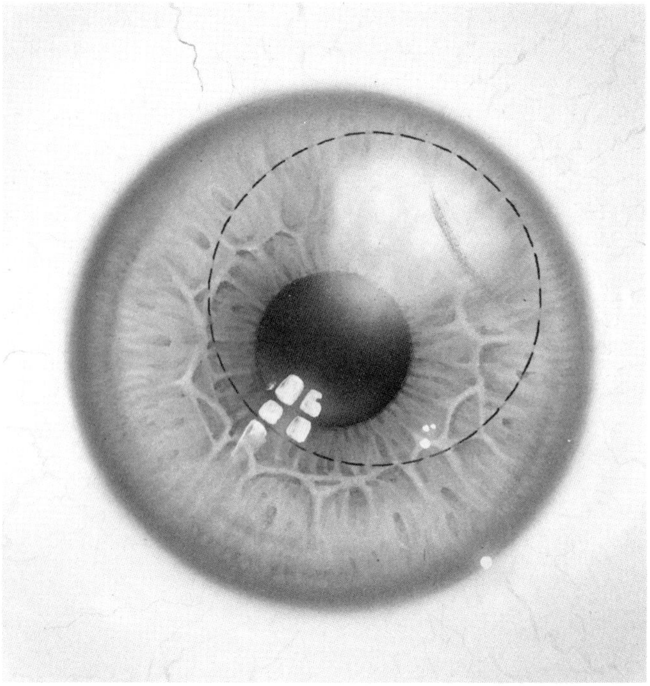

3

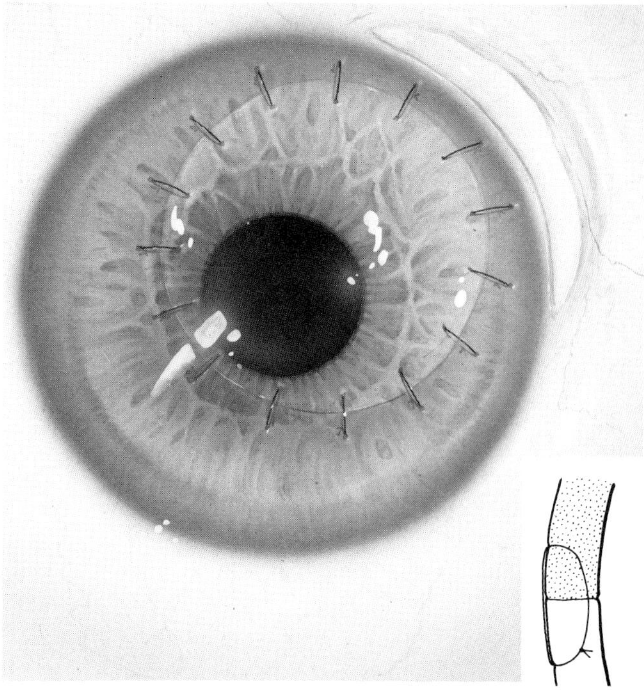

4

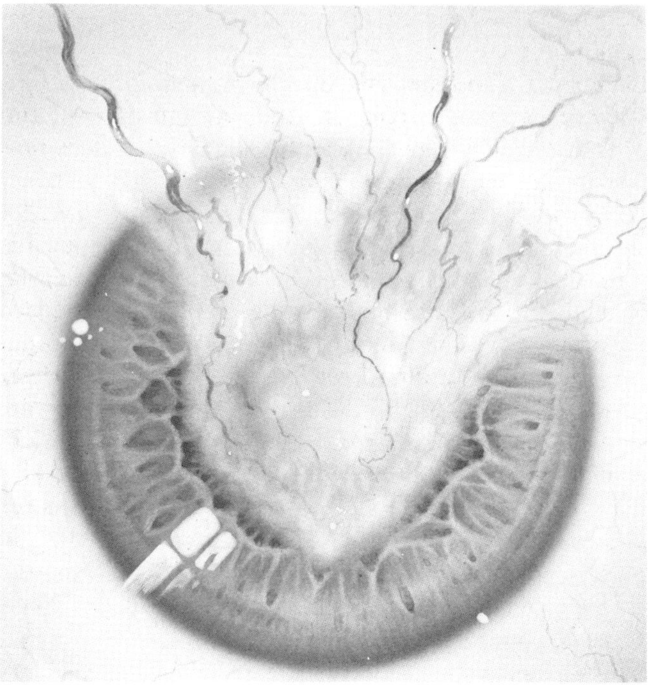

5

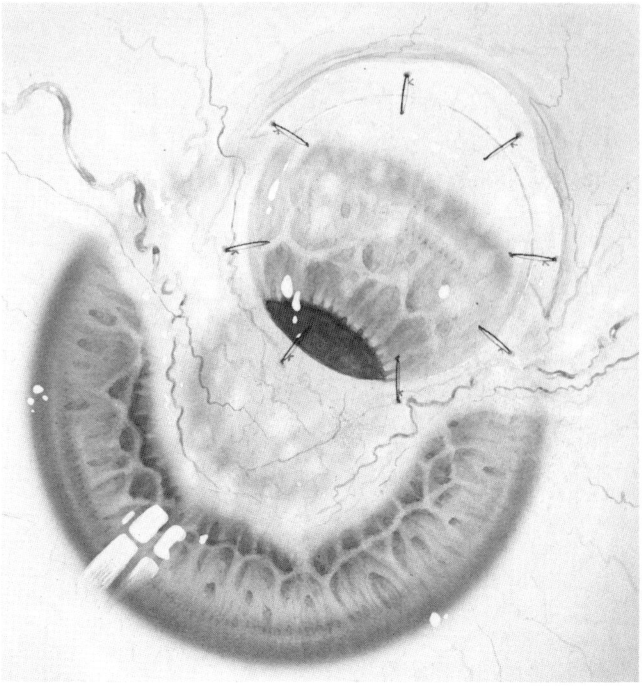

1.**2** and **3** If any portion of the recipient corneal tissue is less than one-half the normal corneal thickness within the optimal recipient zone, delay of healing and occurrence of tissue vascularization at that site are expected complications that can lead to graft failure. Thus, the surgeon must decide in advance of surgery whether he should decenter the graft to obtain a sufficient recipient tissue thickness throughout the circumference of the graft or, alternatively, whether tectonic lamellar keratoplasty to thicken the recipient tissue in the area of the optimal recipient zone should precede a subsequent optical penetrating keratoplasty procedure.

1.**4** to **8** A preliminary tectonic graft may be lamellar or penetrating. Here, a peripheral lamellar graft is used to thicken an area of marked corneoscleral thinning prior to a second operation consisting of a centered penetrating keratoplasty. The indications for penetrating keratoplasty, its prognosis, and variants have been discussed elsewhere.[1]

6
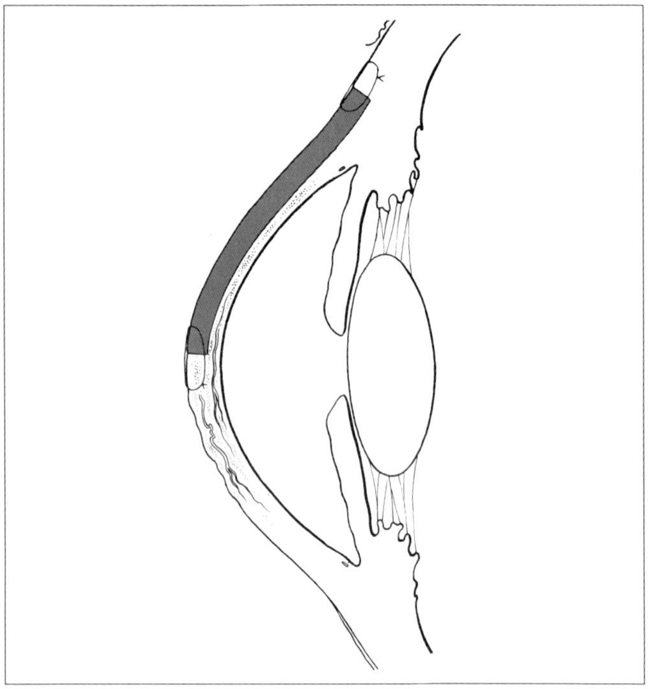

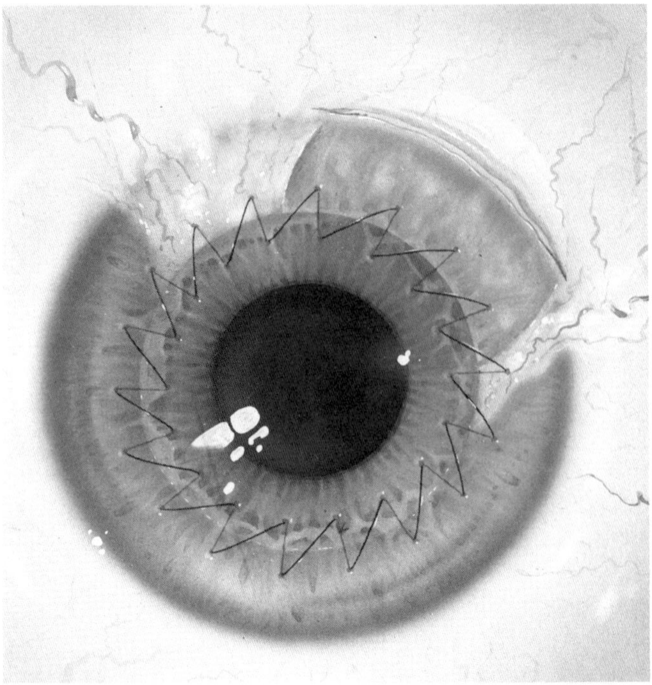
7

8
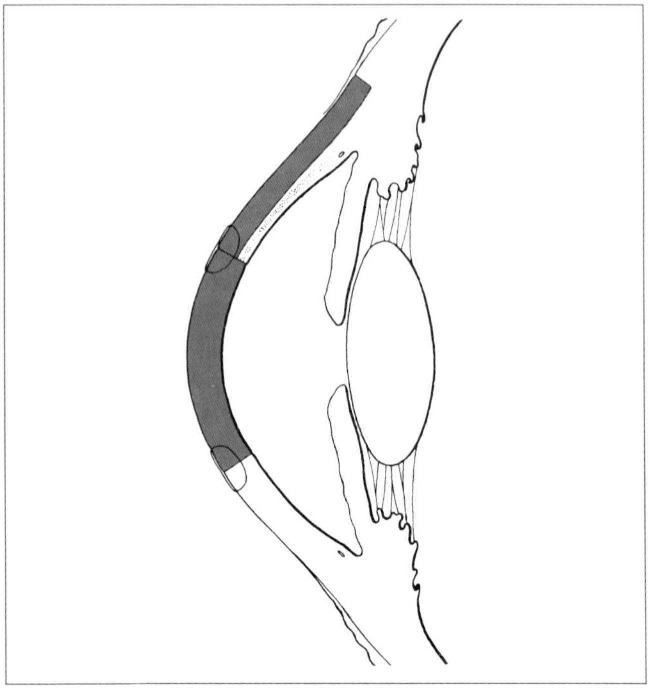

Preoperative Evaluation

Each patient and each eye must be individually assessed with respect to the visual needs of the patient, the potential for visual improvement with penetrating keratoplasty, and alternatives that may be available, such as the use of a contact lens. Intraocular pressure should be determined by an applanation tonometer and, if corneal opacification prevents ophthalmoscopy, the eye must be assessed by B-scan ultrasonography.

It is at the time of slit lamp examination that the surgeon decides upon the size and location of the graft. Most grafts should be centered, and their diameters should be within the confines of the optimal recipient zone. When a decentered penetrating graft is chosen as the first procedure (rather than a tectonic lamellar keratoplasty preceding a subsequent optical keratoplasty), the surgeon may wish to consider an alternative suturing technique to the basic operation described hereafter, as in Fig. 1.**3**.

Surgical Principles

There are some basic premises underlying the technique of penetrating keratoplasty advocated below: microsurgery is essential for precision; donor tissue (and particularly its endothelium) must be viable and carefully protected; and the surgery must be as atraumatic as possible.

The reader is cautioned that modifications in the method to be described may necessitate changes in the routine for postoperative management. For example, a surgeon employing larger grafts or interrupted silk sutures will have to prescribe a somewhat different postoperative management routine from the simple system outlined below.

Preparation for Surgery

A most important factor in patient management prior to surgery is to give the patient and his family an understanding of the requirements for postoperative care. Patient compliance is a vital component of successful keratoplasty.

Preoperative Medication and Anesthesia

Topical or oral antibiotics are not used routinely prior to surgery. A routine face scrub is given on the night prior to and on the morning of surgery. The brows are not shaved, nor are the lashes trimmed. Standard retrobulbar injection and modified Van Lint akinesia with 0.75% Marcaine combined with 4% Xylocaine in equal amounts is employed. No particular preference for preoperative sedation seems essential to the surgical technique, but it is best to avoid a combination of barbiturate and narcotic analgesics in elderly patients.

When penetrating keratoplasty is performed on a phakic eye and no cataract extraction is to accompany the surgery, routine use of pilocarpine 2% is started an hour before surgery and repeated prior to the surgical prep in order to maintain a small pupil, particulary when local anesthesia is employed. When penetrating keratoplasty is combined with cataract surgery, no miotic is employed and rarely is a mydriatic necessary.

Penetrating keratoplasty for children under 14 is always done under general anesthesia, and intravenous mannitol is started one hour prior to surgery to minimize bulging of the iris/lens diaphragm once the cornea has been trephined. A Flieringa ring is always employed with children.

Instruments

An operating microscope with good illumination and variable magnification is essential. After preparation of the donor material, all steps of surgery are performed with the aid of the microscope. Several small hand instruments are most helpful:

1. hollow-bore trephine shaft with a circular disposable blade (Storz, catalog number E 3086)

2. 13 mm Flieringa ring (Storz, E 4043-13)

3. Bonn forceps with 0.12 mm teeth (Storz, E 1809 or E 1811)

4. two tying forceps designed for handling 10-0 nylon suture

5. Barraquer sweep for lysis of iris adhesions (Storz, E 0485)

6. #30 gauge blunt-tipped cannula for reforming the anterior chamber with balanced salt solution

7. microsurgical corneal scissors, right and left; the blades should be small and sharp

8. Teflon punching block (Storz, E 3062).

For keratoplasty in aphakic eyes, one of the automated vitrectomy instruments is strongly recommended rather than the use of cellulose sponges and scissors for vitrectomy. I routinely employ McCarey-Kaufman (MK) medium (Warner Lambert Research Institute, 1970 Tabor Road, Morris Plains, NJ 07950) to which has been added 100 μ/ml gentamicin. The donor material in MK medium is stored at 4°C until used in the operating room. Tissue from donors between ages 5 and 65 is considered optimal. Even if very fresh donor material is available from the eye bank, I strongly recommend that the donor cornea with scleral rim be placed in MK medium for at least several hours prior to surgery; the dextran of the MK medium promotes deturgescence of the cornea, and this is a factor of importance in reducing the likelihood of loosened suture loops and facilitating optimal suture tightening at the time of surgery.

Surgical Technique

9

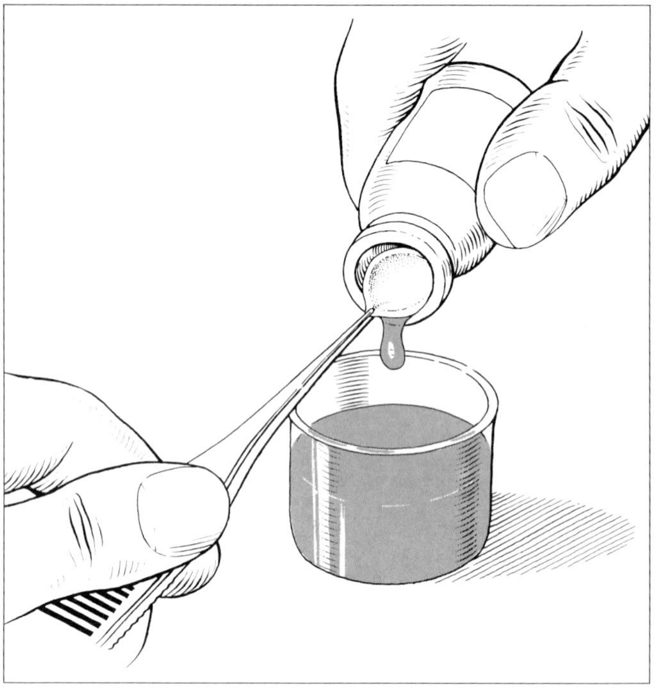

10

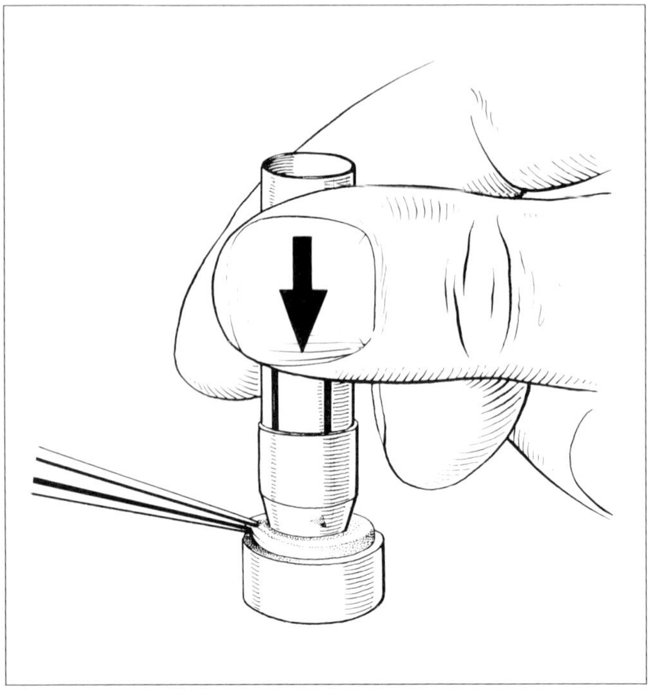

11

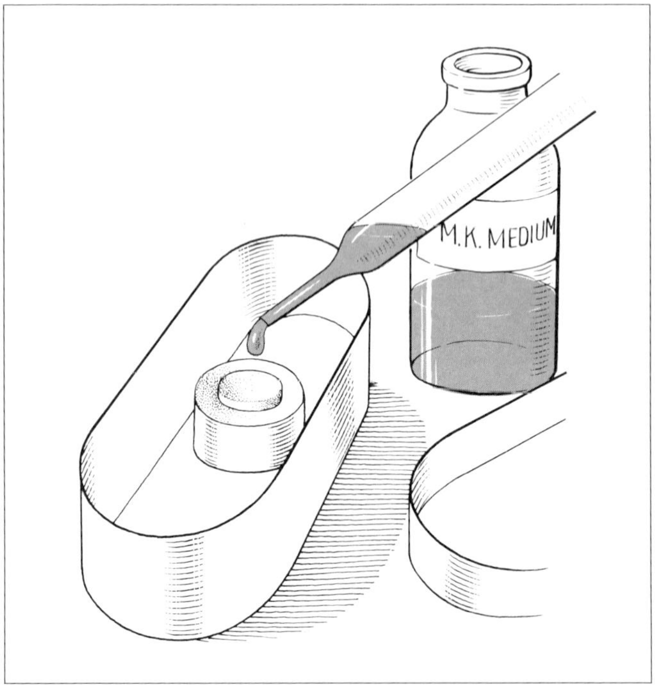

1.9 The stored cornea with scleral rim is emptied into a sterile medicine glass; the surgeon grasps the donor tissue with forceps and delivers it directly to the Teflon punching block. The medium should be cultured.

1.10 The hollow-shaft trephine with disposable blade is hand-held in a vertical position and the donor button is punched (endothelial surface up).

1.11 Rather than using balanced salt solution, a drop of MK medium from the medicine glass is placed on the donor button.

The graft, still on the Teflon punching block, is transferred to a sterile storage container. The top is secured and the container is placed on the tray of the Mayo stand. It is important not to traumatize the graft endothelium, but it is also highly desirable to have the donor epithelium intact, for this will minimize graft edema and will ensure that a continuity of donor and host epithelium covers the suture loops and the wound within 24 hours. The disposable blade of the trephine is exchanged for a new one. (Note that grafts oversized by 0.25 mm to 0.5 mm routinely are employed for phakic and aphakic eyes respectively.) The new blade, when resterilized, can be reused for punching donor tissue at a later operation.

Sterile tape strips are placed over portions of the lid speculum that could catch (and thereby break) a loop of nylon suture.

12

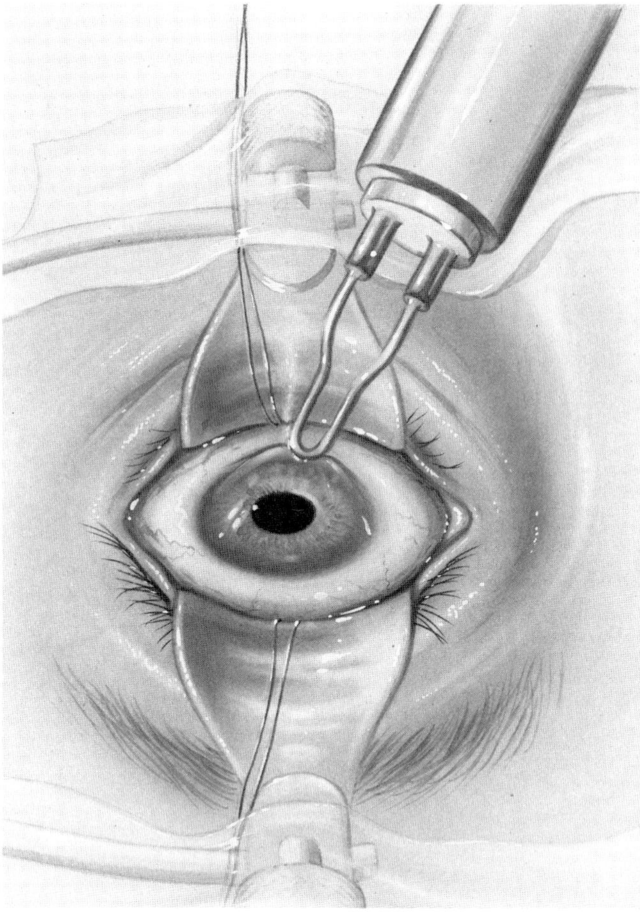

13

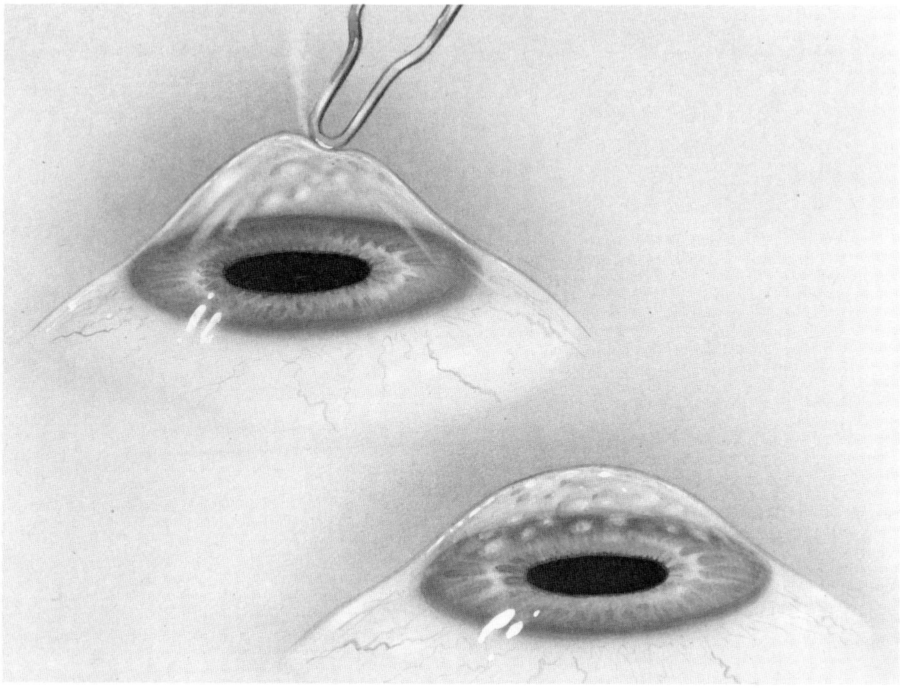

1.**12** and **13** In eyes with keratoconus mild heat applications by a cautery are used on the apex of the cone to flatten the corneal curvature, making the angle of cut in the donor and the recipient tissue more similar. The corneal flattening also facilitates trephining to the desired depth of approximately three-fourths of the corneal thickness.

In cases of surgical aphakia, a *small* (13 mm diameter) Flieringa ring is secured with a minimum of eight interrupted 8-0 black silk sutures to the episclera just peripheral to the limbus.

14

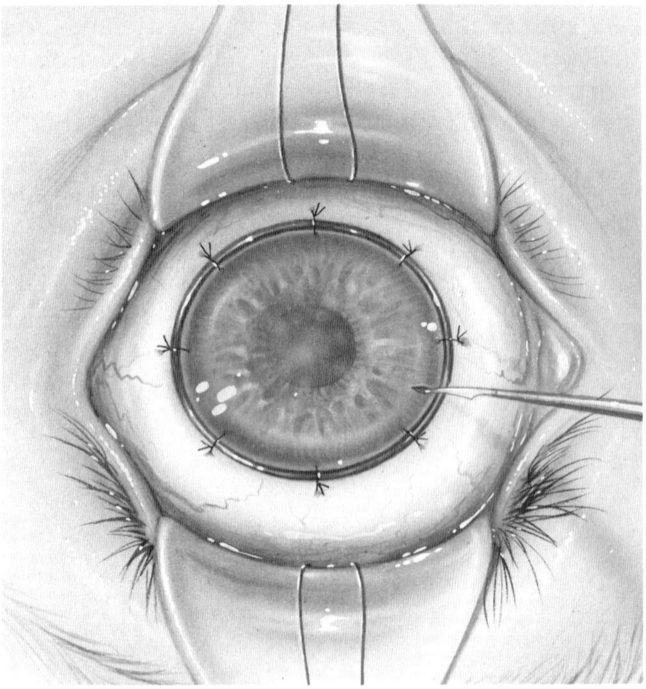

15 a

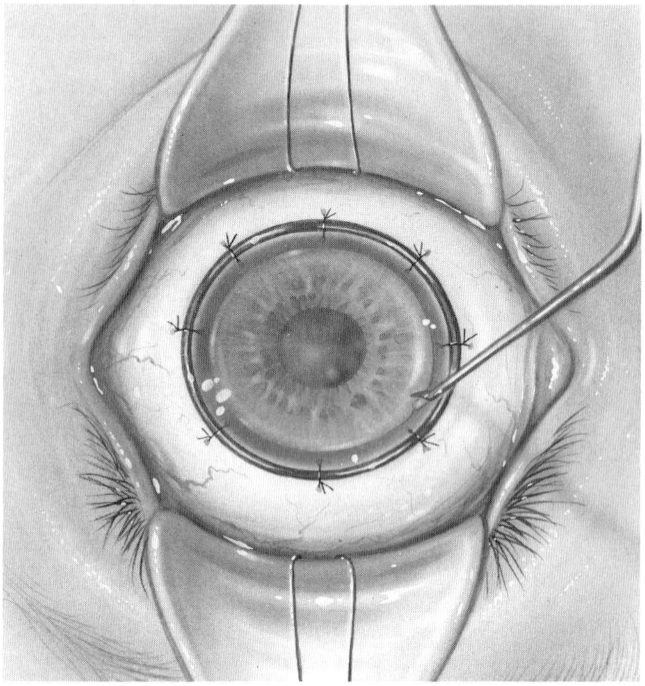

15 b

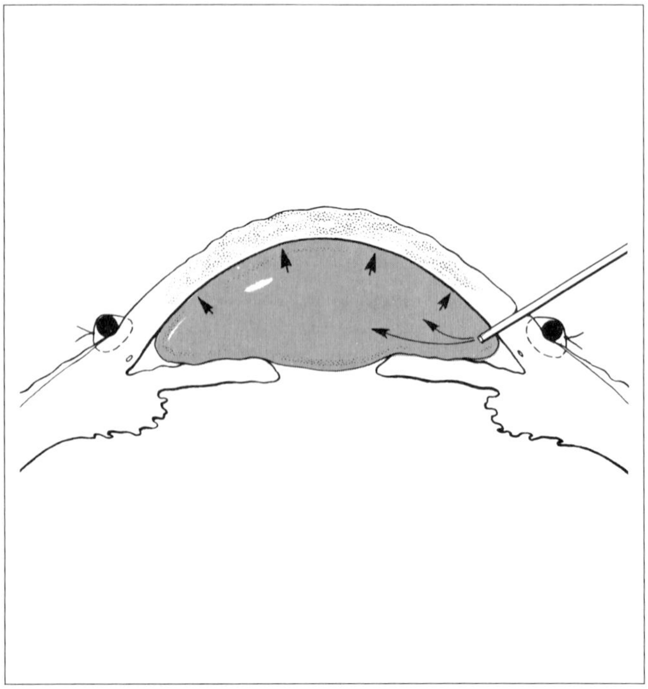

1.**14, 15 a** and **b** Trephining should not be done on an eye with low intraocular pressure; a beveled stab incision is made at the limbus and air injected into the anterior chamber with a # 30 blunt cannula.

16

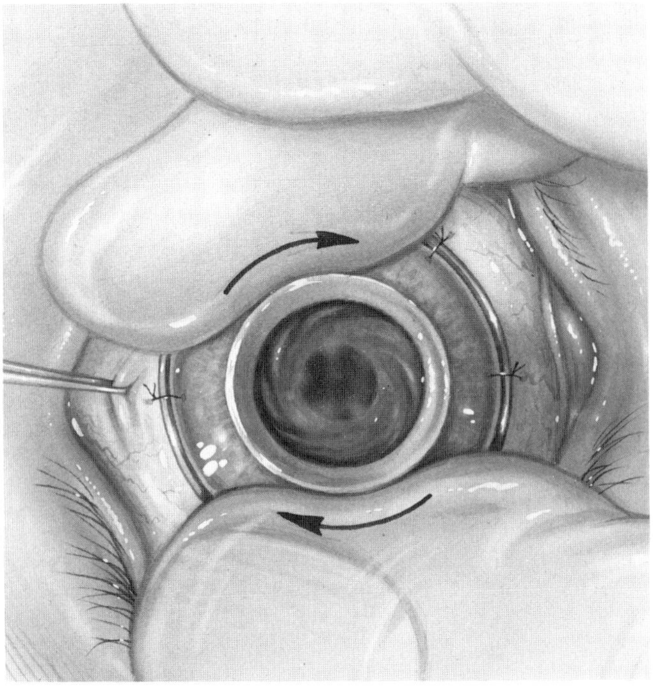

17

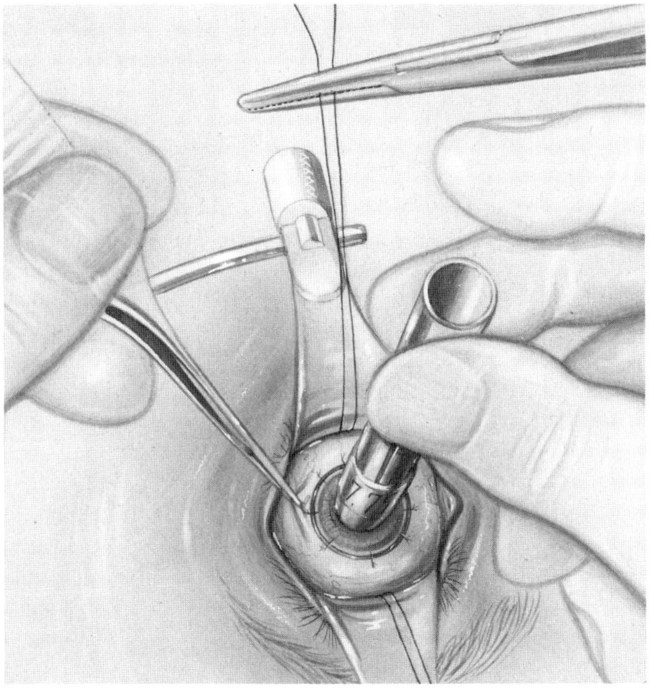

18

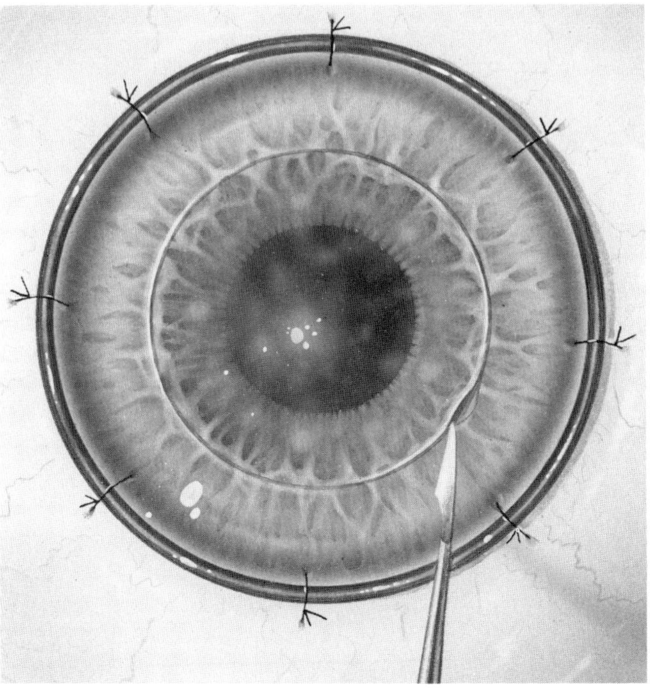

1.16 Trephination of the patient's cornea is done as the surgeon views the cornea through the operating microscope and through the vertically placed hollow-shaft trephine. Precise centering or intentional decentration of the trephination can be accomplished with this simple, inexpensive hand-held instrument.

1.17 While holding the trephine in one hand, the surgeon applies a fixation forceps peripheral to the limbus with the other hand to minimize slight rotation of the globe. Tension on the eye from rectus sutures must be avoided. Trephination is accomplished to a depth of three-fourths of corneal thickness by clockwise or counterclockwise rotation. Whenever possible, a single direction is preferred to a to-and-fro rotation between the thumb and index finger. The trephine must not be tipped from the vertical axis.

1.18 Once the deep groove has been made, the anterior chamber is entered with the cutting edge of a razor-blade chip or a Ziegler knife.

19
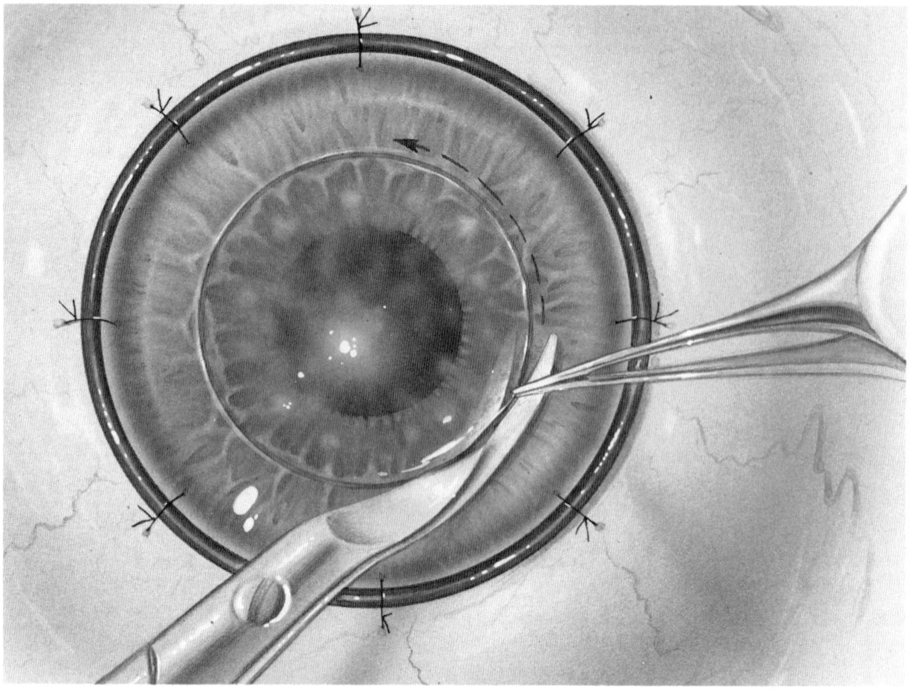

20
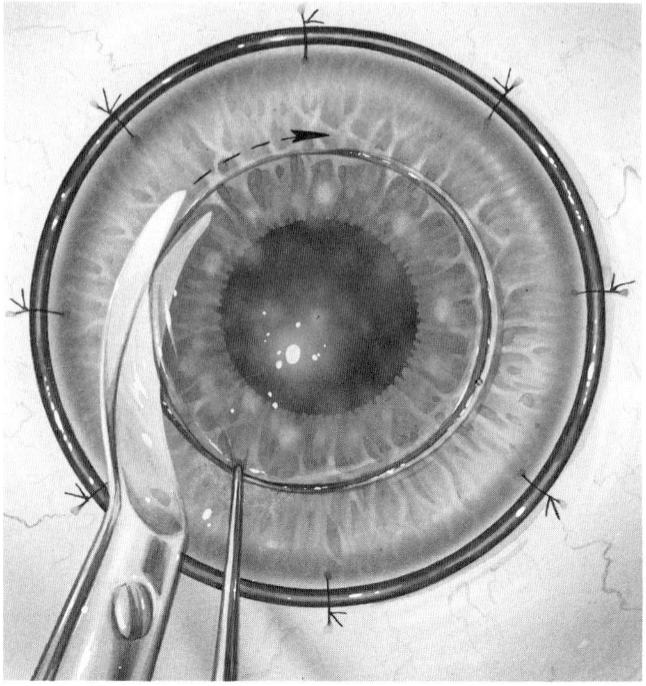

21
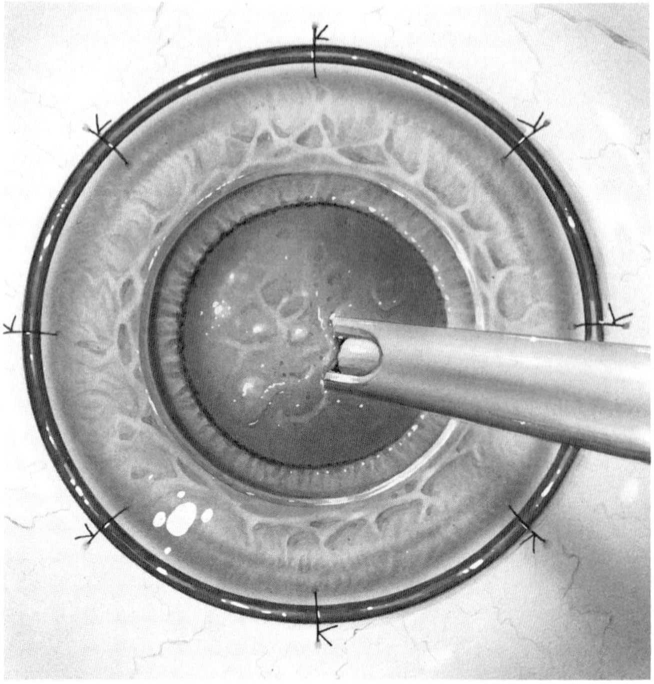

1.**19** and **20** Curved keratoplasty scissors are then employed to excise the central button of tissue. Assuming that the surgeon is right-handed, the left hand uses Bonn forceps to fix the position of the button at its normal location while the right hand uses the scissors.

1.**21** After excision of the button, iris repair, cataract surgery or vitrectomy (illustrated here) are performed according to the needs of the individual eye. If a peripheral iridectomy is desired, it is better to do this before a lens extraction or after a vitrectomy.

22

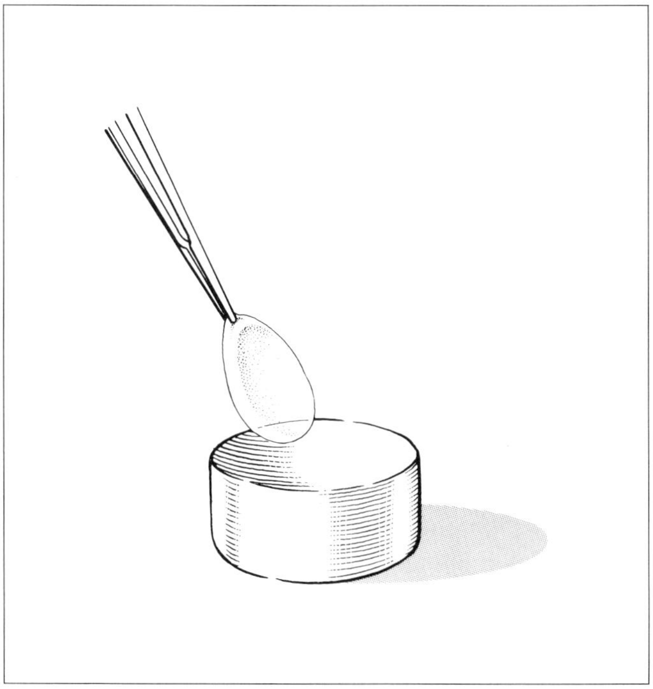

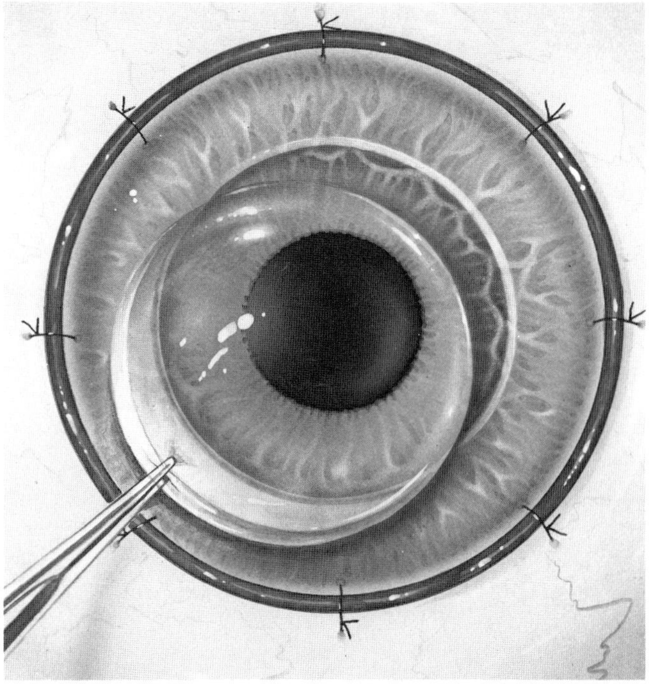

23

24

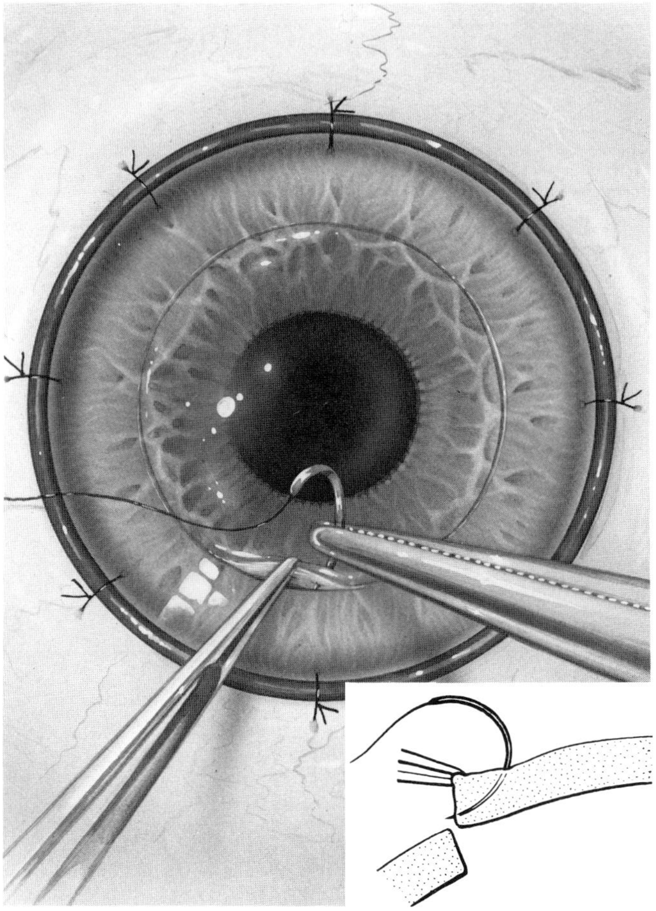

1.22 The container with the donor button is held in the surgeon's left hand and the donor button is grasped with the Bonn forceps in his right hand, taking care not to touch the endothelium.

1.23 The graft is transferred to the recipient eye in a single sequence of motions, including eversion of the graft so that its epithelial surface is facing upward. Note that in the technique recommended here no preplaced suture is employed in the graft.

The surgeon then transfers the Bonn forceps to his left hand and regrasps the button without lifting it. The graft is held in the recipient bed to prevent sliding of its endothelial surface across the iris or the surface of the recipient cornea. If an aphakic eye has a wide pupil and if a vitrectomy has been performed, it is important not to release the graft, for otherwise the donor tissue could sink into the vitreous cavity.

1.24 Positioning of the graft with forceps aided by the "walls" of the trephined wound facilitates placement of the first anchor suture at 12 o'clock. An 8-0 black silk suture with sidecutting needle is recommended. The needle is introduced into the graft and then into the recipient tissue as shown in the inset. The second suture is placed at 6 o'clock, followed by two additional interrupted sutures at 3 and 9 o'clock. Because these fixation sutures will be removed during the course of the operation, it does not matter whether or not they are placed at uniform depth, but they must be radial; if not perfectly equidistant, they must at least position the graft evenly. At times replacement of one of these cardinal sutures helps establish graft-host symmetry before starting the continuous suture.

25

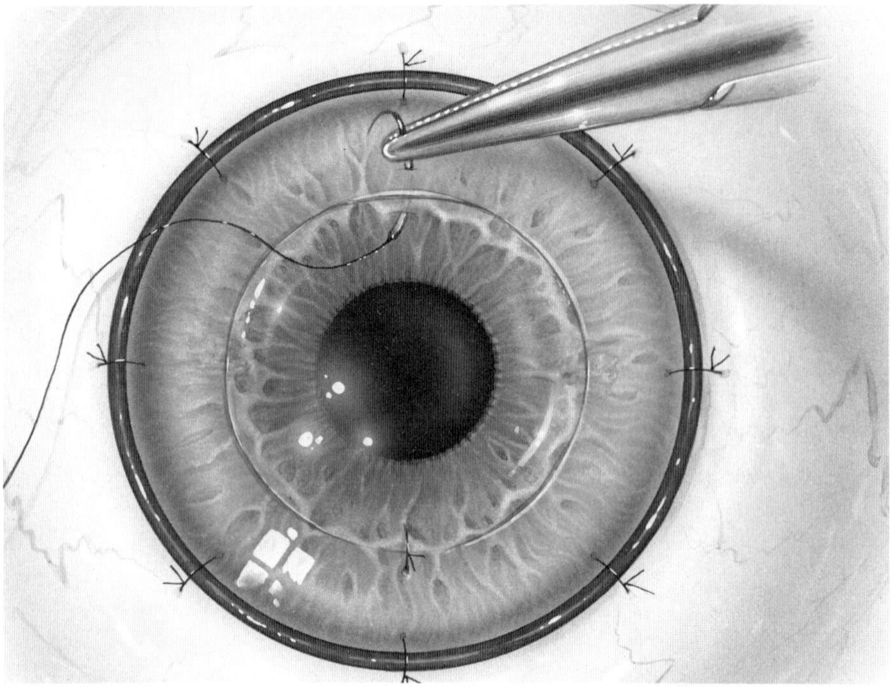

26 a

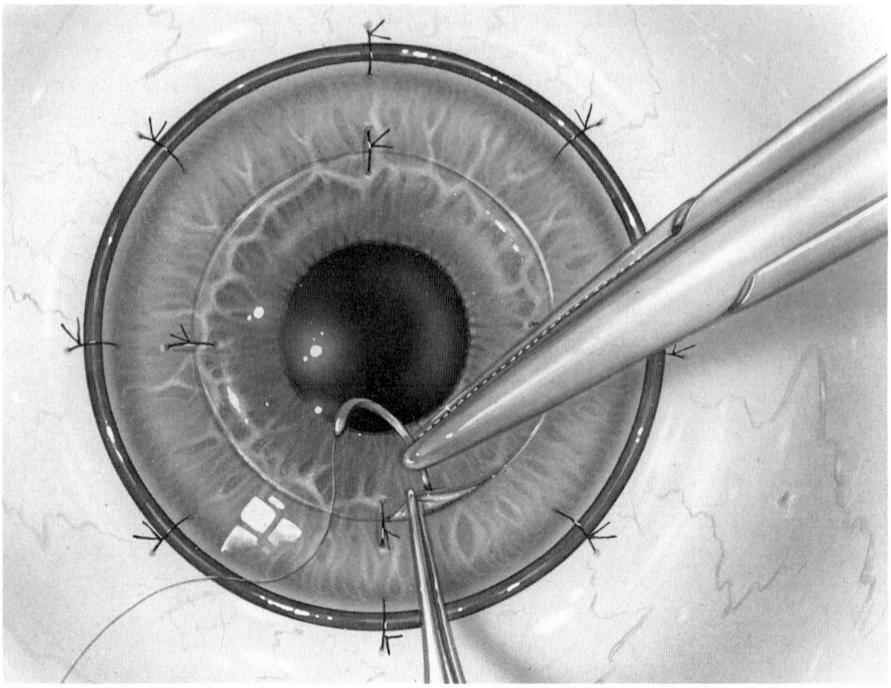

1.**25, 26 a** and **b** A double-armed 10-0 nylon suture with sidecutting half-circle needles is used to secure the graft. Although under usual conditions only one of its needles will be needed, the weight of the second needle will prevent the free end of the nylon suture from rising with convection currents. For the first bite, the suturing needle is waggled from side to side to enlarge the tissue entrance, thereby facilitating burial of the knot of the continuous suture upon completion of the operation.

26 b

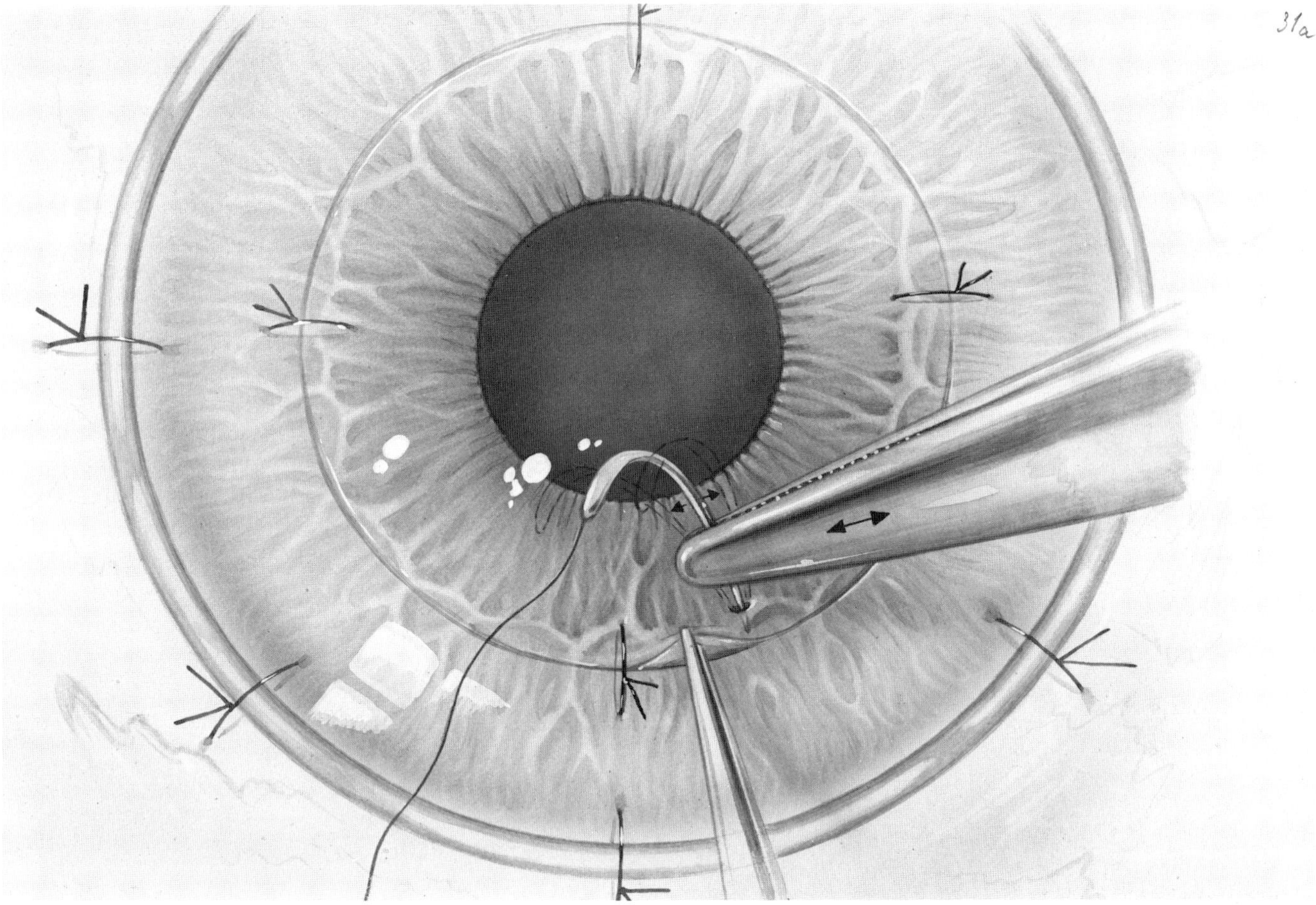

27

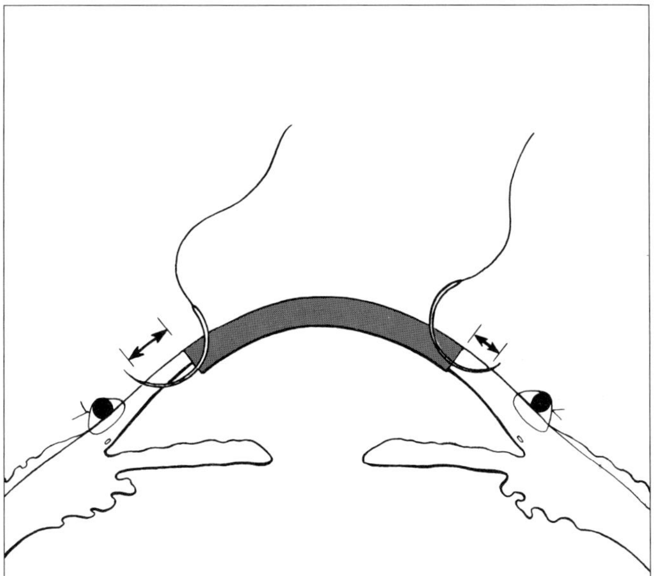

1.27 Many surgeons differ in their opinions as to the length and depth of the suture bites. The author prefers a depth of approximately three-fourths of the corneal thickness with tissue bites slightly longer in the recipient than in the donor tissue. If the recipient tissue is thinner than normal cornea, then longer bites in the recipient are recommended. If the recipient tissue is little more than one-half the normal corneal thickness, then tissue bites as deep as Descemet's membrane may be employed; full-thickness tissue bites are only safe with 10-0 nylon suture material. Each tissue bite should be radial; a graft 7.5 mm in diameter should have approximately five tissue bites per quadrant.

28

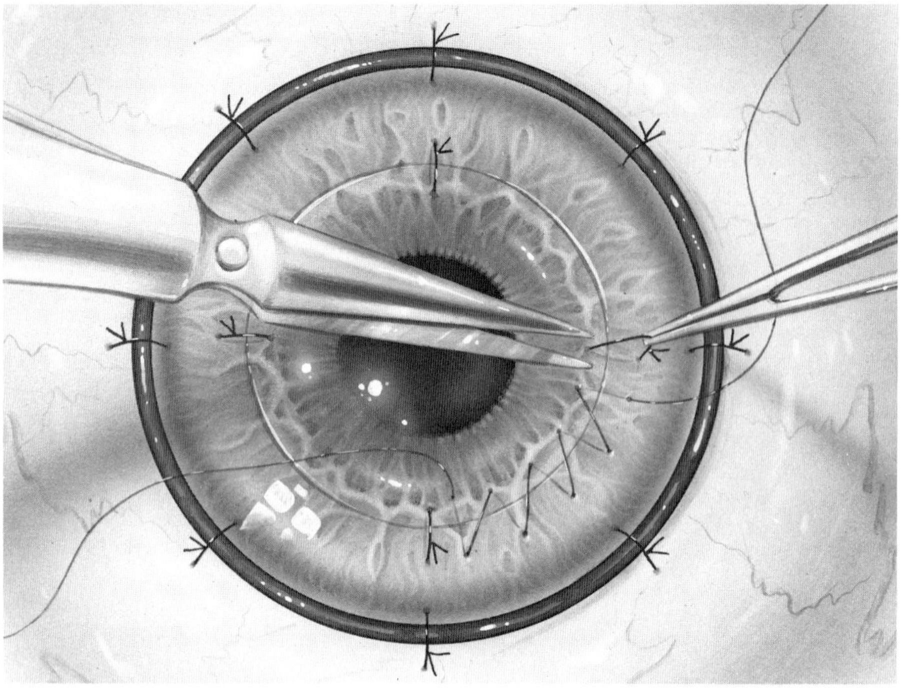

29

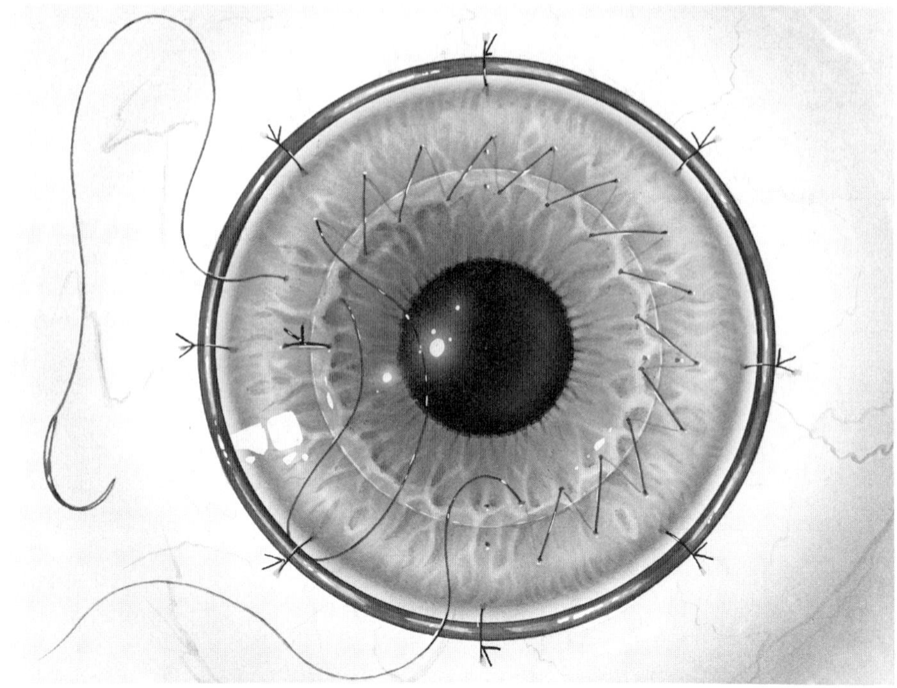

1.28 and **29** As the sutures bring the wound closure to each of the four cardinal fixation sutures, the latter are removed sequentially.

Any suture placed in recipient tissue so near the limbus that the tissue bites include conjunctiva and fascia will loosen. Therefore, because loosening of the continuous suture is a less desirable occurrence than loosening of an interrupted suture, the latter is recommended for suturing grafts intentionally placed in an eccentric position, as in 1.**3**. For interrupted sutures either nylon or silk may be employed. If nylon is selected, the knots can be buried, preferably in the recipient tissue.

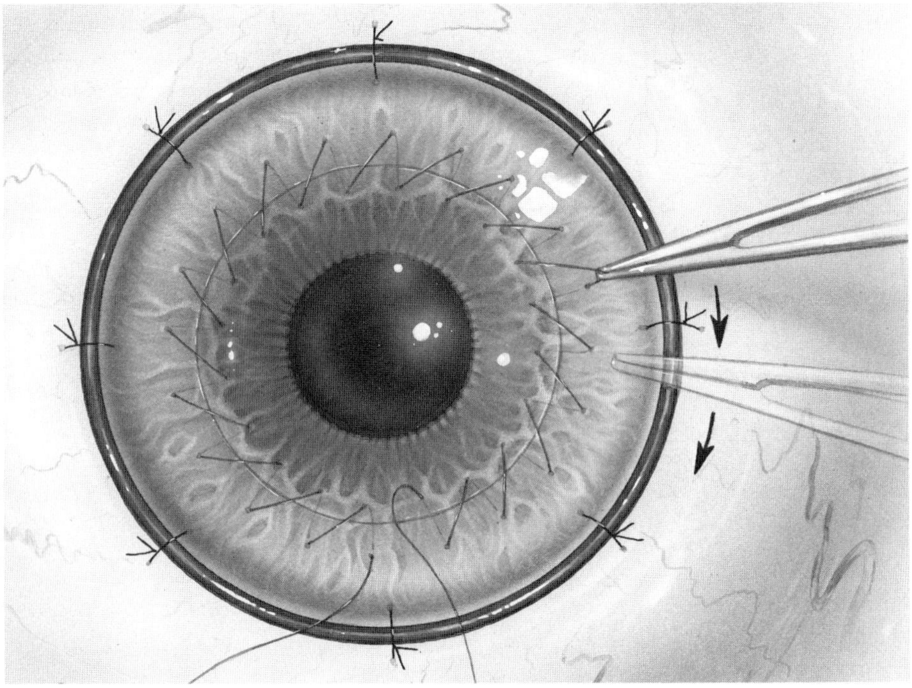

1.30 After completion of bites of the continuous suture, the loops are tightened with the pair of tying forceps starting from the 6 o'clock position and working first clockwise to the free end toward the 11 o'clock position, and then subsequentyl tightening from 6 o'clock counterclockwise to the other free end near the 12 o'clock position. When nylon suture is grasped, it must not be squeezed or twisted, for the suture material is easily damaged by steel instruments and can break at the damaged site either at the time of surgery or in the postoperative period.

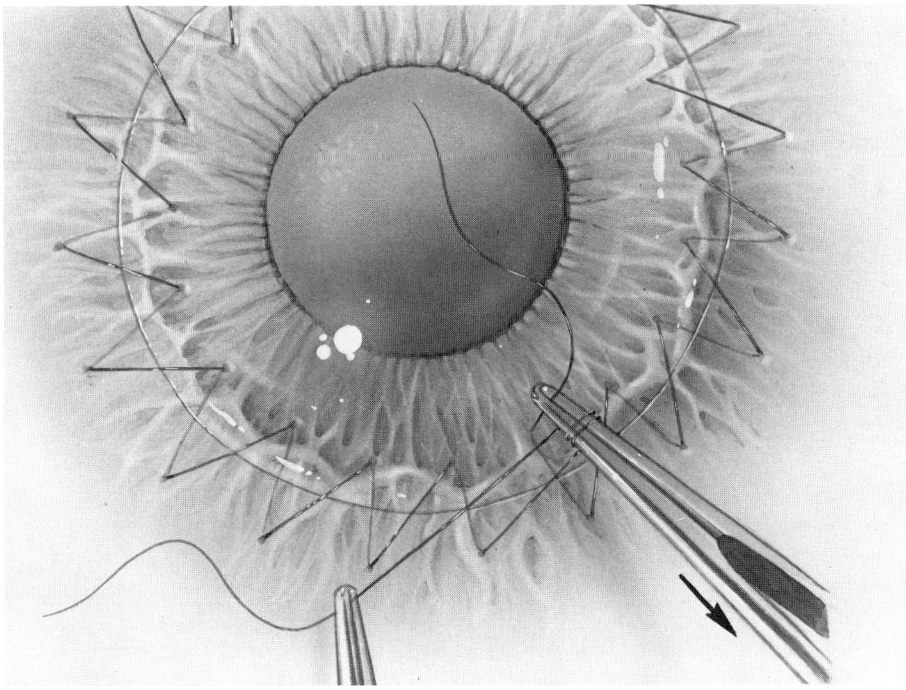

1.31 The ends of the nylon suture are tied together at the 12 o'clock position, employing a preliminary triple throw.

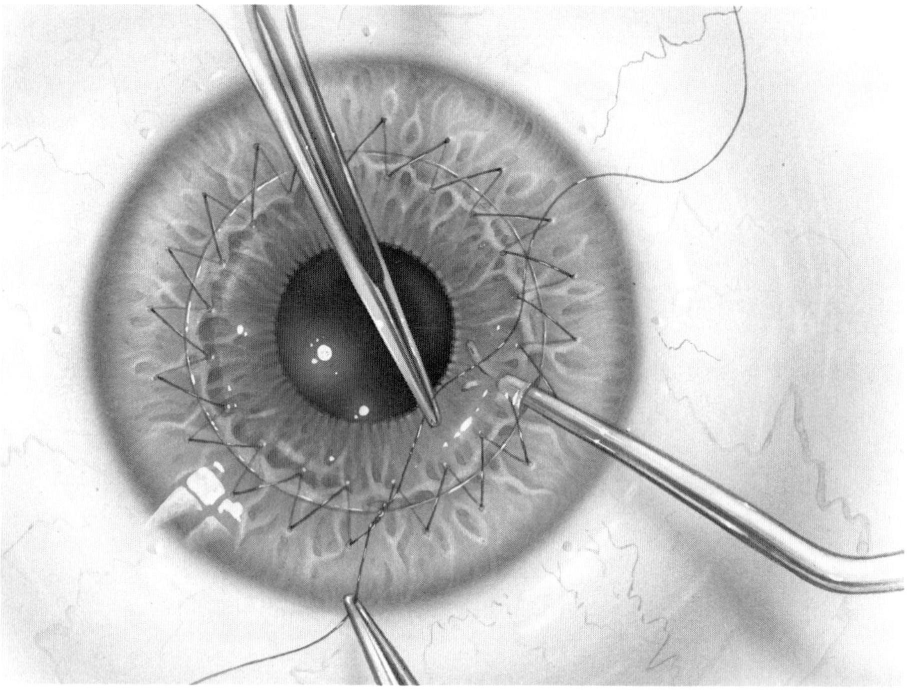

1.32 The anterior chamber is formed by the injection of balanced salt solution, and more slack is removed from the suture by repeating the previously described tightening process, starting again at the 6 o'clock position. Each suture loop should be uniformly tight except for a few loops toward the 12 o'clock position.

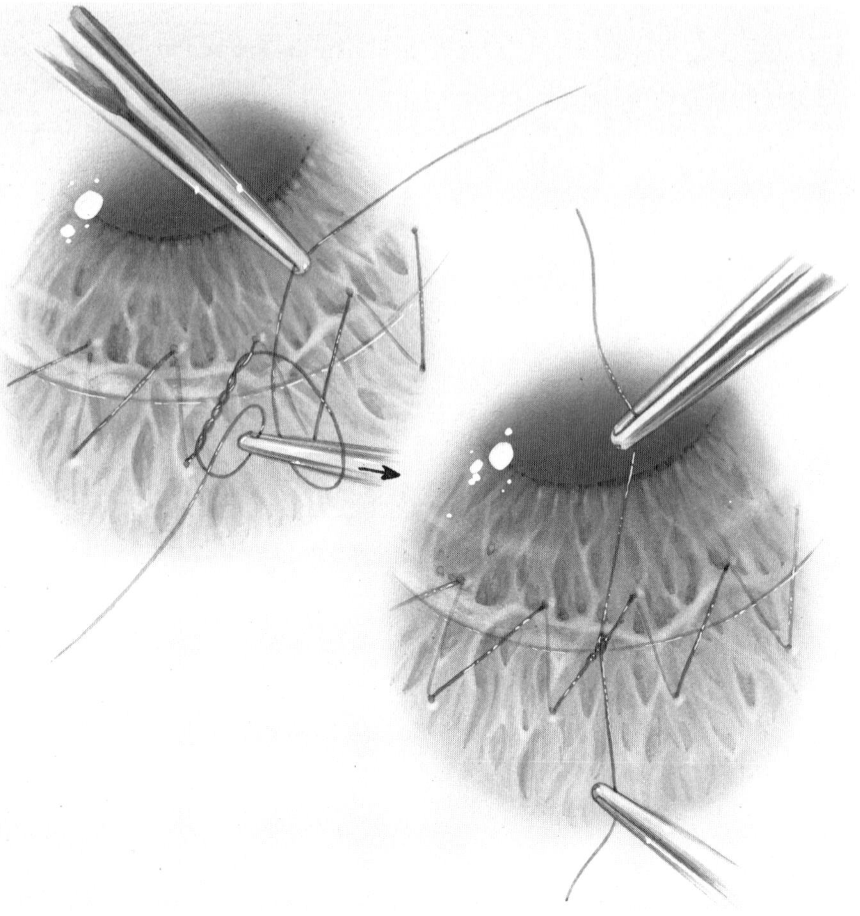

1.33 Once all other slack has been taken up (excessive tightness being avoided), a surgeon's knot is completed.

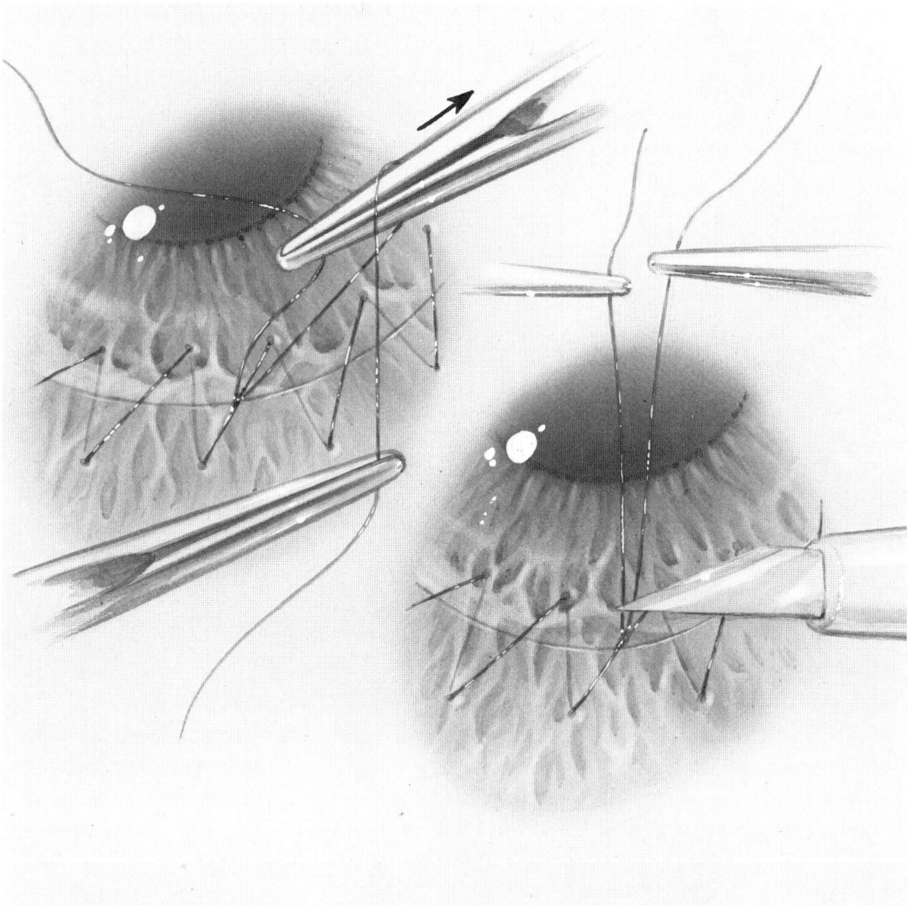

1.34 The ends of the suture are cut flush with the knot using a razor-blade chip or Ziegler knife.

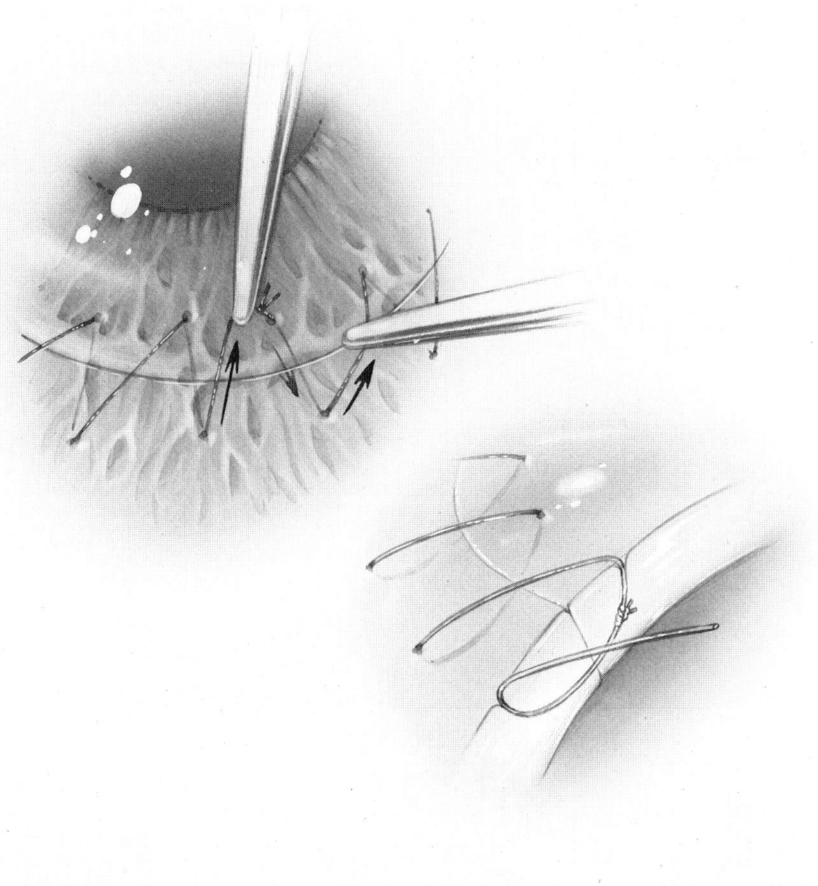

1.35 The tying forceps are then employed to bury the knot in the stroma of the graft. While one forceps slightly elevates and delivers the suture loop on one side of the knot, the other forceps gently drags the knotted suture into the graft stroma.

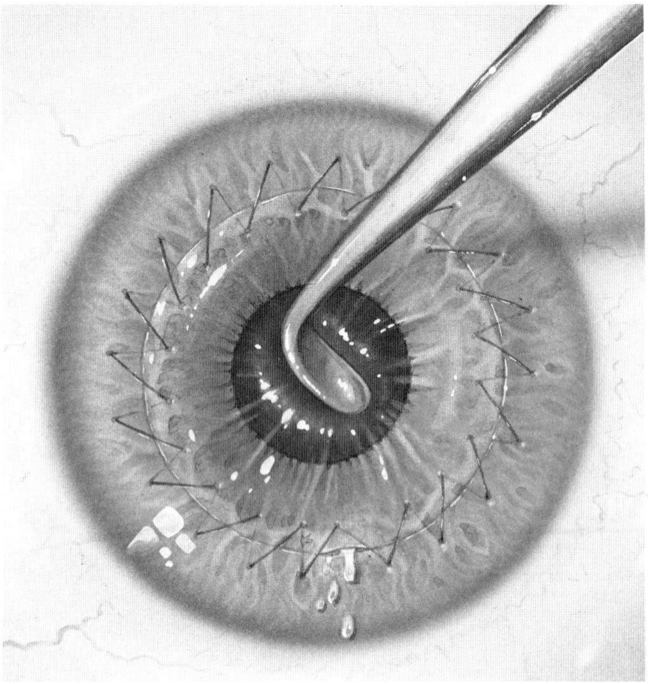

1.36 A muscle hook is then pressed on the center of the graft to elicit sites of aqueous leakage. Note that air is never used to reform the anterior chamber, for it will not provide an adequate test of wound apposition.

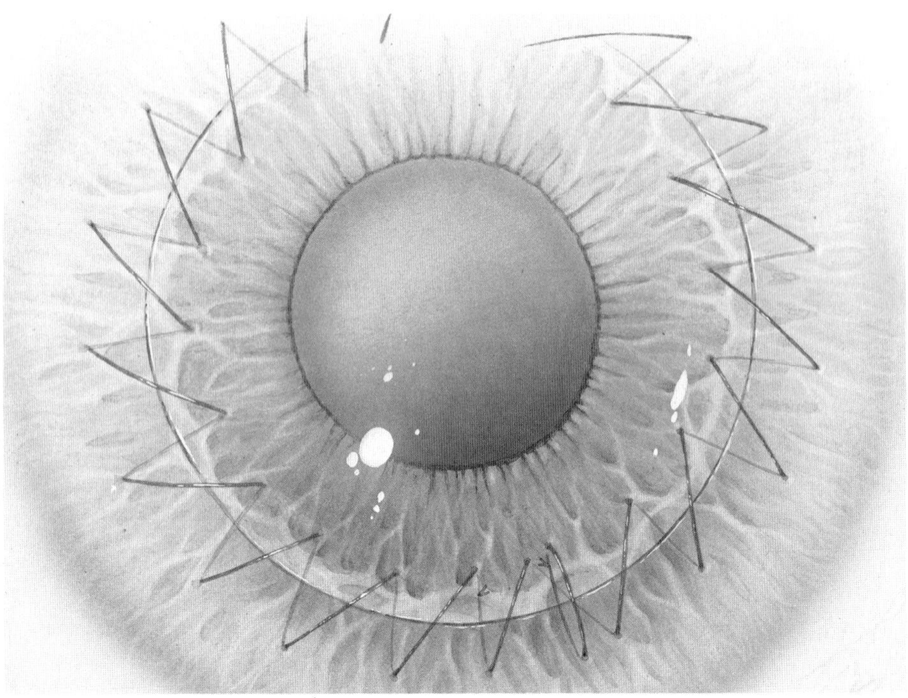

1.37 If any leakage is observed, a single interrupted suture can be placed at that site, taking care not to cut the continuous suture. Such interrupted sutures may be placed either deep or superficial to the tissue bites of the continuous suture. They can be removed within the first two postoperative weeks. An ophthalmic antibiotic ointment routinely is employed. The tightness of wound closure dispels any concern about entrance of ointment into the anterior chamber. A Fox shield protects the eye until the first dressing.

Modifications and Surgical Alternatives

It is usually easy enough to lyse adhesions with a Barraquer sweep using circumferential centrifugal motions of the tip of the instrument. Peripheral corneal and anterior chamber adhesions, however, will have a tendency to recur; if there is postoperative anterior chamber inflammation from iris manipulation or if an anterior vitrectomy has been inadequate, the pre-existing lysed adhesions will reform followed by a "zipper effect" – a slowly progressive closure of chamber angle by adherence of neighboring iris. To limit the possibility of such an occurrence, radial iridotomies or broad peripheral iridectomies are recommended in the iris tissue on the side of the lysed adhesion.

38

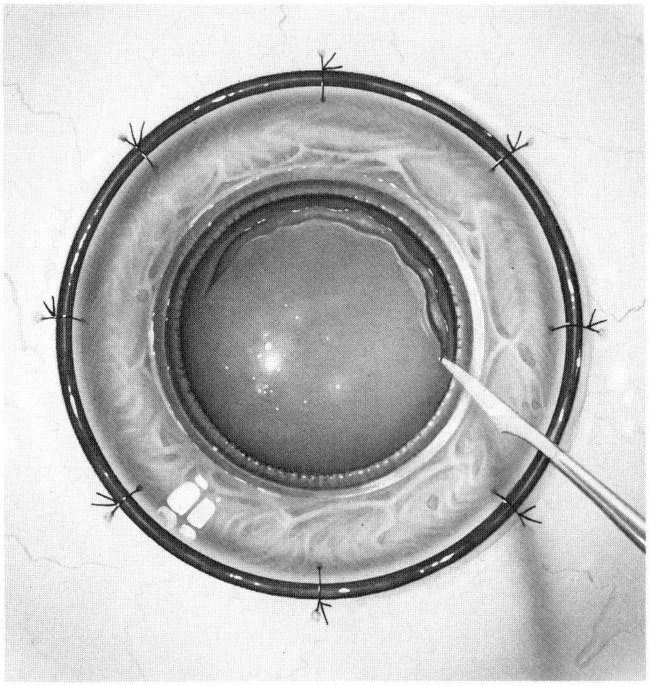

39

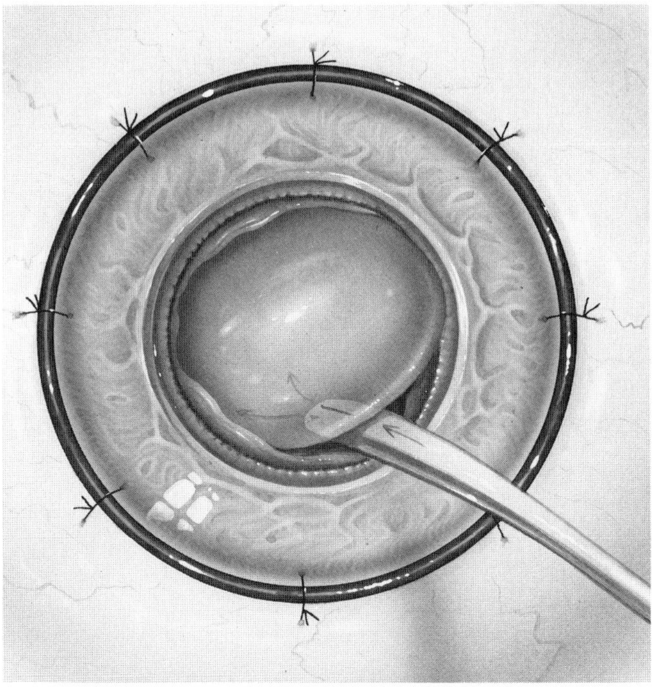

40

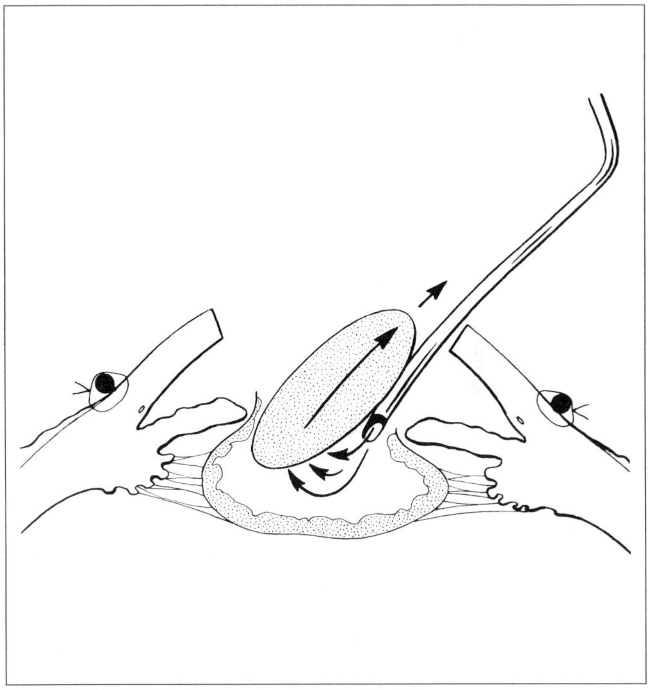

1.**38** to **40** Management of cataract coexistent with corneal opacity is usually done as a "triple procedure" – penetrating keratoplasty combined with extracapsular cataract extraction and posterior chamber intraocular lens implantation. After trephining the cornea a "can-opener" incision is made in the anterior lens capsule, the nucleus is loosened and its delivery facilitated by irrigation.

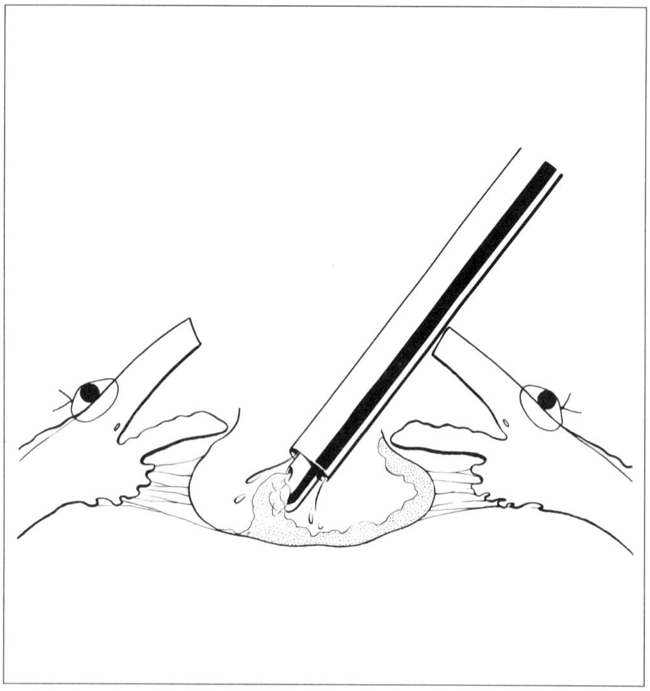

1.41 Cortical material is aspirated by one of numerous methods such as the use of irrigation-aspiration instrument.

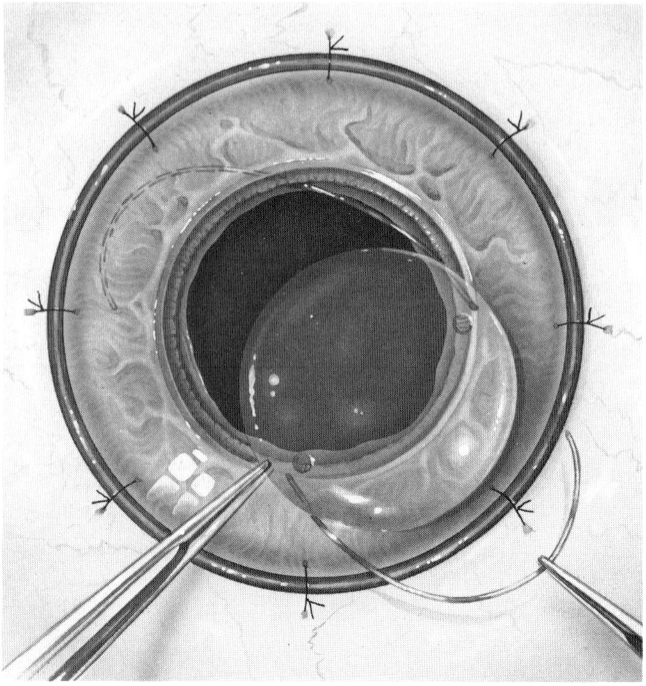

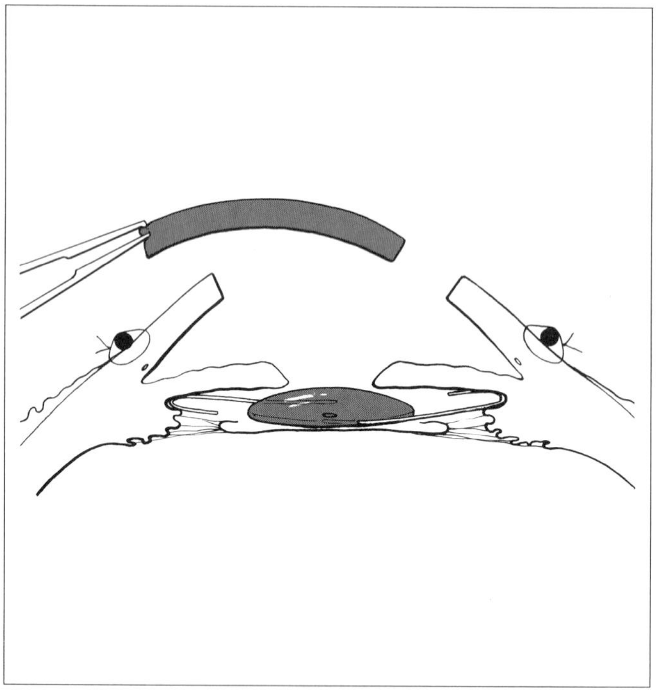

1.42 and **43** After polishing the posterior capsule, a posterior chamber lens is slid behind the pupil and the keratoplasty proceeds as described above. A bubble of air is used in the anterior chamber until completion of the continuous nylon suture.

Complications

Hyphema is an uncommon but troublesome complication usually resulting from excessive manipulation of previously damaged iris. Routine iridectomy is not recommended for cases of routine keratoplasty on phakic eyes.

Primary graft failure usually is the result of poor donor material and is a rare occurrence. Irrigation of the anterior chamber with balanced salt solution should be minimized during surgery, for it can unduly traumatize the graft endothelium. Broken or loose suture loops of the continuous nylon suture must be repaired surgically. Splicing of nylon is not difficult but necessitates the return of the patient to the operating room and a second local anesthesia.

Postoperative endophthalmitis, fortunately very rare, is handled in the same manner as endophthalmitis following other anterior segment procedures.

Admonitions and Suggestions

If there is no backup corneal tissue, be certain not to send from the sterile surgical environment the button that has been excised from the patients's eye until the donor tissue is secured, for loss of donor grafts is a rare but notorious occurrence in busy operating theaters.

Operating time is minimized by the surgeon's familiarity with the sequence of steps of the procedure and the availability of all instruments required. Penetrating keratoplasty generally requires between 20 and 40 minutes of operating time; prolonged surgical procedures are certain to be followed by increased postoperative inflammation and will require increased postoperative steroid therapy above that recommended below.

The importance of recognizing and controlling postoperative ocular hypertension deserves emphasis. Uncontrolled ocular hypertension is the principal cause of graft failure; it occurs most often and is most difficult to measure accurately in aphakic eyes. When medication is not sufficient to control ocular hypertension, cyclocryotherapy is recommended.

When keratoplasty is performed in children, preoperative intravenous mannitol is recommended. In children I routinely use a Flieringa ring at the limbus even with phakic eyes. Keratoplasty in childhood requires a high degree of understanding and compliance on the part of the parents. Very frequent postoperative examinations are required, often necessitating brief general anesthesia.

The allograft reaction can occur in any eye following keratoplasty (except autokeratoplasty), but is more likely in eyes with preoperative corneal vascularization or vascularization that has been induced in the postoperative period by a chronic irritant such as an exposed suture knot or the use of contact lens. Most allograft reactions can be suppressed successfully by steroid therapy if the reaction is recognized promptly.

Postoperative Management

In most circumstances, the eye can be left unpatched within 24 to 48 hours following surgery, for the epithelium is intact over the now buried loops of the continuous suture. Since patching an eye causes vascular congestion, increases bacterial flora (and hence risk of infection), and prolongs postoperative inflammation, it is preferable to have the patient wear dark glasses by day and merely a protective Fox shield taped over the unpatched eye at night. Mild cycloplegia (homatropine 5 %, two to three times a day) and a 1 % topical steroid drop two to four times a day are routinely employed in the first two weeks. Thereafter, the homatropine usually can be discontinued and the steroid reduced to one drop daily.

Postoperatively, oral steroid therapy is not routine, except for a few weeks following surgery if a vitrectomy has been performed. All aphakic eyes routinely are started on acetazolamide or another carbonic anhydrase inhibitor; such medication is continued (if tolerated) throughout the first few weeks of the postoperative course. Routine phakic postoperative eyes rarely require more than topical homatropine and topical steroid. The former is discontinued with the disappearance of aqueous cells and flare, but the latter is reduced to one drop a day for approximately six months and then one drop every other day for the remainder of the first year. This is a low but important dosage for prevention of allograft reaction, and it is not cataractogenic. When grafts larger than the recommended 8.0 mm diameter maximum are employed (except for autografts), more topical and/or oral steroid therapy is required; these patients have a higher incidence of iatrogenic cataract.

44

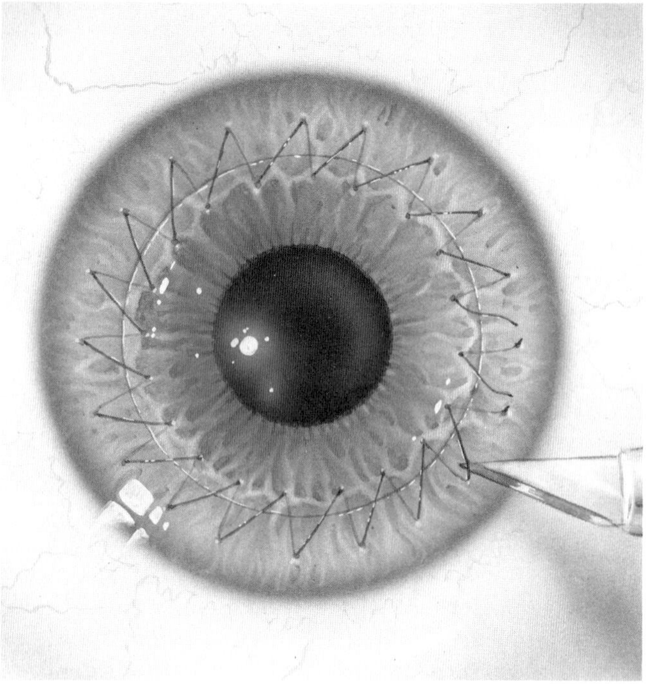

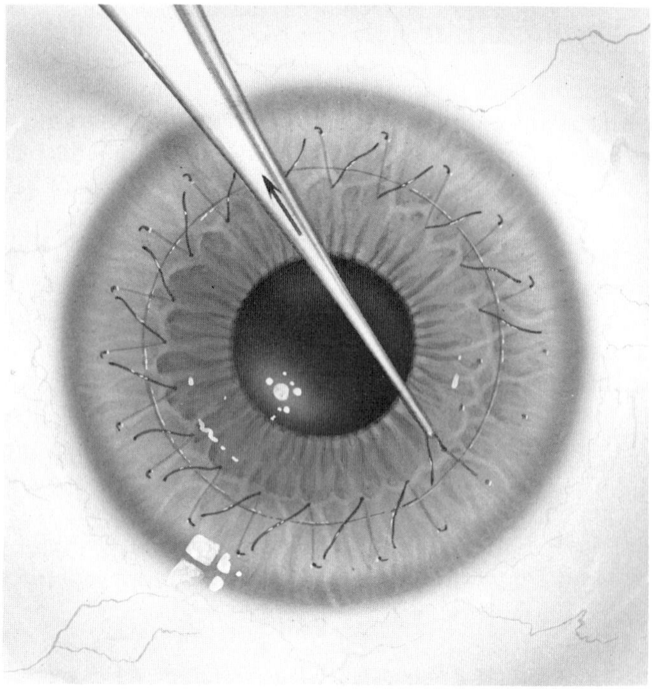

45

1.**44** and **45** Suture removal is performed at the slit lamp (except for young children) using a topical anesthetic, a razor-blade chip, and a jeweler's forceps. In nonvascularized corneas, the epithelium-covered nylon suture is not removed until approximately one year following keratoplasty. After suture removal, the eye is patched for 24 hours, then reexamined to be certain the graft is still in the proper position. Patients who have had bullous keratopathy or keratoconus do not have the suture removed for several years, even though hard or soft contact lenses may have been started as early as six months following keratoplasty.

Recovery of vision following penetrating keratoplasty is extremely variable. Within weeks, excellent acuity may be obtained with spectacle correction alone. In other cases (depending upon the transparency of the graft and the amount of corneal astigmatism), the best corrected acuity may gradually improve over a full postoperative year.

Results

In most cases, the surgeon can give a remarkably accurate estimate of the patient's chances of successful keratoplasty based on the structural changes of the recipient cornea and numerous ancillary factors.[1] Note that an estimate of graft prognosis is not the same as an even more difficult estimate of the patient's chances of gaining normal vision; for other abnormalities, such as cataract, macular edema, optic atrophy and amblyopia, may affect the result of an intended optical keratoplasty. Lastly, a crystal-clear graft showing a high degree of astigmatism and contact lens intolerance is more of a visual satisfaction to the surgeon than a visual aid to the patient. Given the present state of the surgical art, control of postoperative astigmatism is the most important consideration for future research. This is such an extensive topic that it cannot be dealt with here in detail. Various surgical corrections can be done, but are generally postponed until one year following keratoplasty.

Reference

[1] Paton, D.: The prognosis of penetrating keratoplasty based upon corneal morphology. *Ophthalmic Surg.* 7 (3): 36–45, 1976

Lamellar Keratoplasty

Herbert E. Kaufman and
Marguerite B. McDonald

Optical Inlay Lamellar Keratoplasty

Surgical Principles

In optical inlay lamellar keratoplasty, a partial thickness of the recipient cornea is removed and replaced by a partial thickness donor cornea, in order to eliminate superficial scars or other opacities that reduce vision, or to strengthen the cornea. The advantages of lamellar keratoplasty over penetrating keratoplasty, in cases where it is feasible, are that lamellar grafts can be very large – a large as 12 or 13 mm in diameter if necessary – and that lamellar grafts are not generally subject to immune rejection, as are large penetrating keratoplasty grafts. Among the disadvantages are the difficulty of preparing a smooth recipient bed – both free-hand dissection and the use of the microkeratome are difficult – and the considerable risk of perforation in thinned corneas, as in keratoconus.

Preparation for Surgery

Preparation of donor tissue. The donor cornea from which the lamellar keratoplasty graft is obtained need not contain living cells. The graft can be obtained from a cadaver eye that has been frozen at −70 °C or below and thawed just before surgery, or from a whole fresh eye. It is possible to dissect corneal tissue from a specimen with at least 2 mm of scleral rim with the use of an artificial anterior chamber, but it is difficult to hand-cut a lamellar graft from a cornea stored in MK medium. Lamellar tissue is also available commercially, cut to a depth of 0.3 mm and lyophilized (freeze-dried) for storage and transport. All that is necessary is to rehydrate this tissue and trephine the appropriate diameter graft.

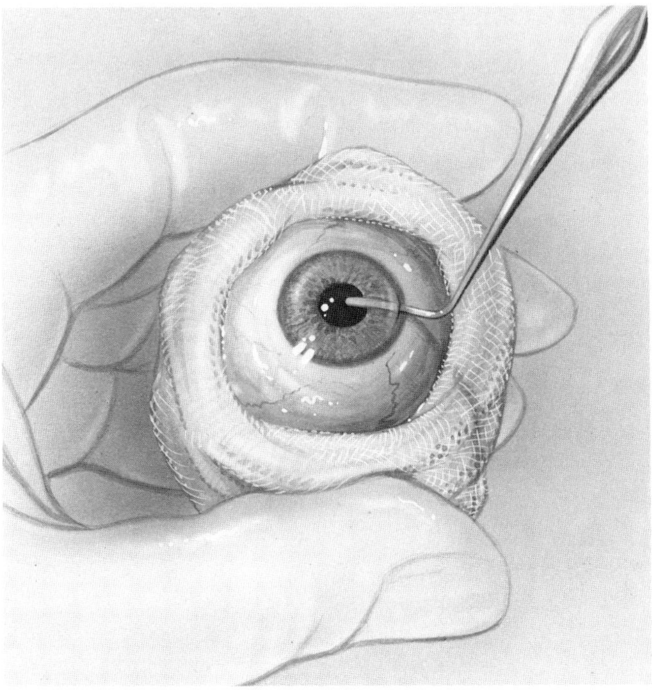

1.46 The lamellar donor button can be prepared in exactly the same way as the recipient bed is made, which is described in detail below. However, this is not the easiest method for working with a whole globe. One of the most popular techniques involves using a razorblade to make a limbal incision in the whole eye, to a depth of approximately two-thirds the thickness of the cornea. The depth of the limbal incision is critical, because it determines the thickness of the resulting lamella. The eye is held by an assistant, while a lamellar splitter is inserted in the limbal incision.

47

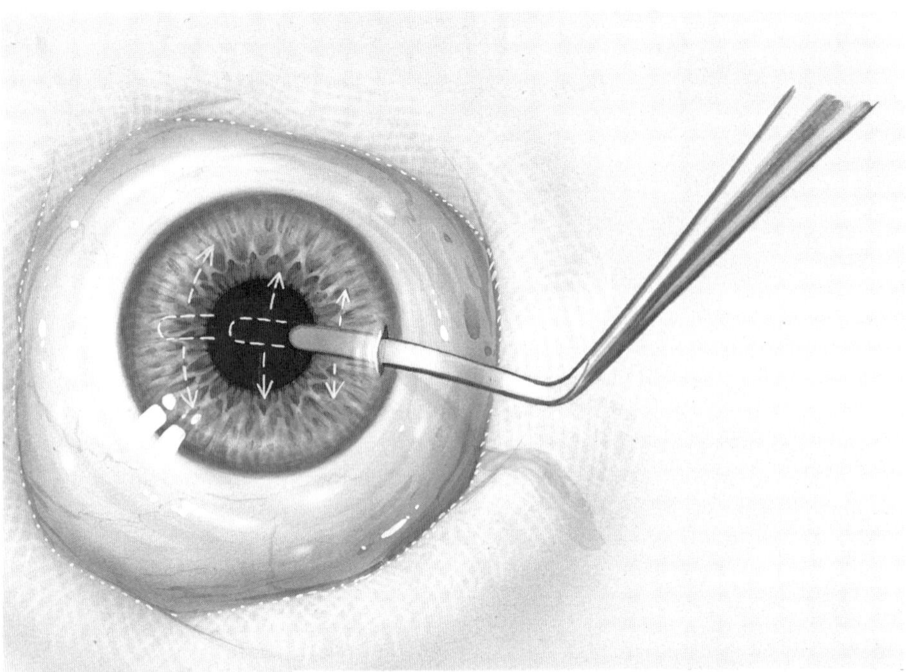

48

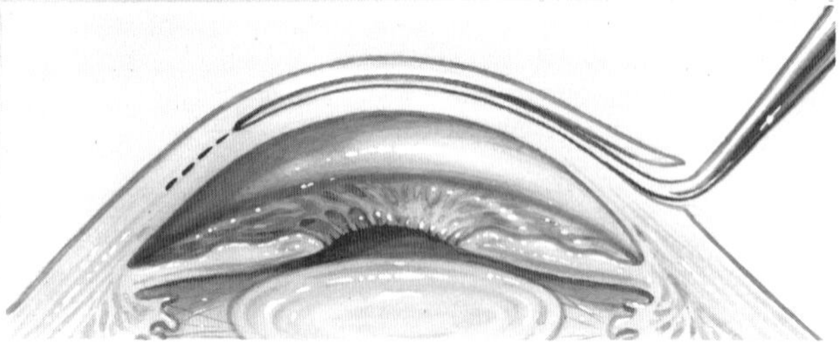

1.47 and **48** The somewhat blunt blade of the lamellar dissector is moved back and forth to divide the lamellar fibrils, but the cornea remains on the eye, because only a small (3 or 4 mm) incision has been made.

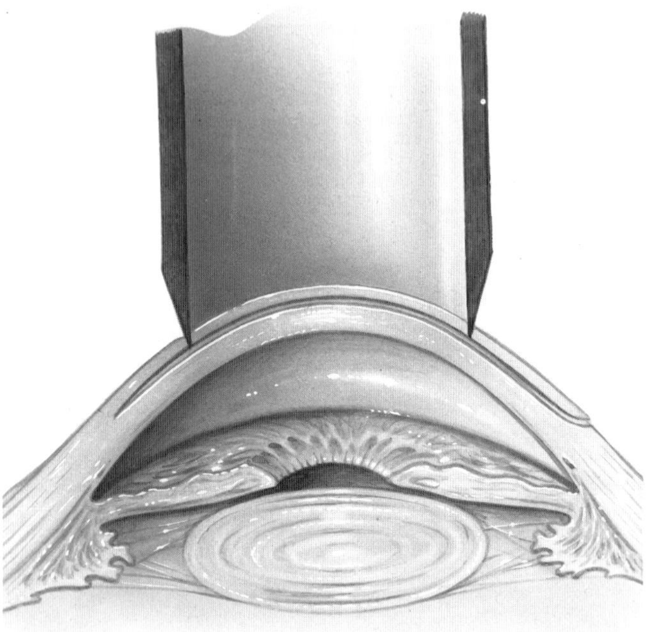

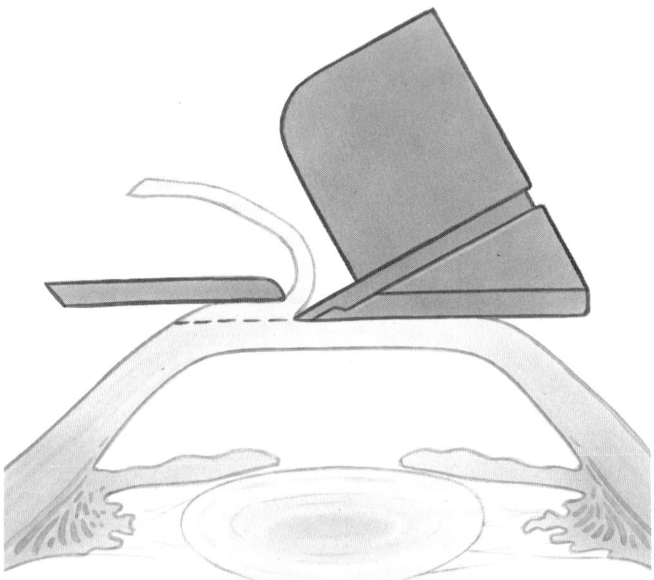

1.49 When the bed is completely dissected, the anterior cornea is separated from the posterior cornea centrally, but is still attached peripherally, except for the area of the incision. In this way, the anterior lamella is stabilized, and the donor disk can be trephined to the appropriate diameter from the center of the cornea.

1.50 Donor buttons of higher quality can be cut with either the Barraquer microkeratome or, perhaps somewhat less precisely, with the Castroviejo keratome. Such machine-cut donor tissue has a smoother posterior surface and apparently results in better vision than a button cut free-hand. Unfortunately, microkeratomes cannot be used safely on scarred tissue or tissue that is ◊

Preoperative Routine

Patient preparation is similar to that for cataract surgery, except that no mechanical or pharmacologic agents, such as mannitol, Diamox, or the Honan balloon, are used to lower intraocular pressure. A soft eye offers too little resistance, and dissection of the bed is therefore much more difficult. Mild sedation, lid block, and retrobulbar anesthesia and topical anesthesia are used, without ocular compression. Any type of local or general anesthesia can be used.

Instruments

A standard penetrating keratoplasty tray is used, with the following additional instruments: permanent or disposable trephines in the various diameters, generally between 7.5 mm and 12.0 mm, the Paufique knife or the angled disposable Grieshaber lamellar dissector, the Desmarres scarifier (optional), the disposable 15° Grieshaber blade (or a shard of razor-blade on a blade breaker), and 10-0 nylon sutures. The CU-5 and TG-160-6 needles are sharp and delicate, ideal for interrupted suturing; the TG-160-6 needle is sturdy and suitable for running sutures.

Surgical Technique

51

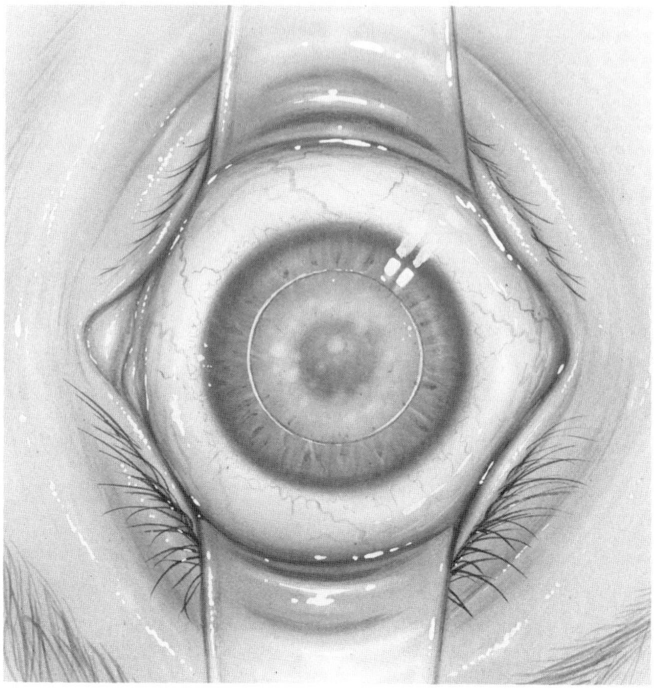

52

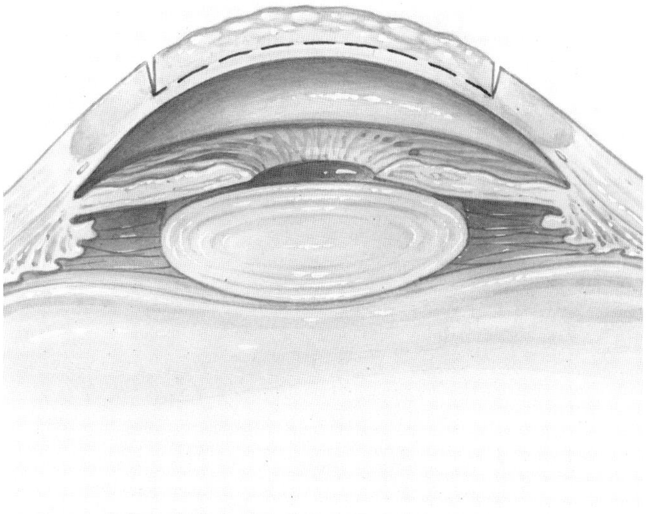

1.51 The speculum is inserted in the eye. Usually, the globe is fixated with superior and inferior rectus sutures. A trephine mark is made to a depth of at least 0.3 mm. If the scarring in the patient's cornea is extensive, the trephine cut can penetrate nearly the entire depth of the cornea, stopping just above Descemet's membrane.

1.52 This trephine cut extends approximately two-thirds the depth of the cornea. The edge of the trephine cut is separated by pulling with a forceps, and an angled lamellar dissector, such as the Paufique knife or one with disposable blades, is used to begin dissection of the lamella.

---

irregular in thickness; they are also difficult to use, and it is almost impossible to cut a donor button larger than 8 mm with these instruments. Commercially-prepared microkeratome-cut or lathe-cut tissue, which is optically and mechanically smooth, is now available.

53
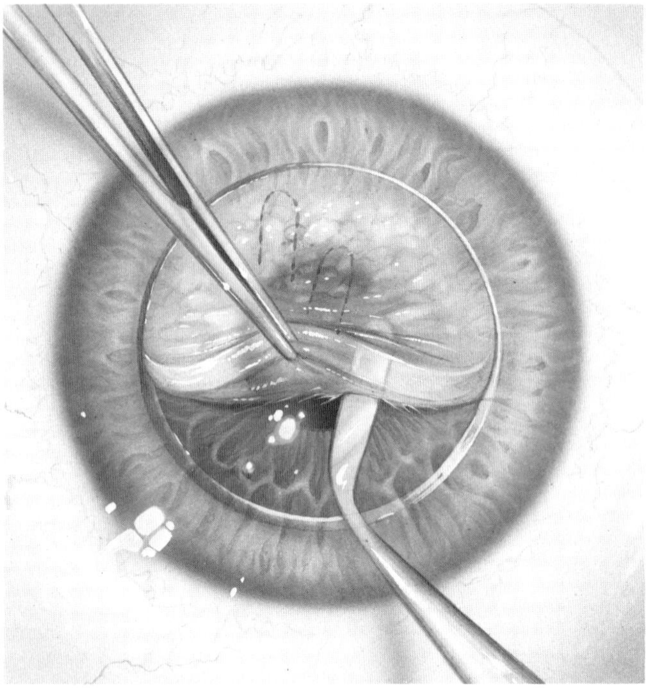

54
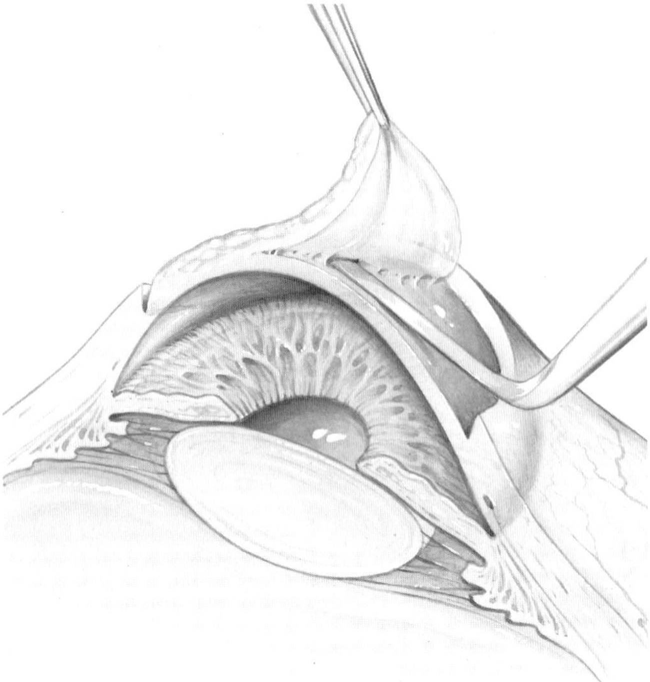

55
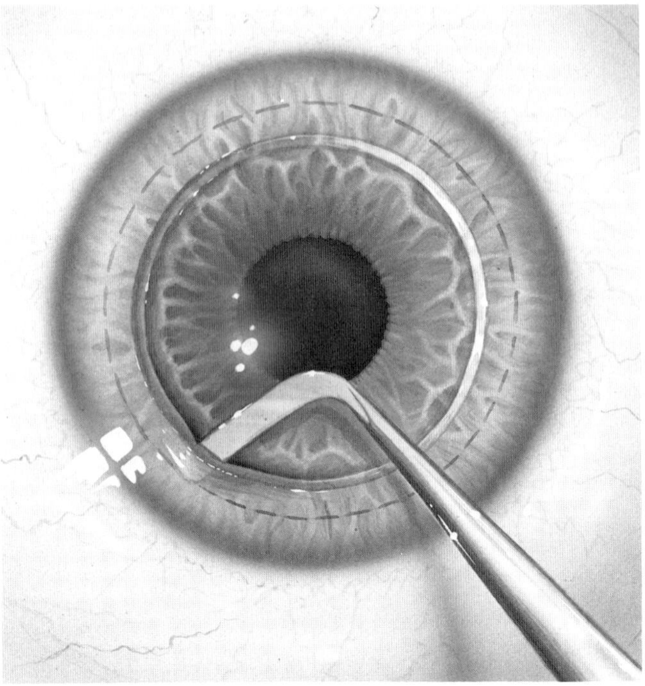

56
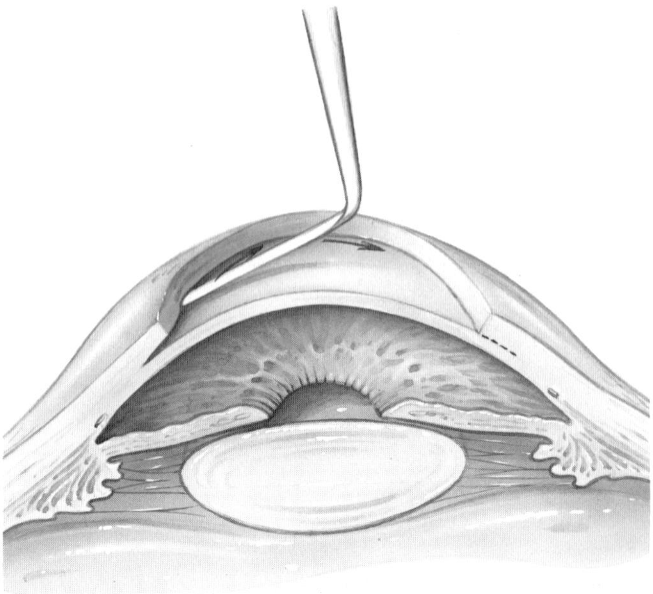

1.53 The lamella is separated from the bed at the depth of the trephine mark. The angled dissector may be replaced with a straight dissector blade, such as the Desmarres scarifier, as desired.

1.54 Lamellar keratoplasty primarily involves pulling and separating the layers of the cornea, rather than extensive cutting. The cornea to be removed is pulled away from the bed, and the small lamellar fibers are divided and cut with the blade. A firm globe facilitates this technique. No fluid should be used for any purpose during lamellar keratoplasty because fluid is rapidly absorbed by the stroma and distorts the tissue, making it difficult to judge depth and maintain the dissection in the proper plane.

If the original trephine cut is not deep enough, the edge can be deepened with a razor-blade. Alternatively, a deeper layer of the bed can be picked up with a fine Colibri forceps or a needle, the dissection extended to the edge of the trephine cut, and the lamella removed with scissors. It is extremely important that the edge of the bed be vertical and not sloping, for good apposition to the edge of the inlay lamellar graft.

1.55 and **56** Sometimes there is a discrepancy between the tickness of the donor tissue lamella and the depth of the edge of the recipient bed. In this case, the edge of the recipient bed can be undermined at the base. This permits the corneal edge to thicken and lift to match the

57

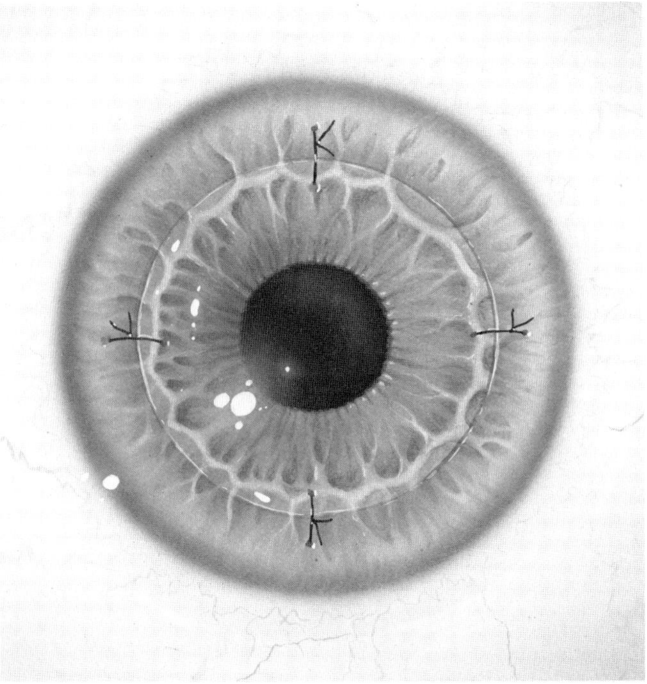

58

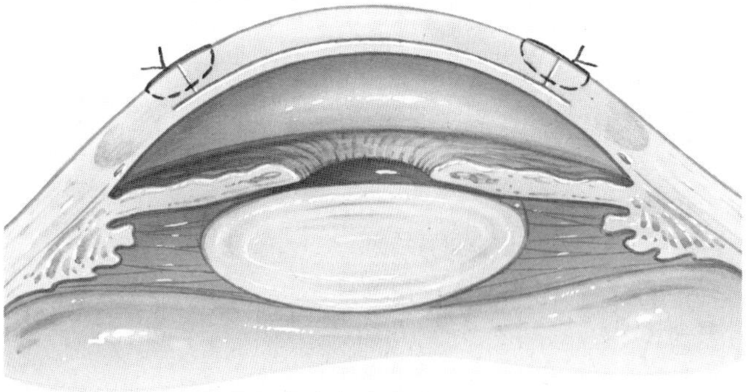

59

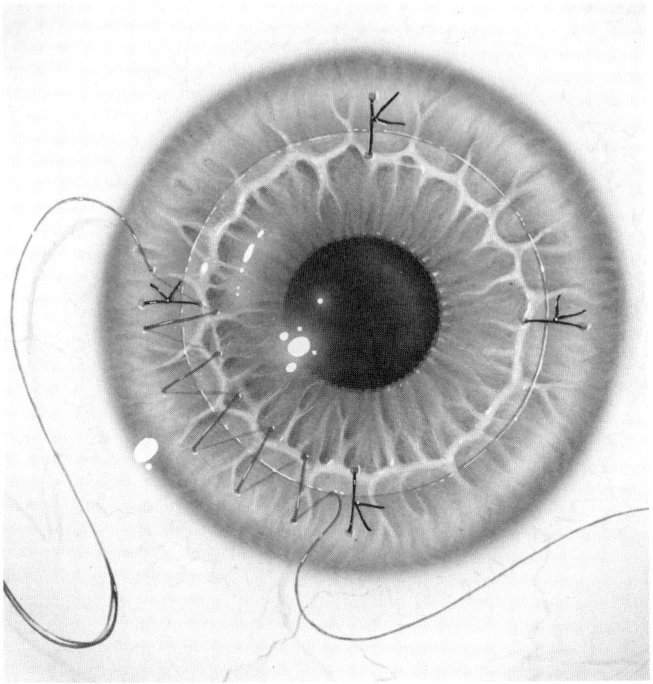

60

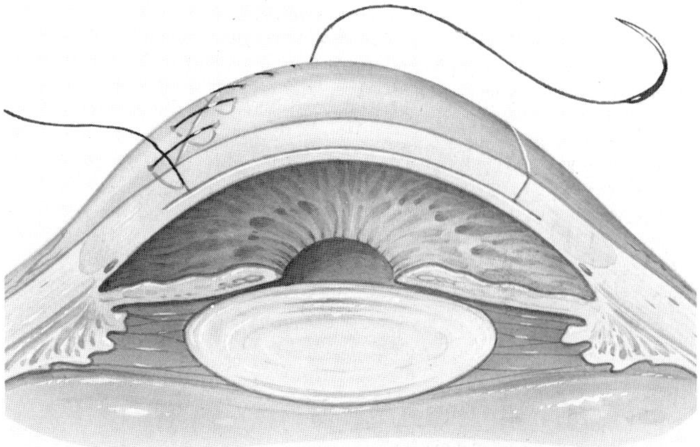

1.57 and **58** Four interrupted 10-0 opposing nylon sutures are placed 90° apart to stabilize and position the graft.

1.59 and **60** A running 10-0 nylon suture is begun within the wound and continued around the graft, with at least four bites per quadrant, for a total of at least 16 bites.

donor, so that the anterior surface at the cornea/donor junction is smooth and level, and will not be bumped by the lids.

61

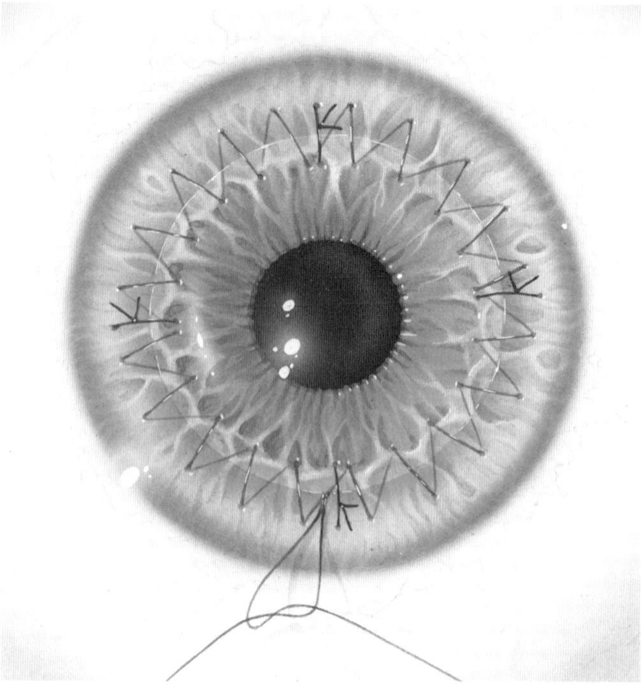

62

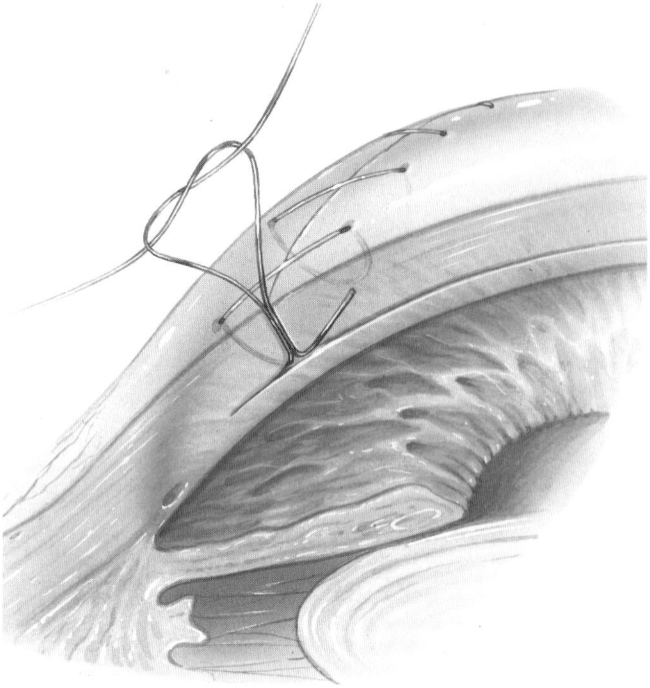

63

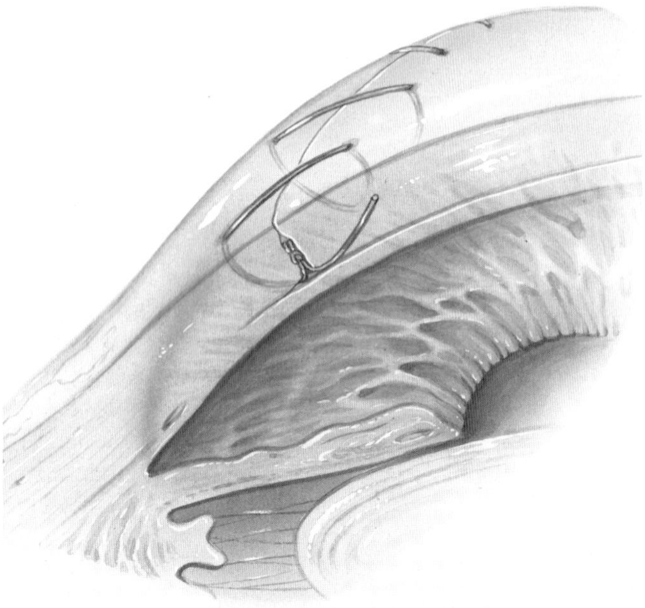

64

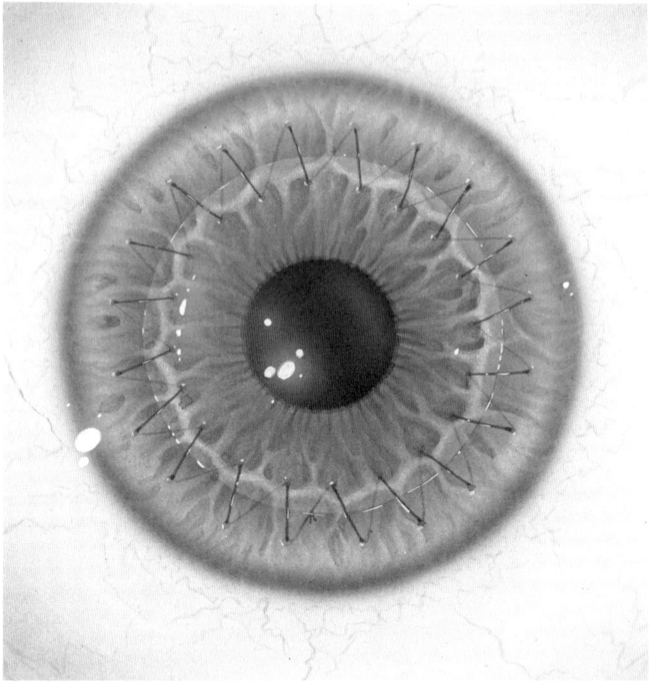

1.61 to **63** The running suture begins and ends within the wound. The ends of the suture are cut short and the knot is buried.

1.64 The four cardinal interrupted sutures can be removed when the running suture is in place.

Modifications and Surgical Alternatives

Interrupted sutures can be use instead of the running suture. Again, at least four sutures per quadrant are needed, and the knots are buried. In cases of unevenly vascularized recipients or eccentric grafts, interrupted sutures permit removal of individual sutures in vascularized areas while other areas heal at a normal pace.

65

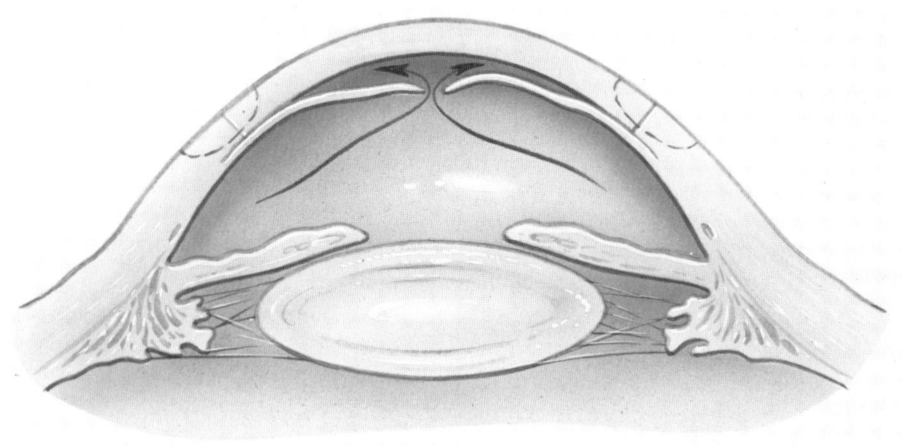

66

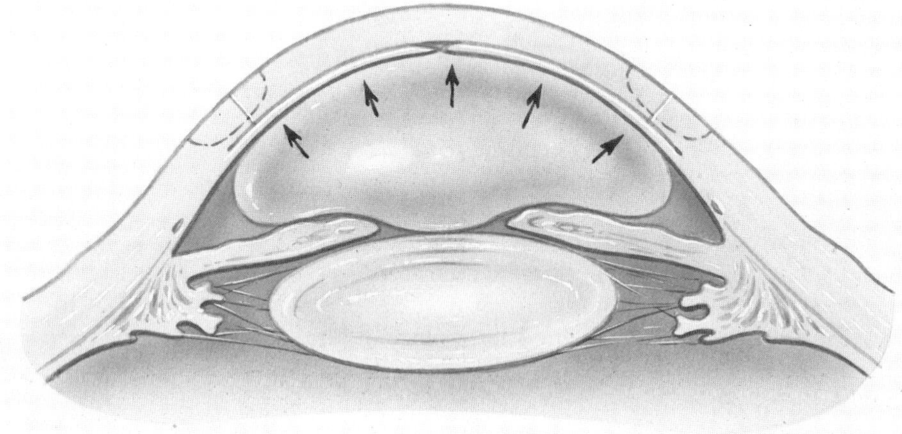

Complications

1.65 If a small perforation develops in the recipient bed, aqueous may accumulate between the bed and the lamellar graft, separating the recipient stroma and Descemet's membrane from the base of the graft. This may resolve spontaneously, but can also persist, resulting in a damaged, cloudy graft.

1.66 To correct the problem, a paracentesis can be performed, and the anterior chamber filled with air to tamponade the hole and maintain the donor and recipient cornea in apposition until a natural fibrin seal forms.

If the tear is very large, a fine 11-0 nylon suture with as fine a needle as possible may be used to close the opening. This suture can be left buried in the deeper layer under the graft. About five minutes after this maneuver, air tamponade can be attempted. In extreme cases, Descemet's membrane can be repaired with a double-arm running 11-0 nylon suture, with the needle brought up through the donor. The knot is tied above the donor in such a way that the base is pulled against the graft.

When the damage to the recipient bed is too extensive and the size of the graft is not too large, the procedure can be converted to penetrating keratoplasty. Because of this possibility, it is safer to plan for simple optical lamellar keratoplasties with small superficial scars no more than 8 mm in diameter.

Admonitions and Suggestions

Small lamellar keratoplasties, 5 mm or less in diameter, are best accomplished when the donor tissue and the recipient bed are cut to the same measurement. With lamellar keratoplasties from about 5 to 9 mm, there is a tendency for the recipient bed to stretch, and the donor tissue should be 0.25 to 0.5 mm larger in diameter. For keratoplasties larger than 9 mm, the donor should be 0.5 to 1.0 mm larger in diameter, to avoid excessive wrinkling of the base and the need to tie the sutures too tightly.

The walls of the recipient bed and the edge of the donor should be cut on the vertical axis, perpendicular to the cornea. Sloping cuts result in poor apposition of donor and recipient, which leads to postoperative astigmatism, increased scarring at the interface, and epithelial ingrowth, in which epithelial cells migrate down into the wound and along the interface, causing the graft to fail.

Postoperative Management

If local anesthesia is used, patients can be discharged the afternoon of the day of surgery; general anesthesia usually requires overnight hospitalization. A pressure patch or bandage lens is necessary until re-epithelialization is complete. A dilating drop (atropine 5% or homatropine 5%) and antibiotic (Garamycin or Sulamyd ointment) are administered twice a day. The pressure patch is changed or the bandage lens checked after twice-weekly slit lamp examination until the graft is 100% epithelialized. Topical corticosteroids are not used routinely except in cases in which there is a marked postoperative iritis or an allergy to 10-0 nylon sutures, evidenced by engorgement of the limbal verssels and collection of opaque white material (white blood cells) where the suture material enters and exits from the cornea. When needed, corticosteroids are applied four times a day for a week and tapered rapidly thereafter.

Normal activity can be resumed on the first postoperative day, with the exception of driving, unless the patient is accustomed to driving with monocular vision.

Postoperative complications are usually minor and easily treated because the procedure is extraocular; the most common problems are the failure of the epithelium to cover the graft within the first three weeks after surgery, and neovascularization of the sutures. Most lamellar grafts re-epithelialize quickly. Occasionally, a chronic epithelial defect will not respond to the wearing of a bandage soft contact lens or patching. In this case, a temporary tarsorrhaphy is performed with three interrupted 5-0 Dermalon sutures. The central Dermalon suture is "bow-tied" so that it can be opened and reclosed for examination of the cornea. Generally, a lamellar graft that has not re-epithelialized after patching or wearing a bandage lens for three weeks followed by a tarsorrhaphy for three weeks will be melted or opaque, at which point it must be removed and a second graft attempted.

In vascularized recipient beds, eccentric grafts, or young patients, the corneal periphery may undergo rapid neovascularization. The vessels can cross the surgical wound and spread throughout the graft, recipient, and interface, causing the graft to fail. Also, the sutures may become loose and collect mucus, which is extremely uncomfortable for the patient. If this possibility is suspected, the surgeon should check the patient more frequently and remove sutures early.

The running suture can usually be removed eight weeks after surgery. The closer the graft is to the limbus, i. e., the larger the graft, the earlier the sutures should be removed to prevent vascularization and graft rejection.

Results

The average patient who receives a lamellar keratoplasty for optical purposes will have reasonable vision if the recipient scar was completely excised during the procedure. Hand-cut lamellar grafts are generally less clear optically than machine-cut lamellar grafts. For example, a patient with a potential for 20/20 vision may have 20/40 to 20/60 visual acuity with a hand-cut lamellar graft and 20/25 to 20/30 with a machine-cut lamellar graft. A 20/20 result with a lamellar graft is unusual. Nonplanar lamellar dissection, which crosses many layers of corneal collagen, results in irregularity and increased scarring at the interface, reducing vision. The recipient bed must generally be cut by hand, as the use of the microkeratome greatly increases the risk of perforation in the presence of excessive scarring. However, machine-cut, preserved donor tissue, which is plano and smooth, improves the visual outcome of optical lamellar keratoplasty.

Onlay Lamellar Keratoplasty for Keratoconus

Surgical Principles

Onlay lamellar keratoplasty involves adding a lamella of donor corneal tissue to the anterior surface of the de-epithelialized cornea, with no dissection of the recipient bed within the optical zone. An annular keratectomy is created peripherally, and the edge of the graft tissue is sutured into this defect. A similar procedure employs a preshaped graft to correct refractive error in the aphakic or myopic eye. In the case of a patient with keratoconus, the plano graft tissue serves to flatten and reinforce the thinned and protruding cone. This reshaping of the anterior cornea enables the patient to tolerate daily-wear contact lenses for optical correction.

Preparation for Surgery

See optical inlay lamellar keratoplasty, above.

Preoperative Medication and Anesthesia

See optical inlay lamellar keratoplasty, above.

Instruments

In addition to the instruments found on a routine penetrating keratoplasty tray, the following additional items are needed: 4% cocaine; blunt-cut cellulose sponges on plastic handles (Weck-Cel sponges can be cut blunt with scissors); infant feeding tube, with the tip cut at an angle and attached to wall suction; 50 ml plastic syringe with a micropore filter between the syringe and the 23 gauge irrigating needle; trephine of the appropriate recipient diameter; Paton spatula (this is usually in the penetrating keratoplasty tray); angled Vannas scissors; disposable or permanent trephine in a size 0.5 mm larger in diameter than the size of the trephine used for the donor.

Surgical Technique

67

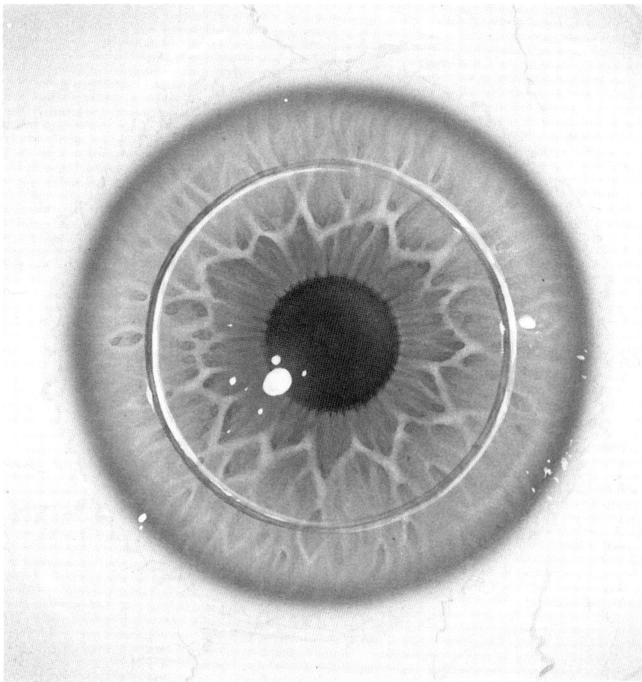

68

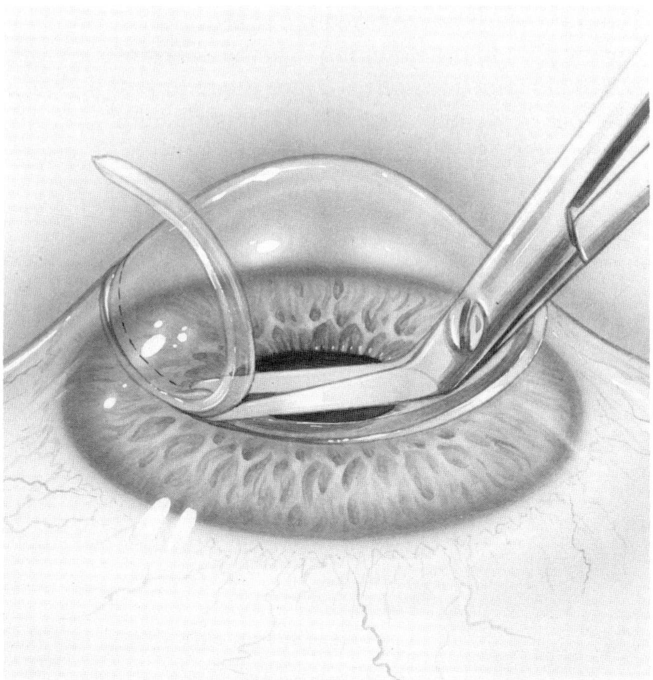

69

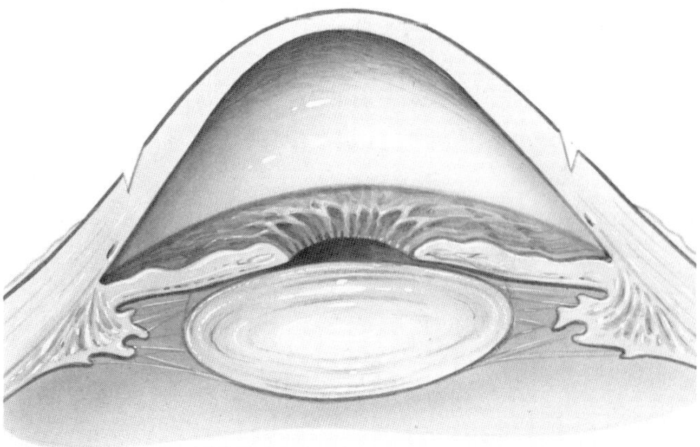

1.**67** The epithelium is removed with a cocaine-soaked, blunt-cut cellulose sponge. A 5 mm cuff of epithelium is left at the corneoscleral limbus, to ensure regrowth of the epithelium over the graft after surgery. A trephine cut is made to a depth of 0.3 mm; the diameter depends on the extent and position of the cone, but can be very large, up to 12.0 mm if necessary. In most cases, a 9.0 mm donor is placed in an 8.5 mm bed.

1.**68** and **69** The inner edge of the trephine cut is grasped in a fixation forceps, such as a Colibri forceps, and a narrow (0.5 mm) wedge of superficial cornea and Bowman's membrane is excised with Vannas scissors. The circular groove or annular keratectomy that is created is well out of the visual axis.

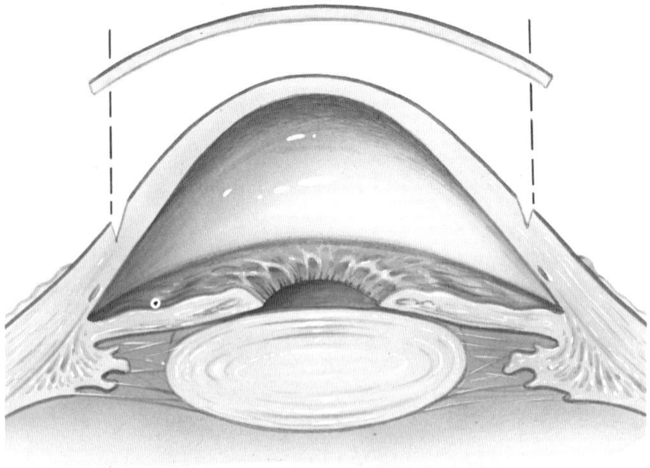

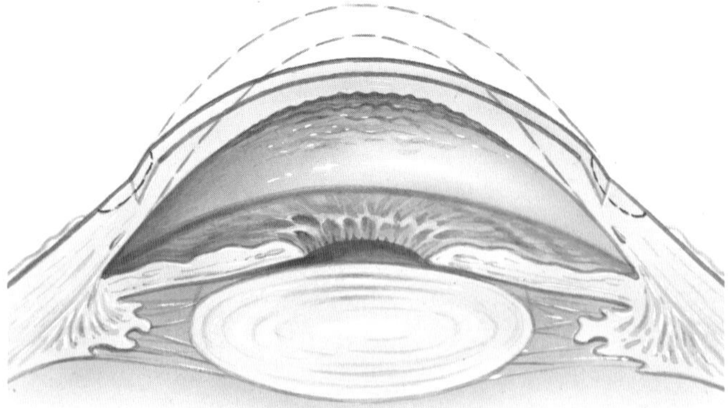

1.70 The onlay lamellar graft for keratoconus is of equal thickness throughout and 0.5 mm larger in diameter than the annular keratectomy.

1.71 The donor tissue is centered over the trephine cut and the edge is sutured into the keratectomy with 20 to 24 interrupted 10-0 nylon sutures. The resulting corneal configuration has two Bowman's membranes – the host Bowman's and the Bowman's on the donor tissue graft. The onlay lamellar graft is cut to the required thickness from the Descemet's side, so that it is machine-smooth. Healing occurs only in the area of the keratectomy, where there is a defect in the host Bowman's membrane.

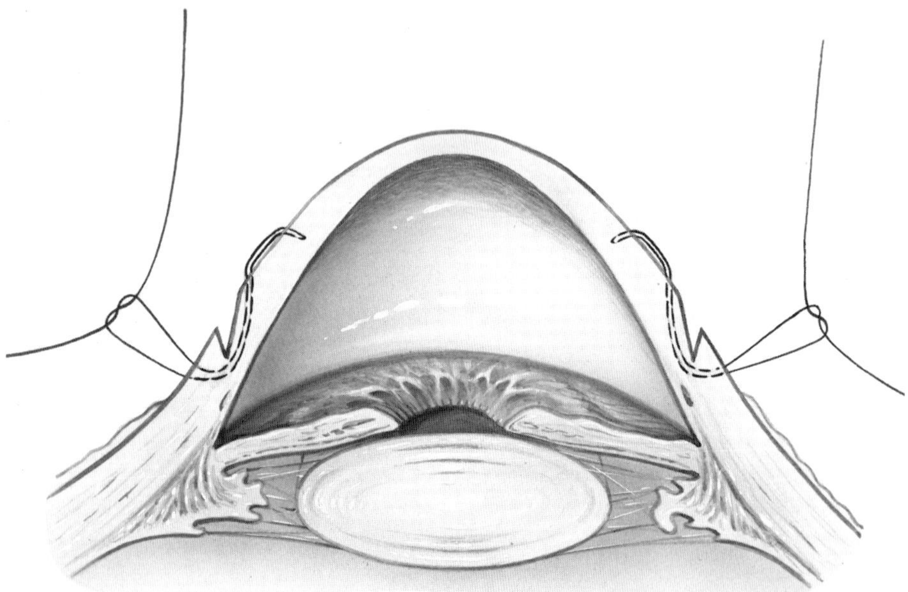

Modifications and Surgical Alternatives

1.72 If there is a keratoglobus with a very large central corneal bulge, the protruding tissue may form large central folds that interfere with vision when the cone is flattened by the graft. In such a case, the folds can sometimes be smoothed out by softening the eye. Often massage is sufficient, but paracentesis can be used if necessary. To reduce the protrusion, sutures can be placed in the middle of the stroma and brought out past the limbus, then tightened to throw the peripheral cornea into folds and smooth out the central cornea. We call these sutures "reefing sutures" because the peripheral corneal tissue is bunched together, much like a reefed sail. Two of these reefing sutures placed 90° apart can move a central recipient scar into a paracentral position before the graft is sewn into place.

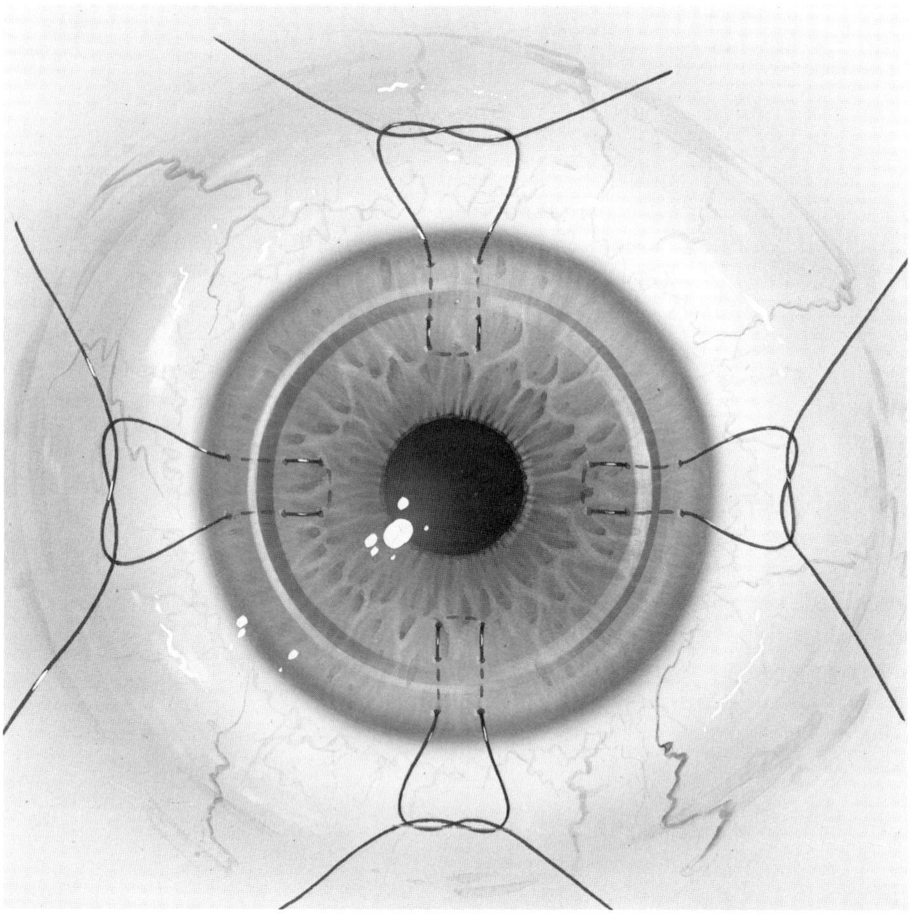

1.73 Four of these sutures at 90° intervals around the cornea can flatten a very large keratoglobus and concentrate the folds in the periphery.

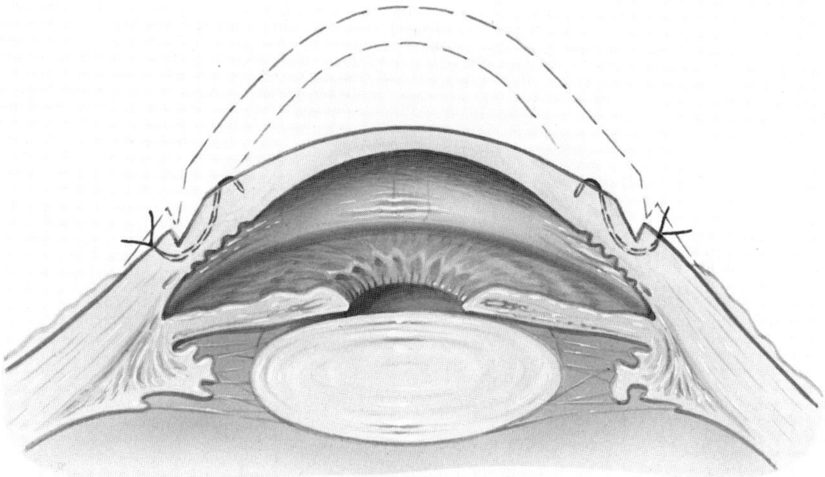

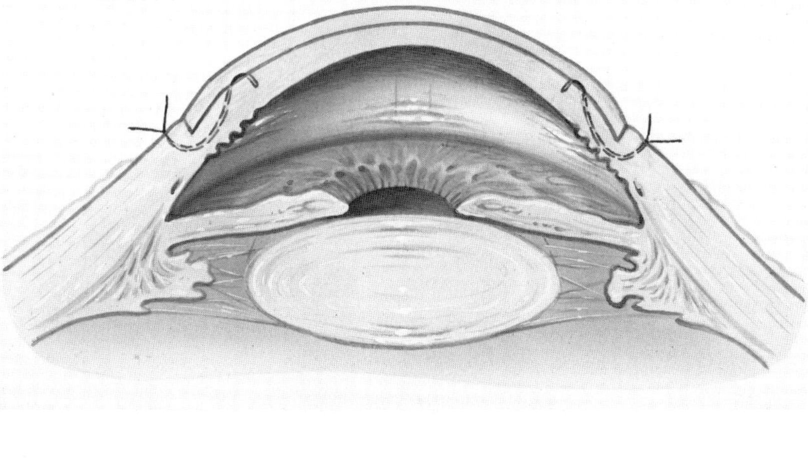

1.**74** and **75** The onlay graft is placed on top of the smooth cornea and sutured into the peripheral keratectomy bed. A keratoglobus usually requires a very large onlay lamellar graft, and donor tissue grafts 10 mm or more in diameter are not uncommon. Antiglaucoma medication should be given for two to three days postoperatively to a patient with a large keratoglobus.

Complications

See optical inlay lamellar graft, above.

Admonitions and Suggestions

We perform onlay lamellar keratoplasty only on keratoconus patients with best corrected visual acuities of 20/40 or better with contact lens correction. The majority of our patients experience a progressive inability to tolerate daily-wear contact lenses, and surgery becomes necessary when decreased wearing time begins to affect their activities. These patients can tolerate the wearing of a hard lens for a few minutes for diagnostic purposes, but are unable to function with the lens in place for long periods of time due to fitting problems and pain. The Takata laser interferometer can be used to measure the potential for acceptable postoperative visual acuity in patients with severely scarred corneas.

With the use of the reefing sutures, patients with keratoglobus and patients with reduced visual acuity due to central scarring become eligible for this surgical procedure, particularly those for whom penetrating keratoplasty is contraindicated because of age (under 12), severe mental retardation or cerebral palsy, or a history of multiple rejection episodes in the fellow eye necessitating frequent application of topical corticosteroids with subsequent cataract formation.

In cases of extreme keratoglobus, with severe scarring and very thin corneas, a very large (from limbus to limbus) onlay lamellar keratoplasty is used to reinforce and thicken the cornea; six months later, when the onlay graft has healed, a penetrating keratoplasty can be done to restore vision, if scarring is severe.

Postoperative Management

See optical inlay lamellar graft, above. Patients with severe keratoglobus should be given timolol maleate, acetazolamide, and pilocarpine for two to three days postoperatively to prevent glaucoma resulting from angle crowding.

Results

Myopia is decreased by approximately 8 D, and regular astigmatism is reduced by about 4 to 4.5 D. Irregular astigmatism is also decreased. Most patients recover, fully or almost fully, their best corrected preoperative visual acuity two to four months after surgery, and all resume full-time contact lens wear with a single lens system; no piggyback lenses are required.

Recurrent Pterygium

Surgical Principles

Lamellar grafts are used only when the pterygium has recurred a number of times in spite of multiple adequate regular excisions. The object of inlay lamellar keratoplasty for recurrent pterygium is to remove the recurrent dysplastic pterygium and to provide tectonic support for the underlying cornea.

Preparation for Surgery

See optical inlay lamellar keratoplasty, above.

Preoperative Medication and Anesthesia

See optical inlay lamellar keratoplasty, above.

Instruments

See optical inlay lamellar keratoplasty, above.

Surgical Technique

76

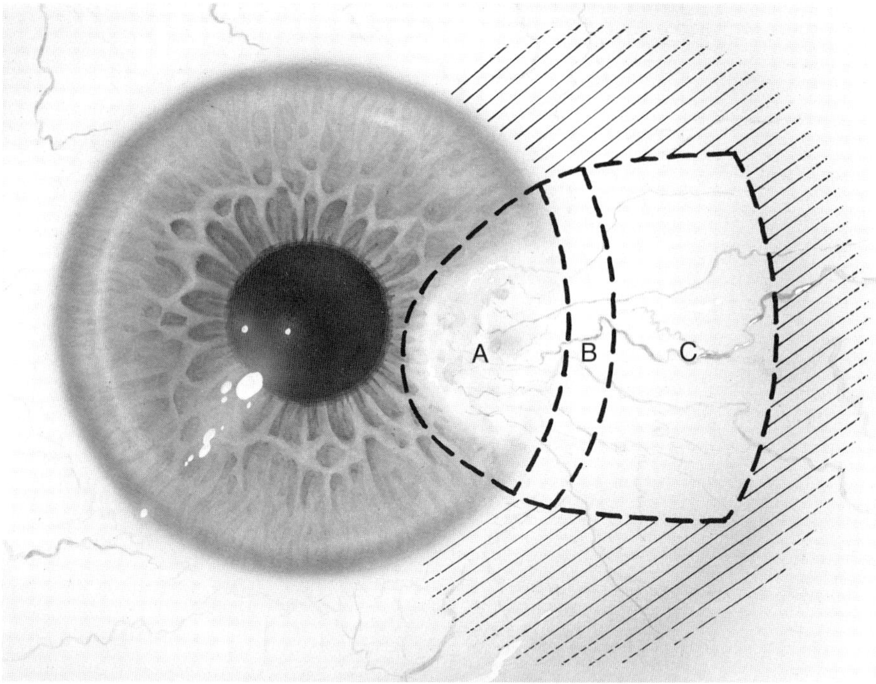

1.76 The first step is to excise the pterygium and the inflamed conjunctiva to which it is attached, leaving an area of bare sclera. The innermost, oval area of the cornea (A) will be covered by an inlay lamellar graft to thicken and reinforce the tissue. The outermost area of bare sclera (C) will be covered by a flap of conjunctiva, in order to prevent excessive scar formation and subsequent limitation of eye movement. A small bare area (B), denuded of conjunctiva and not covered by the inlay lamellar keratoplasty, is left between the inlay graft and the conjunctival flap to minimize interruption of the tear film and dellen formation.

77

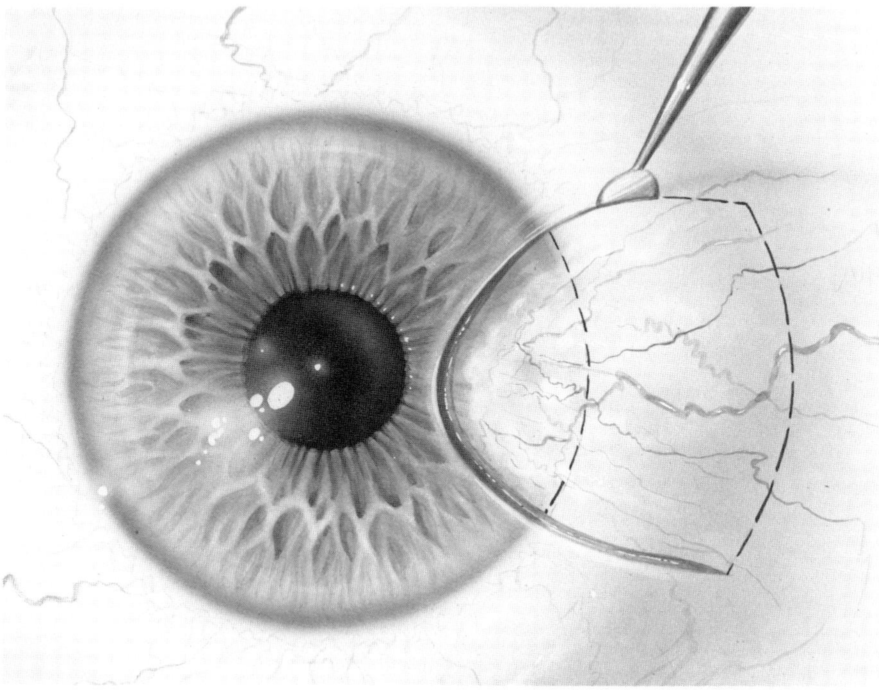

1.77 and **78** Lamellar dissection of the pterygium and its base results in a recipient bed with the leading edge conforming to a semicircle surrounding the head of the growth. Conjunctival excision is performed peripheral to the lamellar dissection.

78

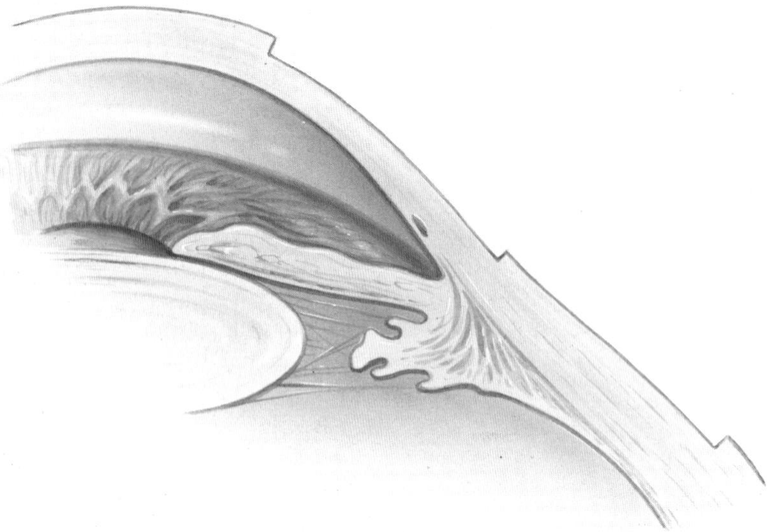

79

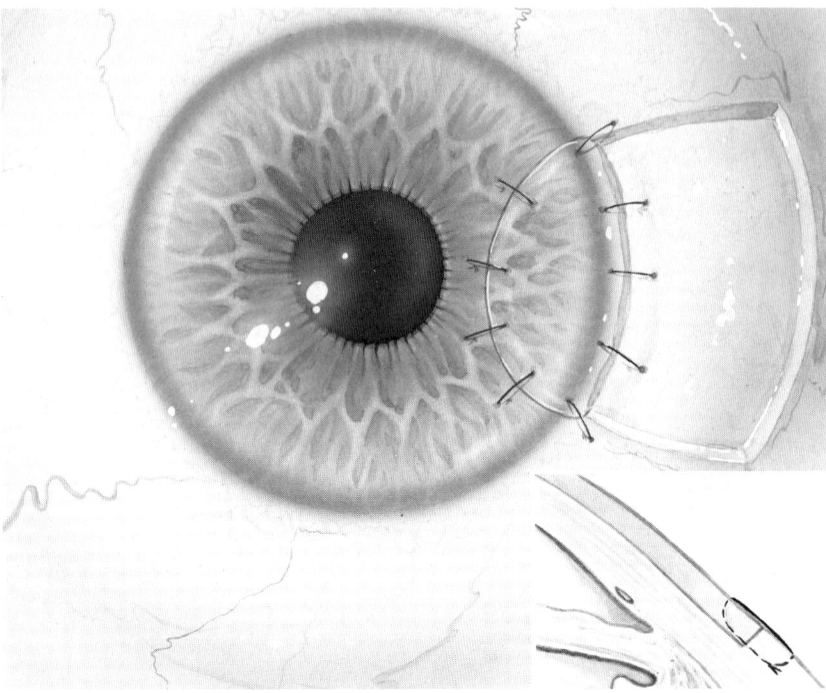

1.79 The graft (obtained from fresh corneal tissue, a frozen globe, or precut preserved tissue) is cut to fit the recipient bed. The donor lamellar tissue is sewn into place with interrupted 10-0 nylon sutures. The knots are rotated into the wound. An area of bare sclera is left, part of which will be covered by conjunctiva from above.

80

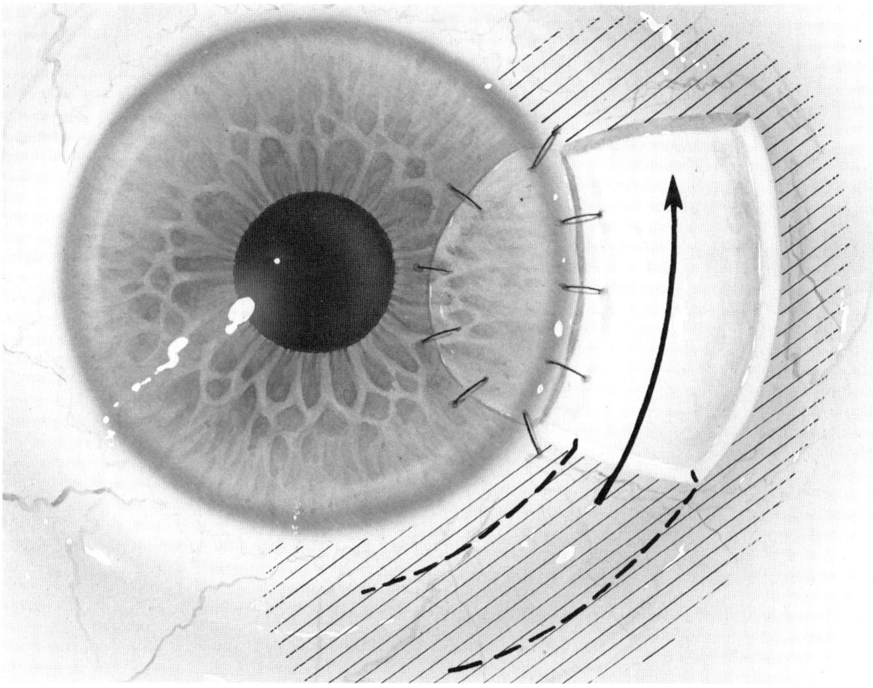

1.80 and **81** Conjunctiva is pulled down to cover some of the bare sclera nasally. A small bare area, denuded of conjunctiva, is left between the sliding conjunctival flap and the lamellar keratoplasty. If this is not done, and too much conjunctiva has been excised, there will be a limitation in the motion of the eye and a greater tendency for the pterygium to recur.

81

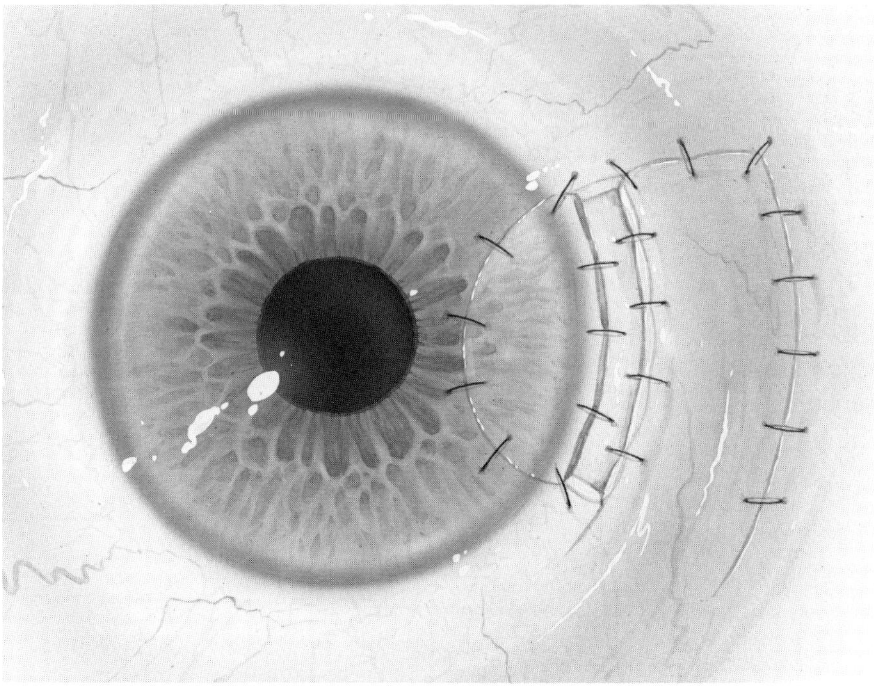

Modifications and Surgical Alternatives

The head of the pterygium can be delimited by a vertical corneal incision through Bowman's membrane into the superficial stroma, extending to the limbus. The area of conjunctiva to be excised is marked, and a semicircular edge is made in the sclera parallel to the limbus. The superficial keratectomy is performed and any rough or infiltrated cornea is excised. The half-moon-shaped recipient bed created by this dissection is easily matched by cutting straight across the circular disk of donor tissue. The donor tissue is sutured into the keratectomy bed and the conjunctival flap prepared as described above.

To avoid dissecting donor tissue during surgery, we frequently use precut preseved tissue that is supplied as a 10 mm diameter disk. It is easy to make a vertical slice through this tissue and sew the vertical aspect of the graft to the vertical cut in the recipient. The 10 mm curve of the donor tissue usually fits quite well into the limbal area.

Complications

Possible complications are those mentioned previously for other forms of lamellar grafts: failure to re-epithelialize, which is rare, and neovascularization. In surgery for pterygium, sutures are placed at the limbus, so vascularization is extremely rapid and the patient must be watched to be sure that the new vessels do not invade the donor, interface, or recipient.

Admonitions and Suggestions

The patient's previous operative history must be examined to determine in advance exactly how much corneal tissue has already been removed. It is possible to dissect what appears to be an extremely thin lamella of recipient corneal tissue that actually is in contact with Descemet's membrane. Once the cornea is excessively thinned, aqueous can penetrate the remaining stroma, and surgical closure becomes extremely difficult.

Postoperative Management

Postoperative management is the same as for the other forms of lamellar surgery described above, except that the sutures must be removed sooner in this case because most of them are located in the limbus. The interrupted sutures at the central edge of the wound are usually removed three to six weeks postoperatively, when a thin white line representing scar tissue becomes apparent, or loosened sutures begin to collect mucus. Sutures in the limbus may be removed as early as two weeks after surgery.

Results

Most patients can see well without contact lenses but require a change in their spectacle prescription. Patients who want to wear contact lenses can be easily fitted. Since this surgery does not involve the visual axis, best corrected acuities preoperatively and postoperatively are the same.

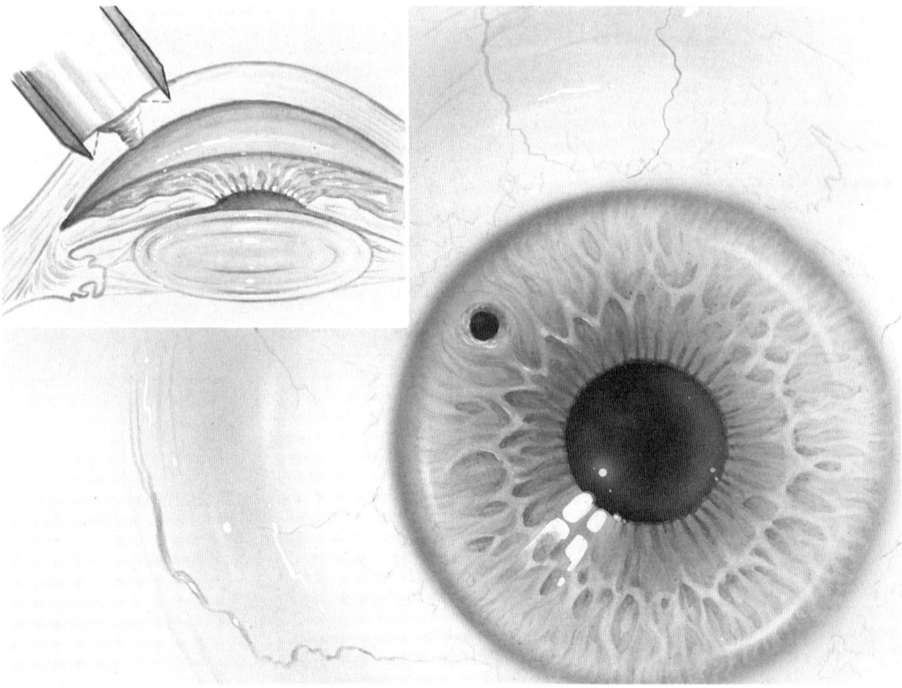

Corneal Perforation

1.**82** In the case of a small peripheral descemetocele, perforation, or even deep ulcer, an onlay transplant can be used. If there is necrotic tissue present, as much as is convenient can be removed. A trephine is placed over the problem area, and a small, 0.3 mm deep peripheral cut is made. The diameter of the trephine should be chosen to keep the trephine mark as far from the thinned area of the cornea as possible, and no dissection of the thinned area is necessary.

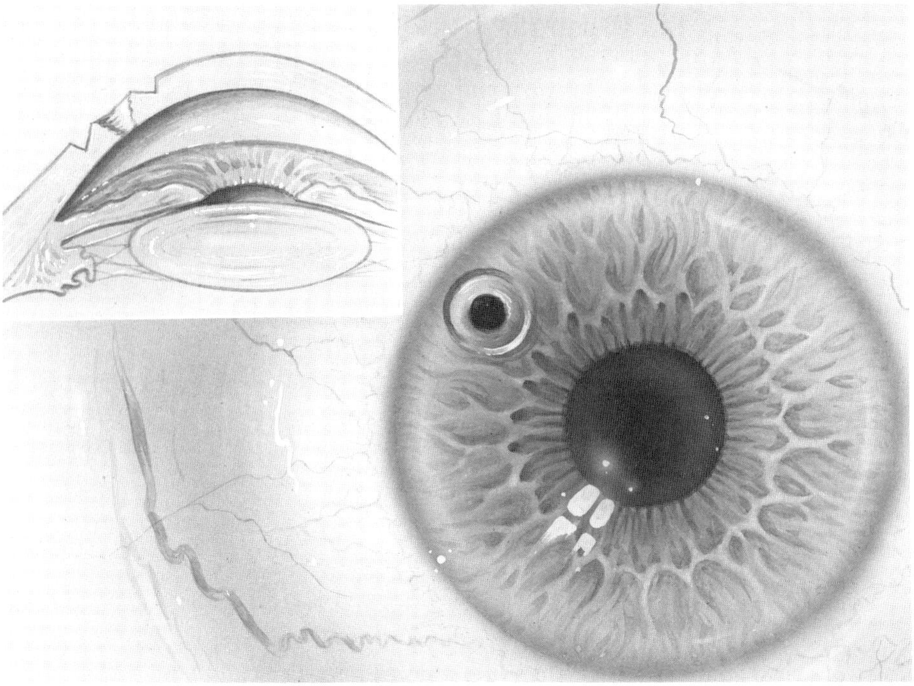

1.83 The inner edge of the trephine cut is dissected to form a small annular keratectomy, much like that used for onlay lamellar keratoplasty for keratoconus. If the eye is soft, the trephine can be used to mark the cornea, and the cut deepened with a razor blade.

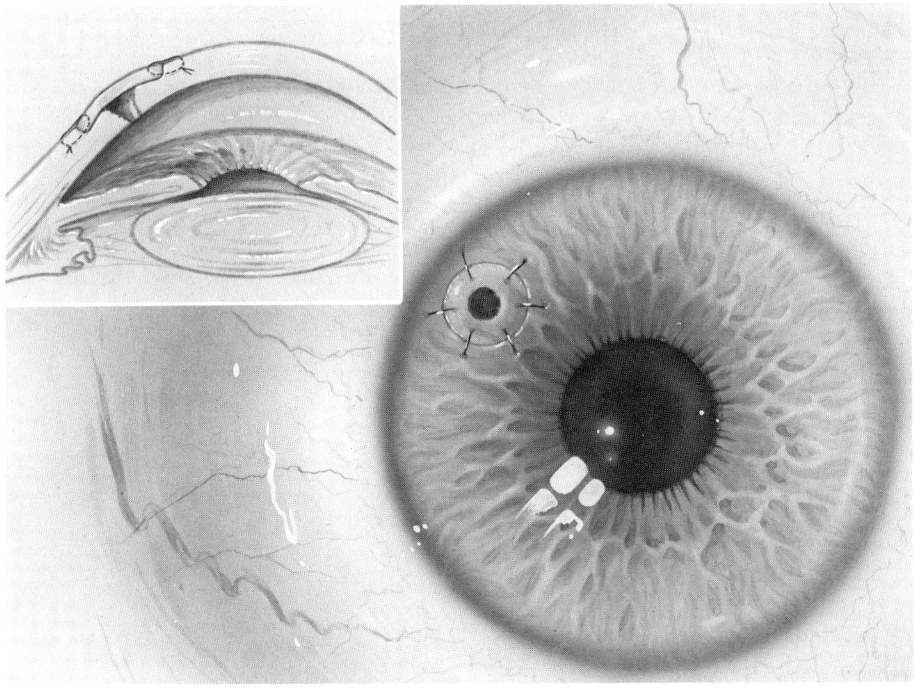

1.84 A thin piece of lamellar tissue, obtained either from a globe, as for lamellar kerato-plasty, or precut preserved tis-sue, is placed over the keratec-tomy and sutured in place to strengthen the thinned and weakened area and seal the eye.

Bibliography

[1] Busin, M., B. L. Halliday, R. C. Arffa, M. B. McDonald, H. E. Kaufman: Precarved lyophilized tissue for lamellar kerato-plasty in recurrent pterygium. *Amer. J. Ophthalmol.* 102: 222–227, 1986.

[2] Kaufman, H. E., T. P. Werblin: Epikeratophakia for the treatment of keratoconus. *Amer. J. Ophthalmol.* 93 (3): 342–347, 1982.

[3] McDonald, M. B., S. B. Koenig, A. Safir, H. E. Kaufman: Onlay lamellar keratoplasty for the treatment of keratoconus. *Br. J. Ophthalmol.* 67: 615–618, 1983.

[4] McDonald, M. B., H. E. Kaufman, D. R. Sanders and the Medical Monitors of the Nationwide Epikeratophakia Study: Epikeratophakia for keratoconus: the nationwide study. *Arch. Ophthalmol.* 104: 1294–1300, 1986.

Radial Keratotomy

James C. Hays and J. Rowsey

Surgical Principles

In radial keratotomy the refracting power of the eye is decreased by flattening the center of the cornea. Incisions are placed radially in the cornea, like the spokes of a wheel, to flatten the central cornea. The amount of flattening will depend upon the depth and number of the cuts and the size of the clear central optical zone. Deeper cuts produce more flattening. A smaller central optical zone will give more flattening than a larger central optical zone. We have found that eight incisions are about 25 % more effective than four incisions.

Preparation for Surgery

The most important surgical preparation is a thorough discussion with the patient about what to expect during and after surgery. The patient may show some anxiety about the operation being performed under topical anesthesia. Reassure the patient that the surgery only takes about 15 minutes and is virtually pain-free.

In the postoperative period, however, the patient should expect moderate to severe irritation and photophobia for the first 24 to 48 hours. Most patients will experience daily fluctuations in vision for several weeks.

The patient should be aware that some eyes are left undercorrected, while some are unintentionally made hyperopic. Patients in their late thirties or early forties should be warned about the possibility of "acute presbyopia" caused by the surgery.

Inform the patient that his visual acuity may decrease at night. As the pupil dilates in a darkened environment, light can enter the eye through the mid-peripheral cornea. The mid-peripheral cornea will not be as flat as the central cornea. This allows a partial return of the original myopia. In addition, the patient will be able to see the ends of the cuts when the pupil dilates, and this may be distressing enough to make night driving difficult for several months following surgery.

Preoperative Routine

The patient should sign a specific consent form which details potential side-effects and complications of radial keratotomy surgery. Topical proparacaine is adequate as anesthesia. Supplemental intravenous diazepam may be added as needed.

The patient will be more comfortable and cooperative if the pupil is not dilated, since the light from the operating microscope can be quite dazzling. A reoperation, however, is technically easier if the pupil is dilated, as the previous incisions will be much more visible. The optical zone will already have been marked from the previous operation, so fixation on the bright light of the operating microscope is not so critical. Two drops of 2 % cyclopentolate about 20 minutes prior to surgery will dilate the pupil adequately.

Instruments

A number of ultrasonic pachymeters are commercially available. In choosing one, remember that a solid-tipped probe is easier to use than a water-filled tip.

Specially designed knives with diamond and steel blades are available for radial keratotomy. Incisions made with diamond knives result in less scarring than those made with steel knives. Properly cared for, a diamond knife should last indefinitely and is the instrument of choice.

Fixation of the globe is difficult using single-pronged, or two-pronged forceps. A fixation ring such as the Thornton fixation ring makes the globe more stable and has the advantage of allowing retropulsion of the globe so that firm intraocular pressure can be maintained.

Surgical Technique

The eye is prepped and draped routinely for ocular surgery. An open-bladed lid speculum is used to minimize the possibility of chipping the diamond blade on the metal of the lid speculum.

85

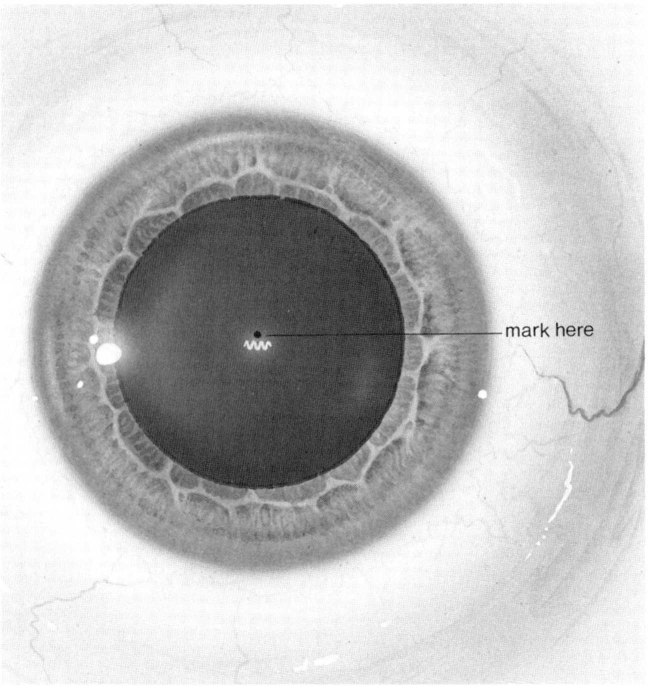

86

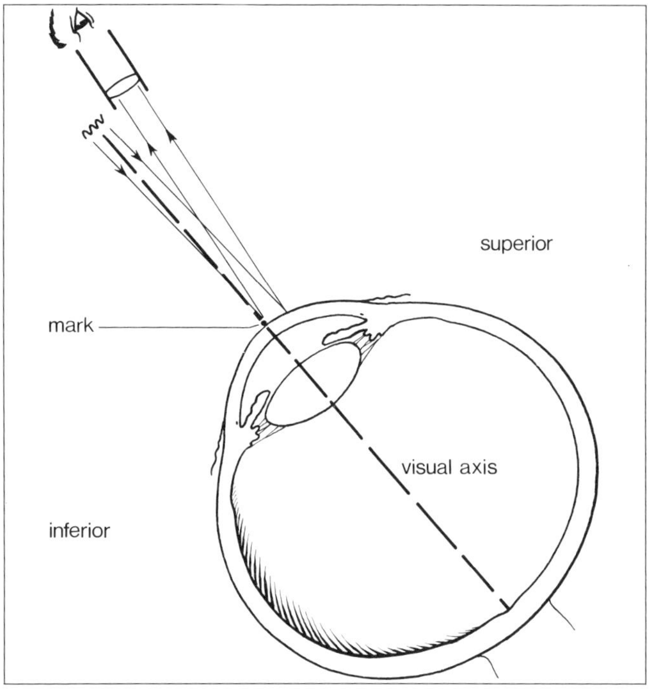

87

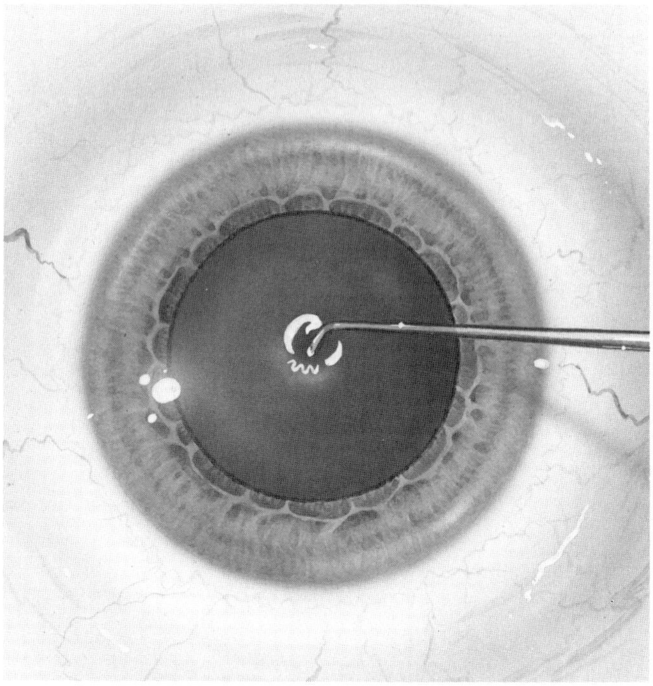

1.85 und **86** The method of marking the visual axis depends upon the type of operating microscope used. The following technique is suitable for the Zeiss OPMI 6-S microscope. With the light on very low intensity the patient is asked to fixate the middle of the filament. Since the light source is not actually coaxial with the eyepieces, but is situated slightly toward the patient's feet, the apparent image of the light reflex seems to move toward the observer. This means that it is necessary to mark lower on the patient's cornea than the light reflex appears. Through analysis of corneascope photos we have determined that the center of the visual axis in the vertical meridian lies at the bottom edge of the light reflex coming from the OPMI 6-S microscope. Since the two eyepieces are equidistant from the center of the light source in the horizontal meridian, the visual axis of the eye is in the middle of the light reflex.

1.87 A small mark is made, using a Sinskey hook, at the bottom of the light reflex (toward the patient's feet) and halfway between the two edges in the horizontal meridian. A drop of fluorescein is applied to the eye and irrigated off to make the optical axis mark more visible.

88 a

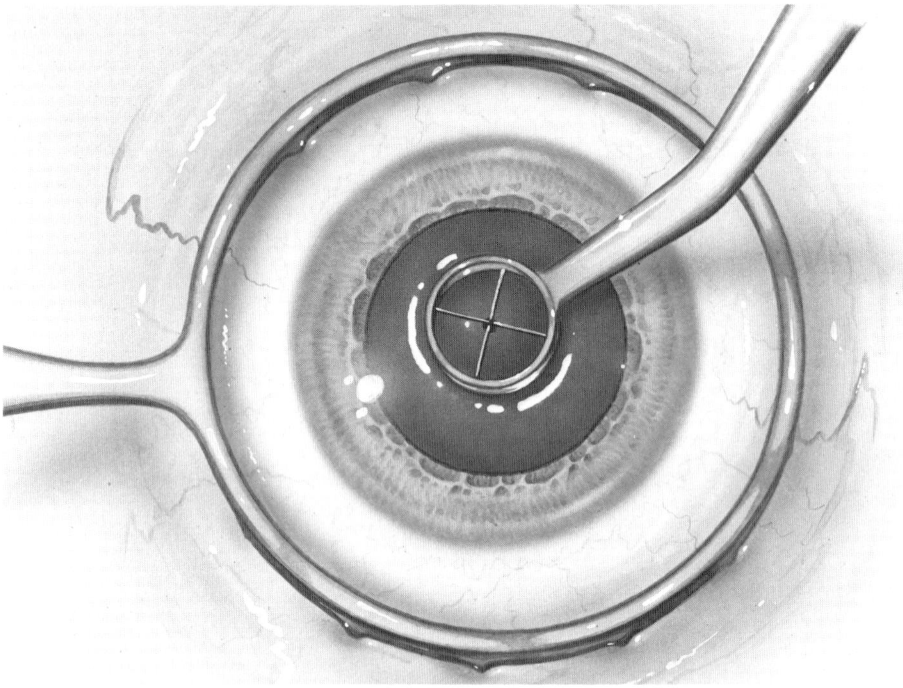

88 b

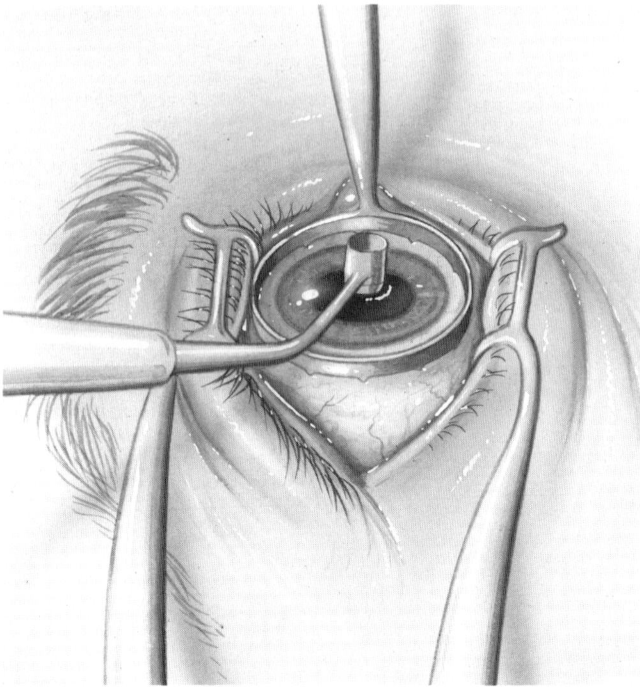

1.**88 a** and **b, 89** The appropriate blunt trephine is selected and the cross-hairs are centered over the fluorescein-stained optical axis mark. After the trephine has been applied to the cornea it is turned through 90° so that the mark is easily visible.

89
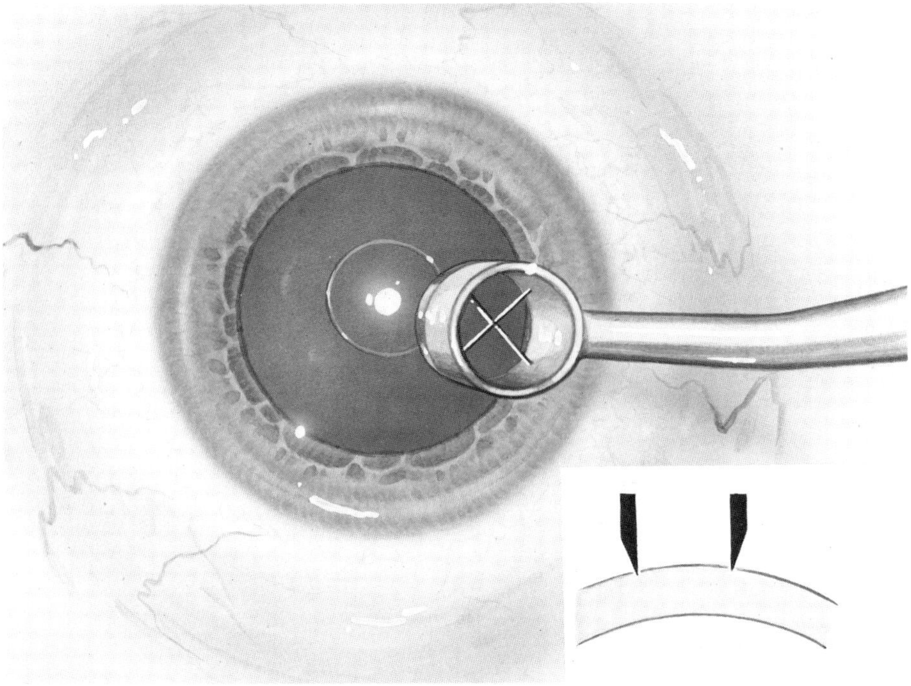

90
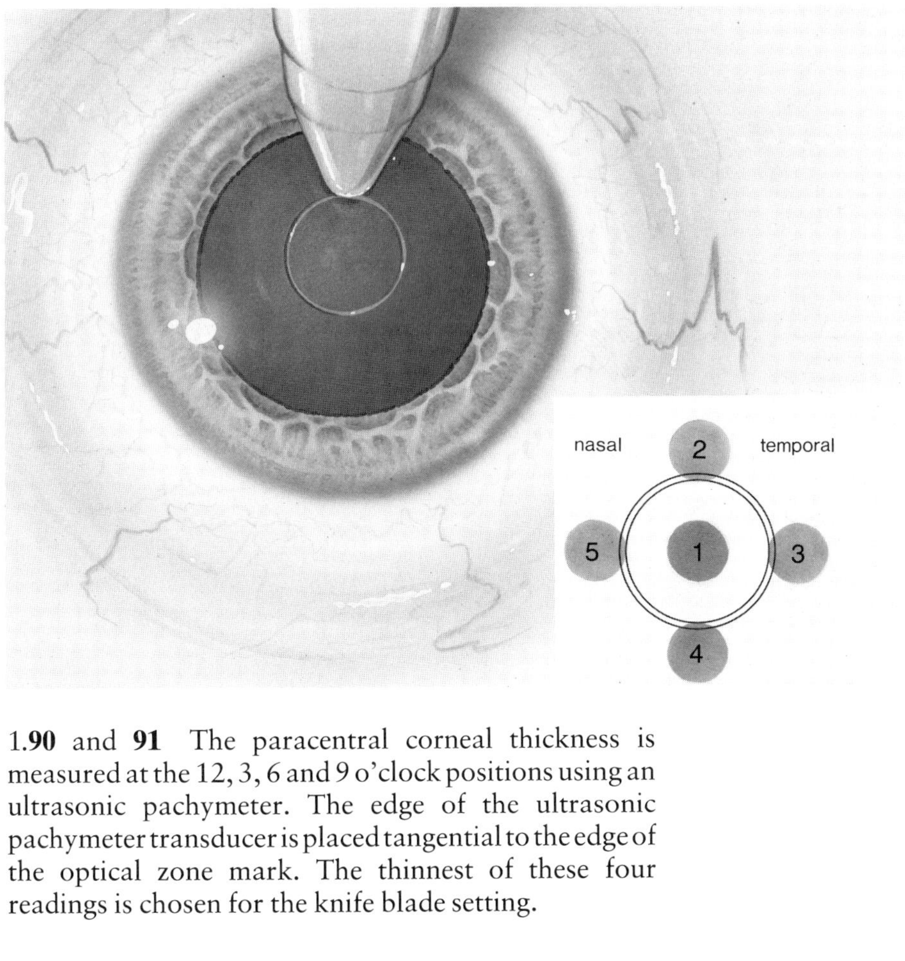

91
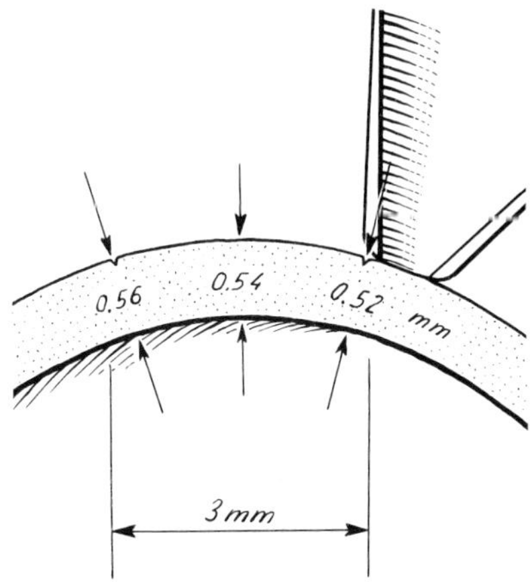

1.**90** and **91** The paracentral corneal thickness is measured at the 12, 3, 6 and 9 o'clock positions using an ultrasonic pachymeter. The edge of the ultrasonic pachymeter transducer is placed tangential to the edge of the optical zone mark. The thinnest of these four readings is chosen for the knife blade setting.

92

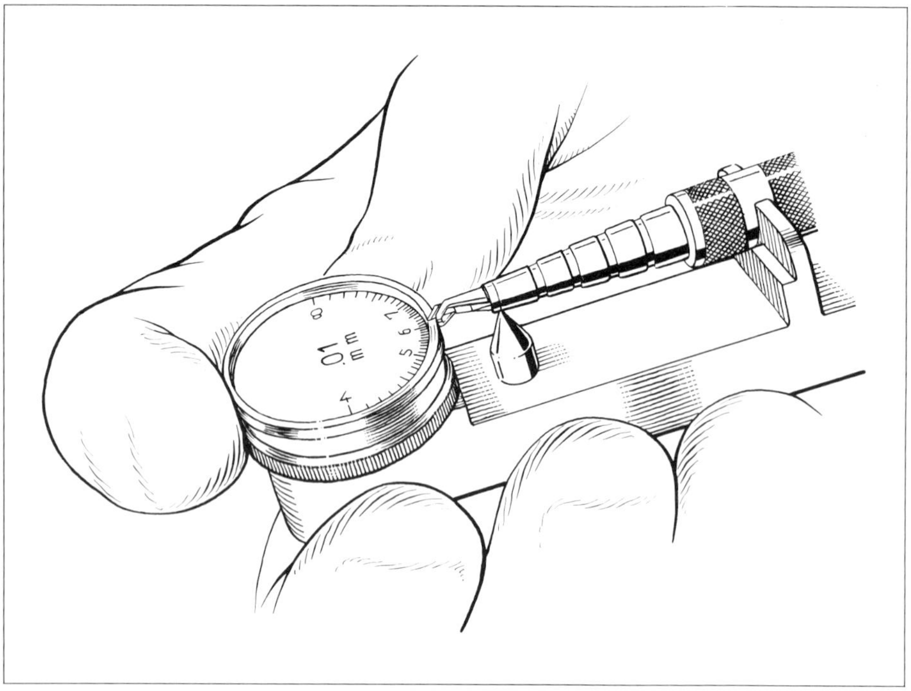

93

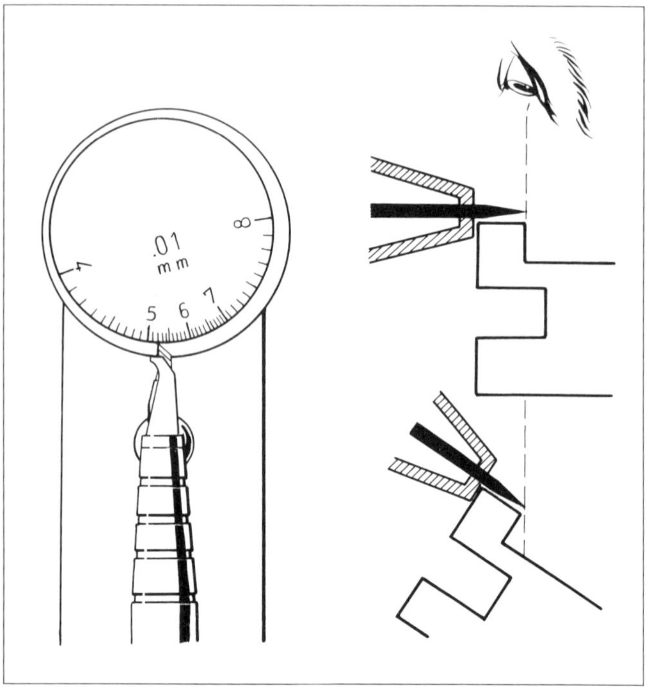

1.**92** and **93** The diamond knife is engaged but not extended. The knife is set into the coin gauge block. The coin gauge is then slid towards the skis on the knife until contact is made. The micrometer handle is turned in a clockwise direction until the diamond advances to the appropriate depth setting. The gauge, block and knife are held perpendicular to the light source and the diamond advanced until the end of the blade is seen to be aligned with the inside edge of the gauge block bevel.

94

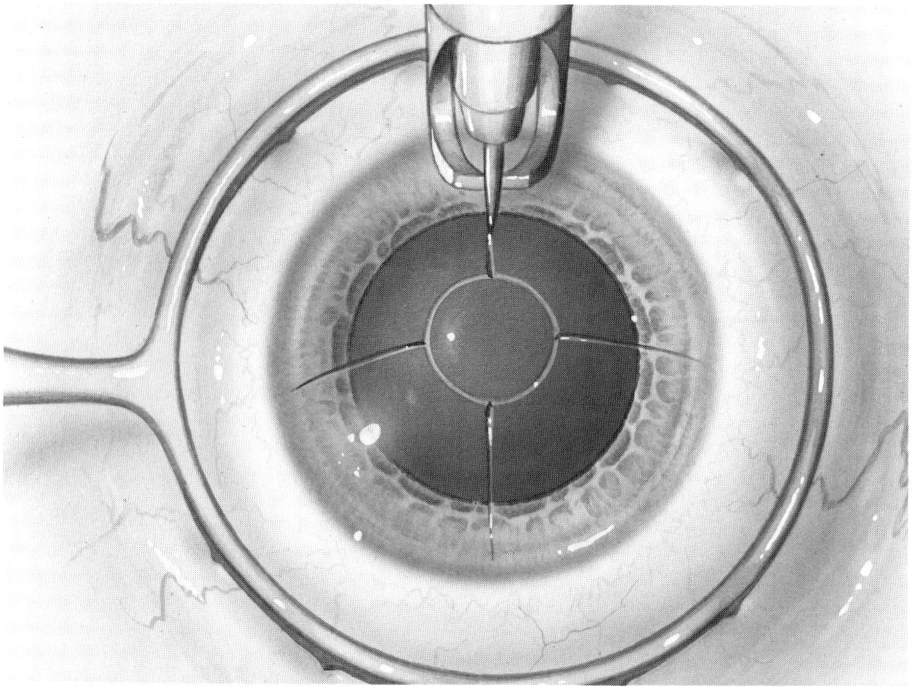

95

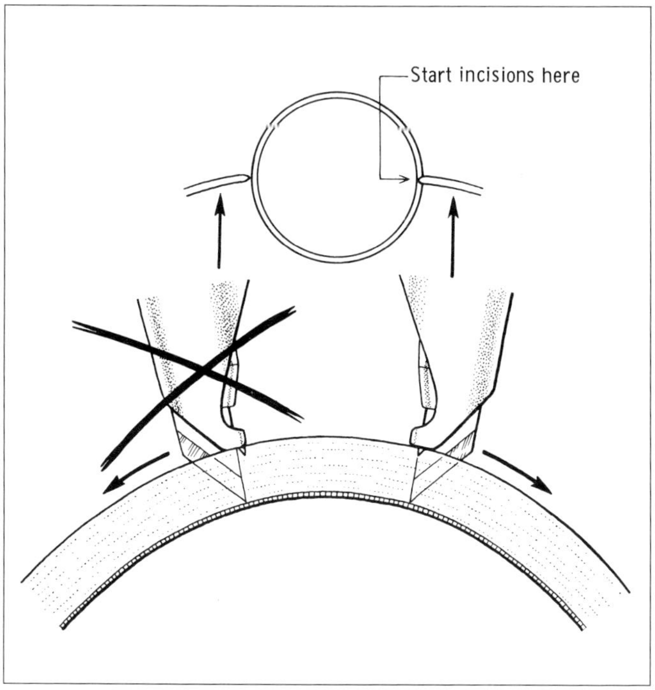

1.**94** and **95** After the knife has been removed from the gauge block, the globe is fixated using the Thornton fixation ring. Use fairly low magnification when making the incisions, as this makes it easier to keep the knife perpendicular to the cornea. Plunge the diamond firmly into the cornea at the optical zone mark. Pause for a moment when the knife is first inserted to allow the cut to achieve full depth. Carry the incision out to the limbus with slight indentation of the cornea. Occasionally there will be a small amount of bleeding from the perilimbal capillaries. If necessary this can be controlled using pressure from a Weck-Cel sponge and 10% Neo-Synephrine.

96 a

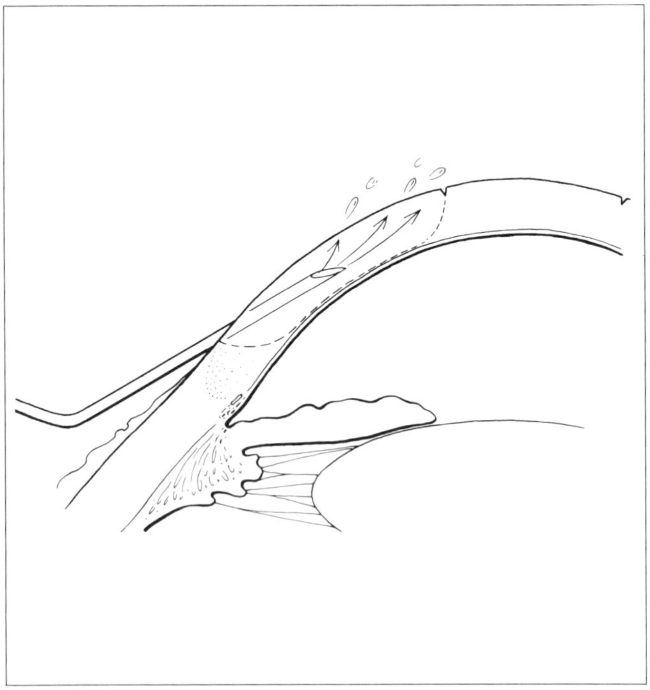

96 b

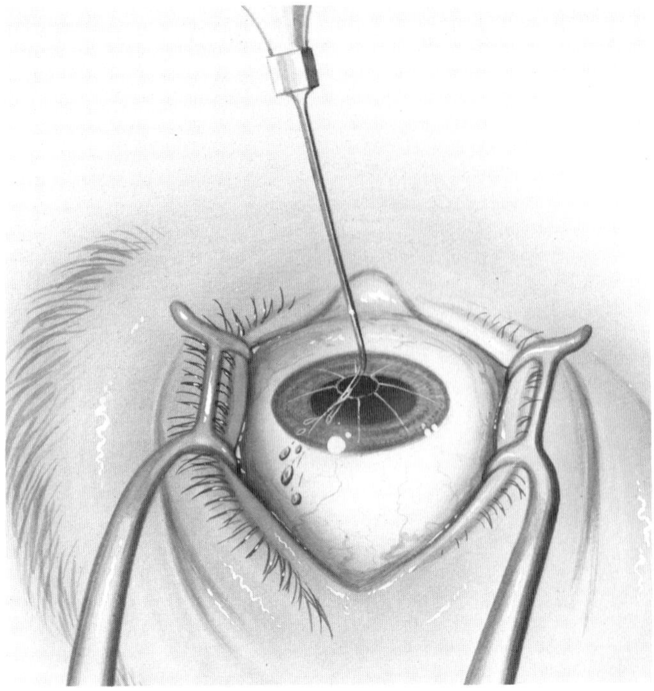

97

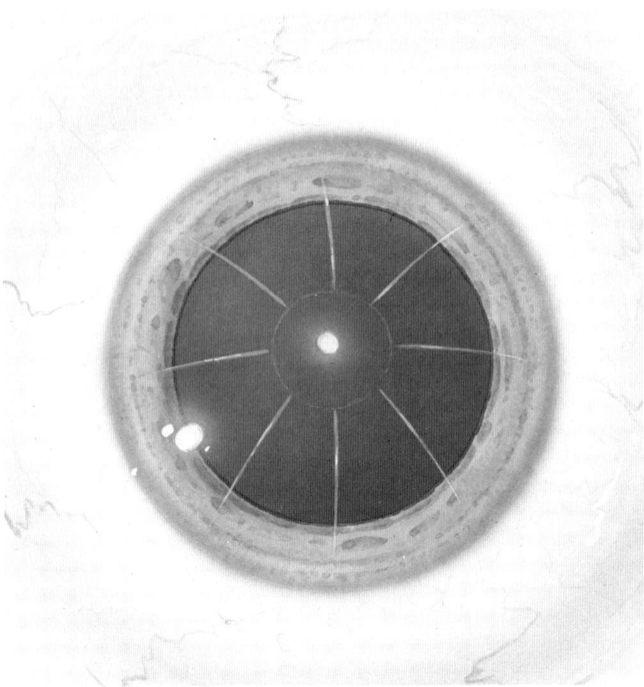

1.**96 a** and **b** Each incision is irrigated using balanced salt solution through a 30 gauge irrigating cannula. This removes epithelial debris from the incisions.

1.**97** Inject subconjunctivally, in the inferior cul-de-sac, 20 mg gentamicin mixed with 0.5 ml 2% xylocaine. Follow this with an injection of 0.5 ml celestone. If the pupil was not previously dilated, instill 1 drop of 2% cyclopentolate. Patch the eye with a light dressing without ointments.

Postoperative Management

The patient is instructed to remove the eyepatch the morning following surgery. Some patients are bothered by the patch on the evening of surgery, and it is more comfortable to remove the patch at that time. The patient uses Maxitrol drops four times daily in the operated eye.

The first postoperative visit is scheduled a week after surgery. If the patient is more than +3.00 D overcorrected at this time, the Maxitrol is discontinued. Otherwise, it is continued four times daily, and the patient is seen three weeks later.

The patient is instructed either to remove the lens from his glasses or to replace the lens with a plano lens. The lens is not changed again until the refraction stabilizes. This is often at the one-month visit.

If the patient remains significantly undercorrected following surgery, reoperation will be considered at the three-month visit.

Admonitions and Suggestions

A technique of redeepening the peripheral part of the incisions has gained some popularity. This technique definitely increases the rate of corneal perforation. Until there is some evidence that this practice improves the results of radial keratotomy surgery, we advise against it.

Cuts made from the periphery of the cornea towards the center have rarely been seen to go all the way to the center of the cornea. Patients with even a single cut through their visual axis are dissatisfied with the surgical result. We believe that it is more appropriate to make incisions from the central optical zone out toward the peripheral cornea.

After marking the optical zone, be sure to have the patient refixate the light filament and check that the light reflection is centered in the optical zone mark. This takes only a few seconds and is reassuring to the surgeon before making the incisions.

Modifications

To ensure consistent results, the technique should be modified as little as possible. We perform the operation with either four or eight incisions. Using just four or eight incisions allows us to reoperate on patients who are left undercorrected. We use 3.0 mm, 3.5 mm, and 4.0 mm optical zones.

In patients with more than 1.5 D of astigmatism, we have performed operations using an oval optical zone, 3.0 mm by 4.0 mm; the 3.0 mm zone is used in the plus axis of astigmatism. Unfortunately, with this technique we have only been able to achieve an astigmatic correction of slightly less than 0.5 D.

Results

We have found that patient satisfaction is directly related to the expectations aroused in the patient by the surgeon preoperatively. We have found that an eight-incision radial keratotomy using a 3.0 mm optical zone gives approximately 5.2 D of refractive change. Eight incisions with a 3.5 mm optical zone will give approximately 3.5 D of refractive change. Eight incisions with a 4.0 mm optical zone will give approximately 3.0 D of refractive change[1].

A four-incision radial keratotomy using a 3.0 mm optical zone will give approximately 4.2 D of refractive change. Four incisions with a 3.5 mm optical zone will give approximately 3.0 D of refractive change. Four incisions with a 4.0 mm optical zone will give approximately 1.5 D of refractive change.

Our results indicate that the patient's age is a significant factor in predicting the effect of radial keratotomy. Older patients will get more benefit from the same operation than younger patients.

Reference

[1] Rowsey, J. J., Balyeat, H. D., Rabinovitch, B. et al.: Predicting the results of radial keratotomy. *Ophthalmology* 90: 642–645, 1983.

2

Chamber Angle

Jörg Draeger, Klaus Heilmann,
Alan L. Robin, Irvin P. Pollack,
George L. Spaeth, Rolf Winter

Trabeculectomy

George L. Spaeth

Surgical Technique

Trabeculectomy is a modification of a standard filtration operation for glaucoma. The creation of a scleral flap which can be used to control the amount of filtration allows the surgeon to determine the amount of flow through the sclera quite accurately. This gives greater control over the final surgical result, with a lower incidence of complications. It is possible to modify the procedure to obtain maximum flow, in which case the incidence of flat anterior chamber rises. It is also possible to suture the scleral flap tightly, in which case the likelihood of flat anterior chamber and malignant glaucoma is reduced to a minimum, but the final intraocular pressure is higher than if a full-tickness filtration procedure had been performed. Thus, when a trabeculectomy is planned, the surgeon must first clearly define his or her goals before deciding upon the technique. If a low intraocular pressure is the most important goal, then copious filtration with little scleral coverage is important; if safety and a higher intraocular pressure is the primary goal, then minimal flow through the scleral flap is appropriate.

Indications for trabeculectomy are the same as for standard filtration procedures. In addition, however, the ability to close the scleral flap tightly, and thus minimize the likelihood of flat anterior chamber, makes the procedure of special value in patients in whom a flat anterior chamber is either expected or would be especially problematical. Thus, trabeculectomy is preferred over a full-thickness filtration procedure in patients who have uncontrolled intraocular pressure following acute angle surgery for glaucoma, but in whom the optic disk is fairly healthy, and in whom a low intraocular pressure is not required postoperatively. It is also the procedure of choice in patients predisposed to malignant glaucoma, as well as in patients in whom cataract is already present, and in whom hypotony and persistent flat anterior chamber would be expected to cause more rapid progression of the cataract.

Preparation for Surgery

If the patient is receiving a long-acting miotic, such as echothiophate, administration should be discontinued at least three weeks preoperatively; a short-acting agent, such as pilocarpine, can be substituted. In patients with marked elevation of intraocular pressure, this should be lowered preoperatively with an osmotic agent. In the inflammatory glaucomas, such as those associated with uveitis or trauma, topical (and perhaps systemic) corticosteroids should be instituted the day prior to the trabeculectomy. It is essential that the surgeon obtain a well-documented evaluation of the visual field and the optic disk prior to surgery in order to permit accurate determination of the possibility of change in the postoperative period.

Preoperative Medication and Anesthesia

The patient is prepared for surgery in a fashion standard for any intraocular surgical procedure. Local or general anesthesia may be employed. An operating microscope or other method of obtaining high magnification is essential.

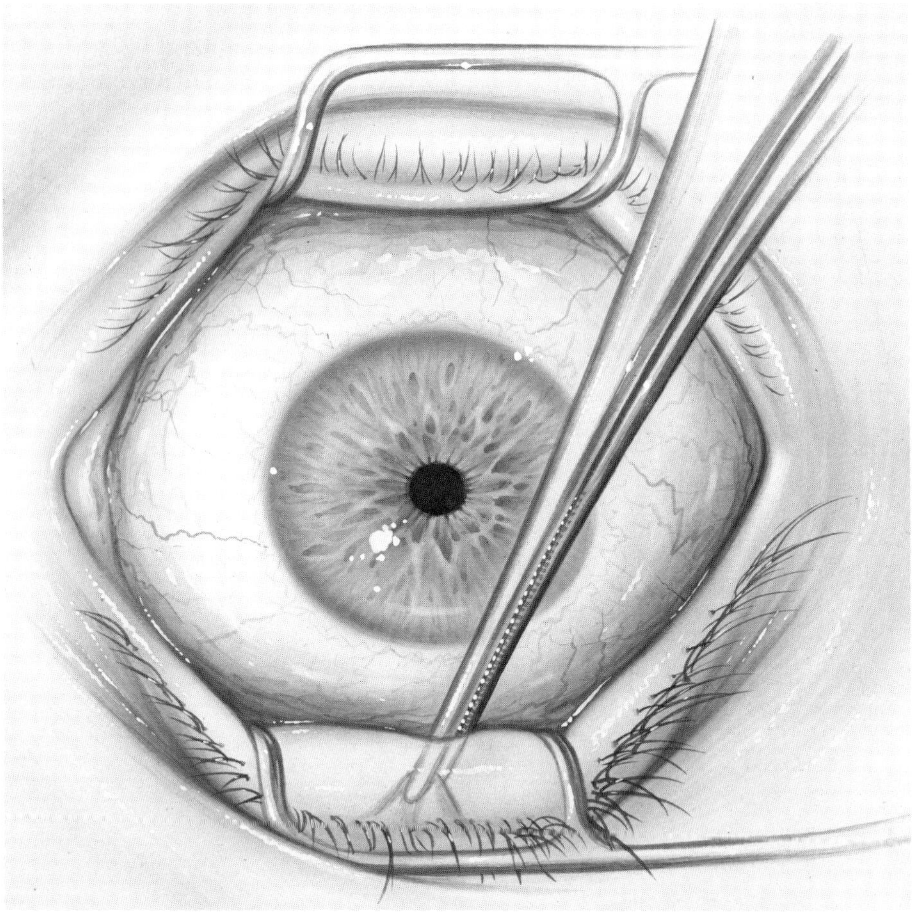

Surgical Technique

2.1 A superior rectus bridle suture is placed, at the beginning of the procedure. To this end, the conjunctiva should be grasped as high in the cul-de-sac as possible, using a forceps with good holding qualities, such as a Lister or Wills Eye Hospital utility forceps. The forceps is pressed firmly against the globe, in a direction fairly perpendicular to the globe, in order to facilitate grasping the superior rectus muscle in its jaws.

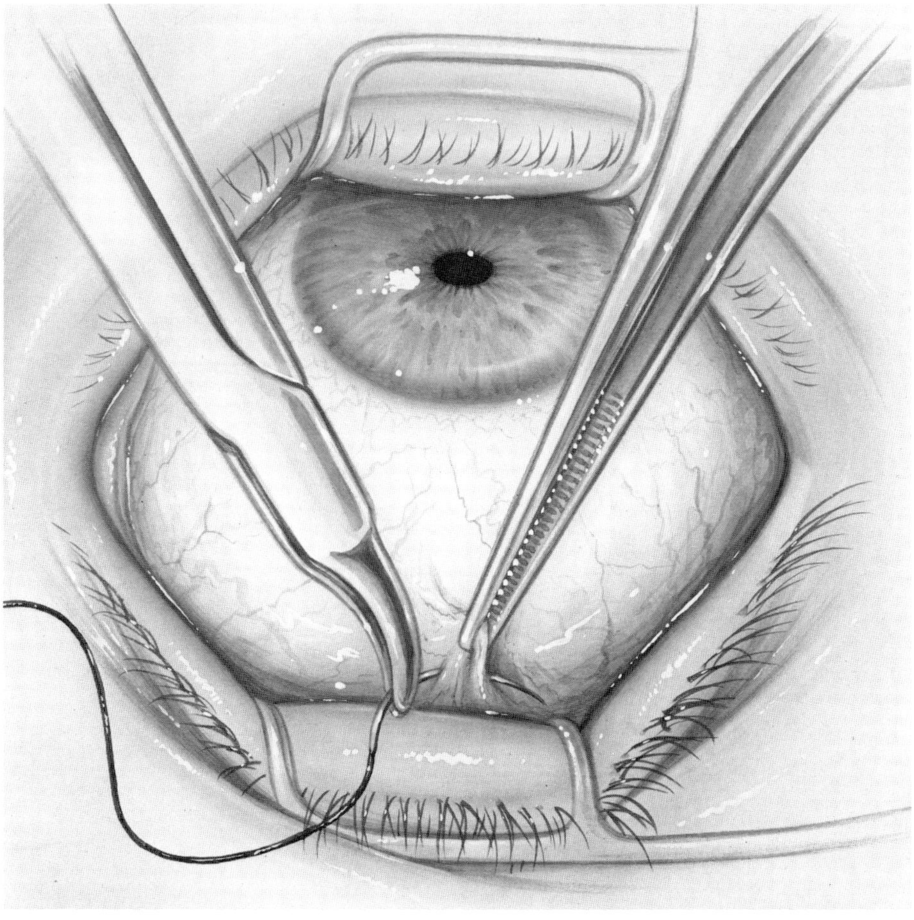

2.2 The tissue is pulled anteriorly and superiorly towards the microscope, and the 4-0 black silk suture placed under the muscle belly with a noncutting needle. In order to avoid perforation, the tip of the needle should never be directed toward the globe.

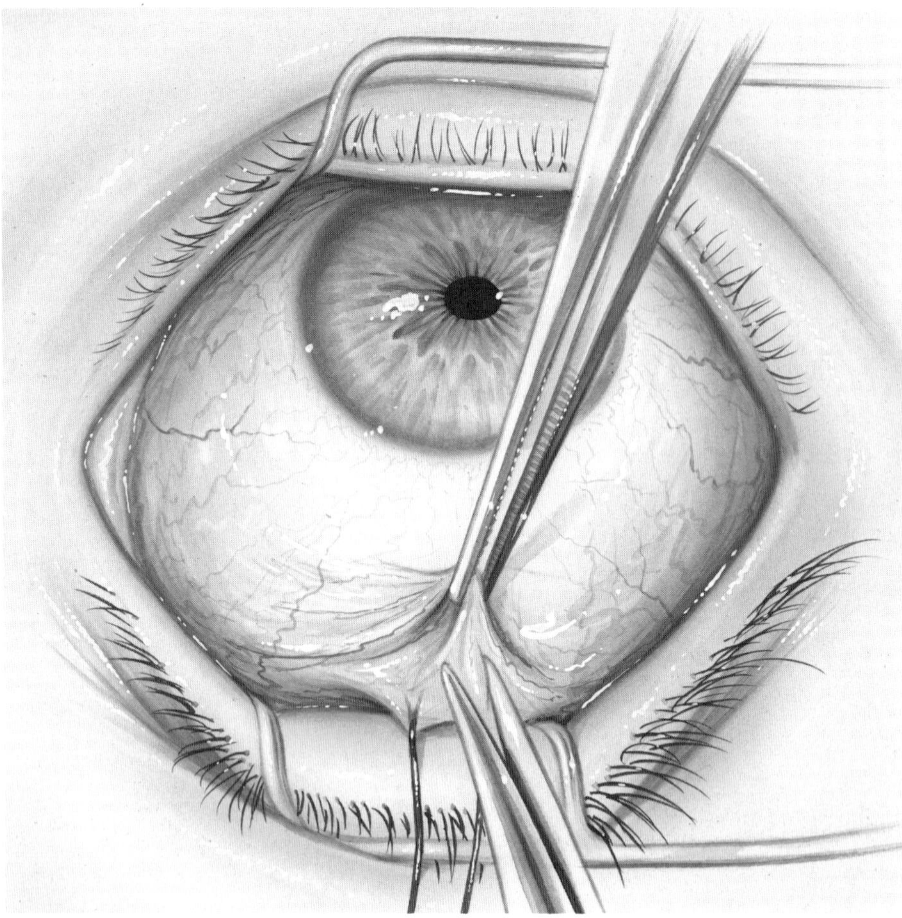

2.3 With the bridle suture in place, the conjunctiva is grasped with a nontoothed forceps, such as a Wills Eye Hospital utility forceps or Pierse-Hoskins forceps, as close to the bridle suture as possible, and pulled inferiorly, using the superior rectus for countertraction. The direction of traction is 180° opposed to the pull of the bridle suture. Blunt-tipped Westcott scissors are used to incise the conjunctiva immediately anterior to the superior rectus suture.

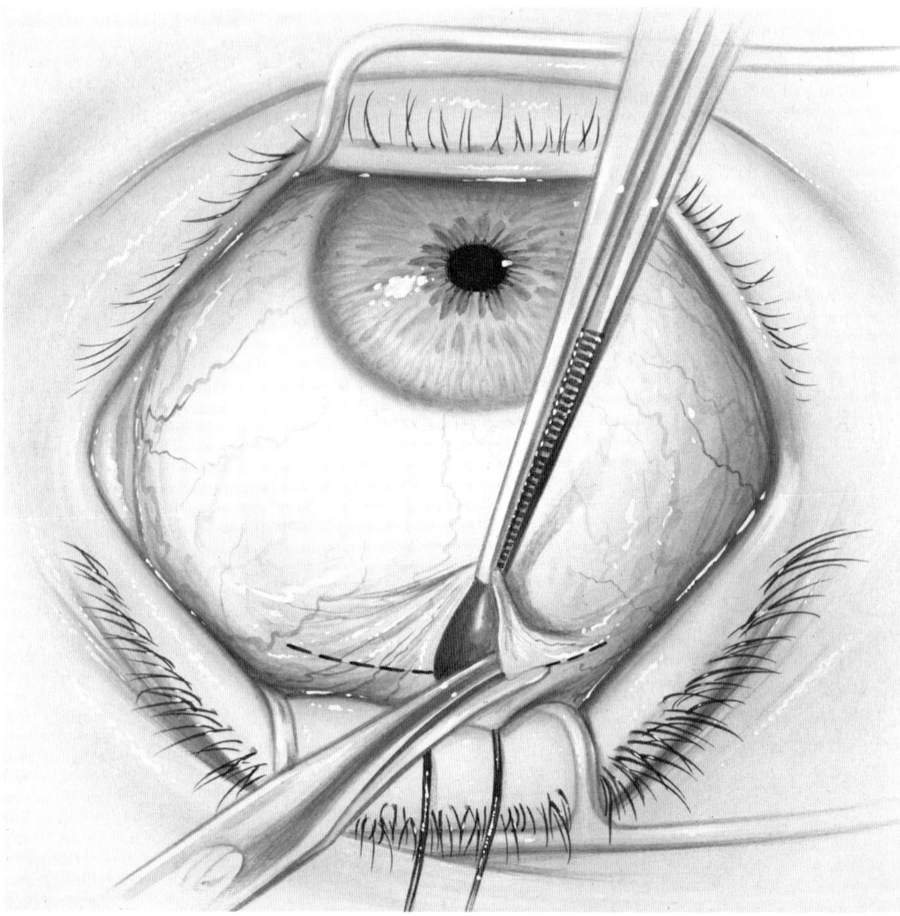

2.4 The incision is extended approximately 8 mm nasally and temporally, as high in the cul-de-sac as possible.

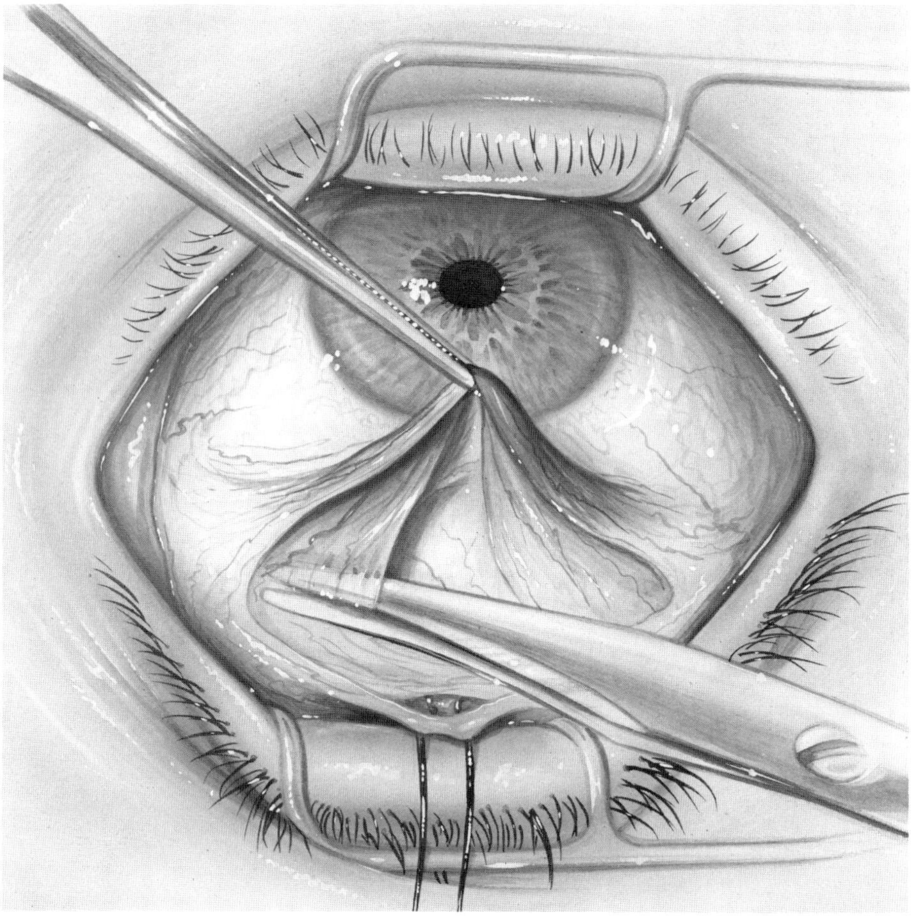

2.5 The thicker, more opaque Tenon's capsule is grasped anterior to the conjunctival incision and buttonholed. The tips of the Westcott scissors are placed in the buttonhole and spread until the bare sclera is visible. Tenon's capsule is lifted away from the globe toward the microscope and put on stretch by pulling it anteriorly. Tenon's capsule is then opened parallel to the previous conjunctival incision for the same distance.

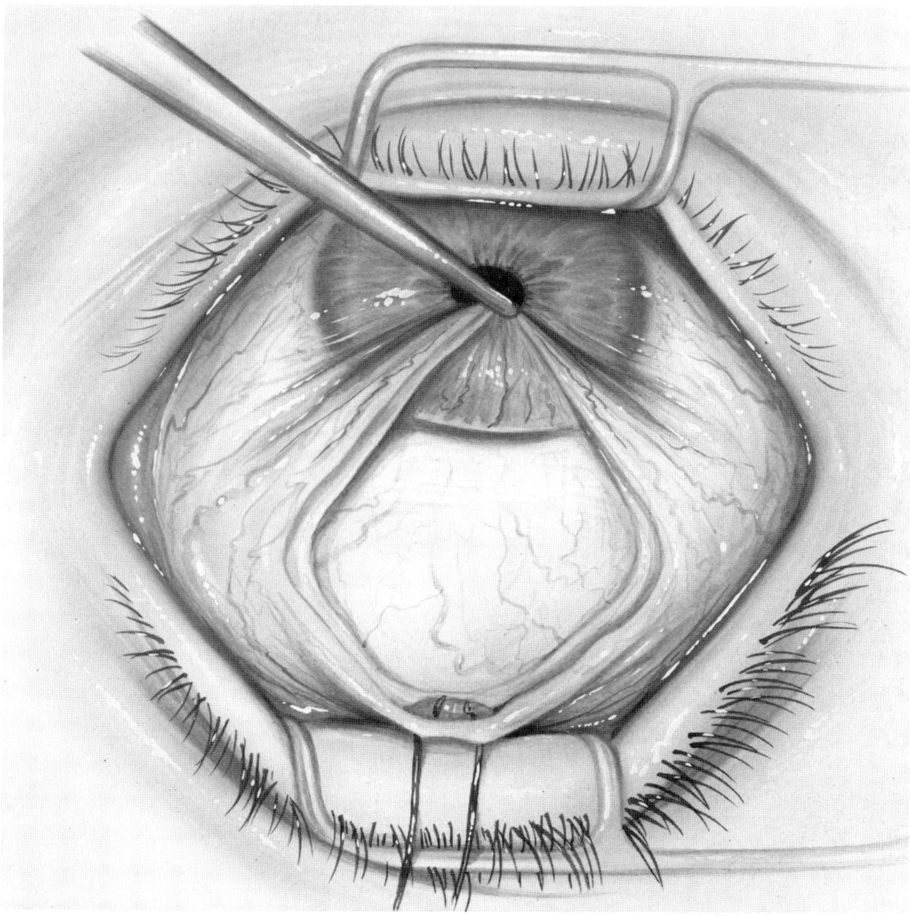

2.6 The flap containing Tenon's capsule and conjunctiva is pulled anteriorly over the cornea, exposing the episclera and the scleral sulcus. If there is a remaining layer of deep Tenon's capsule or prominent episcleral tissue, the tissue is grasped 3 mm posterior to the limbus, lifted up vigorously toward the microscope, and buttonholed with the Westcott scissors. The tip of the Westcott scissors is then inserted circumferentially, incising this deeper layer parallel to the scleral sulcus for a distance of approximately 4 mm on either side of the buttonhole. The tissue is pulled anteriorly and the episclera cleaned well, until there is clear visualization of the scleral sulcus. The deep layer of Tenon's capsule may also be incised here so that only the conjunctiva remains unincised, providing a thin barrier directly at the scleral sulcus.

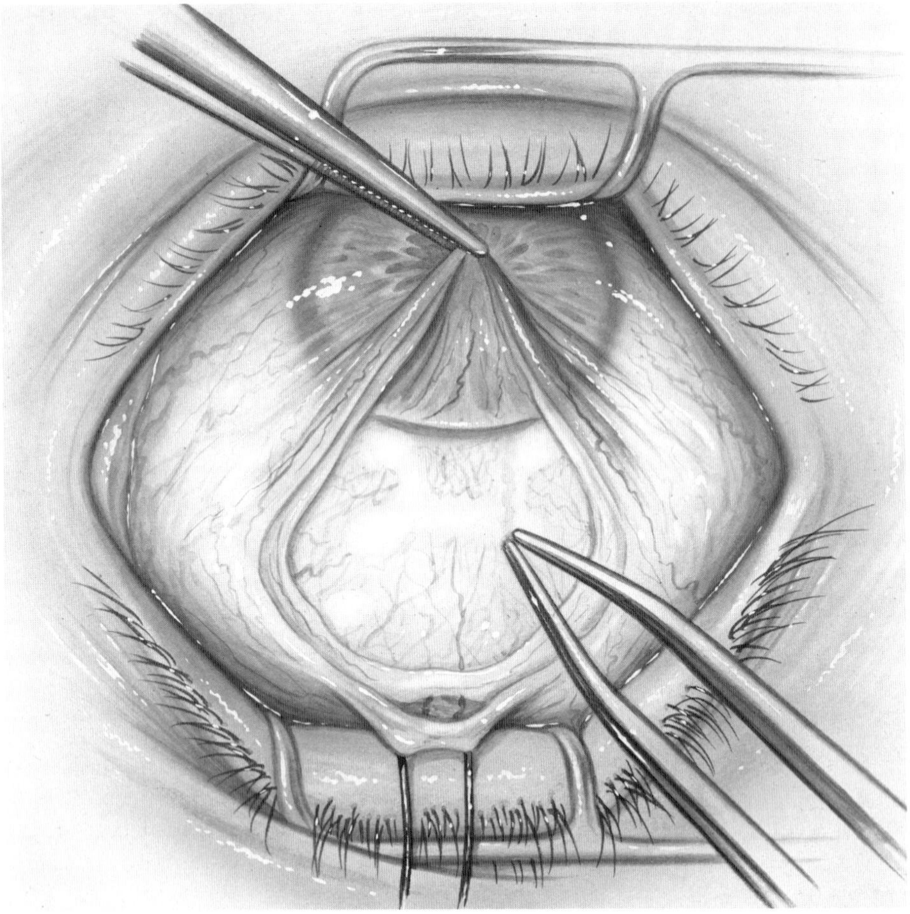

2.7 Bipolar cautery is used to coagulate every vessel which is bleeding, so that all hemorrhage is stopped. Vessels which have stopped bleeding spontaneously are touched with the irrigator and, if they start bleeding again, are cauterized. The surface of the globe as well as the episclera and Tenon's flap must be completely free of bleeding. The area in which the sclera is to be incised is outlined with cautery, and a further outline made just exterior to the flap where the sutures will be placed. This flap is approximately 2–3 mm wide parallel to the equator and extends 3–4 mm posterior to the limbus on the meridian plane.

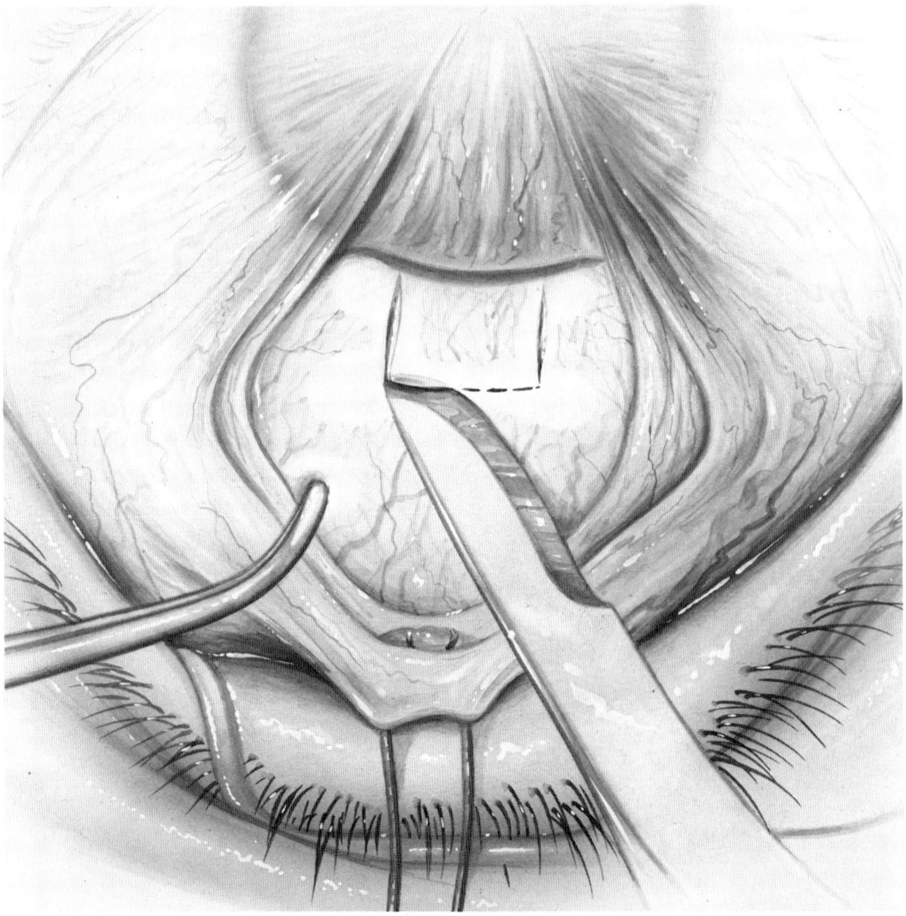

2.8 A Beaver # 67 blade is used to develop the scleral flap. The power of the microscope should be increased at this point, so that the flap can be well visualized. The sclera is fixated with a Pierse-Hoskins or Colibri forceps. The radial grooves of the scleral flap are made first and then connected posteriorly. The depth of the groove should be at least half and preferably three-quarters the thickness of the sclera.

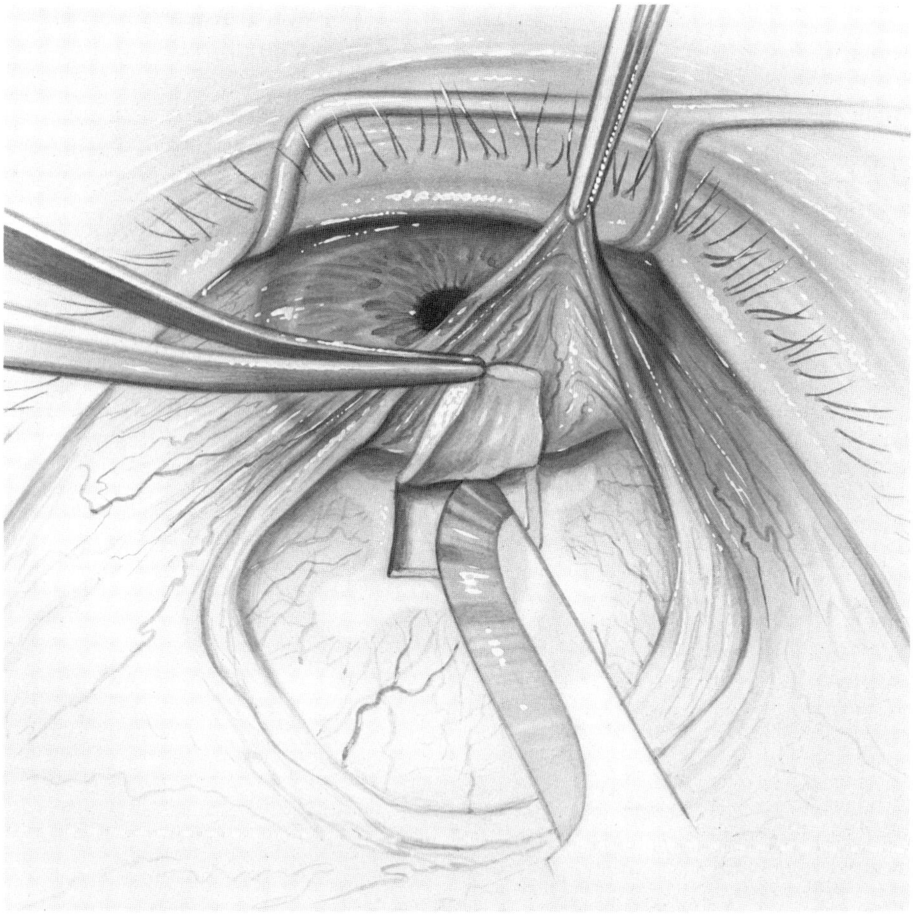

2.9 Initial incisions are made quite steeply in order to ensure that the flap is thick at its posterior edge. It is dissected completely across the posterior edge and kept square as it is dissected anteriorly. The tip of the blade should always be visualized. The scleral flap should be kept on good tension, and as it is developed it can be flipped backward and forward in order to determine if it is the proper thickness. The usual thickness is around one-third of the total thickness of the sclera. The flap should be so thick that it cannot be torn or penetrated by a fine-toothed forceps. I use a nontoothed Pierse-Hoskins forceps to hold the scleral flap. It is essential that the flap be dissected well into clear cornea beyond the scleral sulcus. One has to make sure that the flap extends well anterior to the iris root so that a block of tissue anterior to the iris can be excised. The surgeon should be aware of the need for this anterior extension as dissection proceeds.

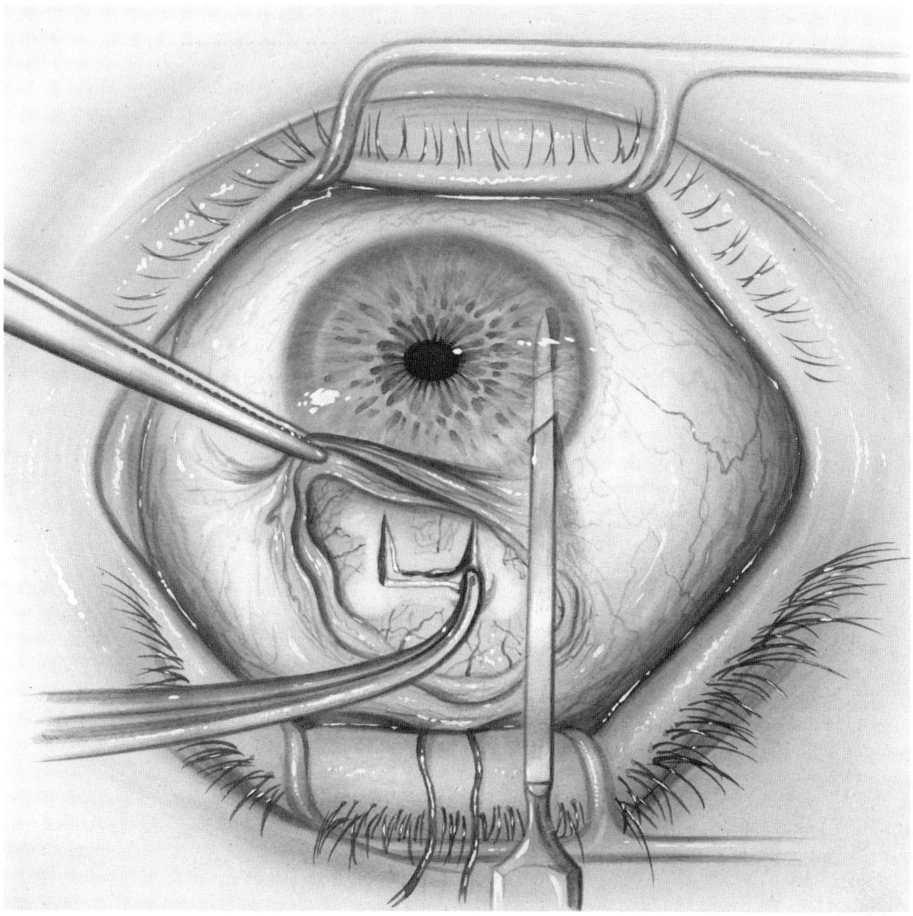

2.10 When dissection of the scleral flap has been completed, a paracentesis track is made. This can be done using a sharp Wheeler knife or, preferably, a disposable, sharp, short # 25 gauge needle. The paracentesis should be performed so that the plane of the knife or needle is always kept parallel to the plane of the iris. The needle should never be pointed toward the iris. Penetration through the cornea is achieved by depressing the handle of the knife or the syringe holding the needle posteriorly so that the cornea is indented. Then, anterior motion of the knife or needle will cause it to penetrate the cornea, permitting a short or long track depending upon the surgeon's wishes. The left hand should fixate the globe firmly throughout this procedure and should pull posteriorly as the knife or needle is gradually and carefully moved anteriorly.

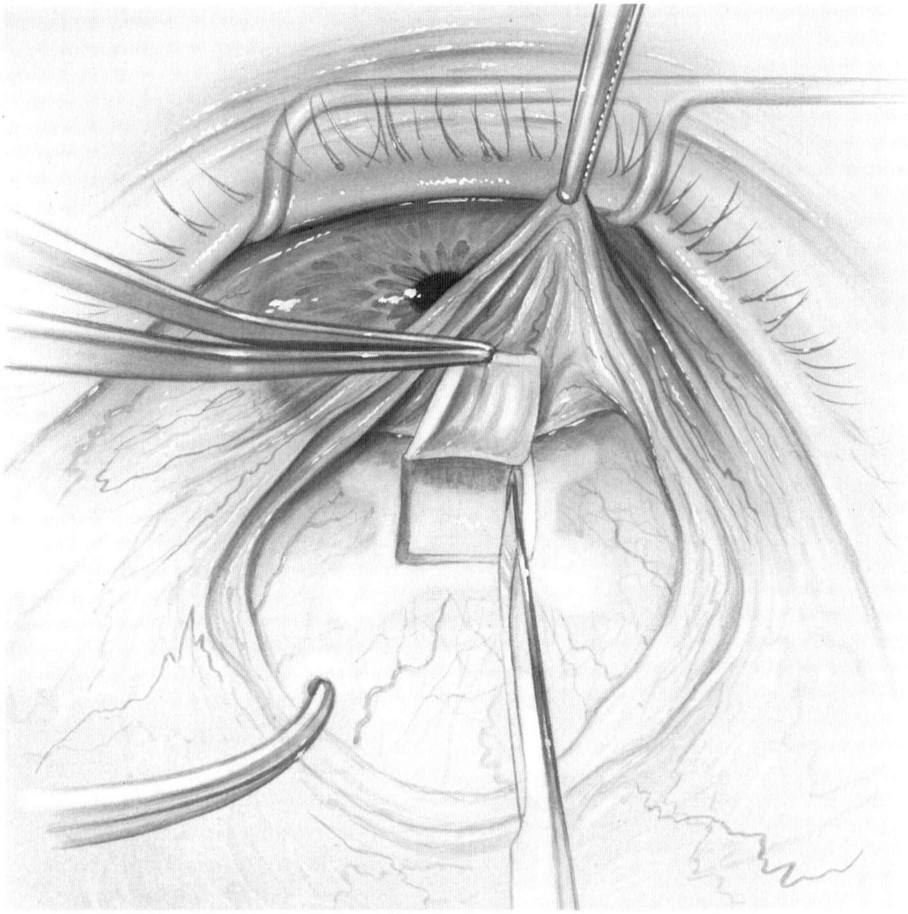

2.11 With the scleral flap firmly fixated and traction applied anteriorly, the right-hand radial incision into the anterior chamber is made, using the # 67 Beaver blade. Entry into the anterior chamber should be achieved as far anteriorly as possible. The radial groove is then extended posteriorly until it reaches opaque, white sclera, just posterior to the position of Schlemm's canal. Atropine 1 % is instilled on the eye several times.

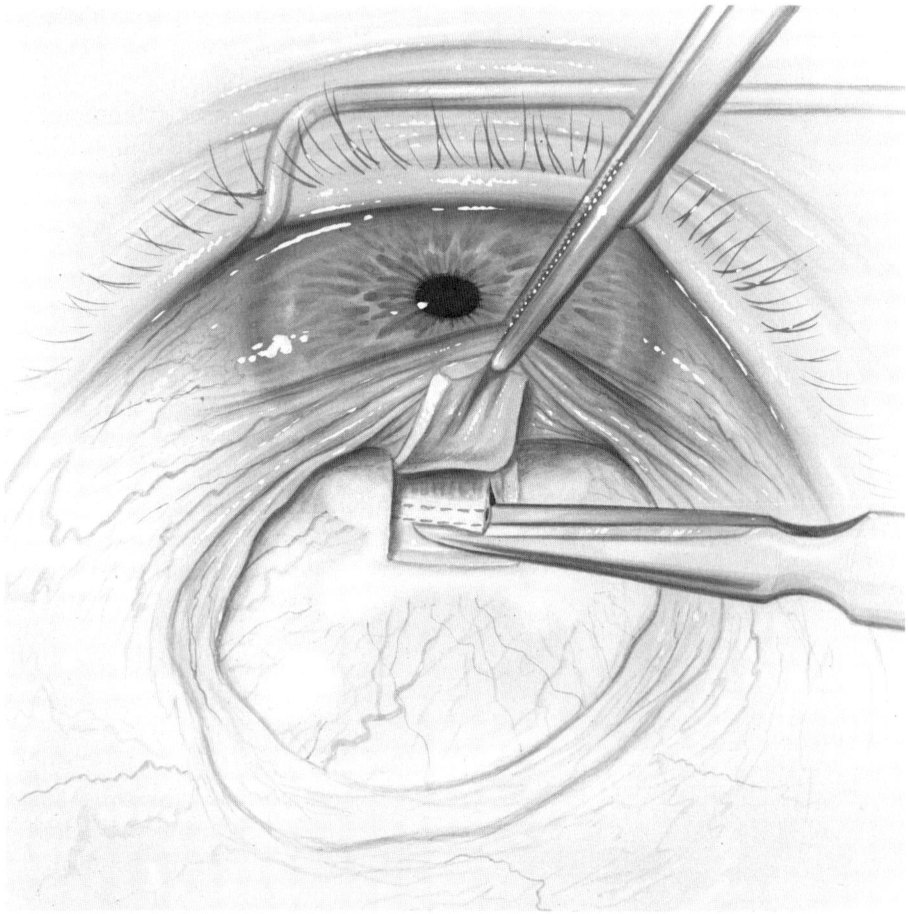

2.12 Vannas scissors are inserted in the area of clear cornea and pulled posteriorly until they stop as they impinge the scleral spur. The posterior edge of the internal block of sclera is then incised with the Vannas scissors.

Holding the posterior edge of the block, the left-hand radial incision is then made, cutting anteriorly, so that the block is hinged at its anterior end. The radial incisions should ordinarily be made so that ledges approximately 0.5 mm wide remain.

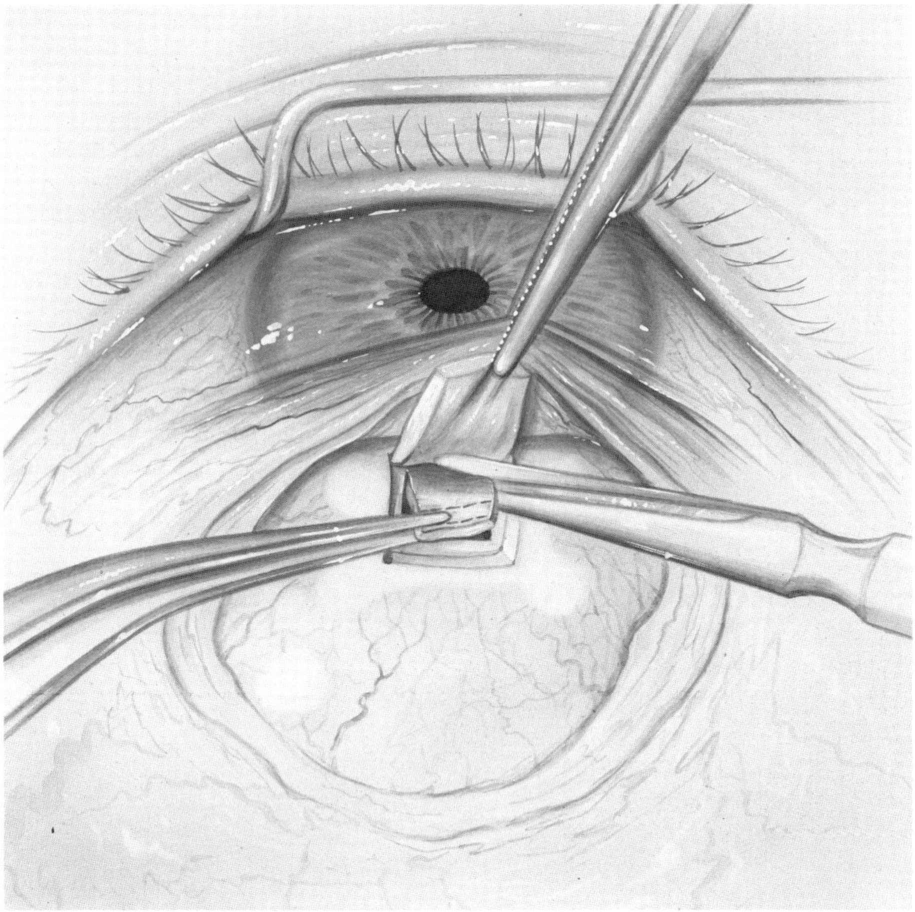

2.**13** Grasping the internal block at its posterior edge, the block is pulled posteriorly with the left hand. The assistant should hold the scleral flap, giving firm traction anteriorly. The Vannas scissors are then inserted under direct visualization so that the tips can be seen. In order to do this, the inner block must be lifted anteriorly, placed in the jaws of the Vannas scissors, and then pulled posteriorly, at which point the lower blade of the Vannas scissors disappears from view. The block is then amputated as far anteriorly and as squarely as possible. Atropine 1% is instilled on the eye.

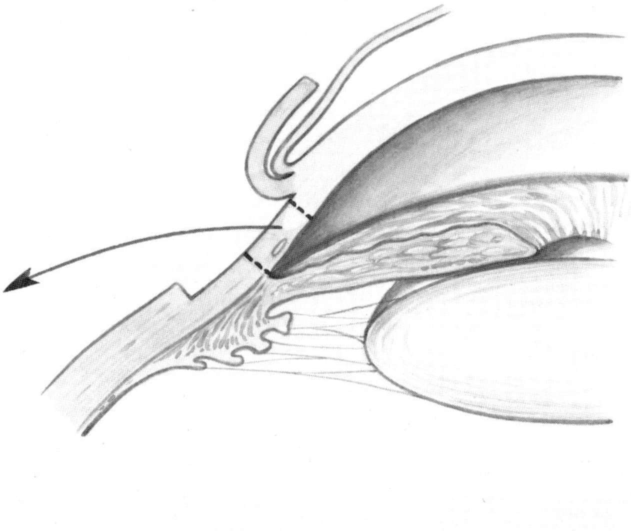

2.**14** Illustrated here are the conjunctival flap, the anterior dissection of the scleral flap, and the portion of internal sclera excised. The sclera should be removed anterior to the scleral spur. The scleral spur should not be disinserted; the ciliary body should not be exposed.

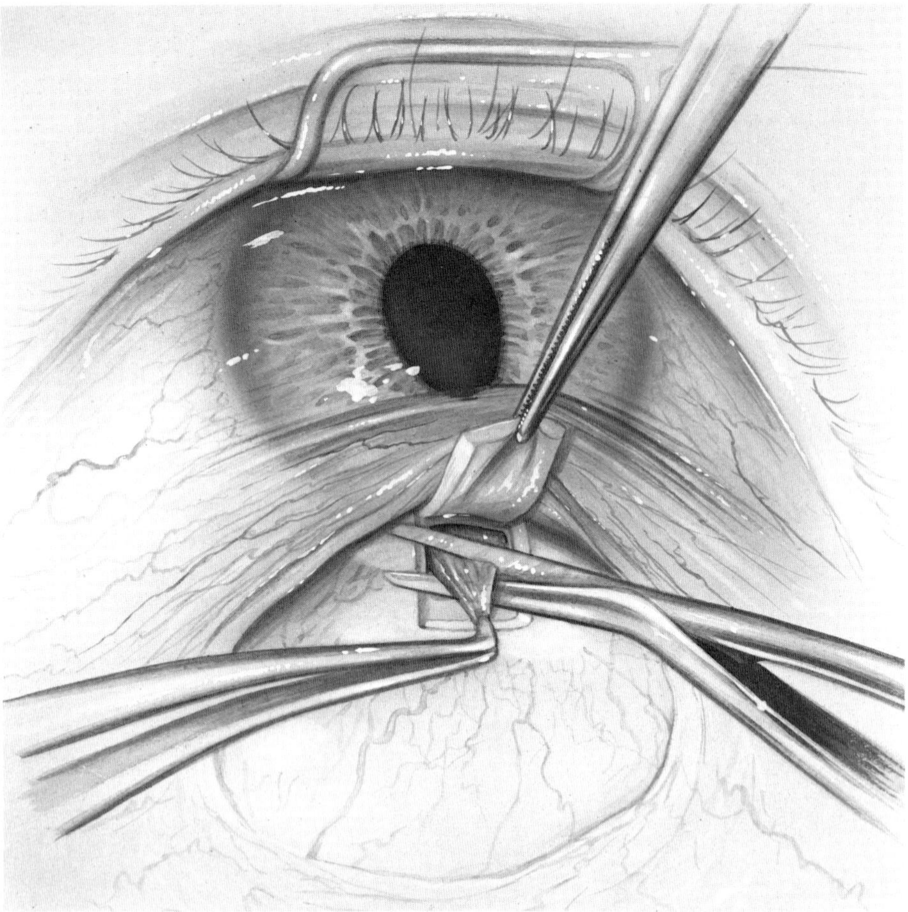

2.**15** A large iridectomy is performed, the iris scissors being held circumferentially so that the iridectomy is broad at its base. The purpose is to make sure that the size of the iridectomy is greater than the size of the internal block of sclera just removed. Atropine 1 % is instilled on the eye.

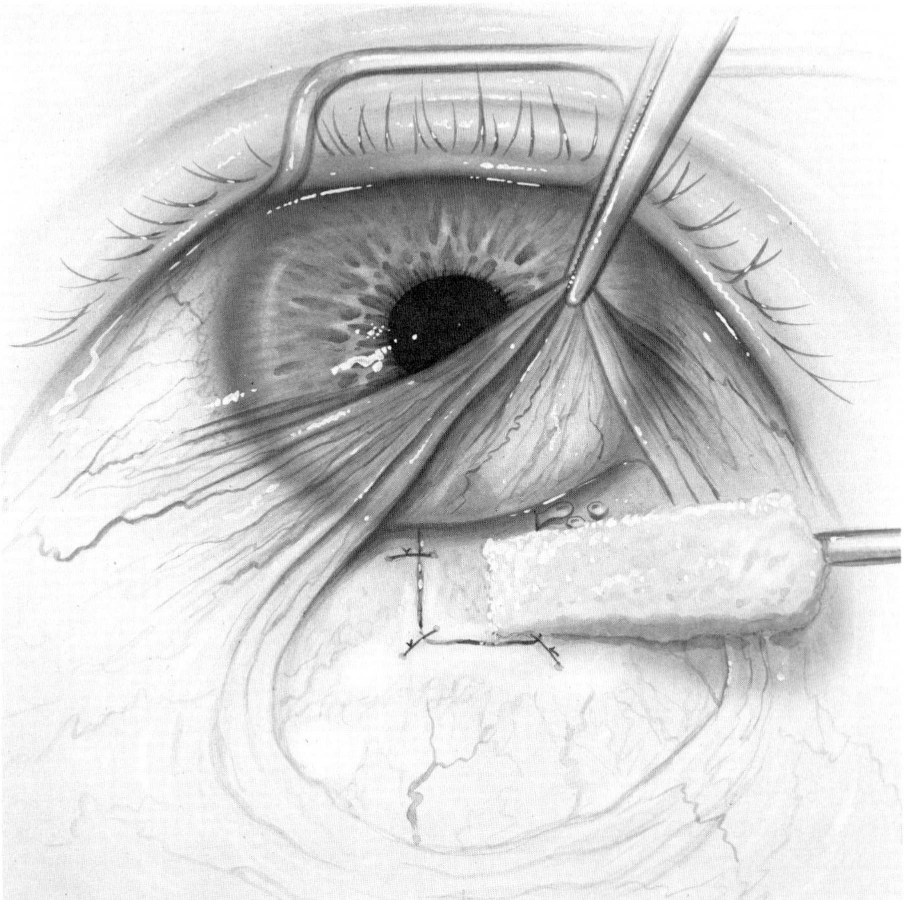

2.**16** The scleral flap is closed with 10-0 nylon sutures. In many cases one suture at each posterior corner will be sufficient. Where cautery has been required to coagulate bleeders at the edge of the flap, where the flap is thin, or where the amount of ledge produced is small, it may in addition be necessary to put sutures in the radial edges of the flap, as shown here. At this point the anterior chamber is filled with balanced salt solution through the previously-placed paracentesis track and the amount of leakage through the scleral flap determined; it can be tested with a cellulose sponge. If leakage is judged excessive, additional sutures are placed. If insufficient, a suture may be removed, or cautery lightly placed at the edge of the scleral flap in order to produce separation of the edges and increase the amount of leakage. I believe

⇨

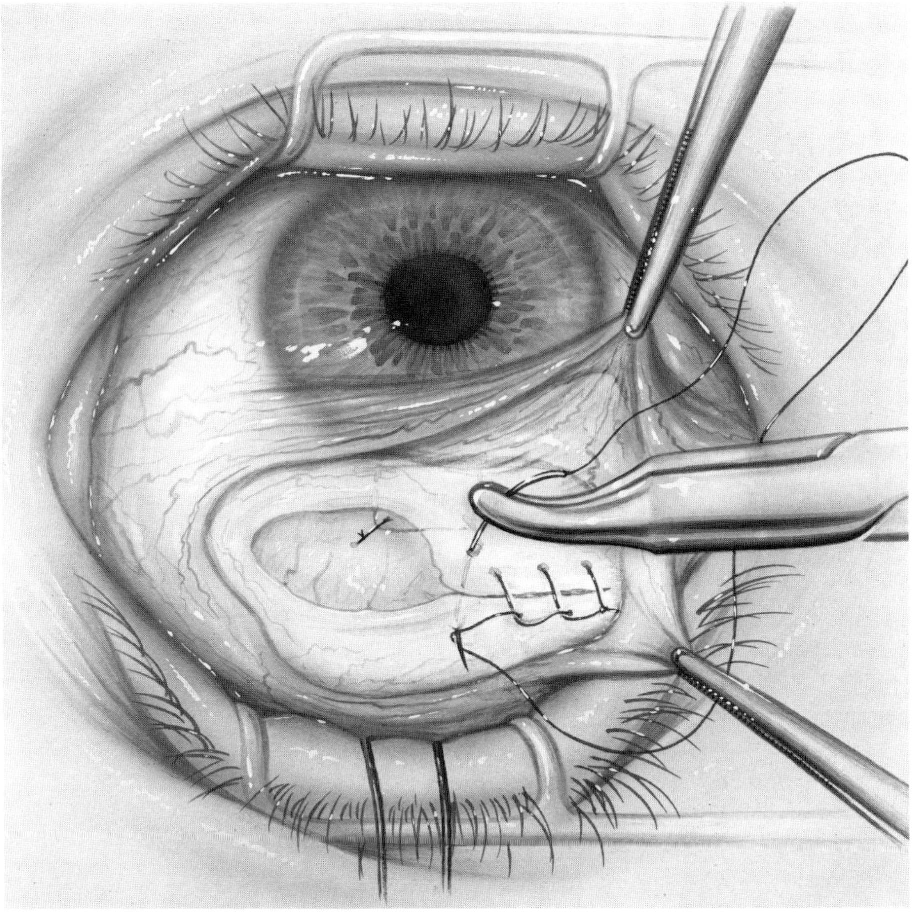

2.**17** Tenon's capsule is closed separately with running, locked 8-0 chromic collagen sutures. The sutures should be sufficiently closely placed that the tissue is well apposed.

this to be an essential part of the trabeculectomy procedure. It can be quite time-consuming. Repeated reformation of the anterior chamber may be required in order to achieve the appropriate amount of leakage. The surgeon should not be satisfied until the anterior chamber is formed and remains formed even when gentle pressure is applied. A finger is held on the globe to monitor the intraocular pressure as the anterior chamber is filled through the previously-placed paracentesis track. Pressure should be restored to a level of around 15 mm Hg. Using a # 30 gauge needle to reform the chamber, it should not be possible to raise the intraocular pressure much above this level. If the intraocular pressure rises to the point that the eye becomes hard, and the chamber remains deep, the amount of leakage through the scleral flap must be inadequate; in such cases one or more of the sutures probably needs to be released. If, after release of the suture(s), leakage is still not adequate, cautery may need to be placed on the sclera at the anterior portion of the radial incision(s). The cautery should be adequate to shrink the tissue, to permit the appropriate amount of aqueous flow through the sclera. If at the time of reformation of the anterior chamber through the paracentesis track the intraocular pressure rises and the anterior chamber simultaneously collapses, then a malignant glaucoma mechanism must be present, and appropriate steps should be taken to correct this. Atropine 1% is instilled on the eye.

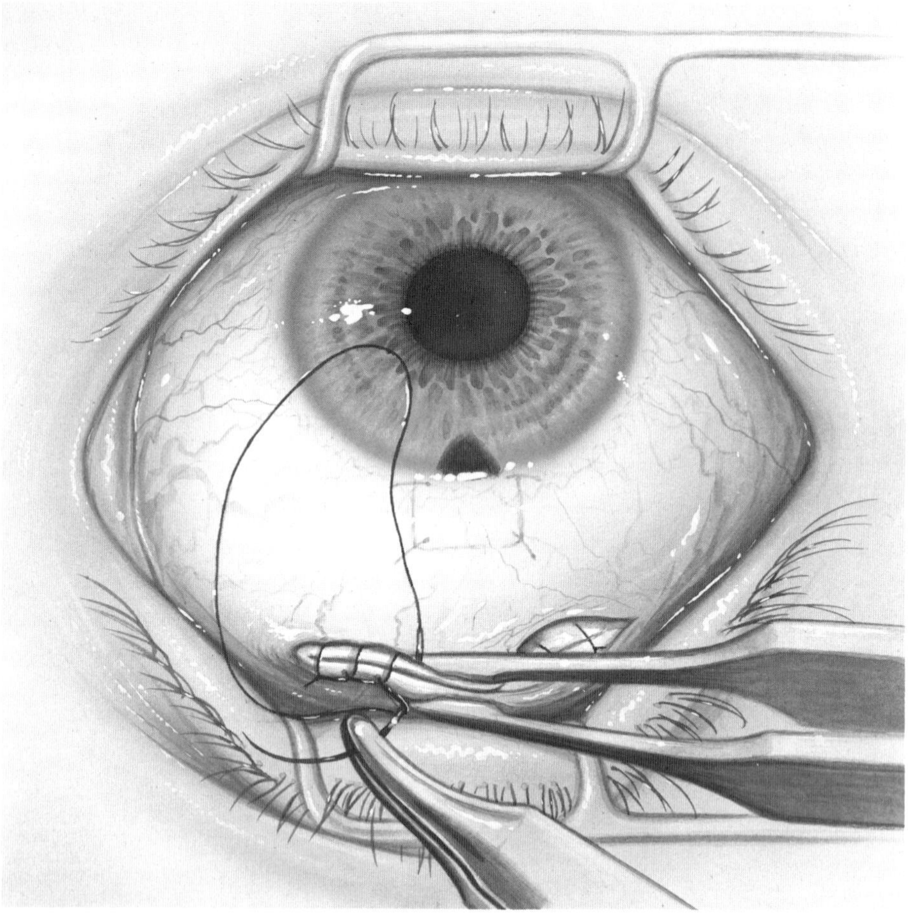

2.**18** The conjunctiva is closed with running 8-0 chromic collagen, placing the sutures no more than 2 mm apart, so that closure is absolutely watertight.

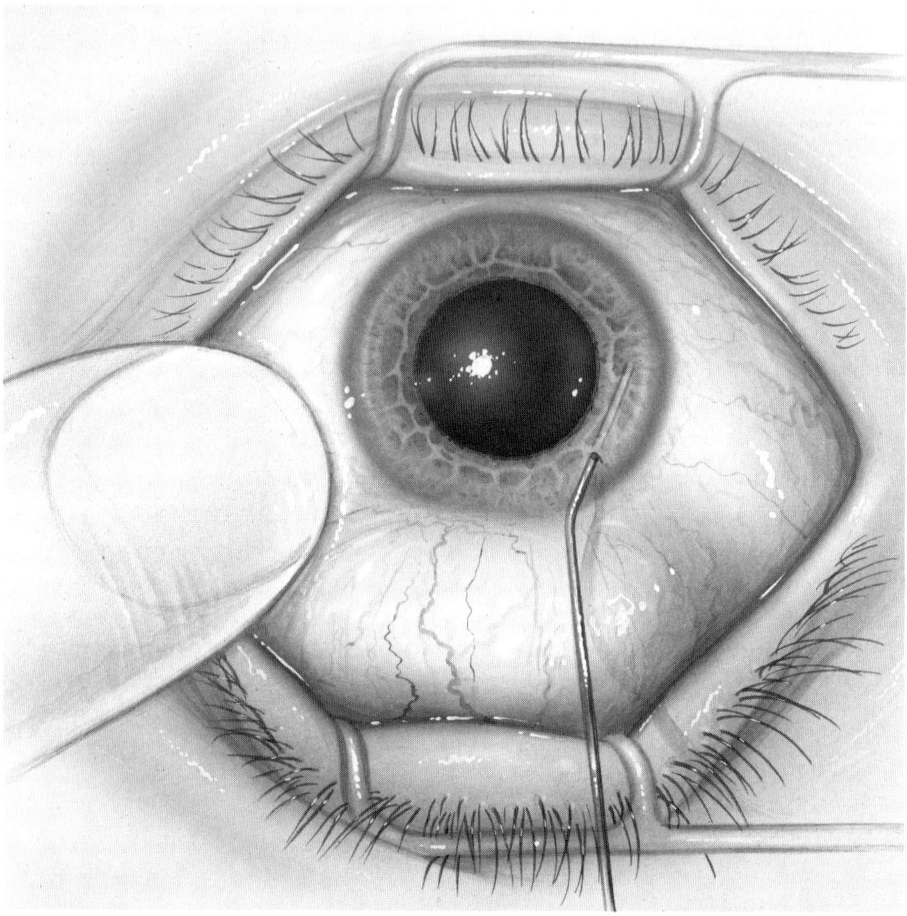

2.**19** By this stage of the procedure, the pupil should be widely dilated. Atropine should have been instilled sufficiently frequently and sufficiently early in the procedure to ensure dilatation by this point. If the pupil is not adequately dilated, phenylephrine 2.5 % is instilled, and the procedure is not concluded until the pupil has been adequately dilated. The anterior chamber is again filled with balanced salt solution through the previously placed paracentesis track, with a finger held on the globe to monitor the intraocular pressure. As the anterior chamber is filled with balanced salt solution, a bleb should develop. At the end of the procedure, the chamber should be well-formed, and there should be a conspicuous bleb present. The anterior chamber should remain formed. Atropine ointment and a combination antibiotic-corticosteroid ointment are instilled, and the eye covered with a light patch and shield.

20

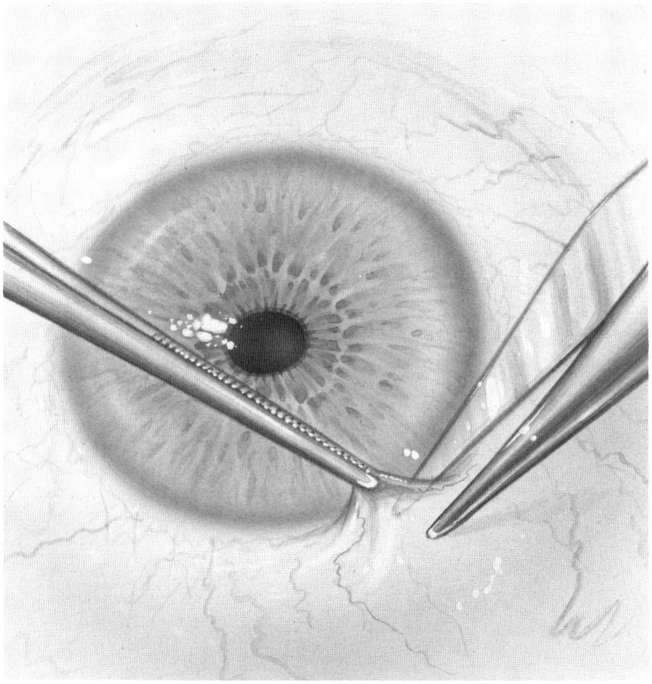

21

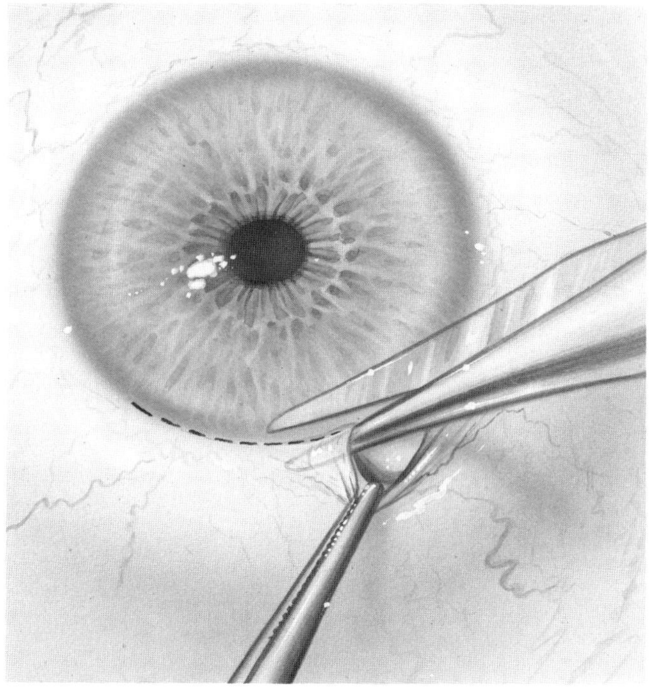

22

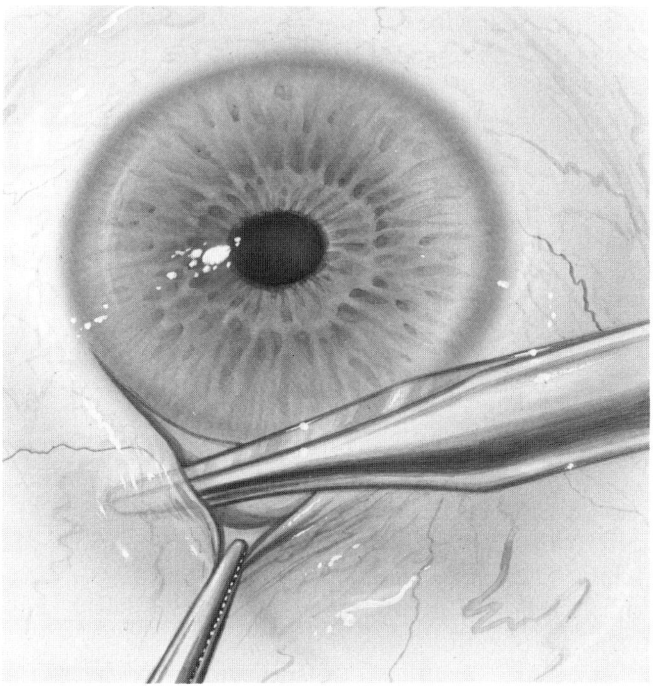

23

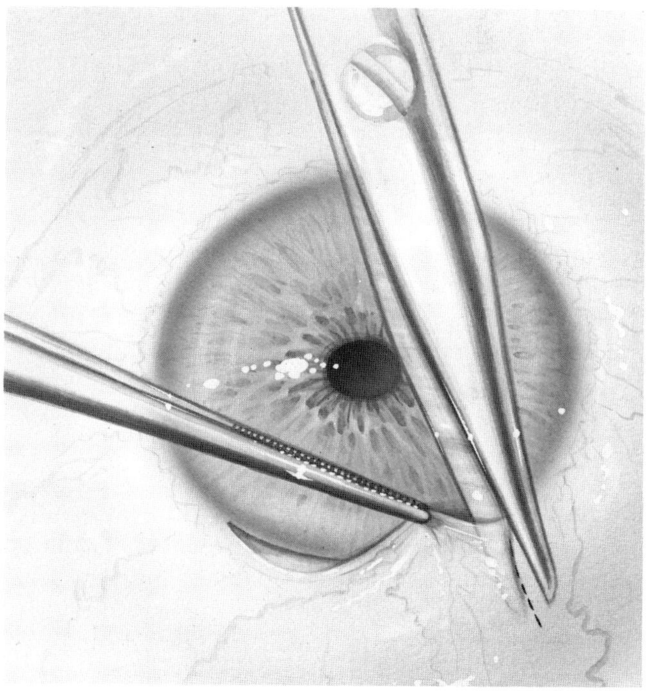

Fornix-Based Flap

2.**20** An alternative method of performing trabeculectomy is to develop the conjunctival flap anteriorly, basing it in the fornix. The conjunctiva is grasped as close to the scleral sulcus as possible and incised a distance of approximately 10 mm.

2.**21** The incision must be made as close to the insertion of the conjunctiva into the cornea as possible. A tag should not be left. A nontoothed forceps such as the Wills Eye Hospital utility forceps or Pierse-Hoskins forceps is most appropriate.

2.**22** The conjunctiva should be separated cleanly from the episclera, carefully freeing it for a distance of approximately 5–7 mm posteriorly.

2.**23** If the conjunctiva is tense, a relaxing incision can be made.

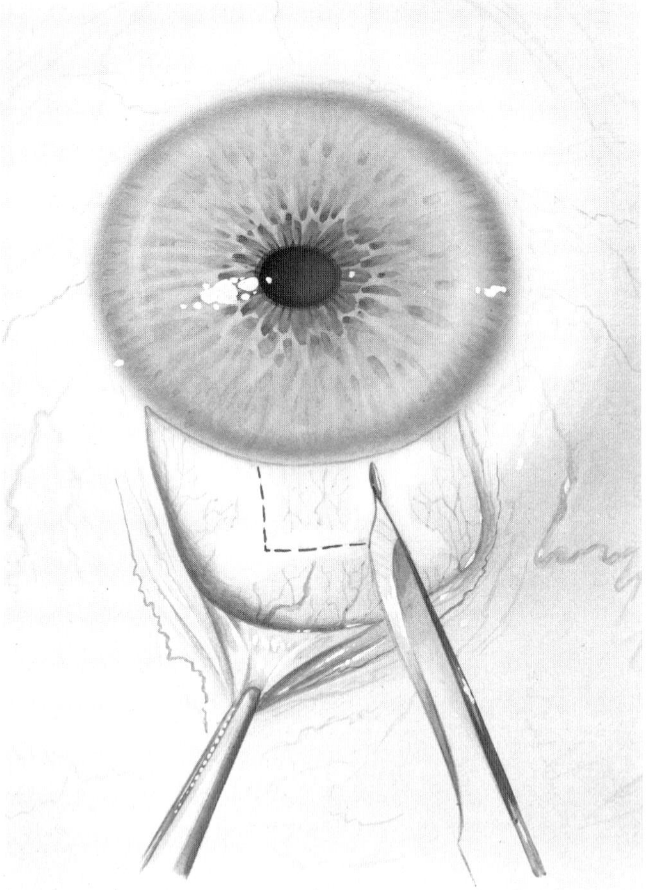

2.24 A trabeculectomy (or other procedure) is then performed. If a filtration procedure is combined with a fornix-based flap, it is usually best to make sure that leakage through the scleral filtration site is minimal.

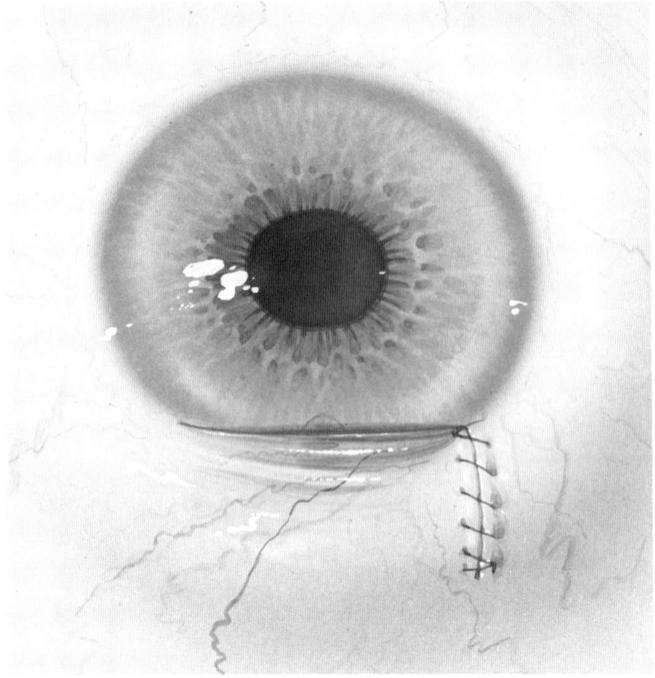

2.25 The cut edge of the conjunctiva is pulled tightly across the corneal surface and sutured securely in place, using fine suture material such as 10-0 nylon or 8-0 chromic collagen. The conjunctiva must be placed on stretch sufficiently tightly to indent the cornea slightly. If a relaxing incision has been made, this is closed tightly with running suture.

Modifications

If the surgeon wishes to obtain a very low intraocular pressure, the amount of filtration produced should be greater. This can be achieved by making a thinner scleral flap, extending the radial grooves farther anteriorly, developing a smaller ledge (that is, making the internal block more exactly the same size as the external scleral flap), placing cautery on the radial edges of the scleral flap, and not employing sutures in the edges of the scleral flap. Where the surgeon's highest priority is to avoid a flat anterior chamber, and achieving a low intraocular pressure is of lower priority, then the flap can be made thicker, the ledge wider, and the scleral flap more tightly closed with a greater number of sutures. The size of the scleral flap and the size of the block excised do not appear to influence the final level of intraocular pressure[10, 21]. The larger the flap, the more dissection is necessary; the worse the trauma, the greater the amount of scarring; consequently, the less tissue disturbed, the better. Furthermore, the greater the area of sclera disturbed, the more difficult is the performance of a repeat filtration procedure.

Where the lowest possible intraocular pressure is desired, it may be advantageous to employ a Simmons compression shell,[16] and not suture the scleral flap at all. Removing Tenon's capsule does not appear to be helpful[9]. Cautery seems to increase filtration, transforming the procedure into one more like a full-thickness filtration procedure.[14, 24]

At the time of surgery, the surgeon should determine where the sclera can be depressed most easily in order to deform the incision and permit a rapid increase in the exit of aqueous through the scleral incision. The location of this point may prove helpful in the immediate postoperative period.[23]

Postoperative Management

The patch is usually removed one to six hours postoperatively, depending upon how urgent it is that filtration develop. Where a low intraocular pressure is desired and much filtration hoped for, the patch is removed promptly and postoperative medications are instituted.[22] These usually consist of a potent anti-inflammatory compound such as prednisolone acetate 1 % at least four times daily, atropine 1 % four times daily, and a topical antibiotic. If further pupillary dilatation is required, phenylephrine 2.5 % or even 10 % is also employed. It is essential to obtain wide pupillary dilatation on the first day. In fact, the pupil should be maximally dilated at the conclusion of surgery.

Where excessive scarring is anticipated, as in younger individuals or reoperations, systemic steroid administration is started prior to surgery and continued postoperatively in full therapeutic doses[22] (20 mg prednisone four times daily for four days, and then tapering off, for approximately one month). As soon as the anterior chamber is seen to be persistently and adequately formed, the atropine can be stopped. This may be around the end of the first week. Pupillary dilatation should be maintained, however, for a period of about one month. Short-acting cycloplegics and mydriatics are adequate for this purpose.

Topical steroids should be stopped as soon as the eye ceases to be inflamed. In most cases dosage four times a day is adequate, and this can be tapered at the end of the first or second week, so that no steroids need be employed following the third or fourth week postoperatively.

If intraocular pressure rises postoperatively, and especially if a "Tenon's cyst" develops, topical epinephrine compound should be employed and further surgery avoided. In almost every case in which there is adequate filtration, the cyst will gradually disappear, and a satisfactory bleb will be obtained. Surgical revision of the bleb is to be avoided; it is rarely successful and is usually unnecessary.

If it appears that the surgical procedure has completely failed, so that there is no filtering bleb, then standard glaucoma medication is again employed.

If successful filtration is present, so that there is a high bleb and a shallow chamber, it is usually adequate to follow the patient's progress carefully, using atropine and phenylephrine vigorously. Where the bleb is collapsing and the intraocular pressure falling due to the development of aqueous shutdown associated with a choroidal detachment, it may be necessary to drain the choroidal detachment and reform the anterior chamber. This is an unusual complication when the anterior chamber has been well formed at the conclusion of surgery. If the eye is soft and there is contact between the lens and the cornea, the anterior chamber will not reform and should be corrected surgically as promptly as possible, preferably the same day. This requires drainage of the choroidal detachment and reformation of the anterior chamber with balanced salt solution. If at the time of reformation the chamber cannot be kept in a formed position, the conjunctival flap should be revised and the scleral flap closed sufficiently to permit the anterior chamber to be maintained with balanced salt solution. Sodium hyaluronate cannot be recommended as a method of ensuring maintenance of the anterior chamber. If, despite all efforts, the anterior chamber cannot be kept formed, the possibility of aqueous misdirection syndrome should be considered. If, rather than this, excessive filtration is the cause, then a large air bubble may be placed in the anterior chamber.

Where filtration is not adequate in the immediate postoperative period, a Traverso maneuver is often immensely helpful.[23] Here the surgeon presses directly on the well anesthetized conjunctiva with an applicator over the area where he or she has previously determined that pressure will be effective in increasing leakage. This is done at the slit lamp and is associated with immediate development of a higher bleb and shallowing of the anterior chamber. The maneuver may need to be repeated as often as twice daily and, when successful, it usually transforms a failure into a successful procedure. It is highly recommended.

Results

Around 85 % of trabeculectomies will be successful in terms of controlling intraocular pressure without significant complication. Final intraocular pressure averages around 18 mm Hg. Where intraocular pressure is lower to start with, the final intraocular pressure is commensurately lower. Trabeculectomy does not lower intraocular pressure as markedly as do full-thickness filtration procedures.

Bibliography and References

1 Bakker, N. J. A., Manku, S. I.: Trabeculectomy versus Scheie's operation: a comparative retrospective study in open-angle glaucoma in Kenyans. *Br. J. Ophthalmol.* 63: 643–645, 1979.

2 Blondeau, P., Phelps, C. D.: Trabeculectomy vs. thermosclerostomy – A randomized prospective clinical trial. *Arch. Ophthalmol.* 99: 810–816, 1981.

3 Cairns, J. E.: The case for early surgery in primary open-angle glaucoma. *Glaucoma* 3: 7–9, 1981.

4 Cairns, J. E.: Trabeculectomy. Preliminary report of a new method. *Amer. J. Ophthalmol.* 66: 673–679, 1968.

5 Drance, S. M., Vargas, E.: Trabeculectomy & thermosclerectomy: A comparison of two procedures. *Can. J. Ophthalmol.* 8: 413–415, 1973.

6 Gloor, B., Niederer, W., Daicker, B.: Operationstechnik, Resultate, Indikationsstellung. *Klin. Monatsbl. Augenheilk.* 170: 241–248, 1977.

7 Heuer, D. K., Gressel, M. G., Parrish II, R. K. et al.: Trabeculectomy in aphakic eyes. *Ophthalmology* 91: 1045–1051, 1984.

8 Jerndal, T., Lundstrom, M.: 330 Trabeculectomies – a follow-up study. *Acta Ophthalmol.* 55: 52–63, 1977.

9 Kapetansky, F. M.: Trabeculectomy, or trabeculectomy plus tenectomy: A comparative study. *Glaucoma* 2: 451–453, 1980.

10 Lalive d'Epinay, S., Remé, C., Witmer, R.: Der Einfluß verschiedener Lokalisationen der Trabekulectomie auf die intraokulare Druckregulation beim primären Glaukom. *Klin. Monatsbl. Augenheilk.* 182: 387–390, 1983.

[11] Lewis, R. A., Phelps, C. D.: Trabeculectomy vs. thermosclerostomy. *Arch. Ophthalmol.* 102: 533–536, 1984.

[12] Luntz, M. H.: Trabeculectomy using a fornix-based conjunctival flap and tightly sutured scleral flap. *Ophthalmology* 87: 985–989, 1980.

[13] Marion, J. R., Shields, M. B.: Thermal sclerostomy and posterior lip sclerectomy: a comparative study. *Ophthal. Surg.* 9: 67–75, 1978.

[14] Schimek, R. A., Williamson, W. R.: Trabeculectomy with cautery. *Ophthal. Surg.* 8: 35–40, 1977.

[15] Shuster, J. N., Krupin, T., Kolker, A. E. et al.: Limbus- vs. fornix-based conjunctival flap in trabeculectomy: A long-term randomized study. *Arch. Ophthalmol.* 102: 361–362, 1984.

[16] Simmons, R. J., Kimbrough, R. L.: Shell tamponade in filtering surgery for glaucoma. *Ophthal. Surg.* 10: 17–34, 1979.

[17] Spaeth, G. L., Poryzees, E.: A comparison between peripheral iridectomy with thermal sclerostomy and trabeculectomy: a controlled study. *Br. J. Ophthalmol.* 54: 783–789, 1981.

[18] Spaeth, G. L.: Complications of glaucoma surgery stressing innovations and trends, in Fasanella, R. M. (ed.): *Eye Surgery Innovations and Trends, Pitfalls and Complications.* Thomas, Springfield 1977, pages 58–82.

[19] Spaeth, G. L., Poryzees, E. M.: Relationship between the technique of surgical trabeculectomy and the final postoperative result. *Glaucoma Update II* 53–57, 1983.

[20] Spaeth, G. L., Joseph, N. H., Fernandes, E.: Trabeculectomy: a re-evaluation after three years and a comparison with Scheie's procedure. *Trans. Amer. Acad. Ophthalmol. Otolaryn.* 79: 349–361, 1985.

[21] Starita, R. J., Fellman, R. L., Spaeth, G. L. et al.: Effect of varying size of scleral flap and corneal block on trabeculectomy. *Ophthal. Surg.* 15: 484–487, 1984.

[22] Starita, R. J., Fellman, R. L., Spaeth, G. L.: Short- and long-term effects of postoperative corticosteroids on trabeculectomy. *Ophthalmology* 91: 107, 1984.

[23] Traverso, C. E., Greenidge, K. C., Spaeth, G. L.: Focal pressure: A new method to encourage filtration after trabeculectomy. *Ophthal. Surg.* 15: 62–65, 1984.

[24] Vorkas, A. P.: Intrascleral thermocautery. *Trans. Ophthal. Soc. U.K.* 98: 20–21, 1978.

[25] Watson, P.: Trabeculectomy: A modified ab externo technique. *Ann. Ophthalmol.* 2: 199–205, 1970.

Corneoscleral Trepanation

Klaus Heilmann

Surgical Principles

The aim of every filtering procedure, i.e., the creation of an extraocular fistula, consists in draining off aqueous humor under the conjunctiva by creating a connection between the anterior chamber and the episcleral space.

It was, in particular, Fronimopoulos et al. who turned the principle of a fistulizing procedure under a scleral flap into a practicable method. Even though any fistulizing procedure is theoretically feasible after preparing a corneoscleral or scleral flap, the method advocated by Elliot, i.e., goniotrepanation, has proved the most satisfactory. The procedure described in the following is known as an Elliot trepanation under a lamellar scleral flap.

Preparation for Surgery

Customary preparation of the patient for a microsurgical operation.

Preoperative Medication and Anesthesia

An antibiotic in drop form is administered to both eyes for a week prior to surgery. If there is any doubt, a conjunctival smear is taken and bacteriologically examined.

If miotics have been administered, they are discontinued and therapy with a beta-blocker and/or acetazolamide is continued up to the time of the operation.

Surgery can usually be performed under local anesthesia. Prior to the operation the patient is sedated; an intravenous approach is created prophylactically in case there are any untoward incidents during the operation. Anesthesiological intervention should be possible.

Instruments

The instruments customarily used for microsurgical procedures are required.

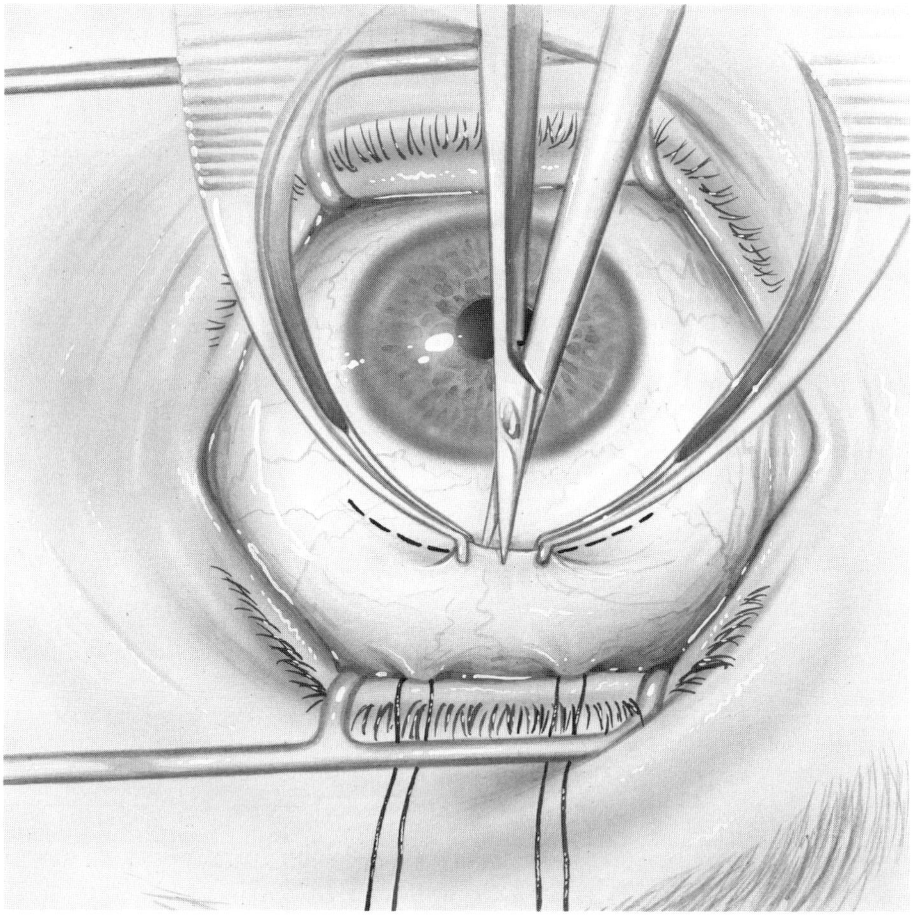

Surgical Technique

2.**26** A bridle suture is placed through the insertion of the superior rectus muscle at 12 o'clock, approximately 8 mm behind the limbus. A Colibri lid retractor after J. Barraquer is then inserted. Following this, the surgical field is flushed with physiological saline solution. The conjunctiva and Tenon's capsule are raised close to the muscle insertion.

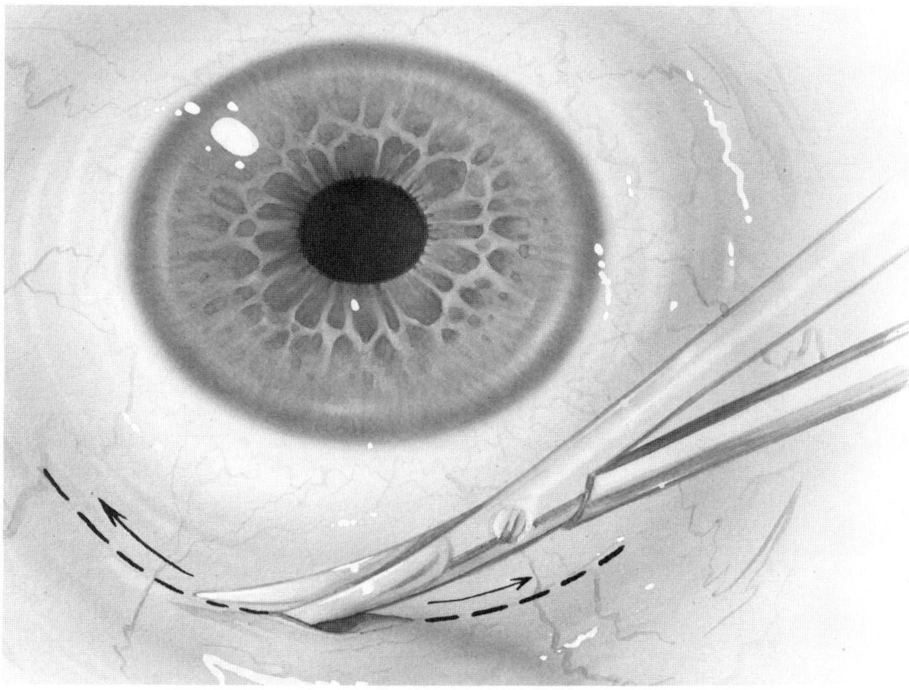

2.**27** The conjunctiva is opened with scissors, and one blade is inserted into the small hole and slid over the sclera, first in one direction and then in the other. The arcuate incision should run approximately from 10 o'clock to 2 o'clock.

28

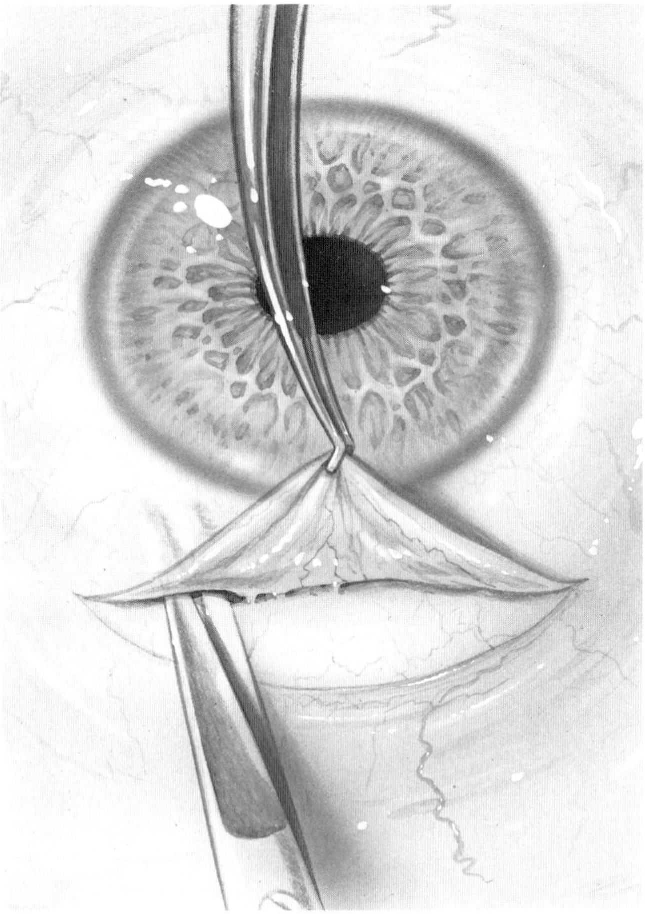

30

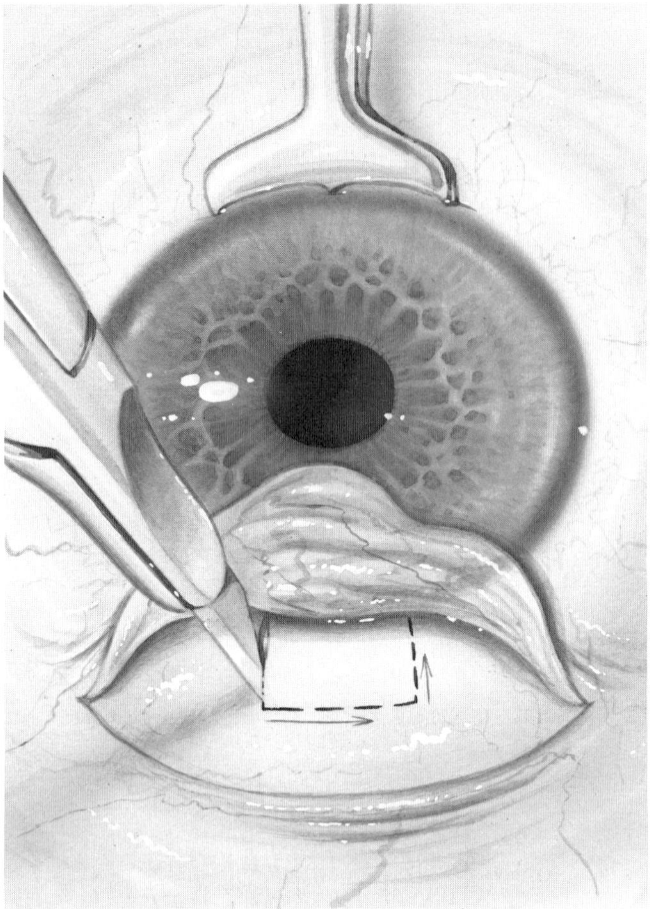

29

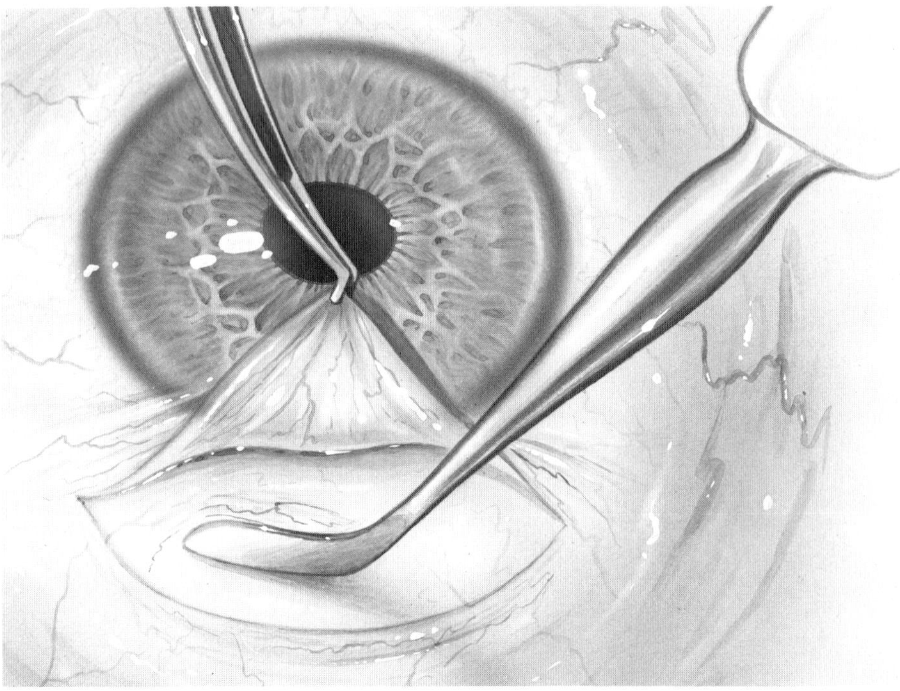

2.**28** The conjunctiva is detached, starting with blunt scissors.

2.**29** The preparations for creation of the scleral flap consist in further cleaning of the sclera using a hockey knife; the blade, attached in vertical setting, is held tangentially and moved toward the limbus. Vessels are obliterated with bipolar forceps.

2.**30** The scleral flap is outlined with a razor blade knife. This author prefers the 3 × 2 mm size.

31

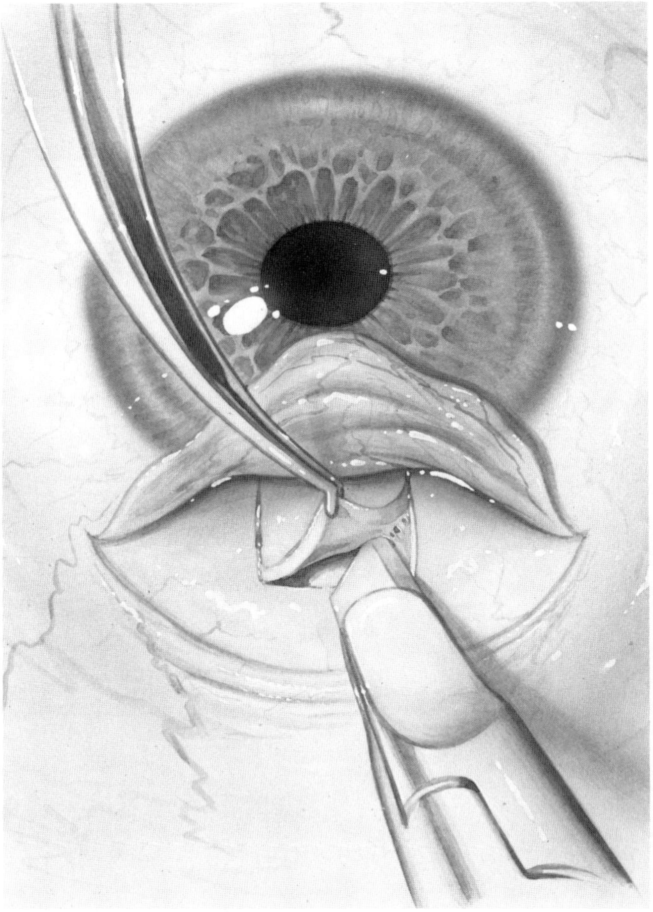

32

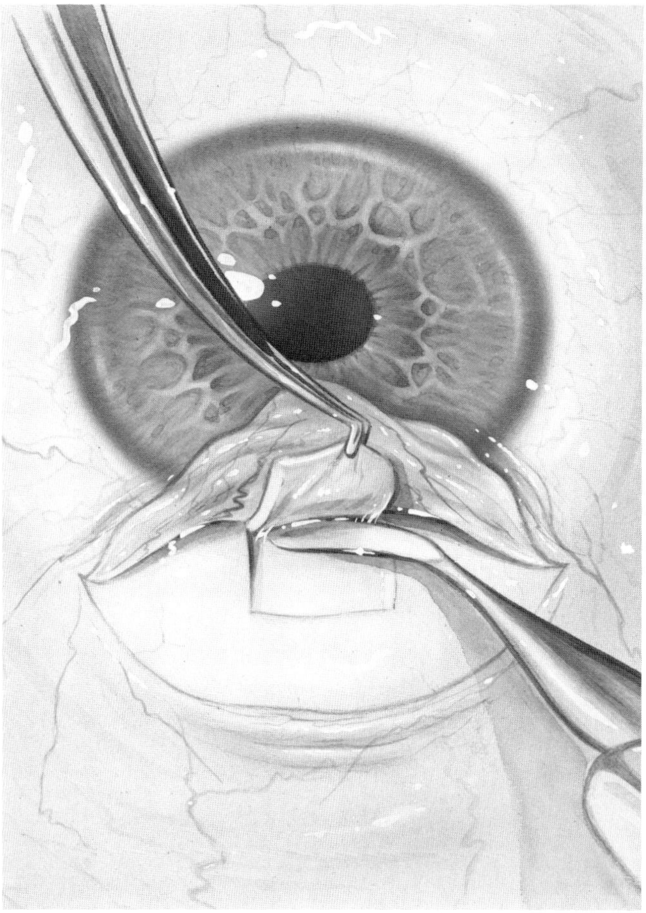

33

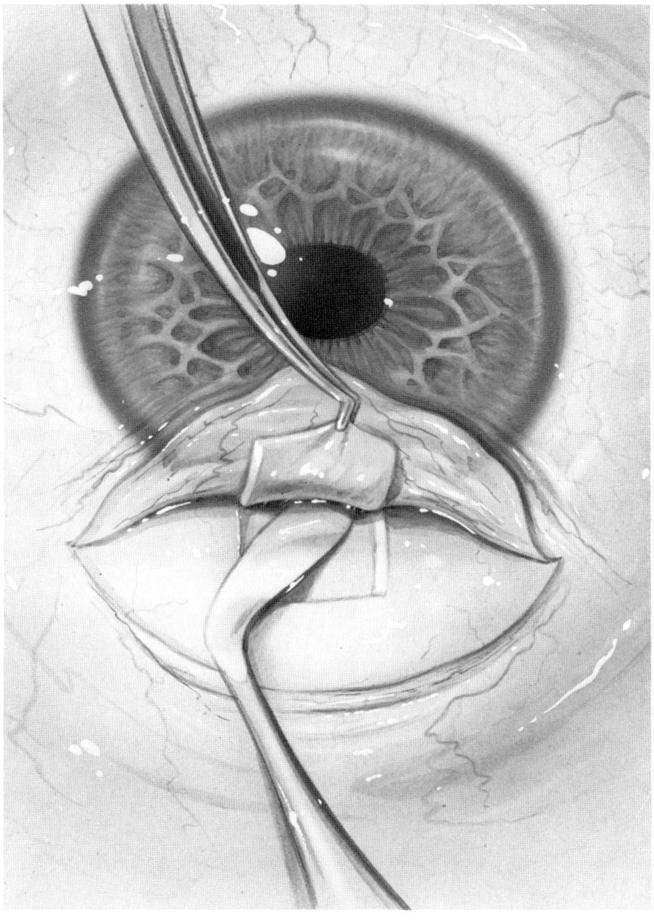

2.**31** The flap is now raised at one edge. When preparing the flap one tries to make it around one-third to one-half the thickness of the sclera.

2.**32** The farther one penetrates into the limbal region the more care must be taken in dissection. The present author prefers to use the less sharp hockey knife for this purpose.

2.**33** It is important to continue preparation of the scleral flap about 1 mm into the superficial layers of the cornea.

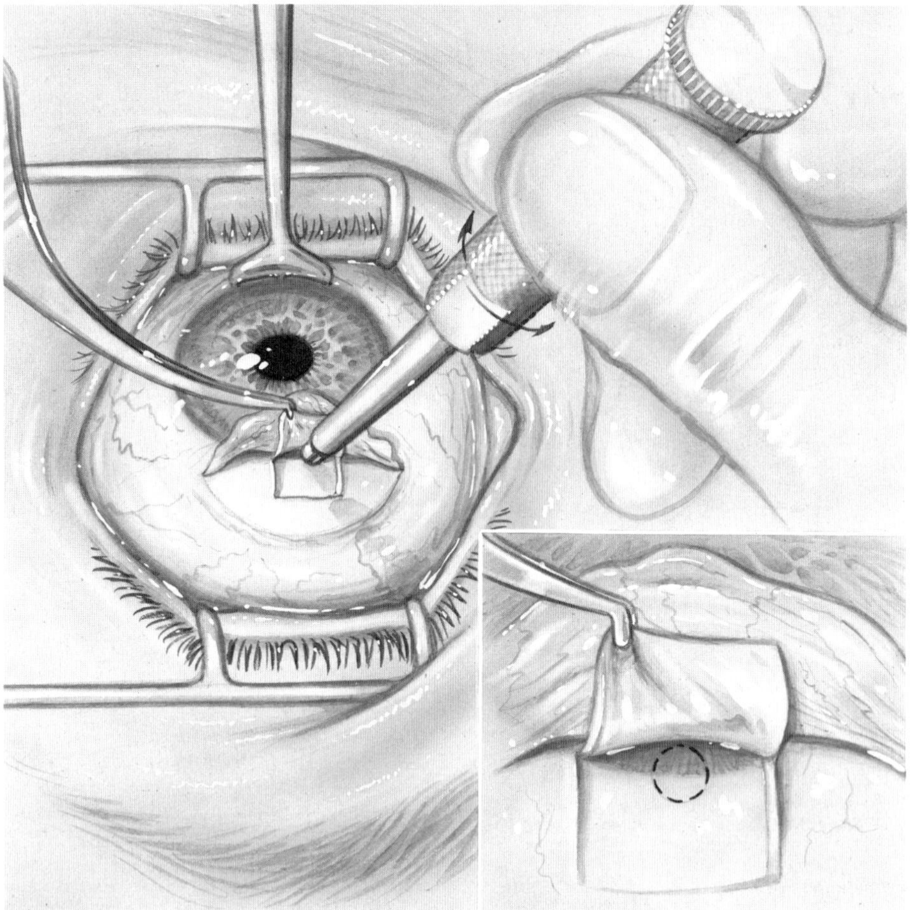

2.**34** The trephine (diameter 1.5 mm) is applied in such a way that one half of it comes to lie on the sclera, the other half on the cornea. The actual trepanation procedure is accomplished by rotating movements and application of uniform pressure. The deeper one goes the less pressure should be applied. By removing the trephine one can assure oneself that the position and depth are correct. It is easy to relocate the trephine in the original circular incision. No force should be used to open the anterior chamber; as soon as there is no longer any resistance the trephine is carefully withdrawn.

35

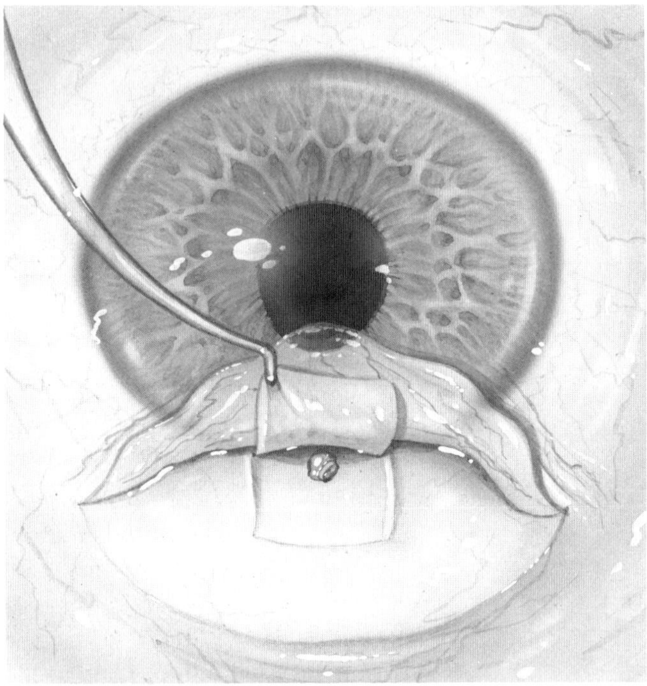

2.**35** Some iris tissue usually prolapses into the trephine hole. The small disk trephined out, which is generally still joined to the sclera, is gripped with the iris forceps and cut off at the edge of the hole using Vannas scissors.

36

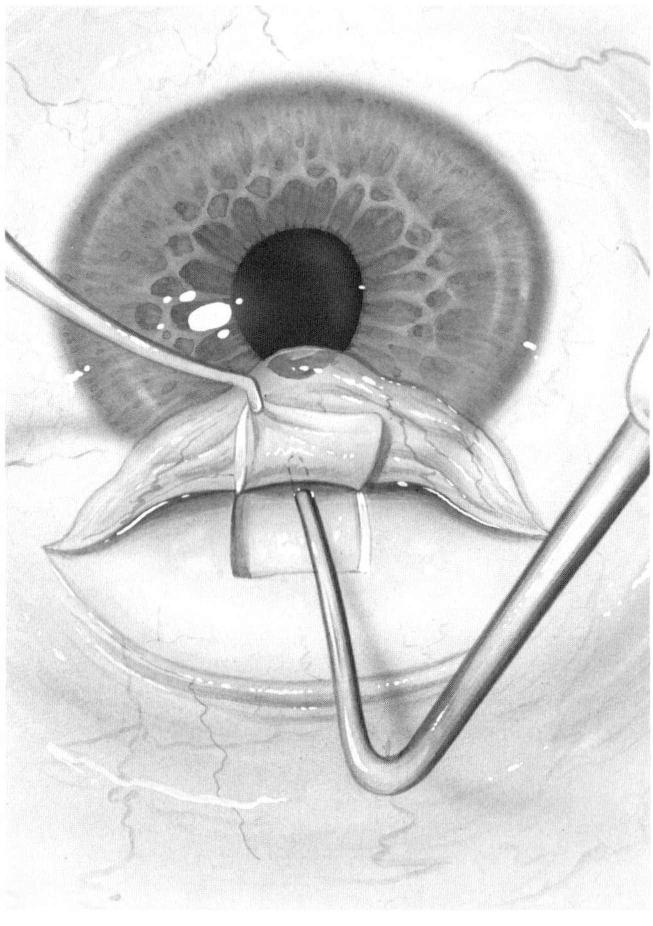

37

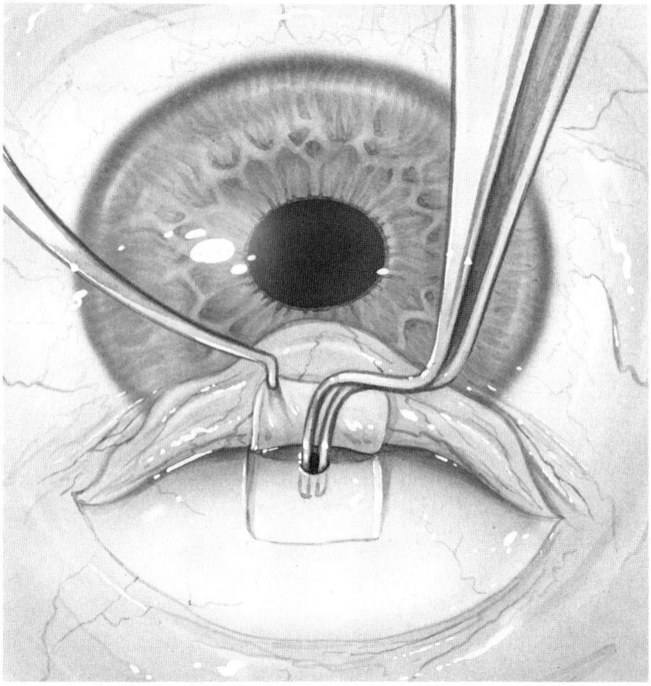

38

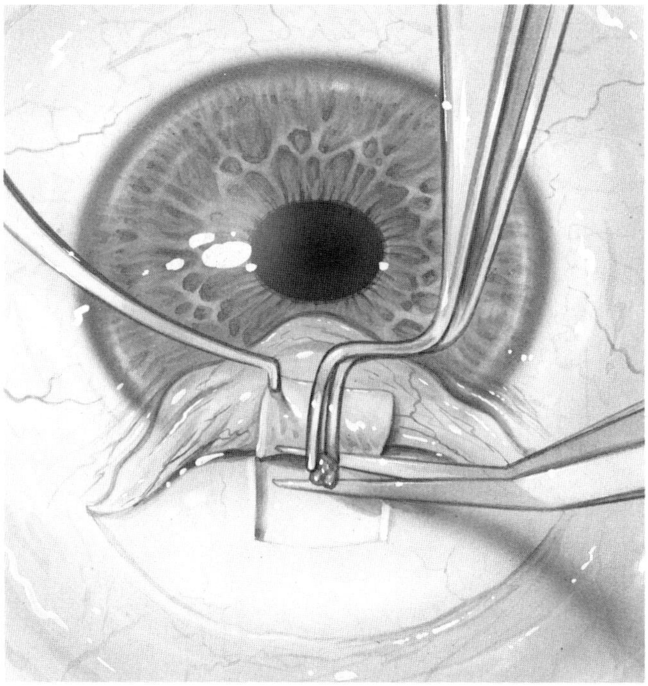

39

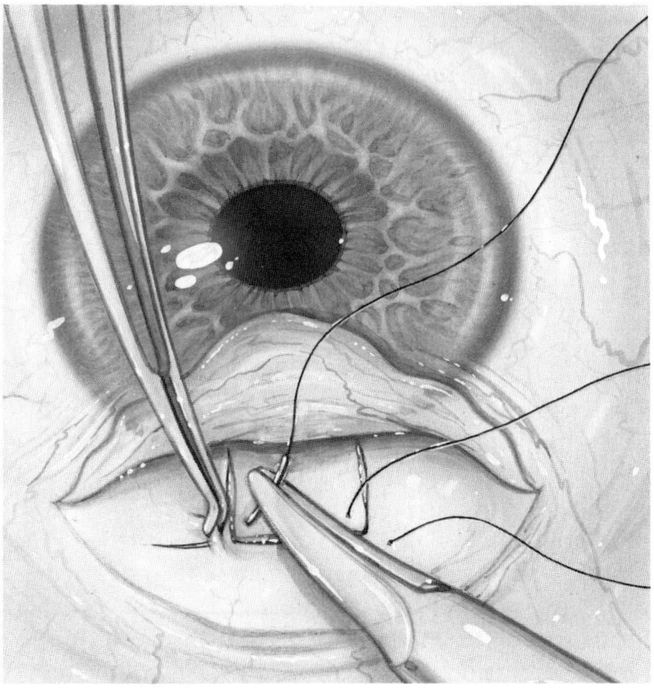

40

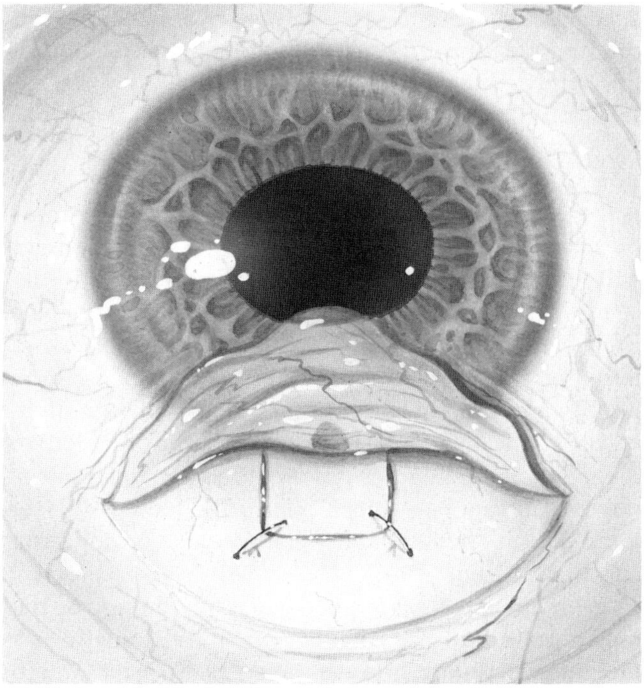

◊ 2.**36** Using a spatula, the prolapsed iris tissue is carefully pushed back into the anterior chamber; the aqueous humor should slowly seep away as this is done. The anterior chamber is subsequently eliminated.

2.**37** After the previously oval pupil has regained its normal shape a pair of sharply angled iris forceps is passed through the trepanation hole. Iris tissue is grasped with them and pulled through the hole.

2.**38** By removing (with Wecker scissors) the iris tissue which has been pulled out the iris retracts: a basal iridectomy has been performed. Even at this early stage dilatation of the pupil is begun, in order to restore the anterior chamber.

2.**39** The scleral flap is folded back into its original bed and fixed at the edges with 2 sutures (monofilament Ethilon 10-0).

2.**40** After knotting the sutures, the knots are buried. The border of the flap usually bulges somewhat.

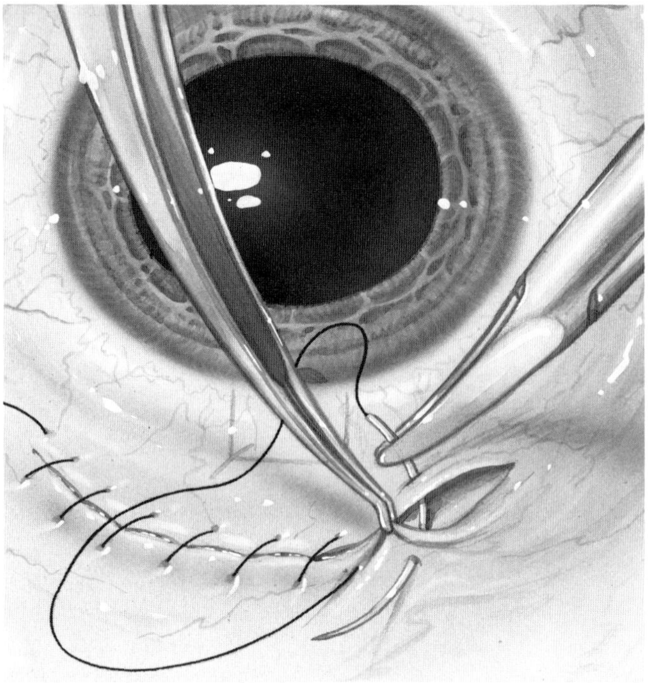

2.**41** After stroking the conjunctiva back into its original position it is carefully closed with a continuous suture (7-0 silk).

Complications

Scleral Flap: When preparing the scleral flap, care must be taken to ensure that it is of uniform thickness as chosen. If it becomes too thin toward the limbus border, it may tear or tear off. If one goes too deep when preparing the flap, the result will be premature perforation and possibly also choroidal bleeding.

Trepanation: The trephine should be applied in such a way that one half of it is on the cornea, the other half on the sclera. If too much of it is on the cornea the resulting hole may be not be covered exteriorly; if it is placed too far over on the sclera there may be bleeding from choroidal tissue.

If too much force is applied when trephining, the flap may recede into the anterior chamber. Usually it is merely folded back and can be carefully gripped with Colibri forceps and folded out. Should it be floating freely in the anterior chamber it has to be removed from it through the trepanation hole. This can be extremely difficult.

Postoperative Complications: The most serious postoperative complication is the continued absence of an anterior chamber and the development of a malignant glaucoma. A shallow or absent anterior chamber *without* elevated intraocular pressure is a sign of choroidal detachment. This occurs relatively frequently and is also noticed by the patient when the dressing is changed, as a shadow or veil. The detachment may be so severe that the pupil is covered.

The more serious complication when there is no anterior chamber and intraocular pressure is elevated is the threat of malignant glaucoma. The lens is displaced anteriorly and the vitreous body follows it. Therapy consists in administering atropine 2 % and phenylephrine 5 % eye drops and infusion of hyperosmotic substances (e.g., Mannitol). If this treatment fails to restore the anterior chamber, a posterior sclerotomy must be performed and vitreous aspirated. The anterior chamber is restored simultaneously by insufflation.

Complications which used to arise, such as a cystic filtering bleb, thinning of the conjunctival flap, and intraocular infection have become rare since the introduction of trepanation under a scleral flap. The scleral flap exerts pressure which counteracts the outflow of aqueous humor; consequently a large filtration area in the conjunctiva is created for the aqueous humor, rather than a conjunctival bleb.

Postoperative Management

Immediately after the end of the operation, atropine 2 % and antibiotics are instilled. Ointments are to be avoided. In order to prevent synechiae and adhesions in the region of the scleral flap, a cortisone depot (dexamethasone) is placed subconjunctivally. The eye is kept under a dressing for a week, after which the conjunctival suture is removed.

In the first few postoperative days the behavior of the pupil and anterior chamber should be kept under close observation. After suture removal dexamethasone and chloramphenicol are administered in combination (in drop form) for one to two weeks.

Results

This author has been practising the method described above for some ten years. On the basis of personal observations the results, with regard to lowering of IOP, can be described as very good; an adequate lowering of pressure is almost always achieved. Even so, in older patients especially, vision gradually deteriorates if there is already some opacity of the lens. Cataract surgery may be necessary at a later date. We know from even longer-term observation that after lowering IOP a slow recovery occurs of the optic nerve fibers which were under pressure, but not completely atrophied. As a result, scotomata may be reduced in size.

Bibliography

[1] Fronimopoulos, J., Lambron, N., Pelekis, N., Christakis, C.: Elliot'sche Trepanation mit Skleraldeckel. *Klin. Monatsbl. Augenheilk.* 156: 1–8, 1970.

[2] Thiel, H.-J.: Filtering Procedures. In: Heilmann, K., Richardson, K. T. (eds.), *Glaucoma. Conceptions of a Disease.* Thieme, Stuttgart 1978, pages 324–329.

[3] Barraquer, J.: Complications after Glaucoma Surgery. In: Heilmann, K., Richardson, K. T. (eds.), *Glaucoma. Conceptions of a Disease.* Thieme, Stuttgart 1978, pages 338–342.

Peripheral Iridectomy with Thermal Sclerostomy

George L. Spaeth

Surgical Principles

The purpose of a peripheral iridectomy with thermal sclerostomy is to develop a permanent fistula in the sclera, connecting the anterior chamber with the episcleral space. The goal is the achievement of a thin cystic bleb and a low final intraocular pressure. Full-thickness procedures of all kinds are associated with a higher incidence of flat anterior chamber, hyphema, and development of cataract than are guarded procedures such as trabeculectomy. However, they are also associated with a lower final intraocular pressure. The advantage of this lower pressure must be weighed against the disadvantage of the higher rate of complications.

An additional indication for a peripheral iridectomy with thermal sclerostomy is when a trabeculectomy has been tried and has failed, or when postoperative scarring is thought to be a possible problem, as in the younger patient.

Preparation for Surgery

The preoperative routine and instruments required are as for trabeculectomy.

Surgical Technique

2.**42** A limbus-based flap is developed as described under trabeculectomy. It is absolutely essential that the flap be dissected as far anteriorly as possible. If this is not done, the incision into the sclera will not be sufficiently anterior. Failure to make the entrance into the anterior chamber sufficiently anterior is a serious and too-frequent error in performing a peripheral iridectomy with thermal sclerostomy. If necessary, the cornea should be split in order to ensure that there is adequate space for entry into the anterior chamber.

Cautery is placed 2 mm posterior to the anterior extent of the conjunctival dissection. The cautery spreads over an area approximately 1 mm wide in a radial direction and 4 mm circumferentially. An incision, using a # 67 Beaver blade, is placed in the middle of the cautery for a distance of 3 mm; the incision must be perpendicular to the globe.

42

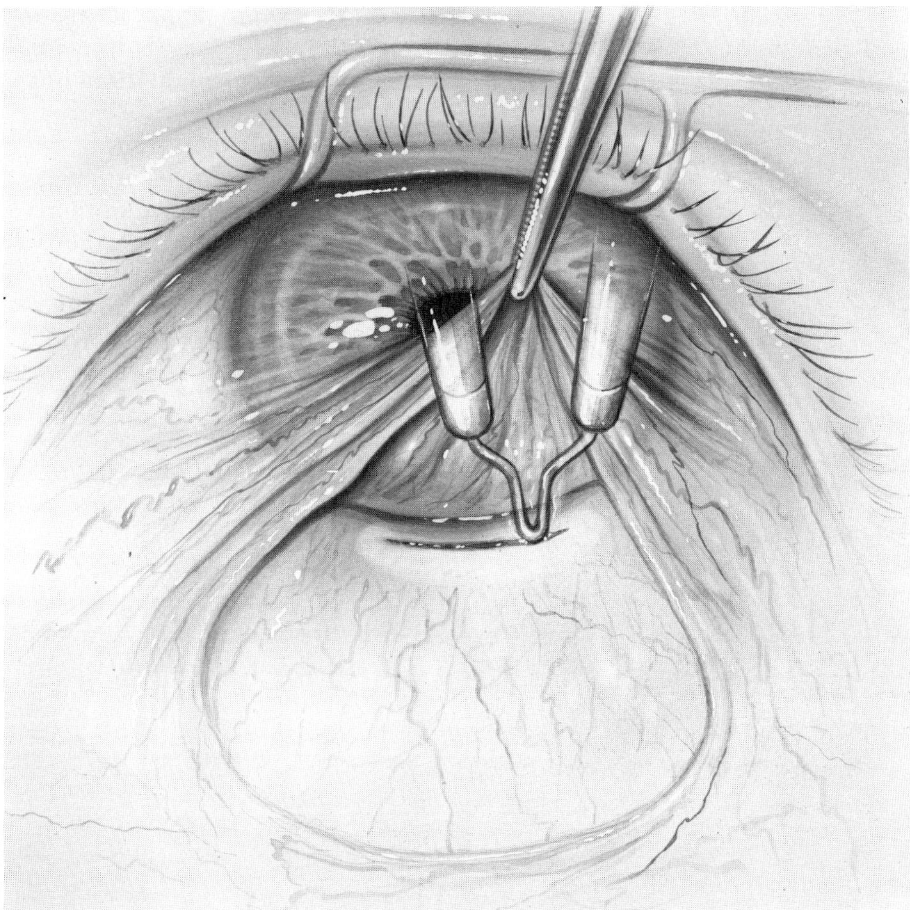

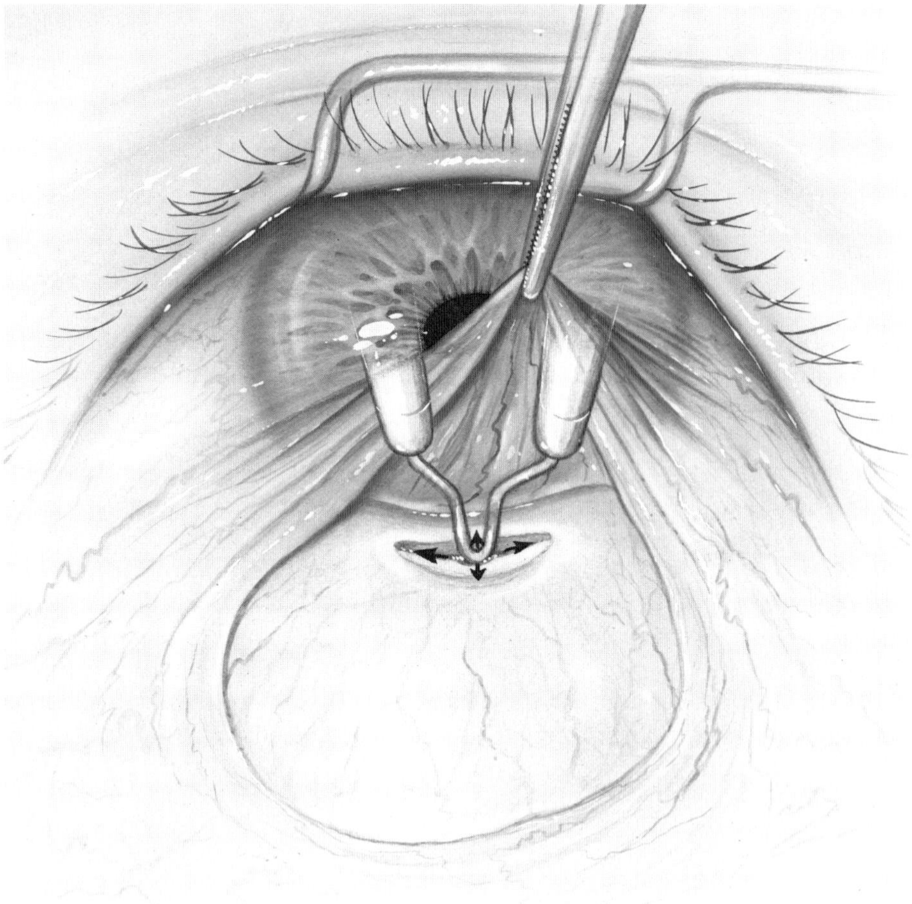

2.**43** The incision is widened by placing a "cool" cautery in the depths of the incision and pulling it posteriorly and pushing it anteriorly. The incision should develop a trough-like appearance. The cautery must not be so hot as to cause browning or charring of the sclera, but just hot enough to cause it to coagulate and shrink.

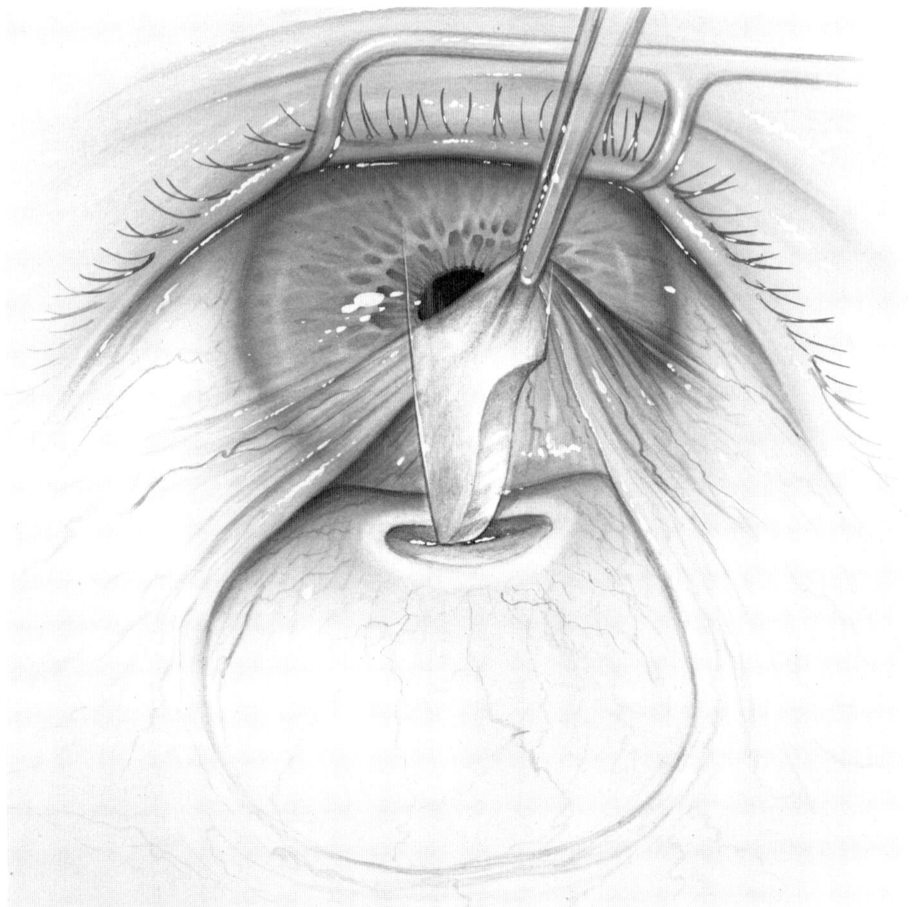

2.**44** After the application of cautery, the incision is deepened over its entire length. It is important to keep the blade perpendicular, and to make sure that the depth of the incision does not vary from one end to the other. The incision should be at the very base of the trough.

This application of cautery followed by partial incision of the sclera should be repeated three to five times. At this point, the anterior chamber can be entered with the knife, making sure that the open incision extends the entire width of the cauterized area. A standard peripheral or sector iridectomy is performed and the limbus flap closed as under trabeculectomy.

Modifications

A 7-0 black silk suture may be passed across the cauterized incision and exteriorized in the cornea. The suture passes deep to the conjunctiva, anterior to the limbus. This suture can then be tightened or loosened to produce less or more aqueous filtration, resulting in a lower or higher bleb, and a greater or lesser likelihood of development of flat anterior chamber. The suture tends to produce quite marked corneal astigmatism while in place. It can be removed when no longer necessary.

Postoperative Management

Essentially the same routines are followed as for trabeculectomy.

Results

The surgeon can anticipate a success rate approximately the same as with trabeculectomy. However, the rate of complications will be higher with peripheral iridectomy with thermal sclerostomy. Specifically, there are usually more hyphemas, synechiae, flat chambers, and postoperative cataracts. The final intraocular pressure averages around 15 mm Hg, which is lower than that usually achieved with trabeculectomy. The blebs are thin and cystic, and patients are therefore predisposed to late endophthalmitis and to other complications of such thin cystic blebs.

Bibliography

[1] Scheie, H. G.: An evaluation of iridectomy with scleral cautery. *Trans. Ophthal. Soc. Australia* 26: 44, 1967.

[2] Scheie, H. G.: Retraction of scleral wound edges – as a fistulizing procedure for glaucoma. *Amer. J. Ophthalmol.* 45: 220–229, 1958.

[3] Shaffer, R. N., Hetherington Jr., J., Hoskins Jr., H. D.: Guarded thermal sclerostomy. *Amer. J. Ophthalmol.* 72: 769–772, 1971.

[4] Viswanathan, B., Brown, I. A. R.: Peripheral iridectomy with scleral cautery for glaucoma. *Arch. Ophthalmol.* 93: 34–35, 1975.

See also the bibliograpy listed under Trabeculectomy, page 2.43

Goniotomy

Jörg Draeger and Rolf Winter

As early as the beginning of this century, Seefelder (1906) discussed the operations performed by de Vincentiis[7] on the chamber angle, under technically adverse conditions. It was not until 1936 that Barkan[1] rediscovered "goniotomy" and performed the operation under direct visualization using a contact lens. His descriptions of his good results in cases of congenital glaucoma[2], which up to then had been considered practically incurable, led a number of clinics to take up goniotomy as a new surgical method.

Surgical Principles

Essentially, the effectiveness of goniotomy is due to two factors. First, mesenchymal tissue, Barkan's membrane, and the chamber angle are, as it were, mechanically displaced and incised, thus reopening the drainage pathways. Second, this method allows a cyclodialysis to be performed *ab interno*. Since Heine[5] it has been known that the latter reduces intraocular pressure, even though the reasons for this still are not fully understood. The procedure may cause a localized trophic disturbance of the ciliary body with reduced secretion or, on the other hand, additional ciliary resorption in the area of the incision.

2.**45** Since the introduction of the manual applanation tonometer[3], it has been possible to establish the diagnosis of congenital glaucoma with greater confidence. This instrument allows pressure to be measured accurately, irrespective of any changes in rigidity, and in any position, even in anesthetized infants.

2.**46** Further progress in diagnosis has been achieved by measurements of the bulb axis length and the recording of growth curves by ultrasonography. In congenital glaucoma, these curves reveal typical changes when compared with normal eye development[6].

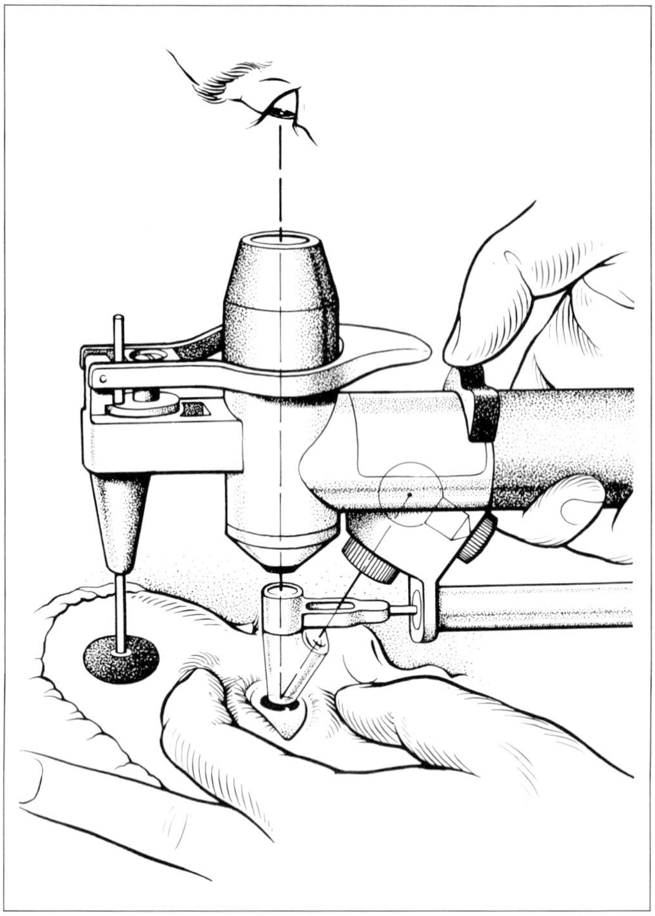

45

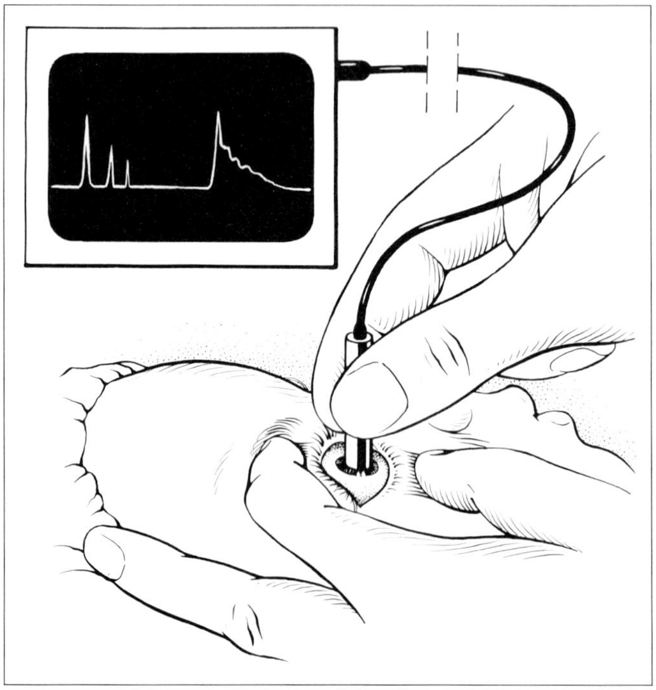

46

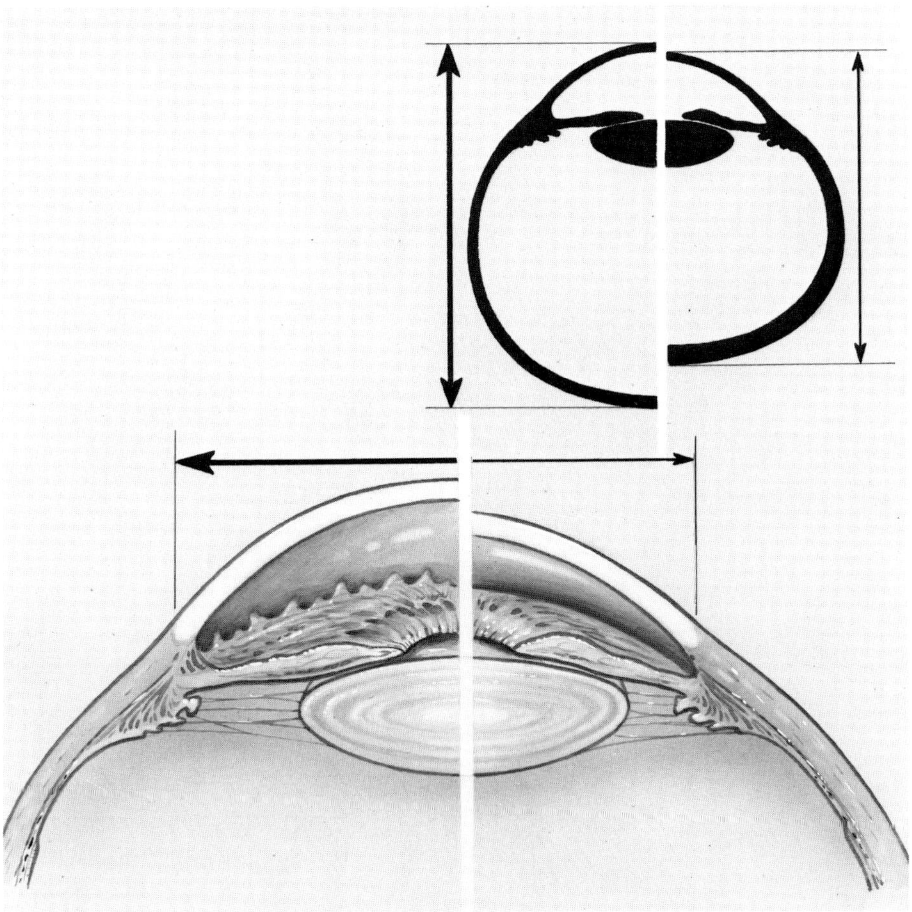

2.47 In addition to the axis length, the corneal diameter is also increased. Appraisal of the chamber angle with its typical abnormal differentiations, and in some cases even with development of a Barkan's membrane, is possible by means of gonioscopy using the slit-lamp or, in infants, the operating microscope.

Once congenital glaucoma has been diagnosed, with increased size of the globe, elevated intraocular pressure, and abnormal differentiation of the chamber angle, surgery is the only possible treatment in the long term. By performing goniotomy under microscopic control, the chamber angle can be incised and cyclodialysis under direct visualization is possible. Furthermore, goniotomy can be performed when only a cyclodialysis is planned, e.g., in cases of precipitations in the anterior chamber, secondary glaucoma, or aphakia. The sole difference from the technique used for congenital glaucoma is that the cyclodialysis effect is given more emphasis than in cases with congenital glaucoma alone.

Preoperative Medication and Anesthesia

Preoperative treatment consists in the administration of a miotic to contract the pupil as much as possible, to widen the chamber angle as much as possible, and at the same time to protect the lens from damage by the goniotomy needle. The procedure can be performed both under general anesthetic, as will usually be the case with infants, and under local anesthetic.

Instruments

Aside from the customary microsurgical equipment the following special instruments are required: lid retractor, Barkan lens, goniotomy needle (if necessary fitted with an infusion system), and needle holder.

It is equally essential that the operation should be performed by an experienced team, properly equipped with microsurgical apparatus if possible.

Surgical Technique

48

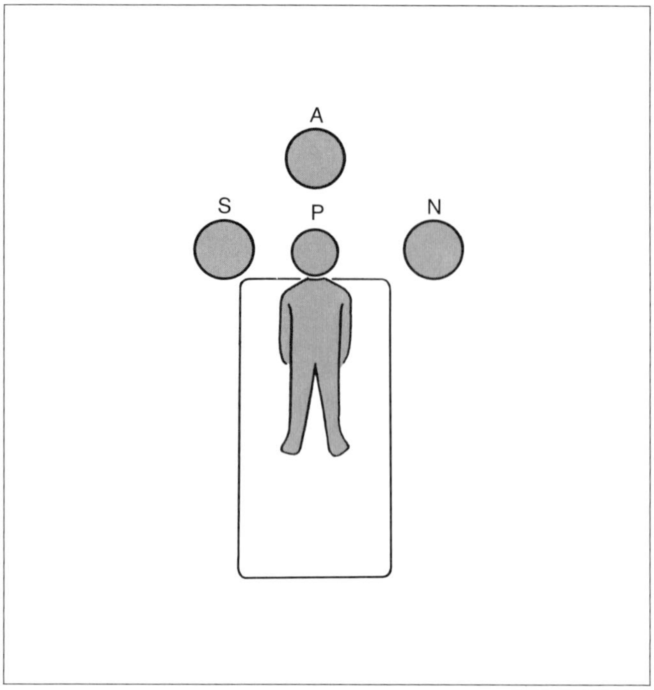

49

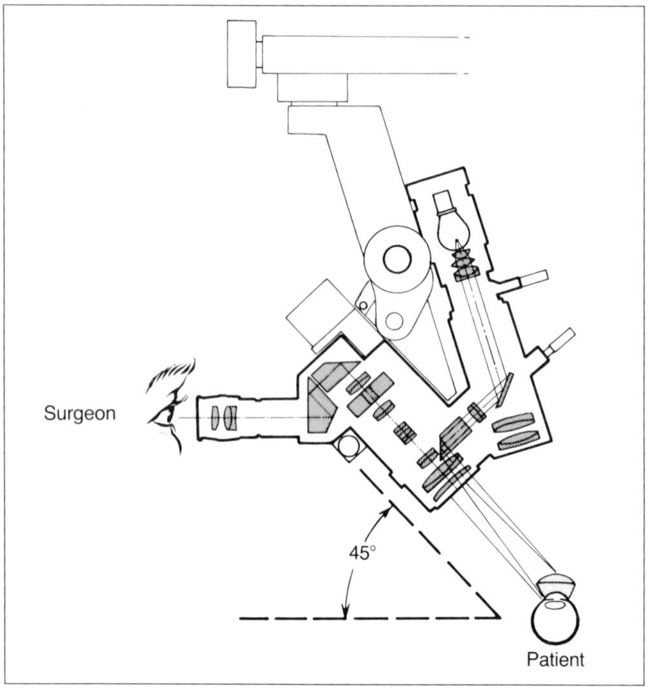

50

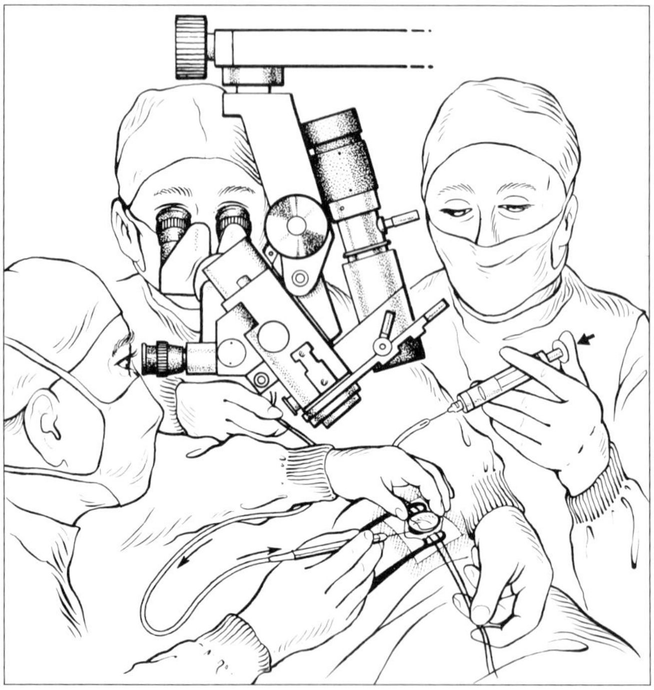

2.**48** Using an operating microscope and a contact lens, the surgeon checks the chamber angle and brings the goniotomy needle into position. At the same time, the assistant guides the globe in the right direction, while the assisting nurse maintains the chamber using an infusion system. The seating arrangement always depends on the eye to be operated on. The surgeon (S) sits on the same side as the eye to be operated on, the assistant (A) next to him, and the nurse (N) on the opposite side.

2.**49** The eye is viewed through the microscope tilted at approximately 45–60°, with coaxial illumination, and a contact lens. Contact lenses made of elastic silicone have been found preferable to those made of PMMA, because they are easier to handle. They adhere better to the cornea, the material is lighter, and the lens can be held better between two fingertips.

2.**50** The microscope, with coaxial illumination, is adjusted so that it is tilted. With the microscope in this position, the operating table must be raised relatively high, so that it is only approximately 15 cm beneath the eye level of the surgeon. Correspondingly, the surgeon's chair must be lowered. Only thus is it possible to see the chamber angle over its entire nasal circumference. A beam splitter enables the assistant to observe through an assistant's microscope, which again is coaxial.

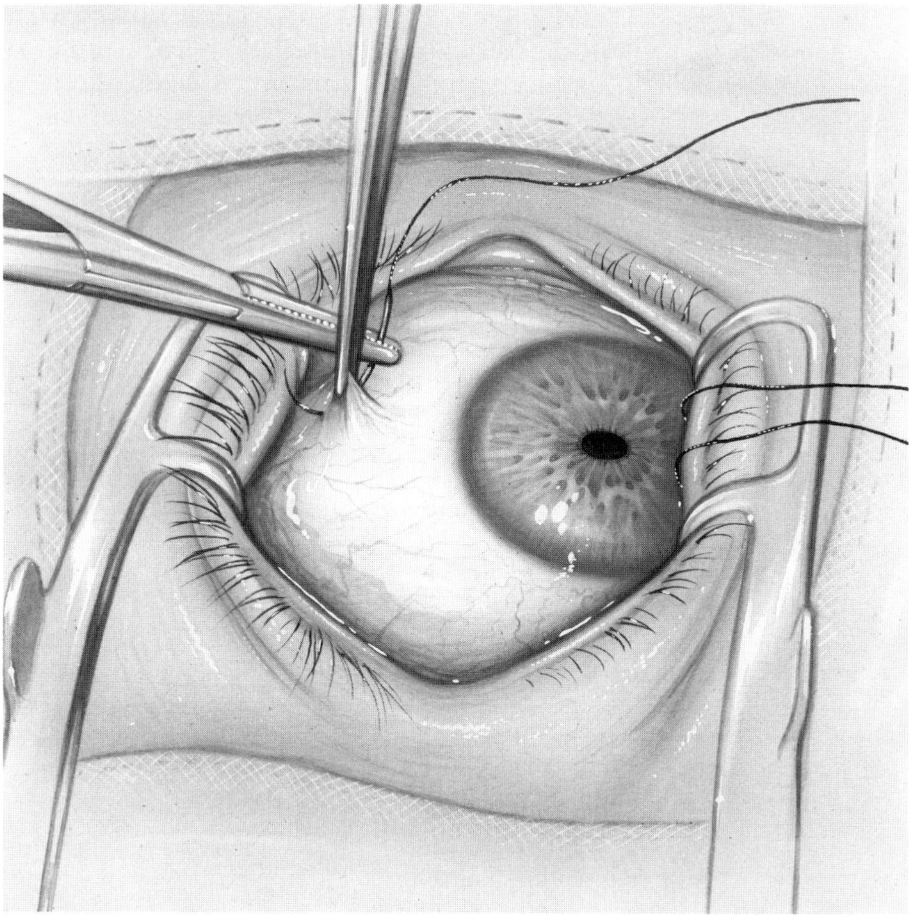

2.51 Fixation of the globe is best achieved by means of two holding sutures passed transconjunctivally through the superior rectus and inferior rectus muscles. In principle the muscle insertions can also be grasped with angled forceps, but when rotation becomes necessary, and especially nasalward, these can be a hindrance because the Barkan lens is between them.

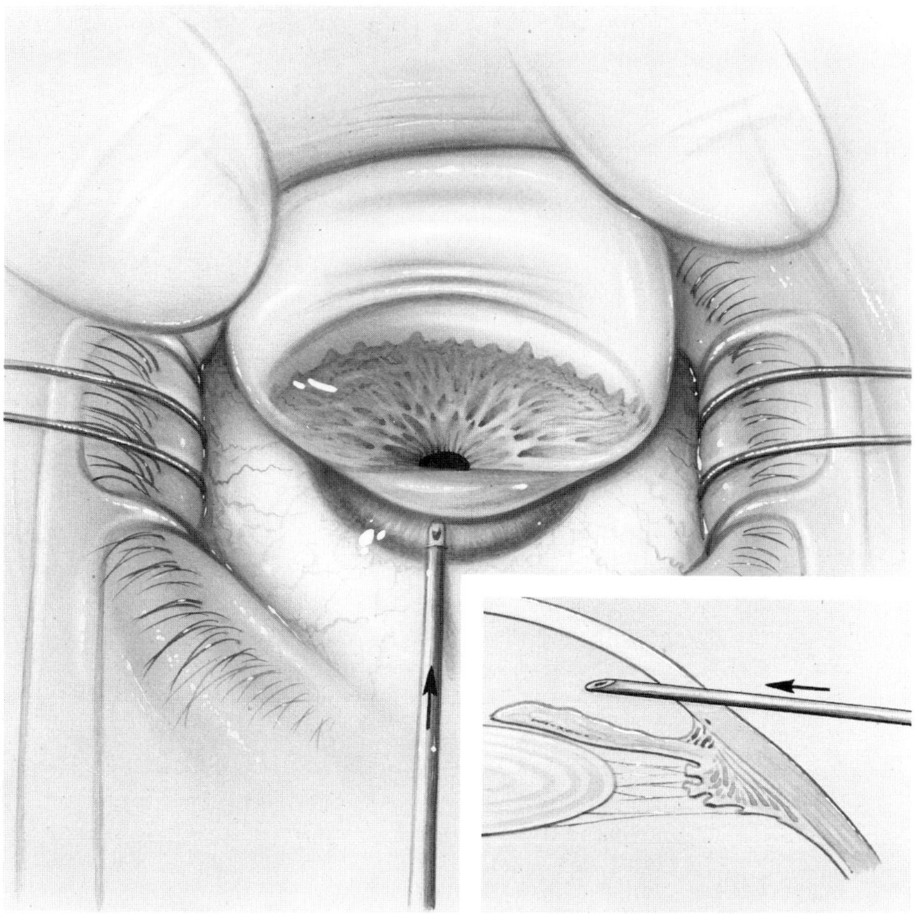

2.52 After perforation of the cornea, a sharp cannulated goniotomy needle is inserted smoothly from the temporal side, immediately at the limbus, at a very shallow angle above the level of the iris. Should a goniotomy knife without an irrigation supply be used, there will be a risk of outflow from the anterior chamber if the knife is turned excessively during the incision. Therefore, as soon as the cannulated goniotomy needle is inside the anterior chamber, normal chamber depth can be maintained by means of the attached infusion tube. At the same time, however, care must be taken to ensure that IOP does not rise to a level which might cause corneoepithelial edema or even dislocation of the lens posteriad. The chamber should merely be maintained at normal depth. By means of the Barkan lens, which is positioned at the same time, the goniotomy needle is maneuvered into the region of the opposite chamber angle.

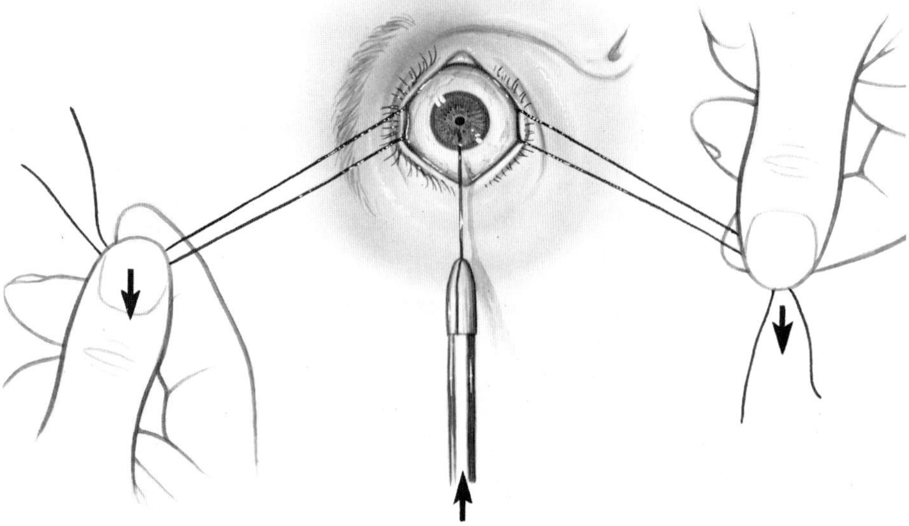

2.**53** The globe is stabilized appropriately by means of the holding sutures. During insertion of the needle it is advisable for the assistant to abduct the globe slightly toward the surgeon.

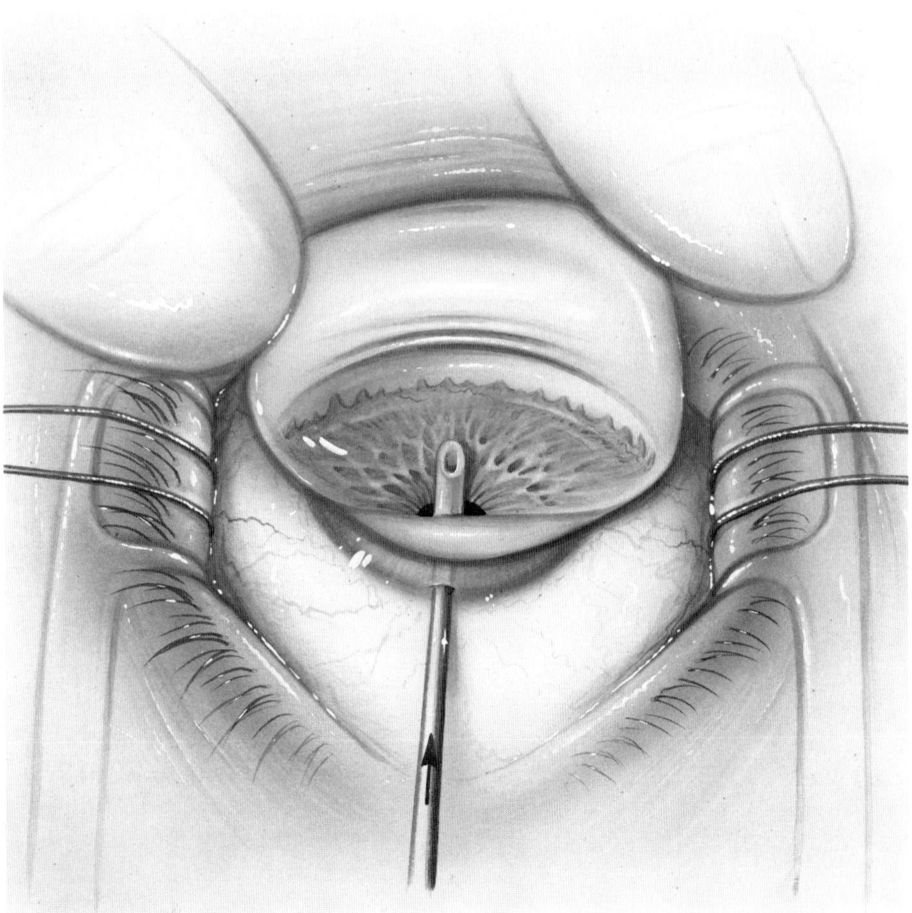

2.**54** Keeping the goniotomy needle in view through the Barkan lens, the surgeon advances the needle to the opposite chamber angle.

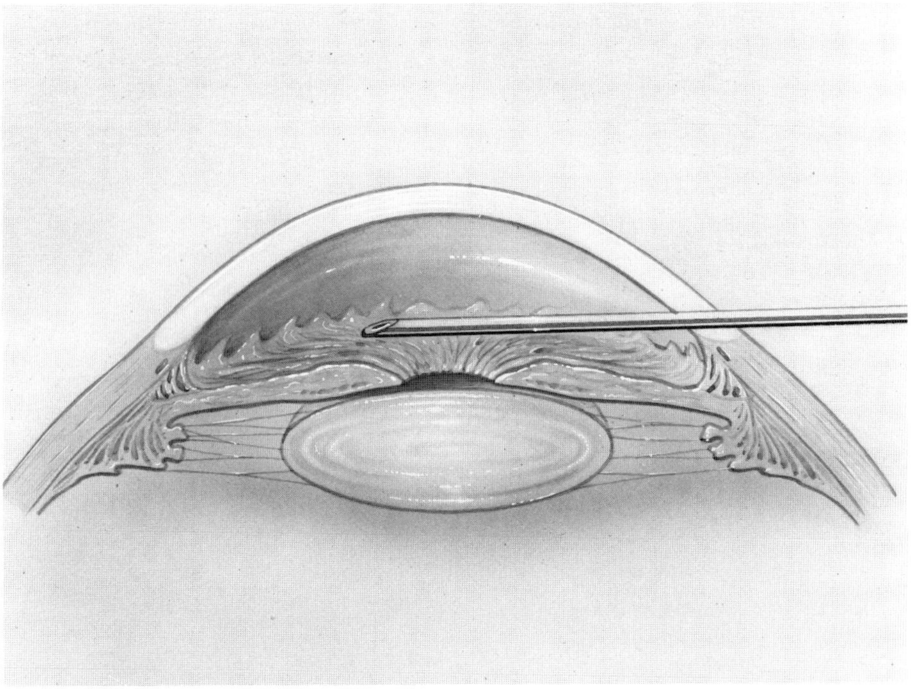

2.55 As he does so, the needle glides levelly over the iris. Miosis should be as extreme as possible.

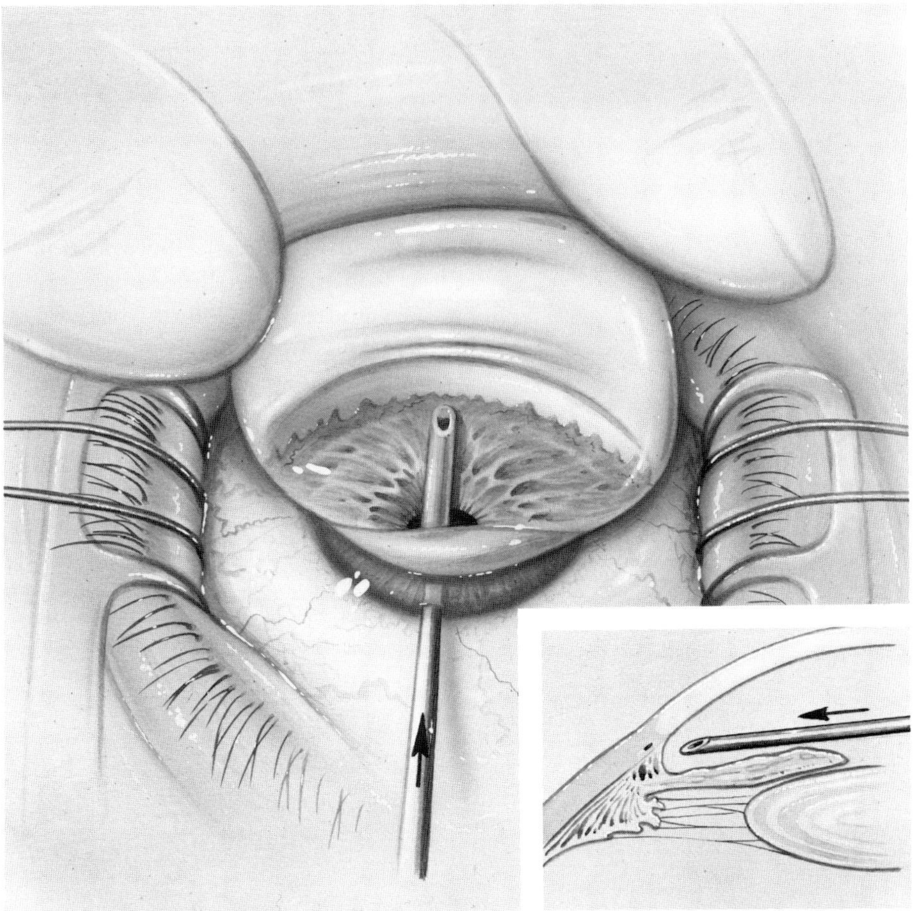

2.56 When infusion is possible, the chamber can be kept at a constant depth. The chamber angle is clearly visible through the Barkan lens.

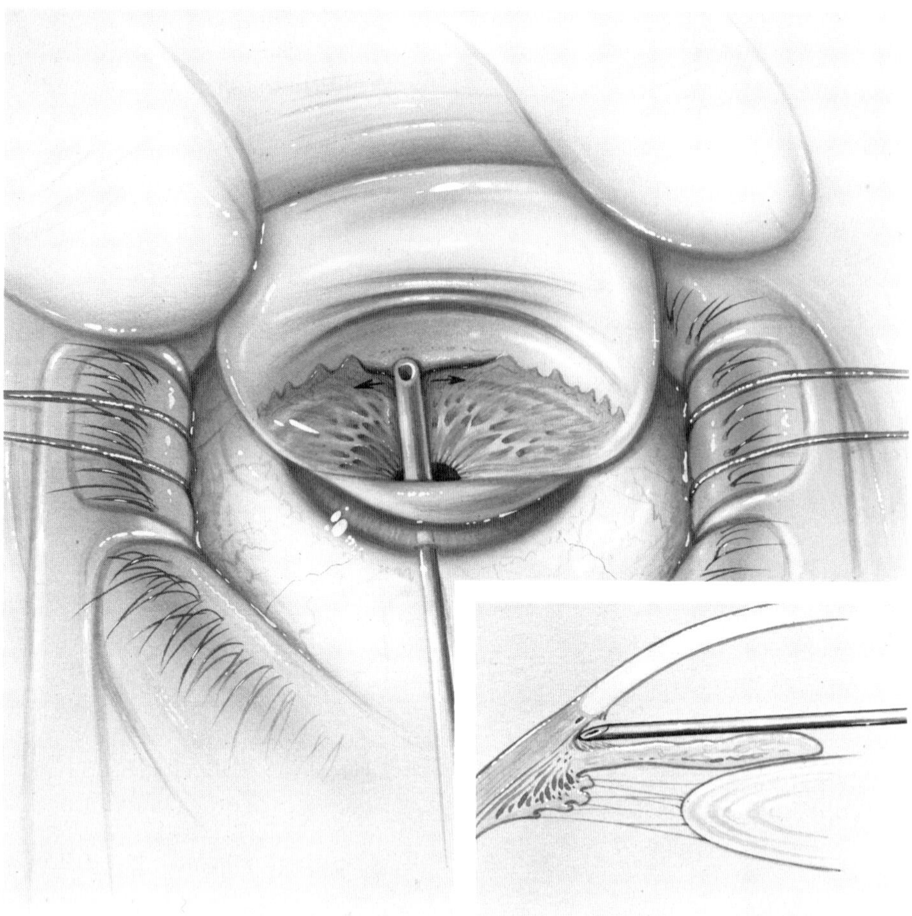

2.**57** As soon as the needle has reached the opposite chamber angle the superficial incision at the anterior margin of the trabecular meshwork is begun.

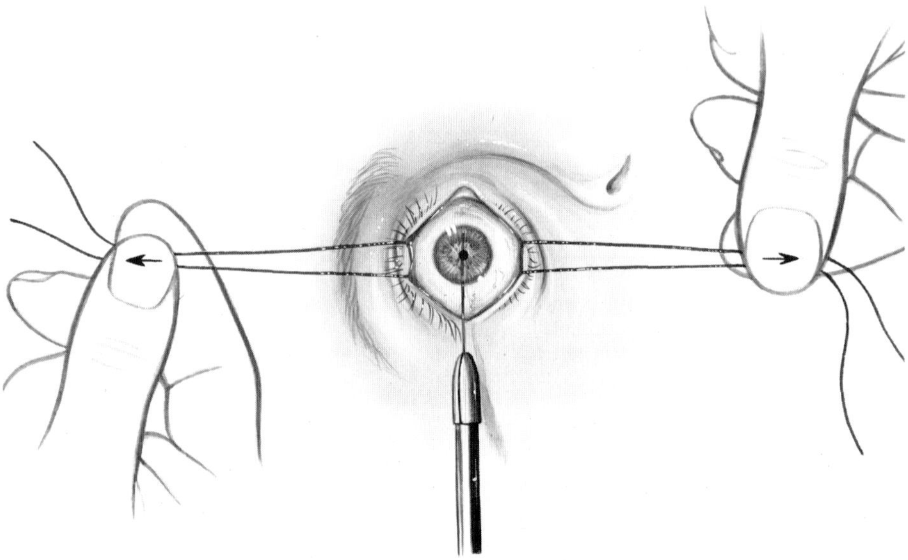

2.**58** During the incision, traction on the two holding sutures stabilizes the globe in a horizontal position. If necessary, it can also be rotated in order to extend the dissection laterally.

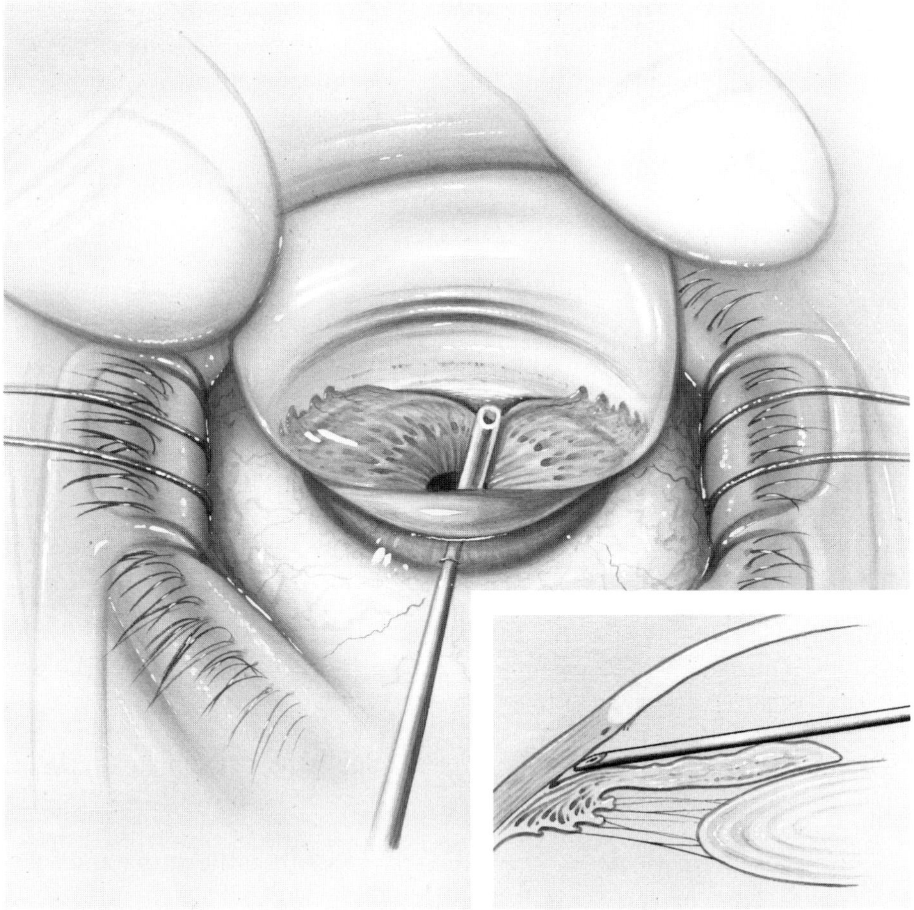

2.**59** If planned, a cyclodialysis is now performed, i.e., incision as far as the ciliary border. The anterior chamber is deepened and the needle is advanced toward posterior along the sclera, using gentle sideways movements.

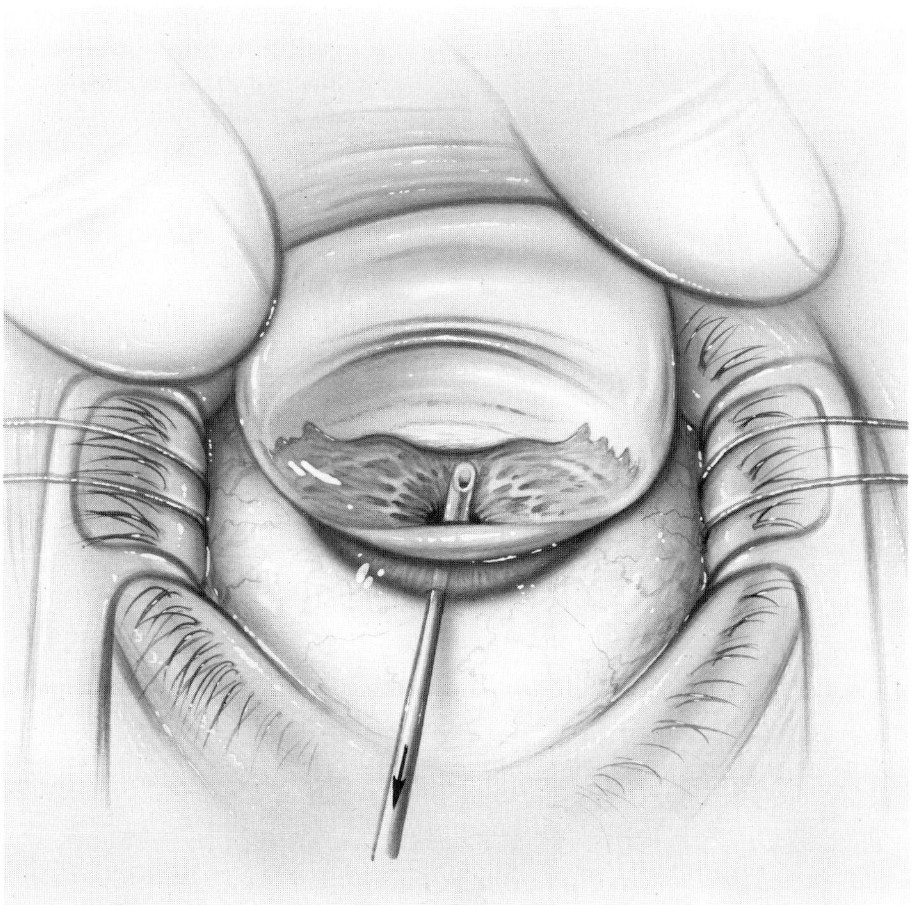

2.**60** It must be kept in mind that the fulcrum of the needle is not at the center of the eye; therefore, sideways (i.e., caudad or craniad) movements also require slight displacement of the needle.

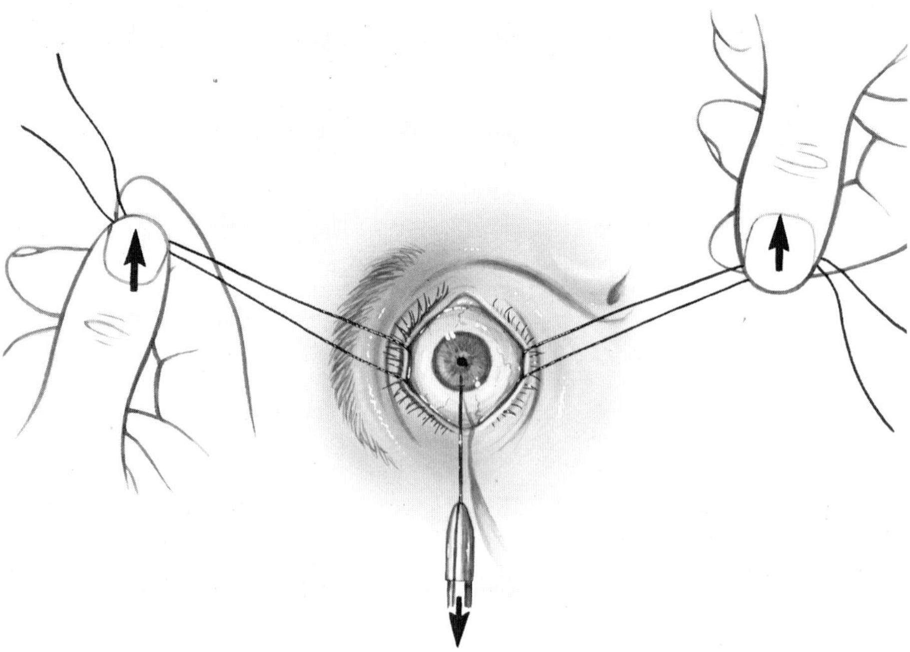

2.61 On completion of the incision the needle is carefully withdrawn, with the chamber still intact.

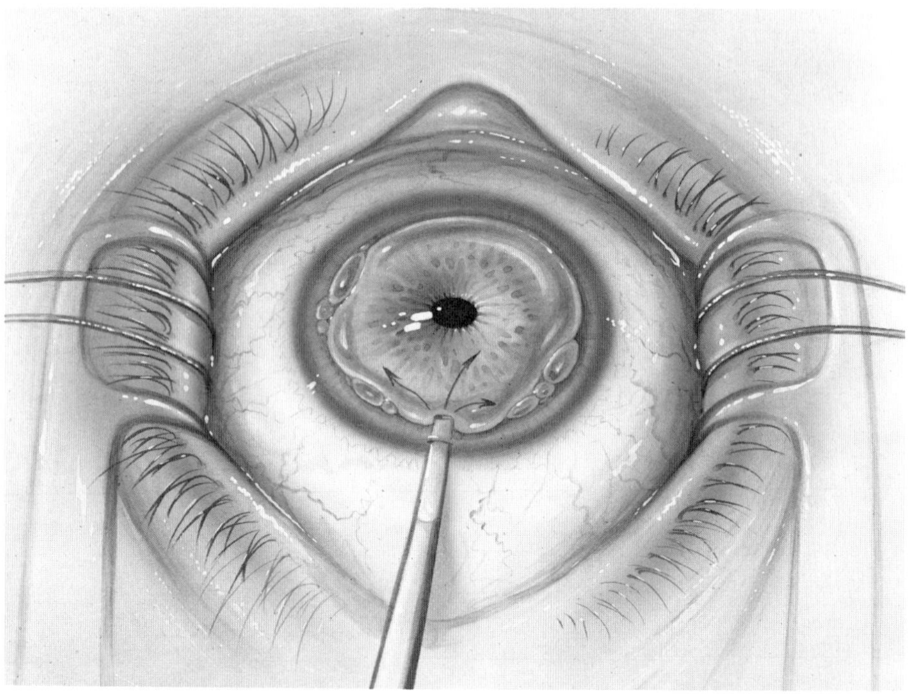

2.62 During this phase the globe must be stabilized by slight traction nasalward.

As soon as the tip of the needle leaves the anterior chamber, pressure on the globe via the holding sutures or the lid retractor must be avoided. Otherwise the anterior chamber may be drained immediately. It is advisable to restore the anterior chamber as soon as the needle has been removed by insufflating an air bubble.

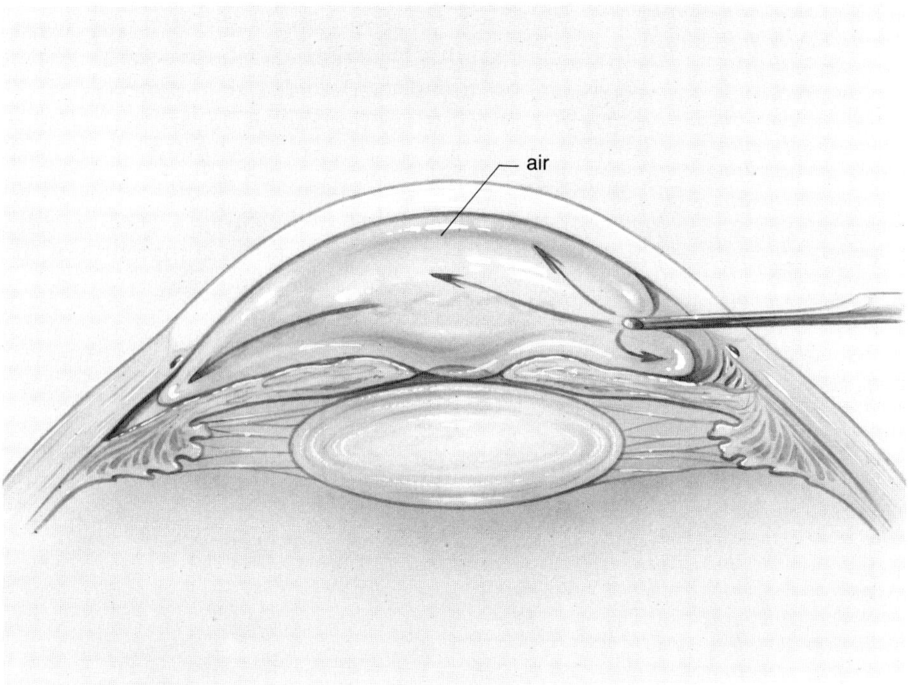

2.63 A compressible buffer under pressure is thus created for the early postoperative phase. In addition, hypotonic hemorrhage is avoided and the incision slit kept open.

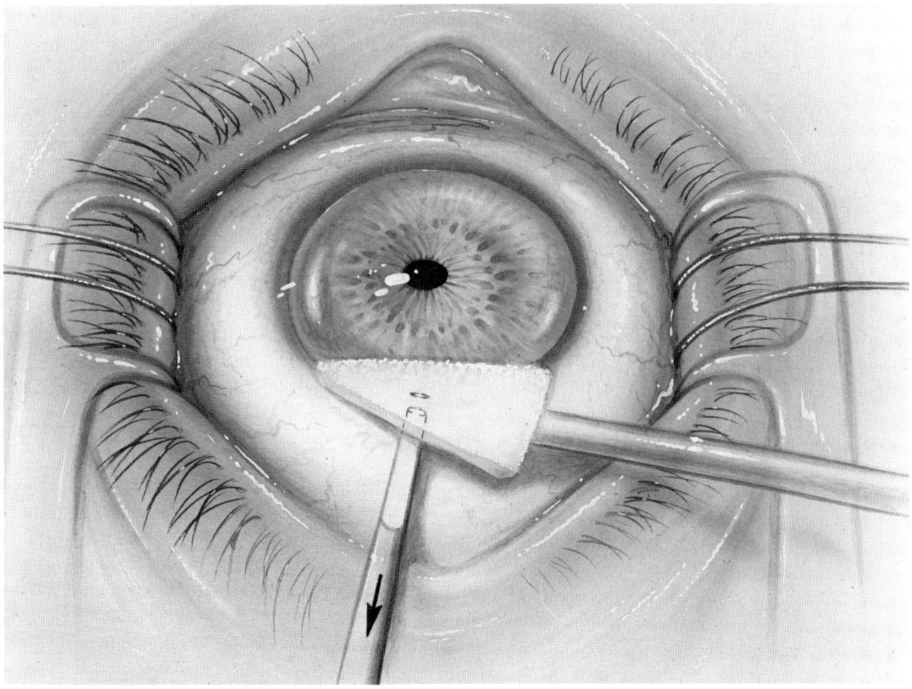

2.64 Air is prevented from escaping by application of a damp swab to the instillation opening after withdrawing the anterior chamber cannula.

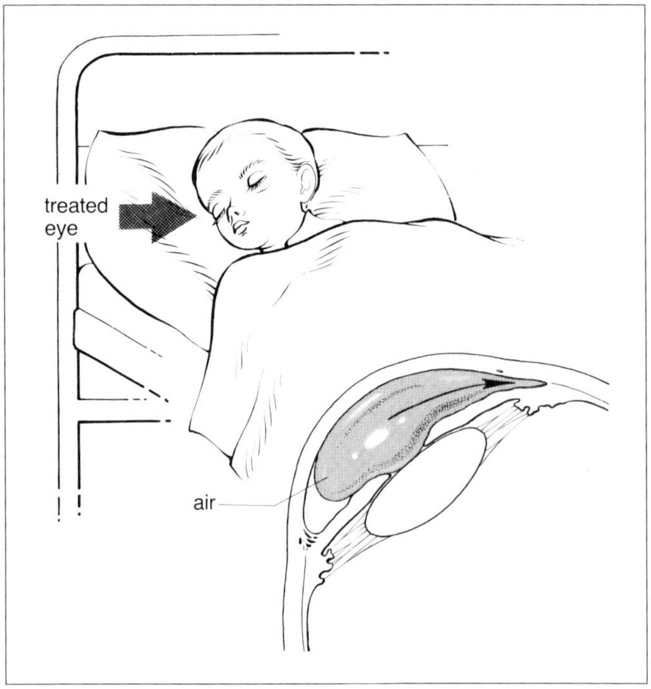

2.**65** The postoperative tamponade effect of the air bubble is most effective if the head is positioned in such a way that the air bubble can rise to the incision area. Therefore, the head should always be turned to the side of the eye which has been operated on. This also will cause any bleeding in the region of the incision to drain into the opposite chamber angle, thus preventing coagulation around the fresh wound. On completion of the operation, a stronger miotic is administered in order to tauten the iris and trabecular meshwork.

Modifications and Surgical Alternatives

Sudden drainage of the anterior chamber can be avoided either by constant irrigation through the goniotomy needle, as described, or by instillation of a viscoelastic substance.

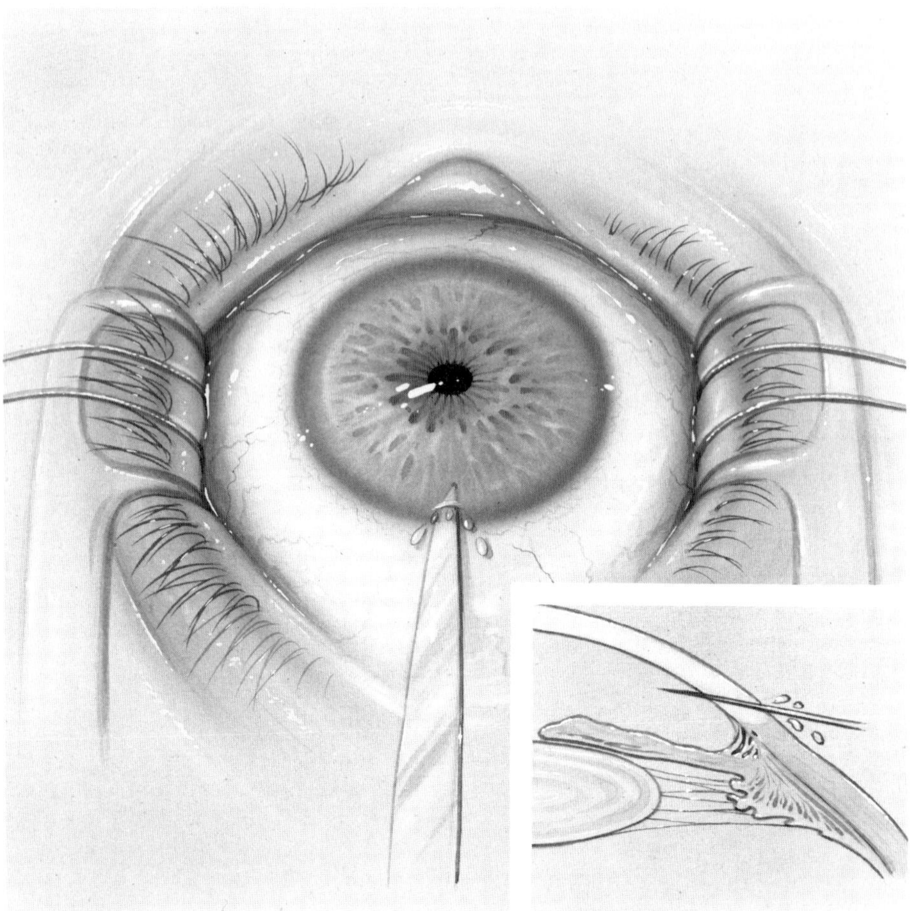

2.**66** In order to do this, some of the aqueous is drained off via a paracentesis at the limbus.

67 a

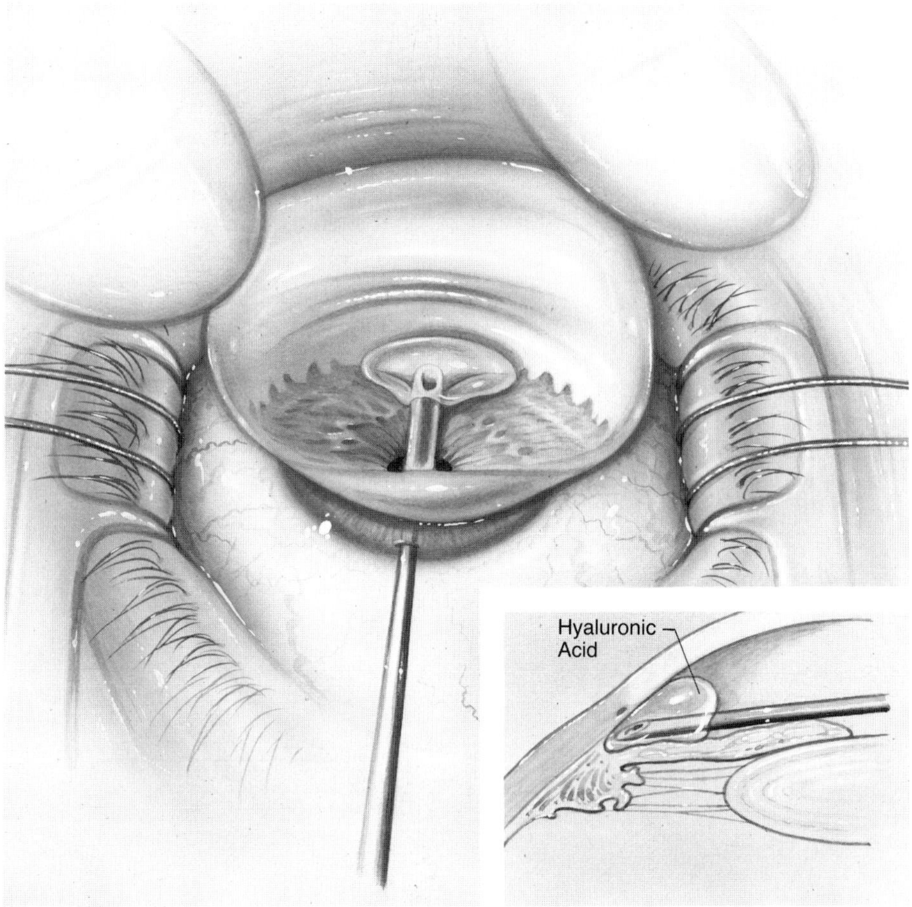

67 b

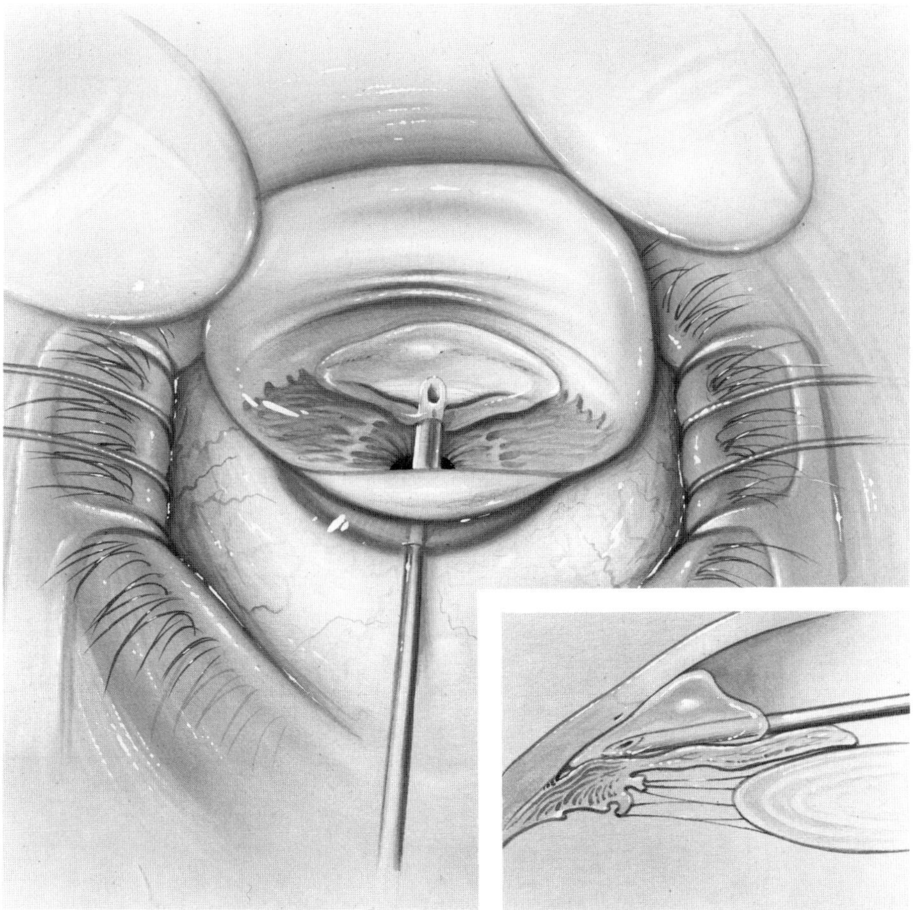

2.**67 a–c** The anterior chamber is then restored to normal depth or slightly deeper by instilling highly viscous hyaluronic acid. The hyaluronic acid will not readily escape via the paracentesis opening.

Following this, goniotomy can be performed in the usual manner as described above, with a deep anterior chamber, even without a cannulated goniotomy knife. In this case there is no need for the assistant to maintain the anterior chamber[8].

However, in some cases the remaining hyaluronic acid may cause elevation of IOP in the immediate postoperative phase. Medication is then necessary to counteract this.

67 c

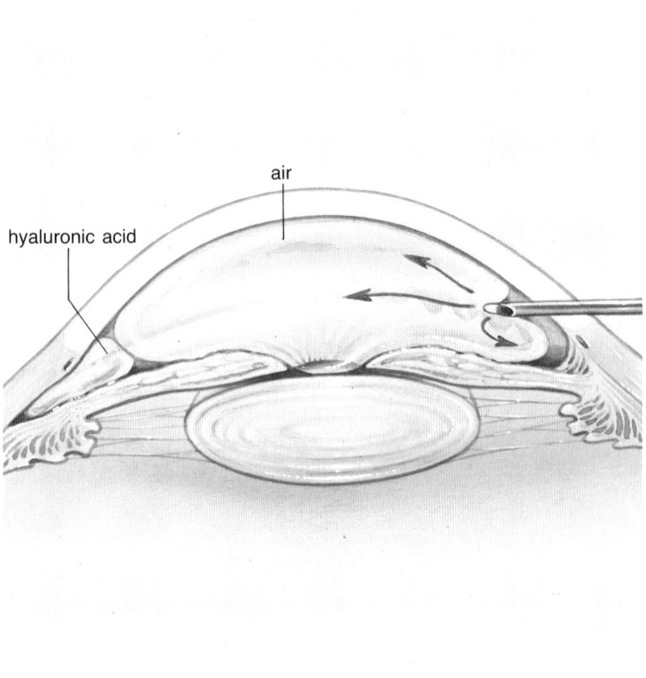

68 a

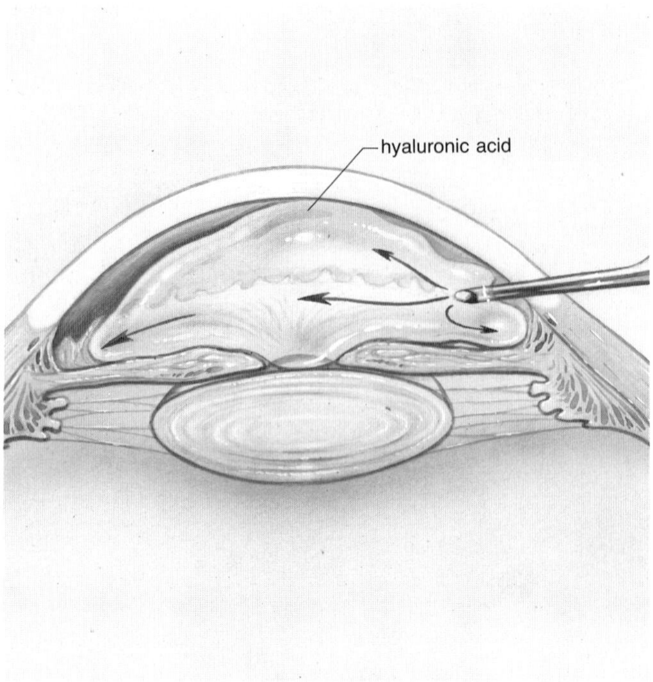

68 b

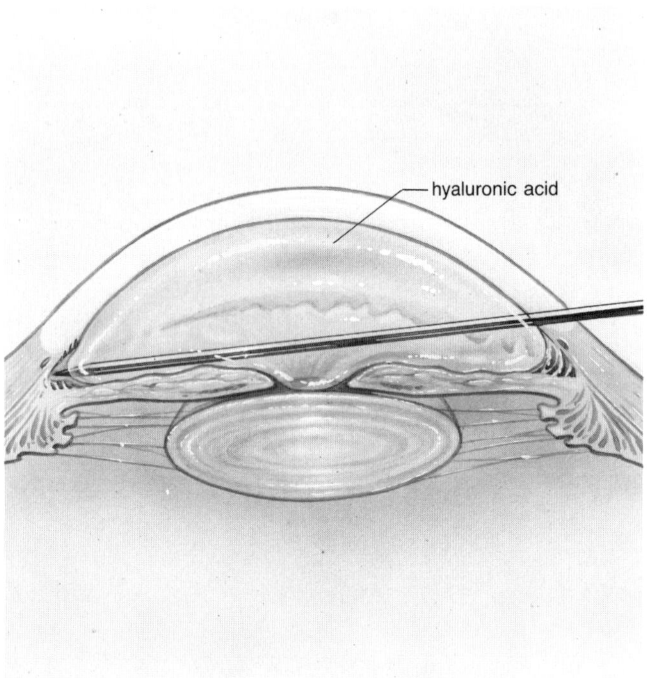

69

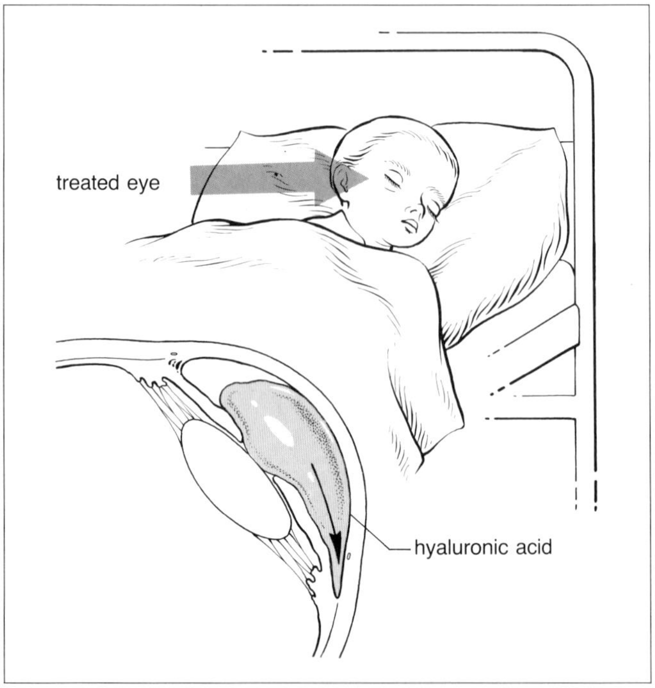

2.**68 a** and **b,** 2.**69** Instead of instilling air as a tamponade at the end of the operation, a small bubble of hyaluronic acid may be instilled through the cannulated goniotomy needle to preserve the newly created chamber angle. In this case, special postoperative positioning of the patient is unnecessary.

Complications

Unintentional fluctuations in IOP are a common intraoperative complication. On the one hand, these might impair the view into the chamber angle due to epithelial edema, or even dislocate the lens posteriad. On the other hand, the chamber may become shallower if too much traction is exerted on the holding sutures and if instillation through the needle is insufficient. Intraoperative bleeding may occur as a result of damage to vessels in the chamber angle. However, with the good visualization provided by the microscope and the Barkan lens, it is easy to avoid this. Reflux hemorrhage owing to hypotension, either at the end of the operation or postoperatively, cannot always be prevented. This complication can be limited by instillation of air or highly viscous hyaluronic acid as described above. In all cases of postoperative bleeding, it is advisable to wait, since it will normally be resorbed within 24 to 48 hours.

Postoperative Management

Initially, the pupil should be kept as contracted as possible in order to spread the incision. Therefore, a strong miotic is administered locally for several days. To prevent premature adhesion of the incision, corticosteroids are administered locally at an early stage. As long as the air bubble is large enough to have a tamponade effect, the patient's head must be kept positioned as mentioned above. Otherwise the patient may move about freely immediately after the operation. A dressing is normally applied for 24 hours only.

Results

One goniotomy will very often not achieve a lasting reduction in intraocular pressure. At the first operation it is practically impossible to estimate the effect surgery will have and so to determine accurately how long and deep the incision should be. However, should the goniotomy prove unsuccessful, the procedure can be repeated several times and "dosed" accordingly. Nevertheless, several weeks should be allowed to pass for the definitive effect. Approximately 80 % of the goniotomies performed for congenital glaucoma are successful[4].

References

1 Barkan, O.: New operation for chronic glaucoma. *Amer. J. Ophthal.* 19: 951–966, 1936.

2 Barkan, O.: Surgery of congenital glaucoma. Review of 196 eyes treated by goniotomy. *Amer. J. Ophthal.* 36: 1523–1534, 1953.

3 Draeger, J.: Ein neues Handapplanationstonometer zur Anwendung am liegenden und sitzenden Patienten. *Ber. Dtsch. ophthal. Ges.* 67: 391–393, 1966.

4 Draeger, J., Wirt, H., Ahrens, V.: Langzeitergebnisse nach Goniotomie beim congenitalen Glaukom. *Klin. Mbl. Augenheilk.* 185: 481–489, 1984.

5 Heine, L.: Zur Therapie des Glaukoms. Erfahrungen mit der Cyclodialyse. *Dtsch. Med. Wschr.* 21, 1905.

6 Sampaolesi, R.: Ocular echometry in the diagnosis of congenital glaucoma. *Doc. Ophthal. Proc. Ser.* 29: 177–189, 1981.

7 de Vincentiis, C.: Incisione del'Angelo iridio nel glaucoma. *Ann. Ottal.* 22: 540–541, 1893.

8 Winter, R.: Technical modification in goniotomy using high viscous hyaluronic acid. *Dev. Ophthal.* 11: 136–138, 1985.

Trabeculotomy

George L. Spaeth

Surgical Principles

Trabeculotomy is, effectively, an external goniotomy (see above). Since a clear view of the anterior chamber angle is an essential requirement for a safe and satisfactory goniotomy, trabeculotomy has the advantage over goniotomy of being possible in patients with hazy corneas, in whom the anterior chamber angle cannot be visualized. It has the disadvantage in comparison to goniotomy of being a far more extensive procedure that requires opening of the eye and causes scarring of the conjunctiva. Since the technique of trabeculotomy is highly similar to that of trabeculectomy, it may also be an easier procedure for the surgeon familiar with trabeculectomy, but not comfortable with goniotomy.

Preparation for Surgery

The preoperative routine is as for goniotomy. The pupil should preferably be miotic, but this is not essential. In many cases surgery will be performed after evaluation of the internal portions of the eye, which requires a dilated pupil. An operating microscope is essential for the performance of trabeculotomy.

Surgical Technique

A standard limbus-based or fornix-based flap is developed as described for trabeculectomy.

70

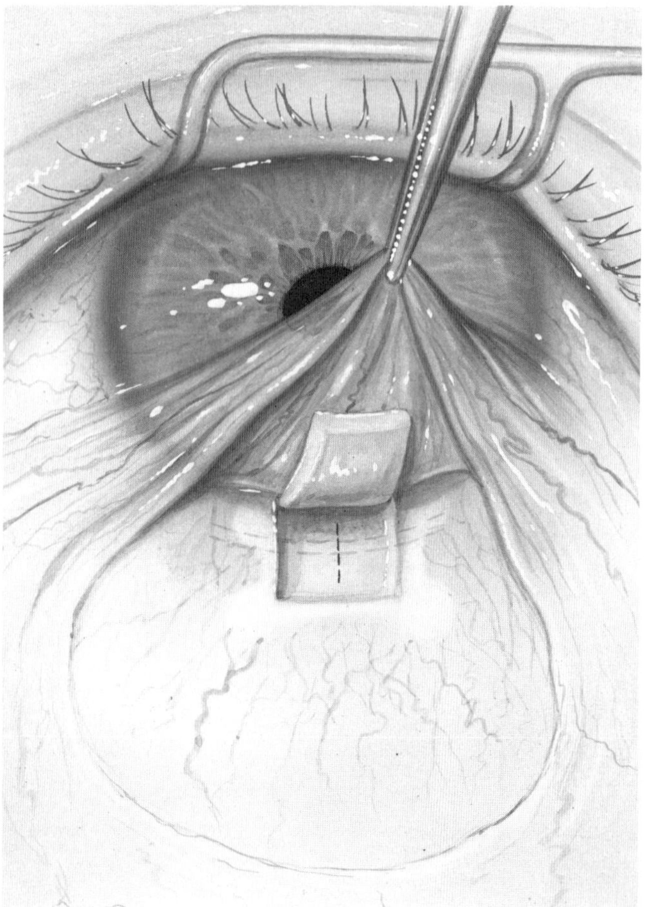

71

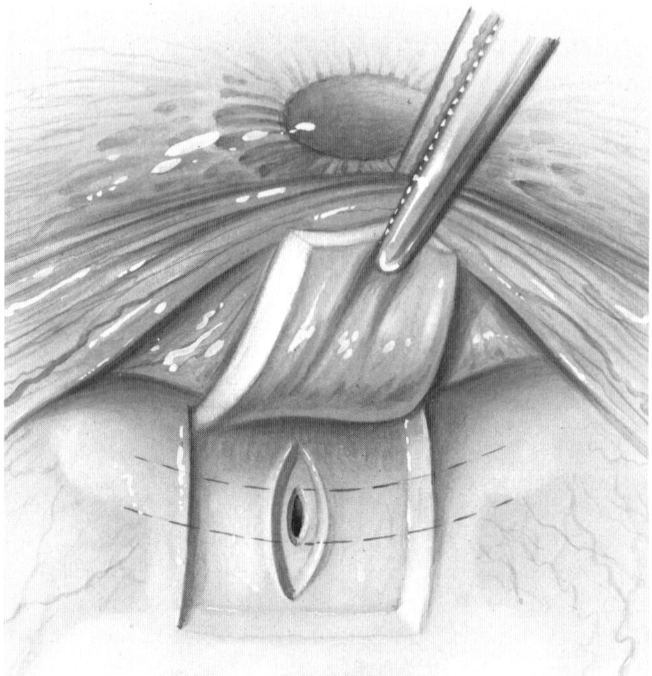

2.70 A scleral flap is developed, similar to the flap created in trabeculectomy. It is hinged at the scleral sulcus. It is not necessary to extend it as far anteriorly as in trabeculectomy. The scleral flap for trabeculotomy should be thicker, being approximately three-quarters the thickness of the sclera, rather than one-third as in trabeculectomy. An incision is made in the scleral bed, deep enough to open Schlemm's canal.

2.71 The edges of the incision are spread, permitting visualization of Schlemm's canal at its base. The microscope should be "zoomed up", so that quite high magnification is employed at this point.

72

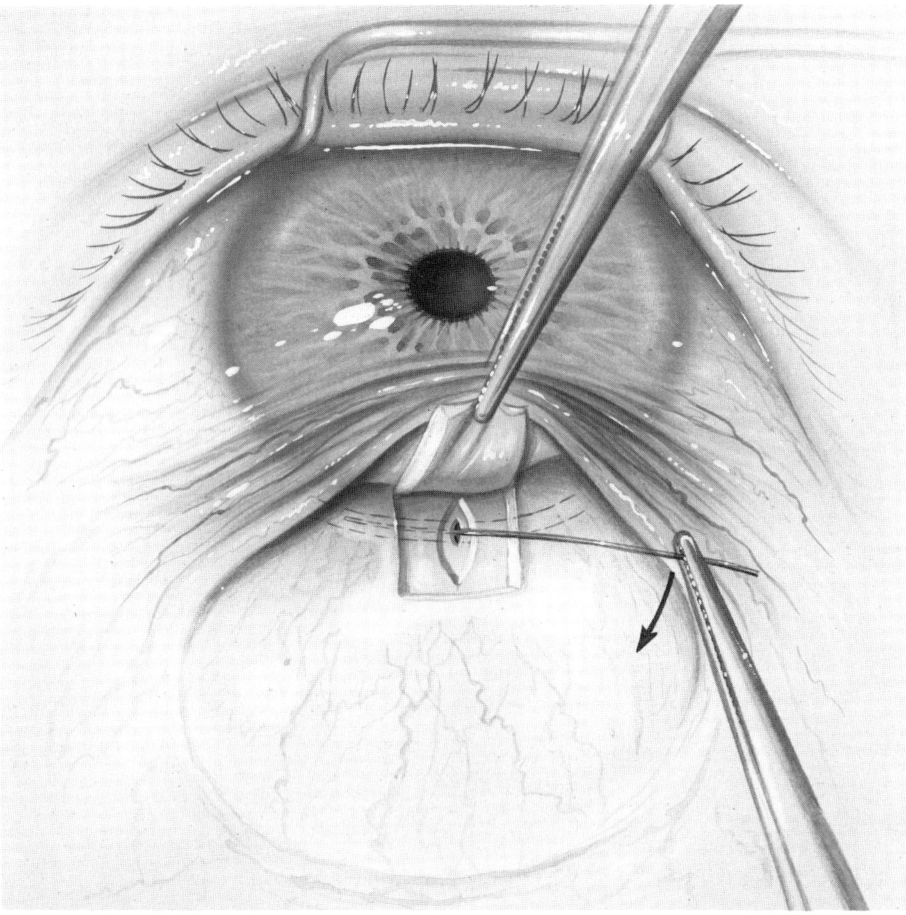

73

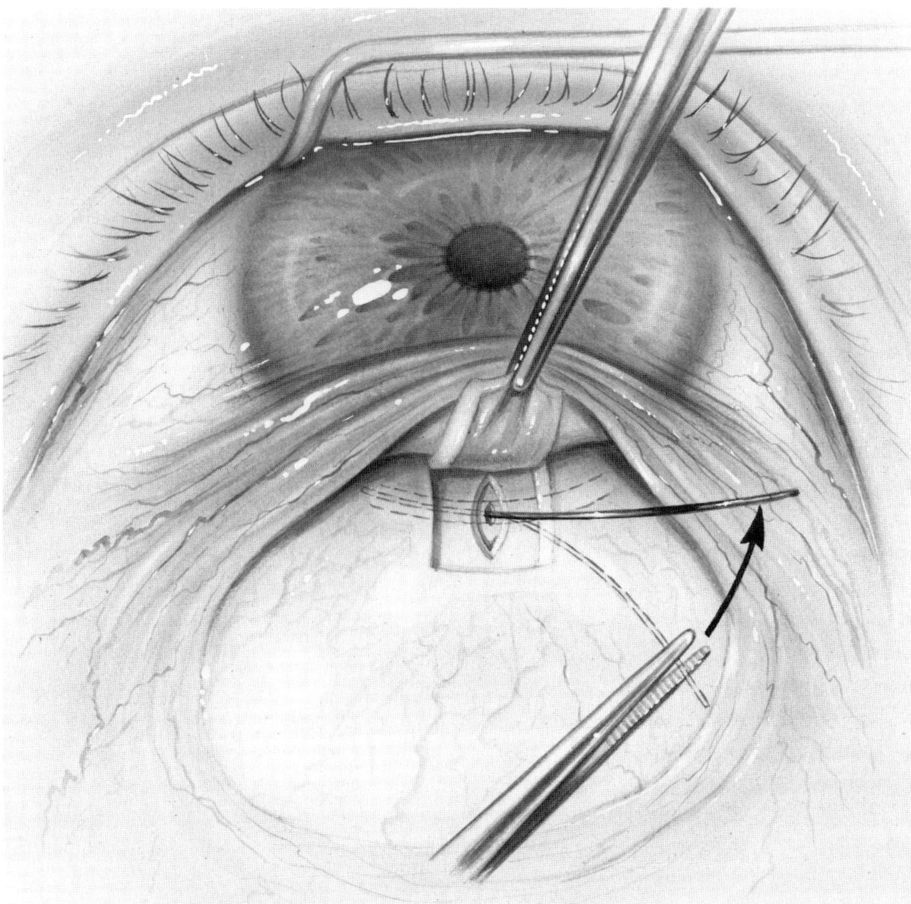

2.**72** and **73** A springy, stiff suture, such as 5-0 nylon, is threaded into what is thought to be Schlemm's canal, is then pulled posteriorly and released. If the suture is within the canal, the released end will spring back crisply so that it is in line with Schlemm's canal.

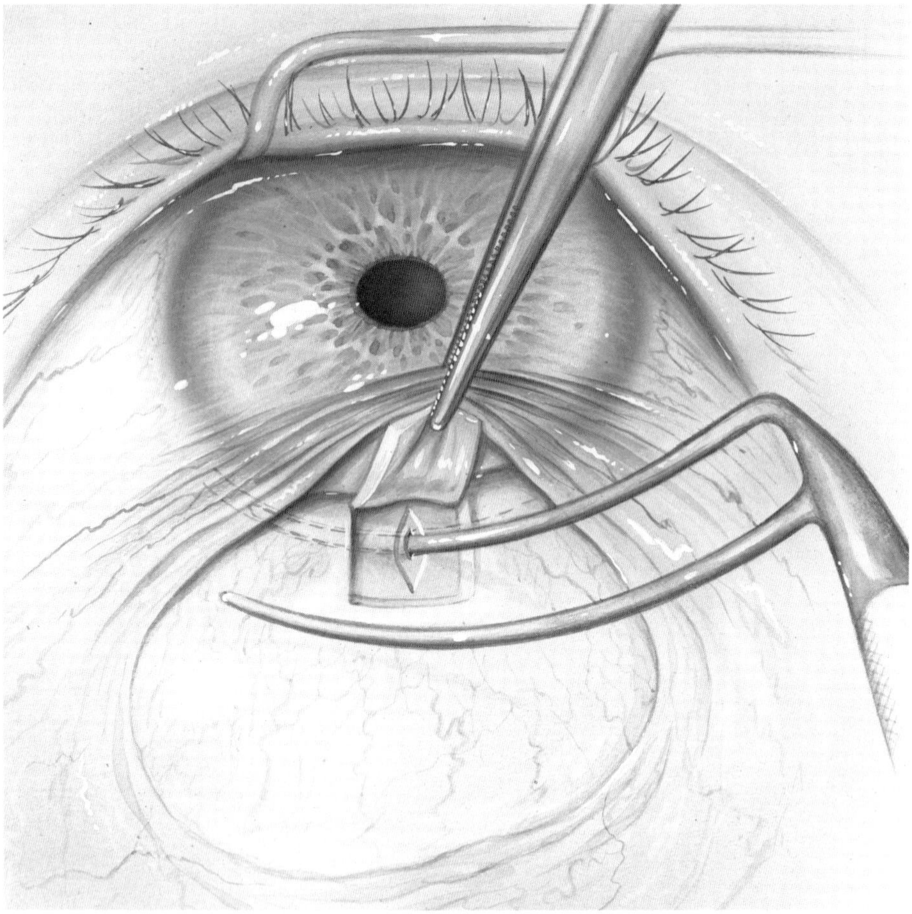

2.74 After Schlemm's canal has been properly identified, Harms trabeculotomes are employed to break open the internal aspect of the trabecular meshwork. The trabeculotome is gently threaded into Schlemm's canal as far as possible; the handle is positioned to make sure that when it is manipulated the probe moves parallel to the anterior surface of the lens, to avoid scratching the corneal endothelium or digging into the lens. The cornea may be split, Descemet's membrane torn, or endothelium traumatized as a result of improper technique.

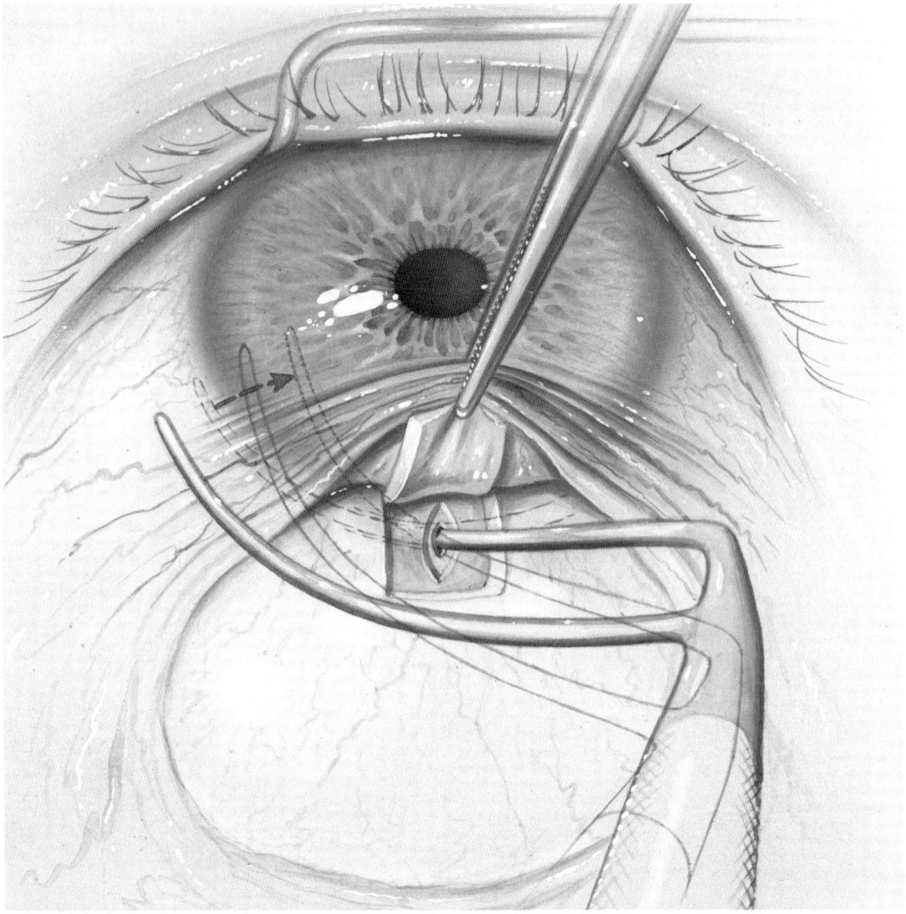

2.75 The trabeculotome is maneuvered so as to tear open the trabecular meshwork. After this has been done on the left-hand side, the procedure is repeated with the right-hand trabeculotome so that around 120° of the angle are treated.

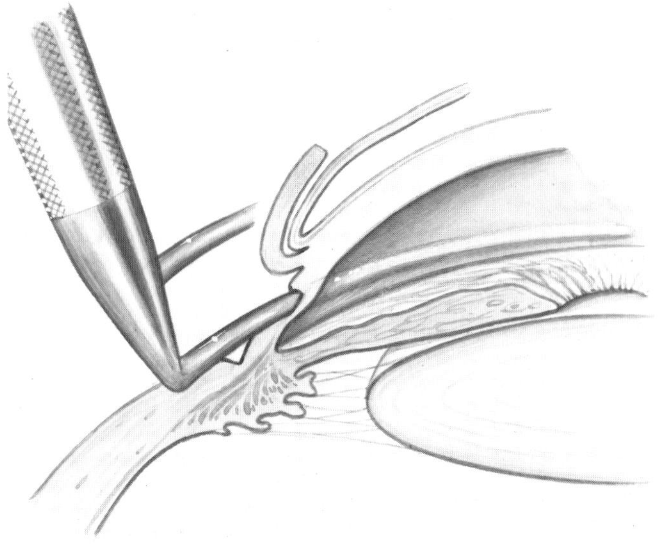

2.**76** The trabeculotome is in position in Schlemm's canal.

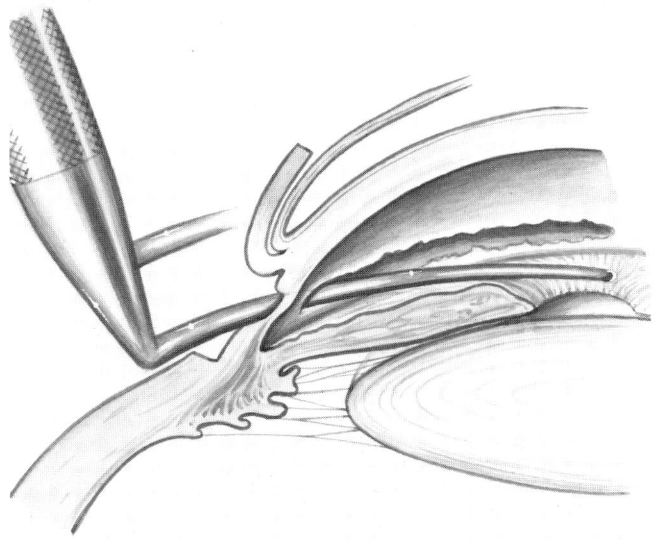

2.**77** As the trabeculotome is turned, it tears the internal lining of Schlemm's canal and the inner wall of the trabecular meshwork. The scleral flap is then closed tightly, so that the anterior chamber is well formed, with no gross leakage of aqueous. The conjunctival flap is closed appropriately.

Postoperative Management

The routine for goniotomy is followed. Topical corticosteroids and pilocarpine are usually employed. Long-term management must consider and appropriately diagnose and treat associated ocular problems, such as the anisometropia that is characteristic of infantile glaucoma, often resulting in a poor visual outcome, even when the intraocular pressure has been satisfactorily controlled.

Results

Results are similar to those with goniotomy, and will vary widely depending upon the initial condition of the eye and the diagnostic entity. Trabeculotomy will be successful in controlling intraocular pressure in most cases of uncomplicated primary infantile glaucoma (trabeculodysgenesis).

Bibliography

[1] Allen, L., Burian, H. M.: Trabeculotomy ab externo – a new glaucoma operation technique and results of experimental surgery. *Amer. J. Ophthalmol.* 53: 19–26, 1962.

[2] Anderson, D. R.: Trabeculotomy compared to goniotomy for glaucoma in children. *Ophthalmology* 90: 805–806, 1983

[3] Dannheim, R., van der Zypen, E.: Klinische, funktionelle und elektronenmikroskopische Untersuchungen über die Regenerationsfähigkeit der Kammerwinkelregion des Primatenauges nach Trabekulotomie. *V. Graefe's Arch. Ophthalmol.* 184: 222–247, 1972.

[4] Dannheim, R., Harms, H.: Technik, Erfolge und Wirkungsweise der Trabekulotomie. *Klin. Mbl. Augenheilk.* 155: 630–637, 1969.

[5] Harms, H., Dannheim, R.: Epicritical consideration of 300 cases of trabeculotomy "ab externo." *Trans. Ophthal. Soc. U.K.* 89: 491–499, 1969.

Argon Laser Iridectomy

George L. Spaeth

Surgical Principles

Indications for a laser iridectomy are essentially the same as those for standard incisional peripheral iridectomy. Specifically, the purpose of the surgery is to create an opening in the iris permitting unfettered access of aqueous humor from the posterior chamber to the anterior. This principle applies to any situation in which there is interference of flow of aqueous humor from the posterior to the anterior chamber. Thus, pertinent indications for laser iridectomy include primary angle-closure glaucoma, pupillary block glaucoma associated with posterior synechiae, pupillary block glaucoma associated with intraocular lenses, etc.

Because of the coagulating effect of argon laser light, iridectomy performed by argon laser offers advantages over iridectomy performed with a knife or with the neodymium:YAG laser in patients predisposed to bleeding conditions, such as those taking anticoagulants or with known blood-clotting disorders. Both argon and neodymium:YAG laser iridectomies are preferred in cases in which entry into the anterior chamber may be expected to be associated with complications, such as in patients predisposed to malignant glaucoma (as would be the case with patients who had malignant glaucoma in the other eye), those with miotic-induced angle closure, or those with high hyperopia or nanophthalmos.

Laser iridectomy is not appropriate where the optical approach to the iris is not clear or where the anterior chamber is extremely shallow.

Preparation for Surgery

As laser iridectomy is frequently associated with a spike of intraocular pressure, the health of the optic nerve must be well understood prior to embarking on surgery. Intraocular pressure is determined with an applanation tonometer prior to performance of the iridectomy. If the optic disk is in jeopardy, appropriate measures must be taken to monitor the intraocular pressure meticulously, and prophylactic and postoperative measures to control the intraocular pressure should be employed.

The pupil should be miotic. Several drops of 1 % or 2 % pilocarpine should be instilled several hours before surgery.

The cornea of the eye to be treated is anesthetized with a topical anesthetic agent such as proparacaine. A facial nerve block is not necessary.

The patient is seated comfortably at the laser, and the instrument is set appropriately. For a brown-eyed individual, utilizing the technique described below, appropriate settings would be: exposure time 0.2 s, power 1000 mW, spot size 50 μm. Settings will vary from instrument to instrument and need to be determined by experience with the individual instrument being employed. If a pulsed laser, such as a Britt, is used, the dials are set to the thermal or "cool" mode, and the power to 25 W.

The oculars should be adjusted to ensure that the laser beam is parfocal with the viewer. This is accomplished by placing a target in the focal plane of the slit lamp of the laser. After selecting a 50 μm laser spot, the slit lamp is focused sharply until the spot is as small and clear as possible. The slit lamp is then locked in place. The procedure should be performed under high power. The 25× magnification is utilized with a Zeiss slit lamp.

Surgical Technique

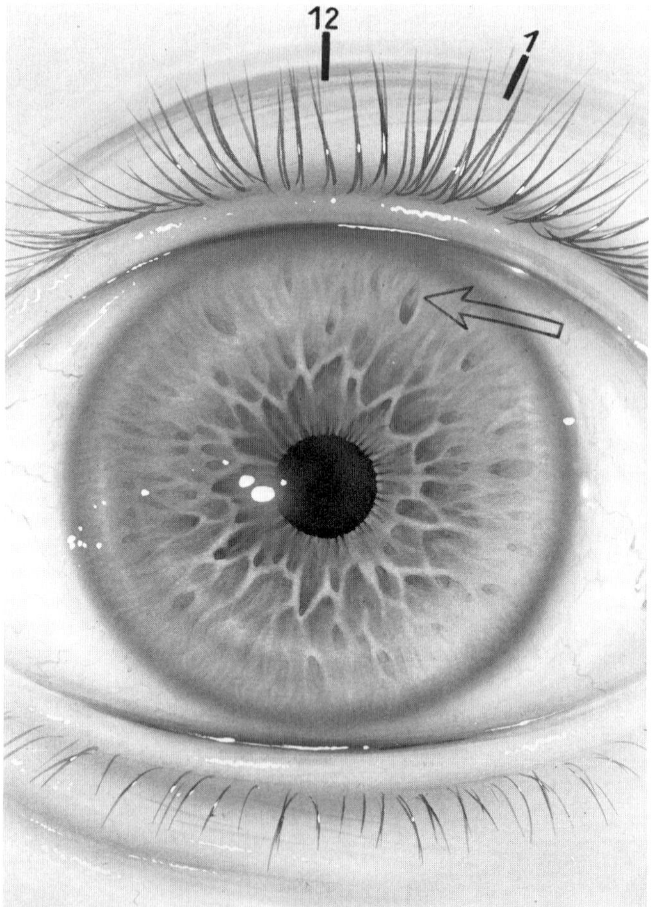

2.78 Making sure that the cornea is clear, an appropriate site in the iris is selected, preferably a crypt just to one side of the 12 o'clock position, as near the iris root as can be visualized. The purpose of locating the iridectomy just to the side of 12 o'clock is to eliminate the presence of obstructing bubbles which may form during the procedure.

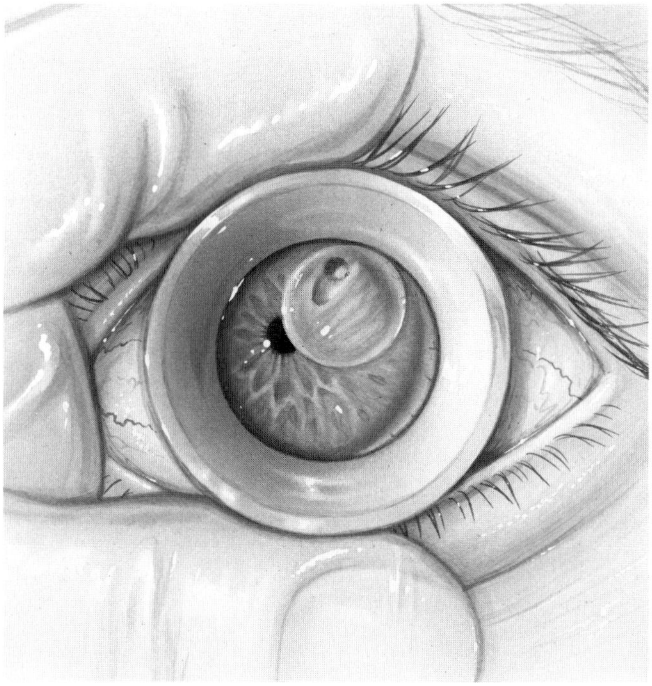

2.**79** The Abraham laser iridectomy contact lens is employed. This goniolens has a comfortable flange for easy manipulation, and a strongly convex (high +) dimple cemented to the front of the lens in order to provide higher magnification and greater convergence of the argon laser beam.

The previously chosen crypt is found and brought into meticulous focus. The patient must *not* be looking directly towards the laser. The gaze can either be slightly up or in, or both, in order to ensure that when penetration of the iris occurs, the laser will not cause a burn on the posterior pole of the retina.

The instrument is readied by flipping the appropriate switch to activate the foot pedal. A test burn is placed in the depths of the crypt. An immediate pit in the iris surface should appear. Repeated applications are placed *exactly* in the same spot, deepening the pit until penetration occurs. If corneal endothelial haziness develops, the power is too high or the exposure too long.

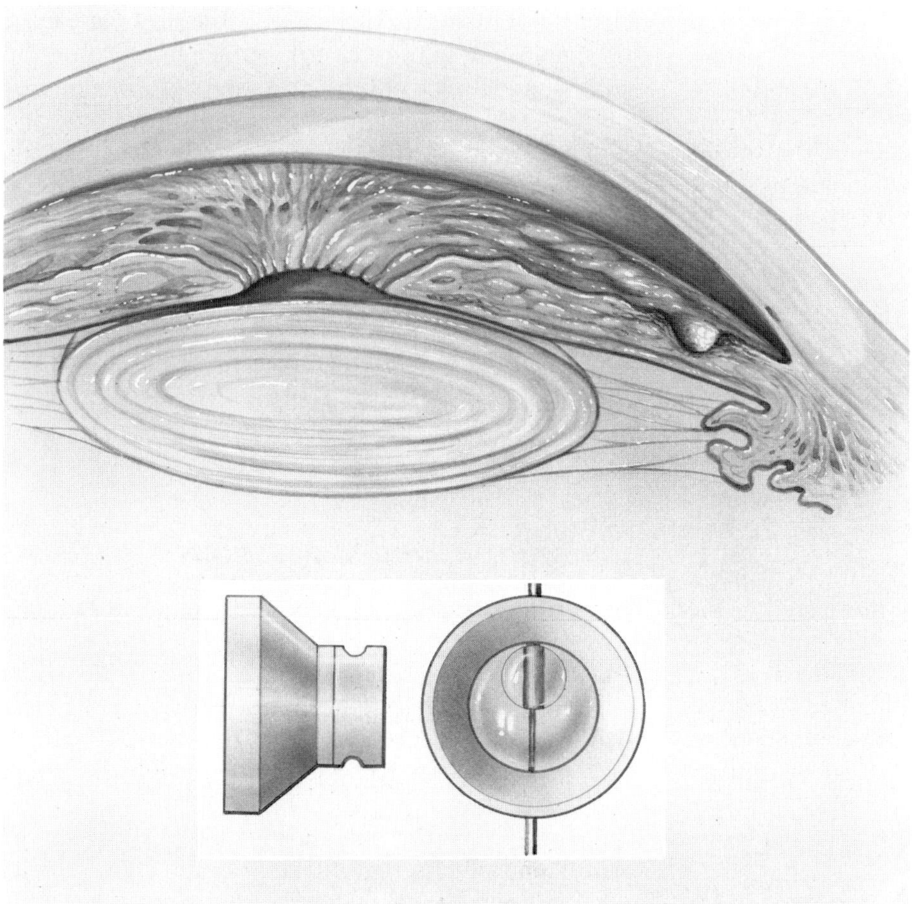

2.**80** The cross-section of the iris shows the peripheral location of the iridectomy and the shape of the pit as it is formed. The Abraham contact lens is illustrated with its magnifying dimple.

81

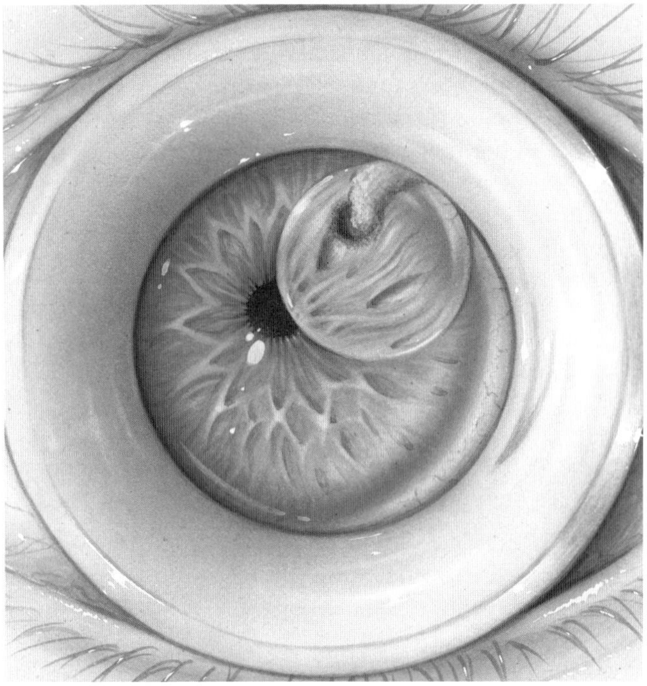

82

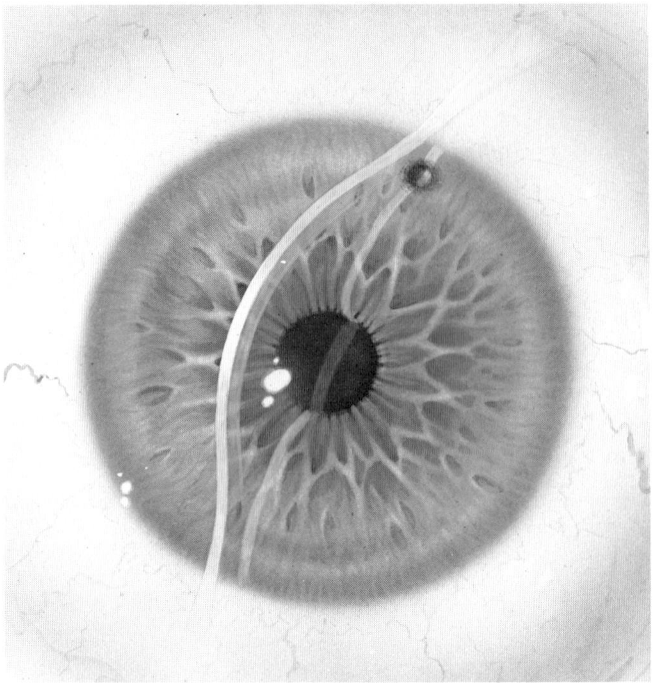

2.**81** When the pit has been deepened to the point that the posterior pigment epithelium is exposed, a further application results in a "smoke signal". This is an explosion of pigment that characteristically floats superiorly towards the angle recess. Once the smoke signal has been seen, the surgeon knows that the next few applications should result in complete penetration of the iris.

2.**82** When the surgeon believes the iris has been completely penetrated, the slit beam is carefully focused on the iris to determine whether or not the iridectomy is, in fact, patent. The presence of a transillumination defect is not an adequate proof of complete patency; a thin membrane may remain, completely blocking the egress of aqueous from the posterior into the anterior chamber, and yet the iridectomy will transilluminate. The surgeon must visualize the anterior lens capsule through the iridectomy site, making sure that the iris has been completely removed and that no tissue remains. This may require asking the patient to change the position of gaze, moving the angle of the slit beam, etc., etc. If the anterior lens capsule cannot be clearly visualized, the surgeon cannot be assured that the iridectomy is complete.

Modifications

Various modifications have been suggested. One method is to reduce the duration of the exposure to 0.01 s and "chip away" at the iridectomy site. This has the advantage of almost certainly avoiding burns to the corneal endothelium, especially if relatively low power is employed. Using low power with a short exposure time requires an increased number of applications. It may take 200 or even up to 500 applications to penetrate the iris using this technique.

Another method is to open the crypt by applying a "stretch" burn immediately adjacent to the crypt prior to starting the iridectomy itself. This stretch burn uses a low power, large diameter, long exposure burn such as 500 mW, 500 μm, for 0.5 seconds. The iridectomy is then performed in the depth of the crypt which has been put on stretch by the initial application; for this part of the procedure a spot size of 50 μm with an exposure time of 0.1 s is employed.

Admonitions and Suggestions

The performance of laser iridectomy requires as much learning as any other surgical procedure. The surgeon comes to learn the responsiveness of iris tissue to the laser burn, and the specific characteristics of the laser being used. Where it is apparent that it is difficult to develop a pit, it is best to cease attempting the iridectomy in that area and move to another portion of the iris immediately. The surgeon must meticulously watch the corneal endothelium to make sure that endothelial burns are not being produced. The position of gaze must be constantly monitored to avoid burns to the posterior pole.

Postoperative Management

Intraocular pressure is measured hourly following the iridectomy for three hours, or more frequently and for a longer period of time if there is concern about potential damage from a pressure spike. Appropriate medication for the lowering of intraocular pressure is used if necessary. Pilocarpine is often helpful when instilled frequently both before and after surgery.

After the surgeon has reassured himself that there is no immediate problem with pressure elevation, the patient is discharged, usually being maintained on previous ocular medications plus a topical anti-inflammatory agent such as prednisolone acetate 1 % four times daily for one week. Depending upon the other clinical aspects, and if there is no reason to fear the development of an intraocular pressure spike, the patient is asked to return one week postoperatively. Since intraocular pressure spikes are common and since they may not be noticed until 24 or more hours following laser iridectomy, patients in whom such a pressure spike could be damaging should be examined frequently and appropriately.

At the first postoperative visit the intraocular pressure is again carefully monitored, and the surgeon determines with certainty that the iridectomy is patent. If so, the pupil should then be dilated order to prevent the development of posterior synechiae. Intraocular pressure is measured following pupillary dilatation, and gonioscopy performed to ascertain the nature of the angle in the dilated pupil. In most cases the topical anti-inflammatory drops can be stopped around one week postoperatively, but pupillary dilatation should continue, the patient using an agent such as tropicamide 1 %, at bedtime once weekly for one month. If the eye is more inflamed, with a greater tendency to posterior synechiae, the corticosteroid may need to be prolonged and the cycloplegic agent used more frequently.

Results

Argon laser iridectomy is successful in most cases. In individuals with extremely dark brown eyes, such as blacks, it is not always possible to penetrate. It is also difficult to achieve patent iridectomies using the argon laser in patients with very light blue eyes, but by modifying the technique the success rate can be significantly increased. The technique is not appropriate in albinos. Penetration at one sitting can be achieved in around 80 % of cases, and at two sittings in most of the remaining 20 %.

Complications include the development of corneal endothelial burns, posterior synechiae, distortion of the pupillary margin, late closure of the iridectomy, persistent iritis, the development of cataract, hypopyon, hyphema, and retinal burns.

Bibliography

[1] Abraham, R. K., Miller, G. L.: Outpatient argon laser iridectomy for angle closure glaucoma: A two-year study. *Trans. Amer. Acad. Ophthalmol. Otolaryngol.* 79: 529–538, 1975.

[2] Anderson, D. R., Forster, R. K., Lewis, M. L.: Laser iridotomy for aphakic pupillary block. *Arch. Ophthalmol.* 93: 343–346, 1975.

[3] Brainard, J. O., Landers, J. H., Shock, J. P.: Recurrent angle-closure glaucoma following a patent 75-micra laser iridotomy: A case report. *Ophthal. Surg.* 13: 1030–1032, 1982.

[4] Cohen, J. S., Bibler, L., Tucker, D.: Hypopyon following laser iridotomy. *Ophthal. Surg.* 15: 604–606, 1984.

[5] Hoskins, H. D., Migliazzo, C. V.: Laser iridectomy: A technique for blue irises. *Ophthal. Surg.* 15: 480–490, 1984.

[6] Rubin, L., Arnett, J., Ritch, R.: Delayed hyphema after argon laser iridectomy. *Ophthal. Surg.* 15: 852–853, 1984.

[7] Podos, S. M., Kels, B. D., Moss, A. P. et al.: Continuous wave argon laser iridectomy in angle-closure glaucoma. *Trans. Amer. Ophthalmol. Soc.* 77: 51–62, 1979.

[8] Pollack, I. P., Patz, A.: Argon laser iridotomy: An experimental and clinical study. *Ophthal. Surg.* 7: 22–30, 1976.

[9] Quigley, H. A.: Long-term follow-up of laser iridotomy. *Ophthalmology* 88: 218–224, 1981.

[10] Ritch, R.: Argon laser for angle-closure glaucoma. *Amer. J. Ophthalmol.* 94: 197–200, 1982.

[11] Robin, A. L., Pollack, I. P.: Argon laser trabeculoplasty in secondary forms of open-angle glaucoma. *Arch. Ophthalmol.* 101: 382–384, 1983.

[12] Robin, A. L., Pollack, I. P.: A comparison of neodymium: YAG and argon laser iridotomies. *Ophthalmology* 91: 1011–1106, 1984.

[13] Rodrigues, M. M., Streeten, B. A., Spaeth, G. L. et al.: Argon laser iridotomy for primary angle-closure or pupillary block glaucoma. *Arch. Ophthalmol.* 96: 2222–2230, 1978.

[14] Schwartz, L. W., Spaeth, G. L.: Argon laser iridectomy in primary angle-closure or pupillary block glaucoma. *Trans. Ophthalmol. Soc. U.K.* 99: 257–264, 1979.

[15] Schwartz, L. W., Spaeth, G. L.: Argon laser iridotomy in the treatment of patients with primary angle-closure or pupillary block glaucoma: A clinicopathologic study. *Ophthalmology* 85: 294–309, 1978.

[16] Snyder, W. B., Vaiser, A., Hutton, W. L.: Laser iridectomy. *Trans. Amer. Acad. Ophthalmol. Otolaryngol.* 79: 381–386, 1976.

[17] Stetz, D., Smith, Jr., H., Ritch, R.: A simplified technique for laser iridectomy in blue irides. *Amer. J. Ophthalmol.* 96: 249–251, 1983.

Q-Switched Neodymium: YAG Laser Iridotomy

Alan L. Robin and Irvin P. Pollack

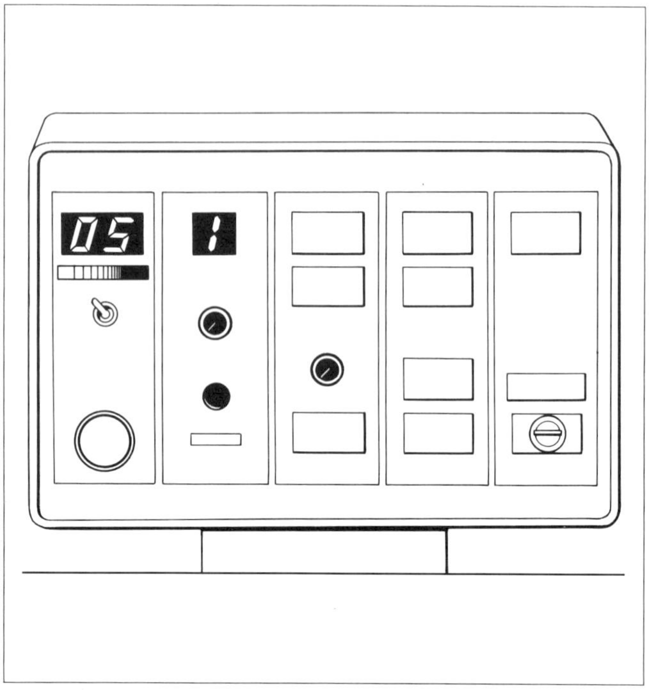

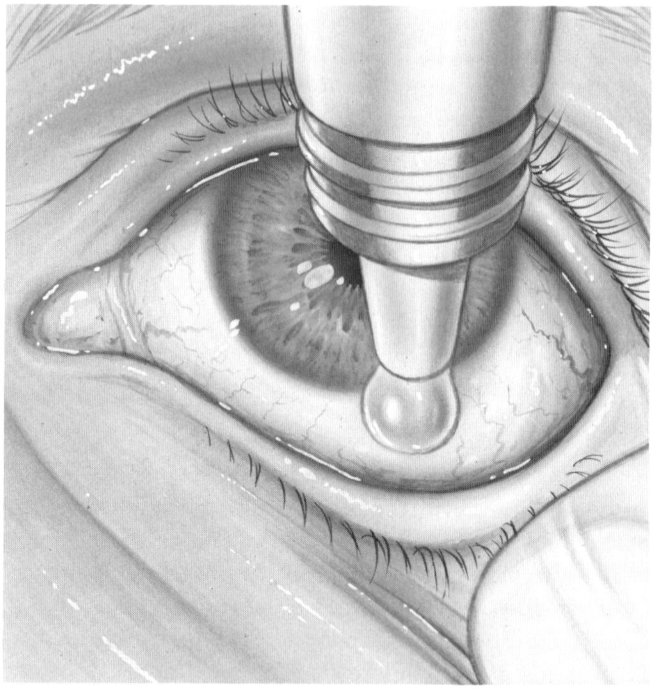

Instruments

2.83 Prior to iridotomy, it is important to be familiar with the Q-switched neodymium:YAG laser system being used. The settings will vary from instrument to instrument. Average settings may be around 5 mJ with a run of one burst. If this setting is not successful in penetrating the iris or makes an insufficient hole, the energy settings can be increased: If the patient is cooperative and fixes well, one may change the laser settings to 5 mJ with a run of three bursts; if the patient is uncooperative or has difficulty with fixation, the next attempt to penetrate the iris may use a setting with an increased power such as 10 mJ and one burst.

Preoperative Medication and Anesthesia

2.84 The patient should be on weak-strength miotics prior to therapy. These should be instilled 30 minutes prior to the procedure, in order to insure that the iris is taut and the pupil miotic. The Q-switched neodymium:YAG laser should be properly aligned, to insure that it is properly focused and the surgeon has an optimal line of vision. Topical anesthesia should be placed on the eye, together with a magnifying contact lens.

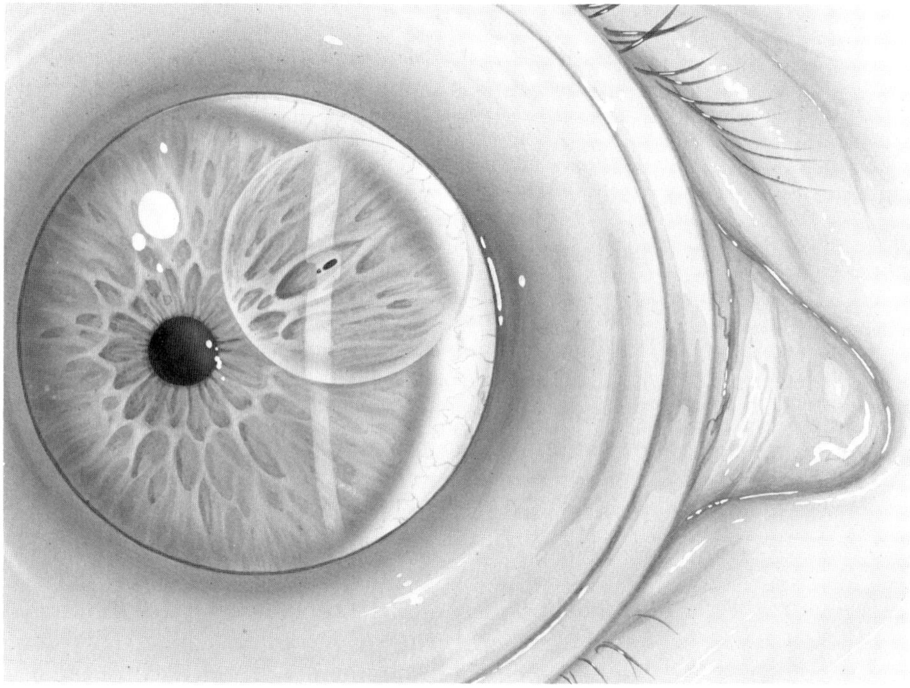

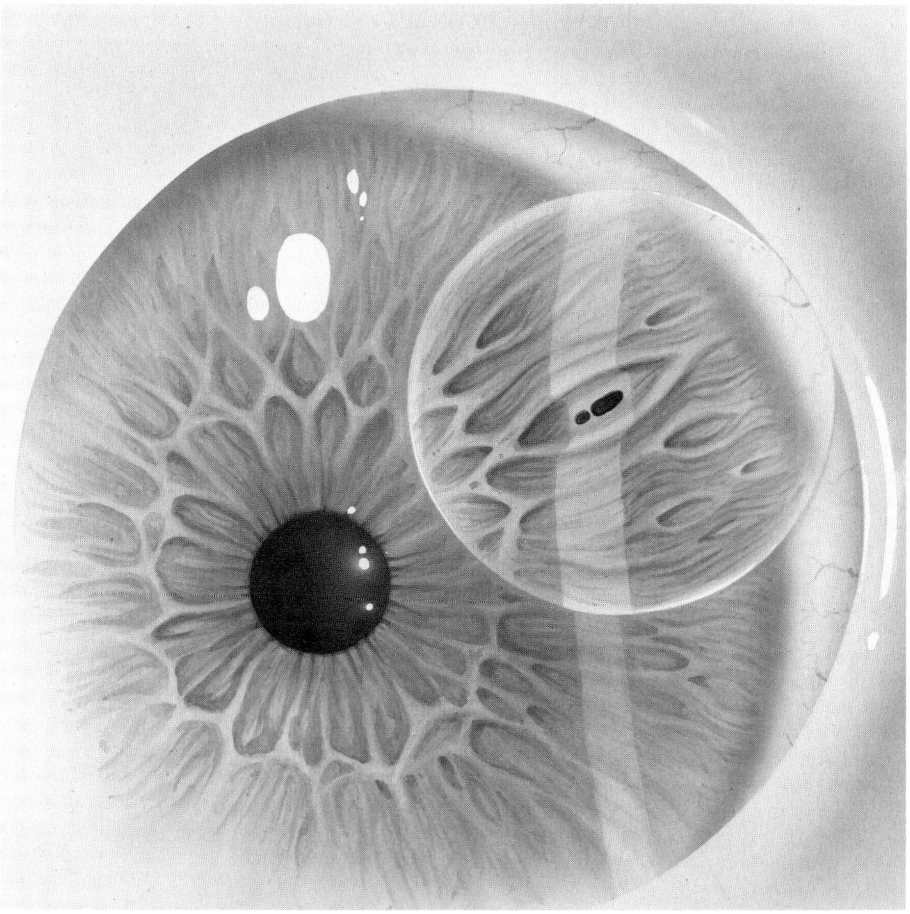

Surgical Technique

2.85 The contact lens should be centered upon the eye to permit clear visualization of the peripheral iris as close to the limbus as possible. The image seen through the magnifying area on the contact lens will, of course, be enlarged. If a peripheral iris crypt is visible, the beam should be focused in the deepest area of the crypt. The most appropriate position to choose is just temporal or nasal to the 12 o'clock position. Keeping the aiming beam focused directly on the anterior surface of the iris helps avoid damage to either the cornea or the lens. The beam should not be focused on an obvious blood vessel. It should not be focused anterior to the iris in the misapprehension that this will increase safety; all this will accomplish is failure to penetrate. It is essential to make sure that the contact lens is held in a position that will allow the entire width of the laser beam to reach the iris; tilting the lens tends to obstruct a portion of the laser beam. *Accurate focusing is probably the single most important aspect of performing a neodymium: YAG laser iridotomy.* The end point of the procedure is a clear view of the anterior lens capsule through the iris opening. A transillumination defect alone is insufficient.

2.86 If one application of the laser beam is insufficient to produce an iridotomy, it is usually safe to return to the same spot for a second application. Failure to achieve penetration is usually a result of faulty focusing, so special attention must be paid to this. If a very small iridotomy is created and one wishes to enlarge it, one should aim just to the side of the iridotomy, making sure that the focus is *not* in the area of the opening. In this way one can minimize the risk to the anterior lens capsule. Q-switched neodymium: YAG laser iridotomies are far less likely to close than are argon laser iridotomies, so that a smaller, but patent, iridotomy is acceptable. If the first burst causes debris to form in front of the area in which the iridotomy is to be made, it may be preferable not to penetrate the first location and to choose a spot well away from the site of the initial application.

87

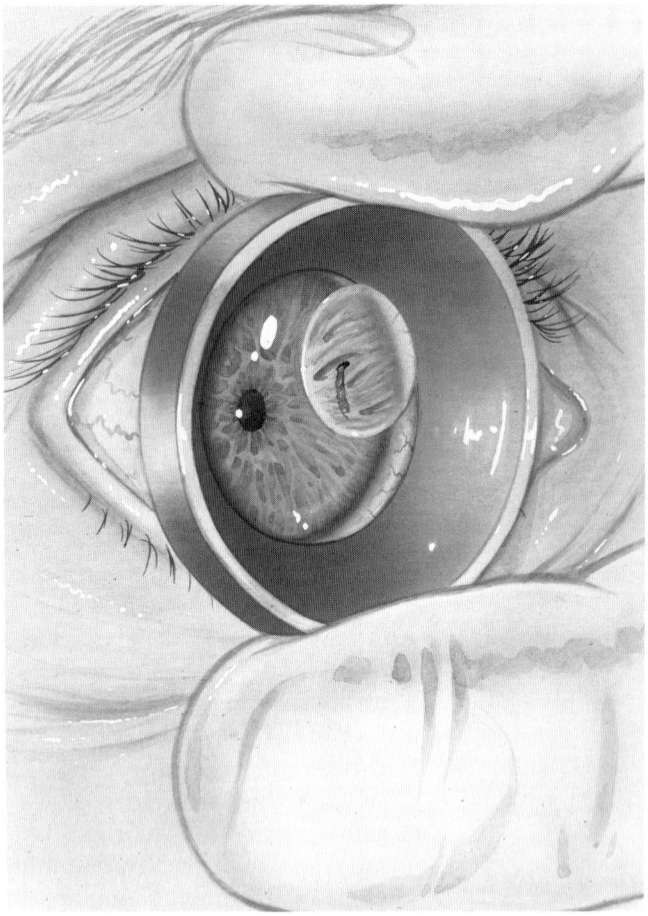

88

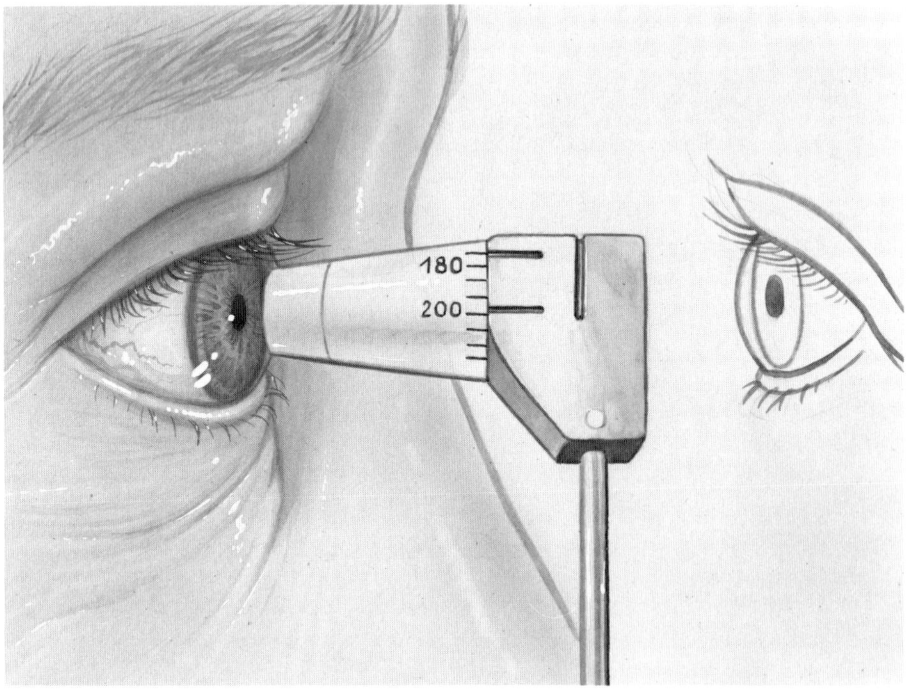

2.**87** Bleeding occurs from the margins of the iridotomy site in approximately 40 % of patients. This usually occurs as a temporary cascade and can be easily controlled by forward pressure upon the contact lens. This pressure usually stops all bleeding within a matter of seconds. Hyphemas are rare, but are more frequent in eyes with chronic inflammation or with neovascular glaucoma.

2.**88** After therapy it is important that topical corticosteroids and glaucoma therapy be continued until the inflammation has stopped and the iridotomy is patent. In addition, one should monitor the intraocular pressure to insure that if an intraocular pressure spike occurs, this can be blunted promptly with appropriate topical, oral, or intravenous medications. After it is clear that the iridotomy is open, pilocarpine should be stopped whenever possible. With all patent iridotomies the pupil should be widely dilated, not only to test the iridotomy, but also to prevent posterior synechiae. Dilatation should usually be continued with a medication such as tropicamide 1 %, once daily for one week; the pupil should be periodically dilated during the first month for the same purpose.

Argon Laser Trabeculoplasty

George L. Spaeth

Surgical Principles

Argon laser trabeculoplasty (ALT) is used to lower intraocular pressure in patients in whom this is required. Up to now it has mainly been used after medical therapy has failed, prior to filtration-type surgery. However, recent studies suggest that trabeculoplasty may in certain instances be used as primary therapy, or early in the treatment of disease after mild medical therapy has been found ineffective. The availability and effectiveness of ALT have resulted in many ophthalmologists moving to ALT, even in those cases where medical treatment is effective in controlling pressure, but is associated with bothersome side-effects.

The effectiveness of ALT is strongly related to the nature of the eye treated. ALT is more effective in the therapy of primary open-angle glaucoma than in any of the many other diagnostic entities. Furthermore, the older the patient, the higher the pretreatment intraocular pressure, and the greater the pigmentation of the posterior trabecular meshwork, the more satisfactory the results tend to be. ALT is also highly likely to lower the intraocular pressure in patients with the exfoliation syndrome and the pigment dispersion syndrome, especially in more elderly patients where the intraocular pressure is higher. It appears to be less effective in secondary glaucomas, especially those associated with inflammation or with structural abnormality of the angle. Some authors have reported success with the Sturge-Weber syndrome, but we have not found the procedure to be of value. Trabeculoplasty is of little or no use in the juvenile types of glaucoma. ALT is only of value in cases where the anterior chamber angle is sufficiently open for clear visualization of the posterior trabecular meshwork to be possible. Obviously, the anterior optical aspects of the eye must be clear enough to permit excellent visualization of the posterior trabecular meshwork.

Preparation for Surgery

Obviously, the nature of the patient's glaucoma and the need for ALT must be determined preoperatively. The angle must be examined meticulously through 360°. The cornea must also be evaluated to eliminate conditions that would make it unwise to proceed with ALT, or would require modification of the technique. If an anterior membrane dystrophy is present, the likelihood of significant corneal de-epithelialization must be considered; an especially gentle technique, or perhaps a soft contact lens may be necessary in such patients. If the cornea is edematous or unclear, it may not be possible to visualize the trabecular meshwork properly, and the power of the laser beam will not be adequately delivered. Marked corneal endothelial dystrophy may make ALT unwise. The aqueous humor in the anterior chamber should be clear; the presence of significant flare or cells or even of significant amounts of fluorescein can limit the effectiveness and safety of ALT.

The patient is seated at the laser; the cornea is anesthetized with proparacaine or a similar agent. A facial nerve block is unnecessary. The instrument is prepared for use. The exposure time is 0.1 s, spot size 50 μm, and power 700 mW; the mode is set at thermal for instruments which have both a "cool" and a "thermal" mode. The slit lamp is set for high power (25×). The beam of the slit lamp is positioned centrally between the oculars.

The laser beam is made parfocal with the viewer's gaze (see above "Argon Laser Iridectomy"). With the patient seated comfortably, the eye is anesthetized, the instrument readied, and the gonioprism placed on the eye.

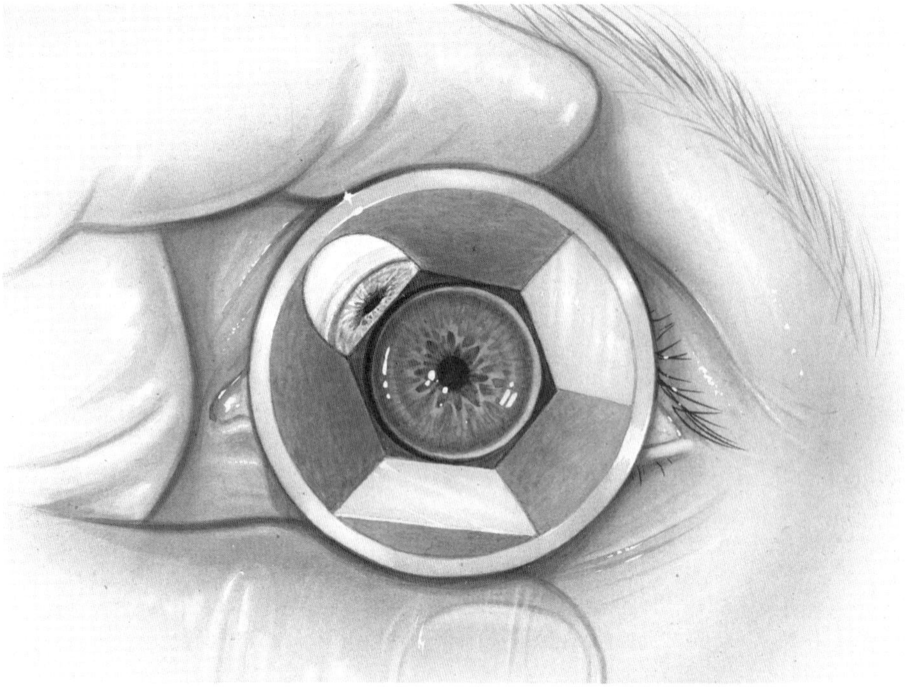

Surgical Technique

2.**89** The trabecular meshwork is visualized through the appropriate mirror; it is essential that all landmarks be identified with certainty. The entire angle has been examined by the surgeon preoperatively prior to deciding upon trabeculoplasty. At this point the landmarks are again identified and the mirror held at the 12 o'clock position so that the 6 o'clock portion of the angle is being examined.

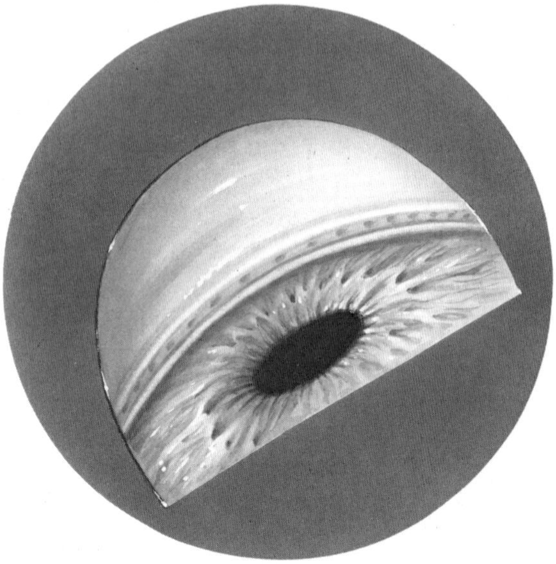

2.**90** The laser beam is meticulously focused by reflecting it from the mirror at 12 o'clock into the angle at 6 o'clock. The prism should be held so that the reflections from the viewing light shine directly back into the surgeon's eyes. This technique is entirely different from that utilized in standard gonioscopy. However, if the laser beam hits the mirror at an angle, as is the usual procedure in standard gonioscopy, it will be reflected in an oval shape onto the surface of the trabecular meshwork, resulting in dissipation of energy and an inconsistent burn. Furthermore, if the energy is not perfectly focused, the power will be diffused, also resulting in inconsistent burns which are larger than the surgeon intends. The position of application of the burns is important. The more posterior the burn, the greater the reaction, the greater the tendency to peripheral anterior synechia formation, and the greater the likelihood of postoperative pressure rise. The more anterior the burn, the slighter the reaction, the less likelihood of a pressure spike postoperatively, and the smaller the chance of producing posterior synechiae. I prefer to place the burns just anterior to the pigmented portion of the posterior trabecular meshwork, so that the application is made posterior to Schwalbe's line in the area of the anterior trabecular meshwork. The application should certainly not be anterior to Schwalbe's line or posterior to the scleral spur.

A test burn is applied at 6 o'clock and the tissue reaction carefully observed. Sufficient power is present when a tiny, transient bubble appears. This bubble should be just faintly visible and requires constant observation with a properly focused instrument in order to be visualized. If the reaction appears too intense, the power is decreased and further test burns applied until the appropriate response is obtained. If the reaction is inadequate, the power is increased until the appropriate reaction is obtained, or until the power reaches 1200 mW, above which the power is not usually increased. The more angle pigment, the less power is usually required.

Burns are then placed in the proper positions proceeding in a clockwise fashion toward 12 o'clock, separating the burns by several degrees so that 25 equally spaced applications are made in each quadrant. The lens is turned after every two to three burns, in order to ensure the clearest view and the best focus. If the lens is not rotated frequently, the applications will not be applied properly. The surgeon may elect to treat merely the right-hand 180° of the angle (the patient's right) with 50 applications, or may prefer to treat 360° with 100 applications. There are advantages and disadvantages to each technique.

Modifications

The position of the applications, the number of applications, and the intensity of power applied can be modified according to the surgeons's intentions. According to the initial protocol of Wise and Witter, 100 burns for 360° were applied in the posterior trabecular meshwork. Placing the burns more anteriorly appears to decrease the postoperative pressure spike without decreasing the effectiveness of the treatment, and is thus recommended. Fewer burns have also been recommended, but appear to have less effect.

The surgeon will need to individualize the amount of treatment depending upon the clinical characteristics of the patient under consideration and his or her experiences with the instrument employed.

If the anterior chamber angle is not sufficiently deep to permit a clear view of the trabecular meshwork, it may be possible to perform a trabeculoplasty by deepening the angle with an iridoplasty first (see below).

Admonitions and Suggestions

Argon laser trabeculoplasty appears to be remarkably safe. As mentioned earlier, it is effective in lowering intraocular pressure in most individuals with primary open-angle glaucoma. However, it is unusual that the intraocular pressure is lowered to the extent that it is possible to stop medical therapy entirely. Patients should be instructed that they will probably need to continue medical treatment even after ALT has been performed, even when it is successful.

Surgeons may wish to try ALT in conditions other than primary open-angle glaucoma, but the patient should be cautioned that the procedure is less likely to be successful. It may also be repeated; where initially successful, it is prone to be beneficial when repeated once or even twice. However, the likelihood of a pressure spike developing increases following repeat trabeculoplasty, and consequently the repeat procedure should be performed with special precautions for monitoring the postoperative intraocular pressure.

An uncommon but important problem with ALT is the occasional occurrence of a spike of intraocular pressure, which persists. In patients with badly damaged optic disks, this can result in further damage to the optic nerve, which may occur rapidly and result in sudden and serious visual loss.

Patients with low intraocular pressure may have smaller drops in pressure following trabeculoplasty. However, this does not mean that the procedure is not indicated. Lowering intraocular pressure from 14 mm Hg to 12 mm Hg may in some individuals be sufficient to permit stabilization of visual field loss and may eliminate the need for filtering surgery, which in such cases might have a tendency to cause "wipe-out". Thus, though of limited value, ALT is not contraindicated in patients with low intraocular pressure. Similarly, in cases of far-advanced glaucoma, whether the pressure is low or high, ALT may be especially valuable because of its ability to lower intraocular pressure without the need to open the eye.

The major problem with trabeculoplasty has to do with the fact that the effect on intraocular pressure is frequently less than desired. In such cases it may be tempting to continue the patient on medical therapy, during which time progressive visual loss develops. To avoid this problem, it is usually advisable to set a definite pressure-lowering goal which the surgeon and patient wish to achieve. If intraocular pressure following ALT fails to fall to that level, the surgeon and patient will in many instances wish to go ahead directly with a standard filtering procedure, rather than wait for the development of further visual loss.

It normally takes around four weeks for the effect of ALT to become maximally apparent. In some individuals it may take a bit longer than this, up to six or even, rarely, seven weeks. After that the intraocular pressure is usually stable, though the duration of stability has *not* been established. It should be assumed that the beneficial effect on intraocular pressure of ALT will gradually diminish with increasing time. Patients with the exfoliation syndrome tend to show a greater initial success, but then a more rapid diminution of the pressure-lowering effect of ALT. Thus, patients with the exfoliation syndrome need to be especially carefully observed for late rise in intraocular pressure following ALT, even when the procedure was initially successful. In many individuals, including some with the exfoliation syndrome, intraocular pressure can remain stable for years following ALT. If the pressure has fallen adequately, medications may be cautiously withdrawn, one at a time, in order to determine whether or not they continue to be necessary.

Postoperative Management

Patients are continued on the same glaucoma therapy as before and, in addition, treated with a mild anti-inflammatory compound such as fluoromethalone, 1 % four times daily for one week. There is rarely a significant postoperative inflammatory response, and it is extremely rare that anti-inflammatory therapy must be continued for longer than a week. If so, the possibility of a steroid-induced glaucoma is enhanced.

Results

Around 50 % of patients with primary open-angle glaucoma can expect to experience a drop in intraocular pressure greater than 20 % following ALT. Another 25 % will have a smaller, questionably beneficial fall. In around a quarter of the cases the effect is minimal. Significant, lasting pressure rises appear to occur in around 1 % or less of patients with primary open-angle glaucoma. The success rate is lower and the complication rate higher in other forms of glaucoma. The intraocular pressure-lowering effect of ALT appears to be long-lasting, in many cases continuing for two years or more. However, more data are needed before the actual duration of the effect of argon laser trabeculoplasty can be stated with authority, and before the factors influencing this duration are better understood.

Bibliograpy

[1] Greenidge, D. C., Rodrigues, M. M., Spaeth, G. L.: Acute intraocular pressure elevation after argon laser trabeculoplasty or iridectomy: A clinicopathologic study. *Ophthal. Surg.* 15: 105–110, 1984

[2] Greenidge, D. C., Spaeth, G. L., Fiol-Silva, Z.: Effect of argon laser trabeculoplasty on the glaucomatous diurnal curve. *Ophthalmology* 90: 800–804, 1983.

[3] Pollack, I. P., Robin, A. L.: Argon laser trabeculoplasty: Its effect on medical control of open-angle glaucoma. *Ophthal. Surg.* 13: 637–643, 1982.

[4] Ritch, R.: Argon laser for angle-closure glaucoma. *Amer. J. Ophthalmol.* 94: 197–204, 1982.

[5] Rodrigues, M. M., Spaeth, G. L., Donohoo, P.: Electron microscopy of argon laser therapy in phakic open-angle glaucoma. *Ophthalmology* 89: 198–210, 1982.

[6] Schwartz, L. W., Spaeth, G. L., Traverso, C. et al.: Variation of techniques on the results of argon laser trabeculoplasty. *Ophthalmology* 90: 781–784, 1983.

[7] Spaeth, G. L., Fellman, R. L., Starita, R. J. et al.: Argon laser trabeculoplasty in the treatment of secondary glaucoma. *Trans. Amer. Ophthal. Soc.* 81: 325–332, 1983.

[8] Spaeth, G. L.: Laser treatment is surgery. *Ophthal. Surg.* 14: 123, 1983.

[9] Stiegler, G.: Laser-Trabekulotomie und Laser-Iridektomie. Drei Jahre Erfahrung mit dem Glaukom-Research-Laser (Britt). *Klin. Monatsbl. Augenheilk.* 175: 333–340, 1979.

[10] Thomas, J. V., Simmons, R. J., Belcher, C. D. III: Argon laser trabeculoplasty in the presurgical glaucoma patient. *Ophthalmology* 89: 187–197, 1982.

[11] Weinreb, R. N., Ruderman, J., Juster, R. et al.: Immediate intraocular pressure response to argon laser trabeculoplasty. *Amer. J. Ophthalmol.* 95: 279–286, 1983.

[12] Wickham, M. C., Worthen, D. M.: Argon laser trabeculotomy; long-term follow-up. *Ophthalmology* 86: 495–503, 1979.

[13] Wilensky, J. T., Weinreb, R. N.: Low-dose trabeculoplasty. *Amer. J. Ophthalmol.* 95: 423–426, 1983.

[14] Wise, J. B., Witter, S. L.: Argon laser therapy for open-angle glaucoma: a pilot study. *Arch. Ophthalmol.* 97: 319–322, 1979.

[15] Wise, J. B.: Long-term control of adult open angle glaucoma by argon laser treatment. *Ophthalmology* 88: 197–202, 1981.

[16] Worthen, D. M., Wickham, M. G.: Argon laser trabeculotomy. *Trans. Amer. Acad. Ophthalmol. Otolaryngol.* 78: 371–375, 1974.

Argon Laser Iridoplasty

George L. Spaeth

Surgical Principles

2.**91** In some eyes the iris bulges anteriorly, tending to cause closure of the angle, or impeding the view of the trabecular meshwork. It is possible to flatten this iris bulge with the application of argon laser energy. The flattening, called iridoplasty, is usually temporary and, as such, iridoplasty is not useful as a permanent treatment for narrow angles. This technique has also been termed gonioplasty. There may be a temporary lowering of intraocular pressure, but a permanent effect is not to be expected.

The major use of iridoplasty is to deepen the anterior chamber angle to permit the performance of argon laser trabeculoplasty in a patient in whom the angle is so narrow that trabeculoplasty would be either difficult or inadvisable without such angle deepening.

91

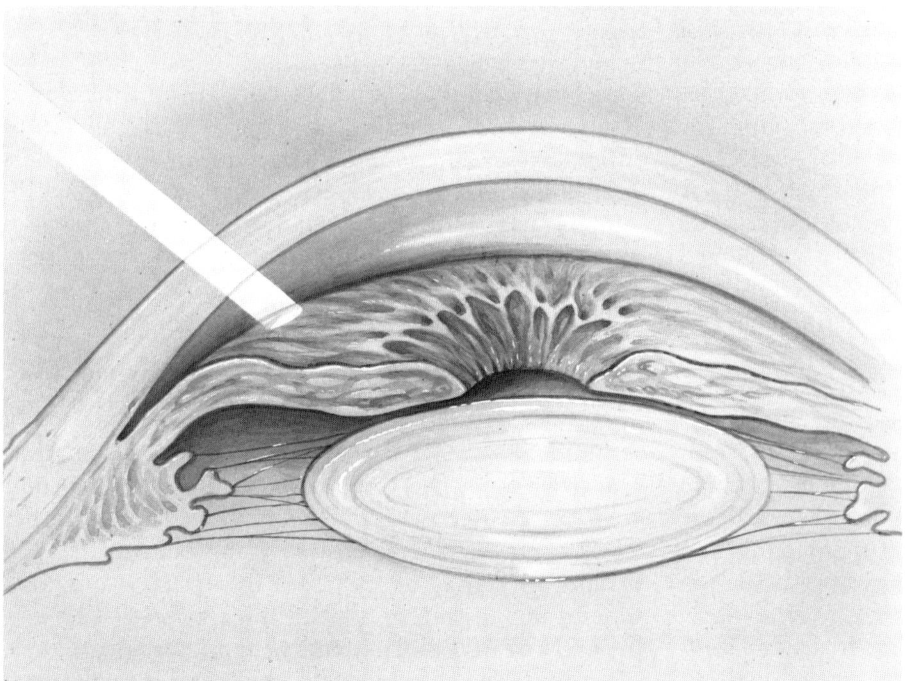

Preparation for Surgery

The procedure is performed under topical anesthesia, employing an agent such as proparacaine. A facial nerve block is not necessary. The cornea must be clear. The chamber may be shallow, but should be sufficiently deep that laser energy can be applied to the iris without burning of the corneal endothelium.

The laser is set for a large spot size with low power and a long exposure. Suggested settings are 500 μm spot size, 200 mW, and an exposure time of 1 s.

92

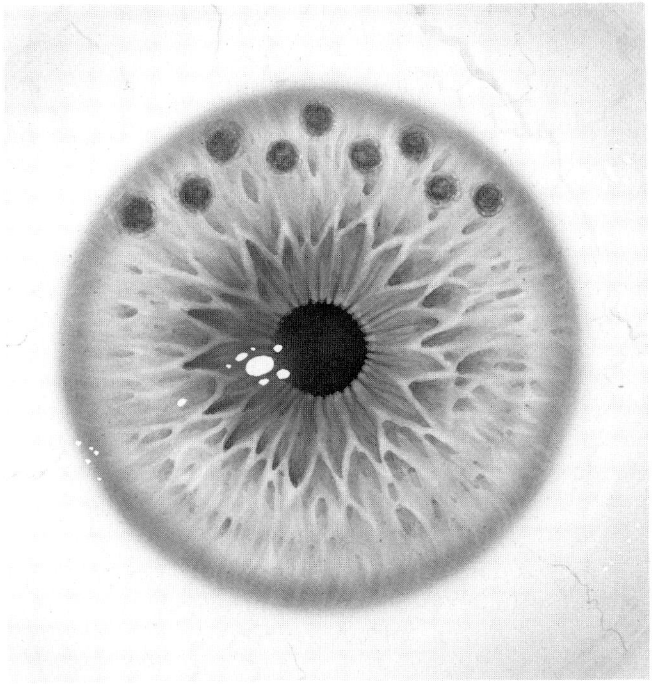

Surgical Technique

2.**92** With the patient seated at the slit lamp and the cornea anesthetized, the iris is brought into clear focus, showing the anterior bulging of the iris. No gonioprism is required. Relatively low magnification can be employed, e.g. 16 ×.

An application is placed as far in the iris periphery as can be visualized. The power should not be high enough to cause charring or burning. Rather, the surgeon should see coagulation, with shrinkage of the tissue, and a flattening of the iris bulge in the area of the application. If insufficient flattening is achieved, the exposure time may be increased. A row of applications is then placed in the area in which the surgeon desires to flatten the iris. If inadequate flattening is achieved, an additional row can be placed further from the angle root, but still well in the periphery.

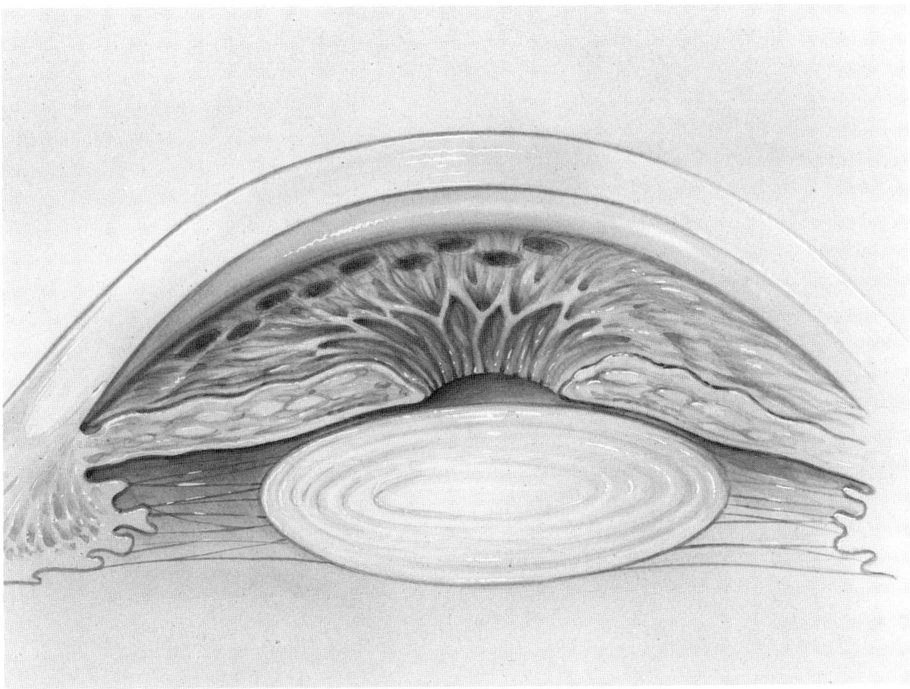

2.**93** The peripheral coagulations should result in a marked flattening of the iris bulge, permitting visualization of the angle structures.

Admonitions and Suggestions

Iridoplasty is of great value in a few cases. It cannot be recommended for long-term treatment of narrow anterior chamber angles, or for attempting to lower intraocular pressure in patients with such angles. When applied judiciously, there is minimal release of pigmentation and minimal inflammatory response; it is usually possible to proceed directly with argon laser trabeculoplasty immediately after iridoplasty has been completed.

Postoperative Management

Patients should continue on their medications as before with the addition of a mild anti-inflammatory compound such as fluorometholone 0.1 % four times daily for one week. Intraocular pressure spikes are uncommon, but the intraocular pressure should be measured 1–2 hours following iridoplasty.

Bibliography

[1] Blumenthal, A., Floman, N., Triester, G.: Laser iris retraction for narrow-angle glaucoma. *Glaucoma* 4: 47–49, 1982.
[2] Ritch, R.: Argon laser treatment for medically unresponsive attacks of angle-closure glaucoma. *Amer. J. Ophthalmol.* 94: 197–204, 1982.
[3] Belcher, C. D., Thomas, J. V., Simmons, R. J. (ed.): Laser Photocoagulation in Glaucoma and Anterior Segment Disease. *Williams & Wilkins, Baltimore* 1984.

3

Ciliary Body

G. O. H. Naumann

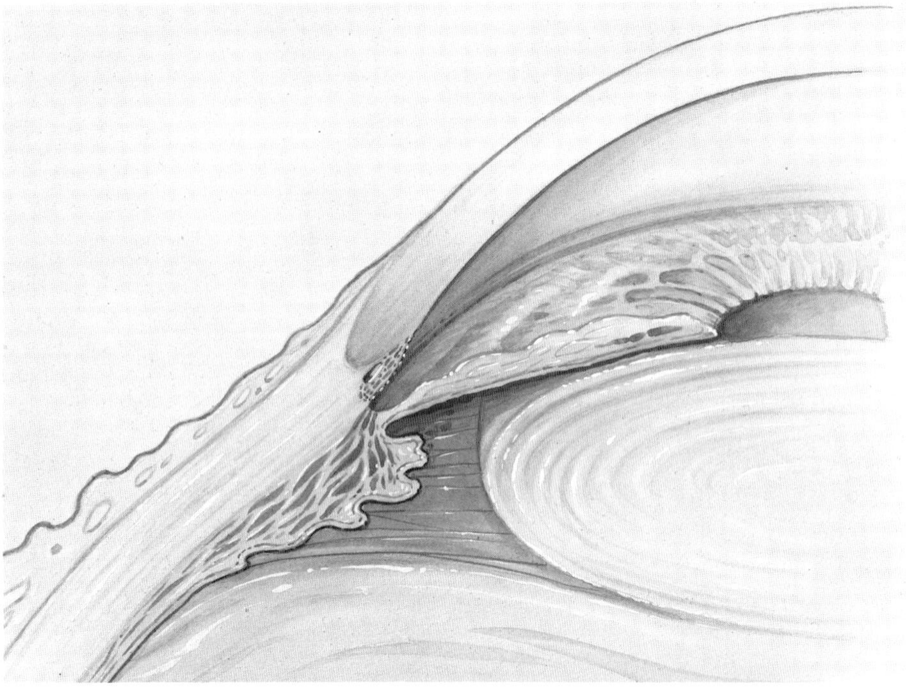

Introduction

3.**1** Of all ocular tissues, the ciliary body is the least accessible to direct observation and examination. The following essential functions are located here:

1. Optically the ciliary body plays a part not only in accommodation, but also in "retinal stretch".
2. Extravascular intraocular circulation: along with aqueous humor, which controls intraocular pressure, the vitreous is supplied with hyaluronic acid by the ciliary epithelium.
3. The ciliary muscles apparently play an essential role in the control of aqueous outflow through the trabecular meshwork and also in the control of uveoscleral outflow.
4. The nutrition of the cornea and the lens depends on the aqueous secretions originating in the ciliary body.
5. The blood-aqueous barrier is located at the level of the zonulae occludentes of the nonpigmented ciliary epithelium. There is probably a "physiological defect" between iris root and ciliary body in the transition zone between iris and ciliary body, i.e., between the nonfenestrated endothelial lining of the iris vessels and the fenestrated endothelium of the ciliary vessels.

Due to these difficulties, the ciliary body is the last "taboo zone" for surgical interventions – although Zirm removed a malignant melanoma by iridocyclectomy as early as 1911.

In all standard intraocular procedures of the anterior segment, the surgeon tries to avoid touching the structures of the ciliary body with his instruments. Even minor injuries to the ciliary processes can lead to unwanted hemorrhage, which can only be stopped with some difficulty. The individual variations of the major arterial circle of the ciliary body and its branch vessels are not yet well understood. The relationship between the lens equator and the pars plicata of the ciliary body cannot be observed with standard clinical examination techniques and is not accessible to observation during standard intraocular surgery of the anterior segment. Therefore, ophthalmic surgeons are generally reluctant to consider surgical procedures involving the ciliary body directly.

However, I hope to show that there are indeed indications for direct manipulation of the ciliary body aside from the indirect transscleral approaches usually used for the treatment of refractory secondary glaucomas with rubeosis iridis.

Direct Cyclopexy for Traumatic Cyclodialysis with Persistent Hypotony Syndrome

Surgical Principles

Persistent ocular hypotony leads to irreversible morphologic and functional damage within the retina and optic nerve. Although the details of the mechanism leading to persistent ocular hypotony in traumatic cyclodialysis are poorly understood, reapposition of the ciliary muscle to the scleral spur cures this pressure anomaly. Direct cyclopexy is indicated in cyclodialysis exceeding 60° and/or with more than six weeks' duration of hypotony, when intensive local corticosteroid therapy has failed to raise intraocular pressure.

Preparation for Surgery

Conjunctival bacterial cultures are obtained on the day before surgery. Only if there is bacterial growth local antibiotics are given.

Preoperative Medication and Anesthesia

Cyclopegics such as cyclopentolate hydrochloride and atropine (1 %) are given preoperatively. For phakic patients with a clear lens, general anesthesia is advised. The anesthetist should be prepared to use controlled arterial hypotension to reduce vis a tergo. In aphakic patients local anesthesia is adequate.

Instruments

A standard instrument tray is required as for lamellar keratoplasty and anterior segment surgery, including a Flieringa ring.

Optional extras are sodium hyaluronic acid, a diamond knife (which facilitates scleral incision of the very soft eye despite intraocular injection of air and/or hyaluronic acid), and an automated vitrectomy instrument (in case anterior vitrectomy should be necessary).

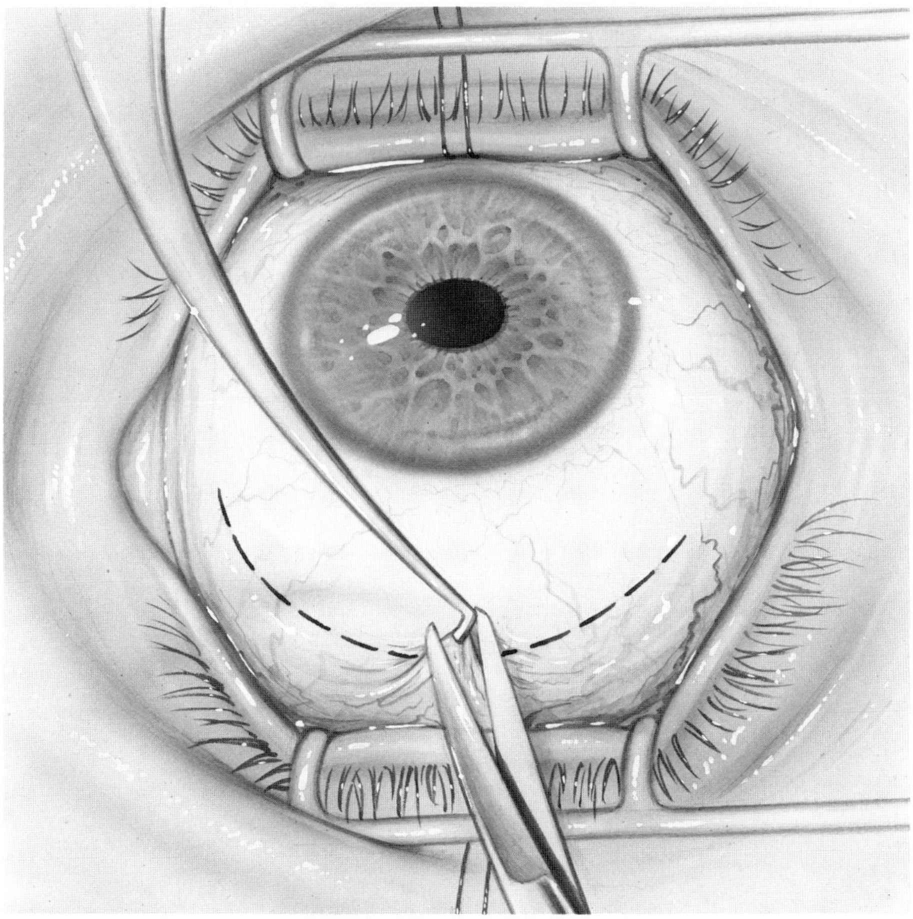

Surgical Technique

3.**2** Traction sutures through the rectus muscles are recommended. A Flieringa ring is mandatory in aphakic patients and in those with manifest or suspected vitreous prolapse due to traumatic dislocation of the lens.

3

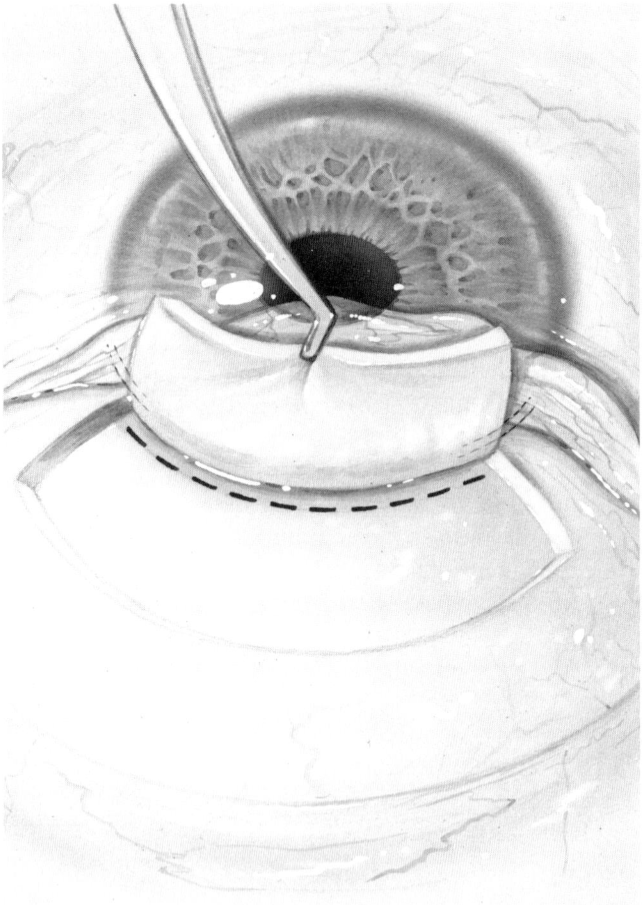

4

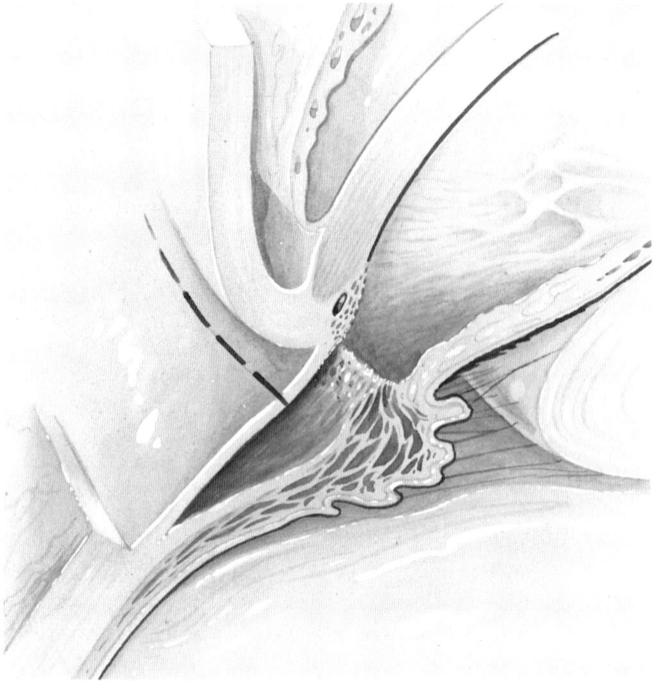

3.**3** A limbus-based deep lamellar scleral flap is created, extending 4 mm behind the limbus over the area of the traumatic cyclodialysis.

3.**4** The remaining scleral lamella is incised parallel and 1 mm posterior to the scleral spur.

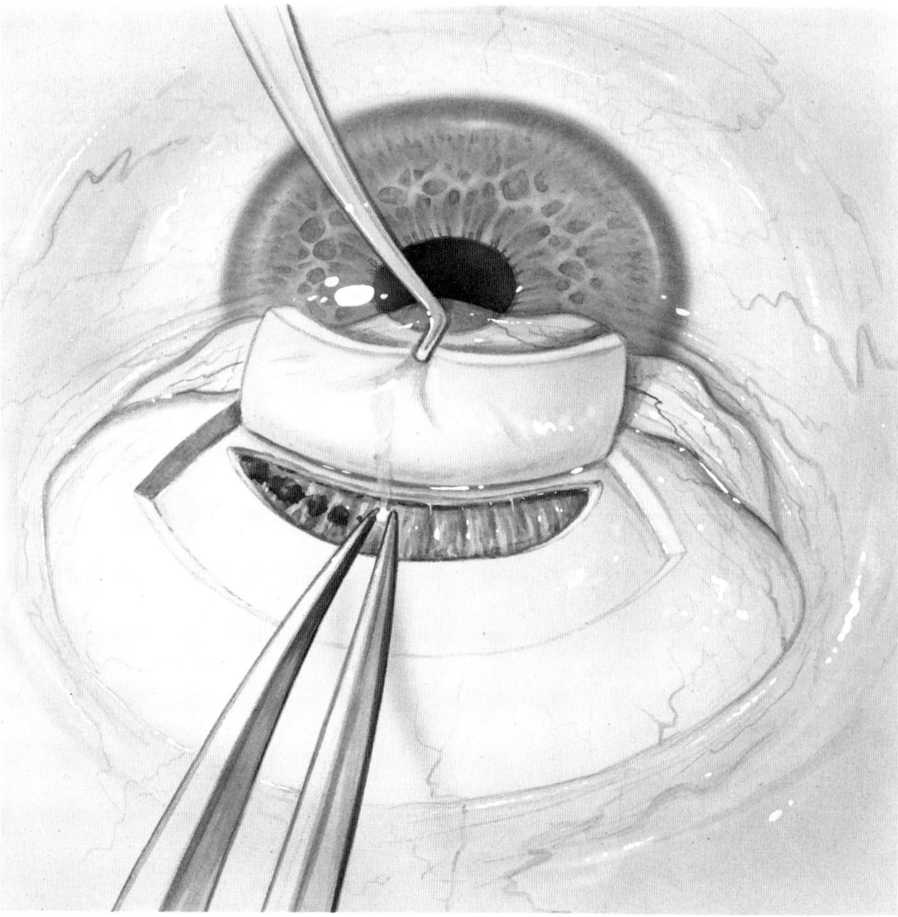

3.**5** Direct bipolar cautery is performed on the ciliary muscle behind the fine gray line indicating the beginning of the insertion to the scleral spur.

6

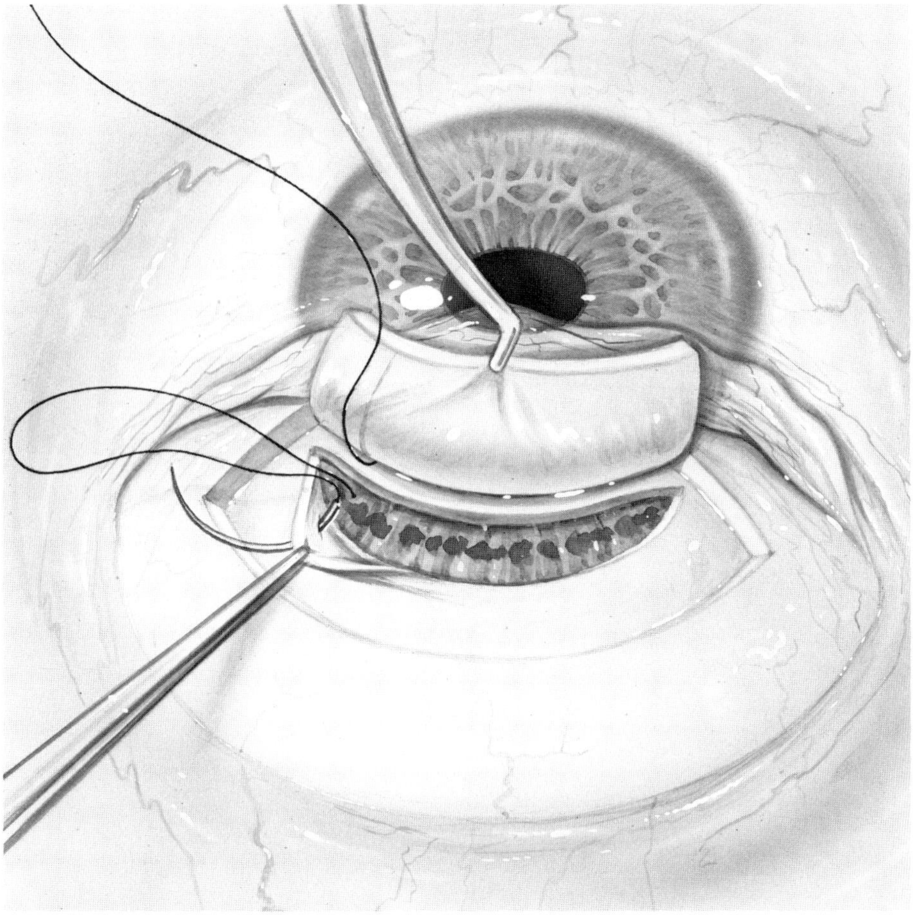

7

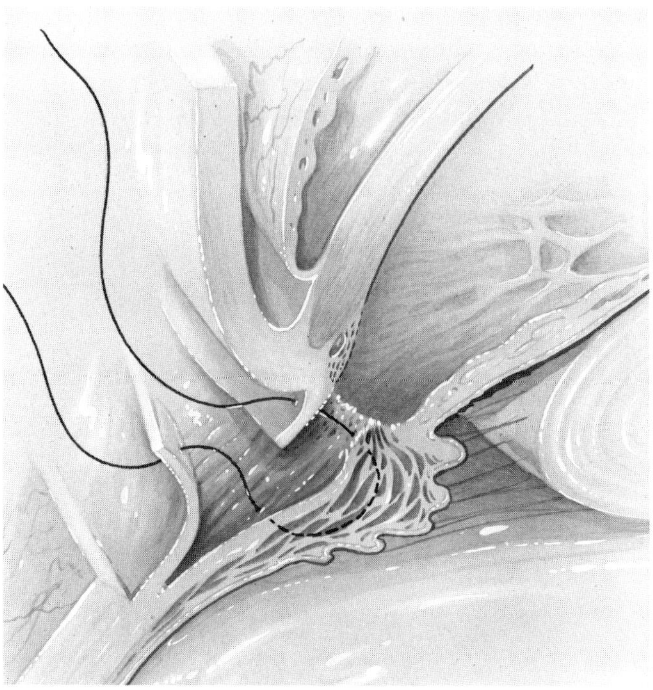

3.**6** and **7** Direct suturing is done through the scleral lamella anteriorly, the ciliary muscle, and the scleral lamella posteriorly, under direct microscopic surgical control.

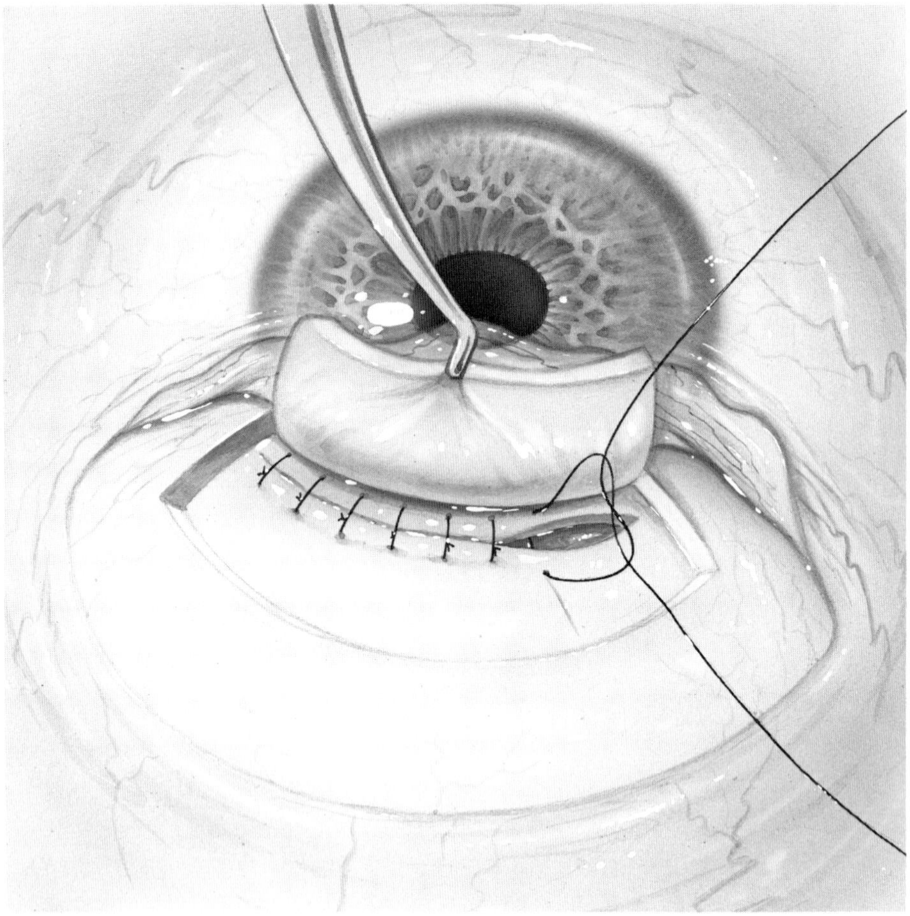

3.**8** The incision is closed with interrupted sutures.

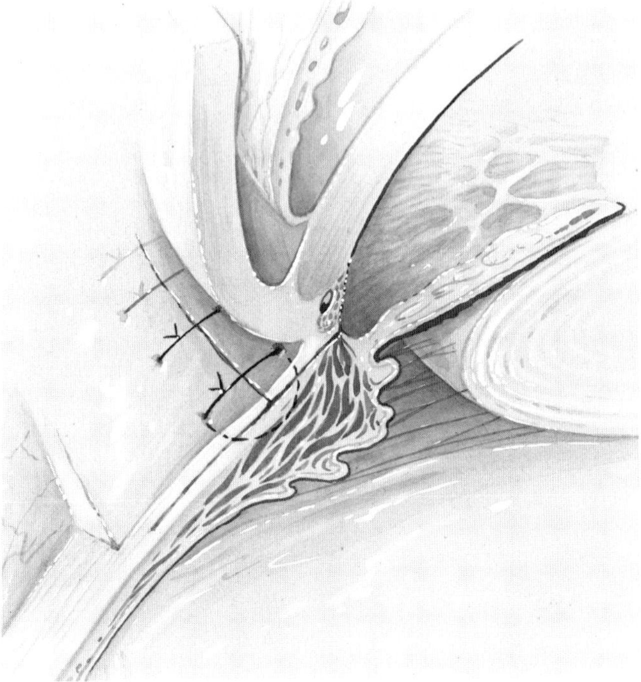

3.**9** A good reapposition of the ciliary muscle to the scleral spur is obtained, corresponding to the original anatomy.

10

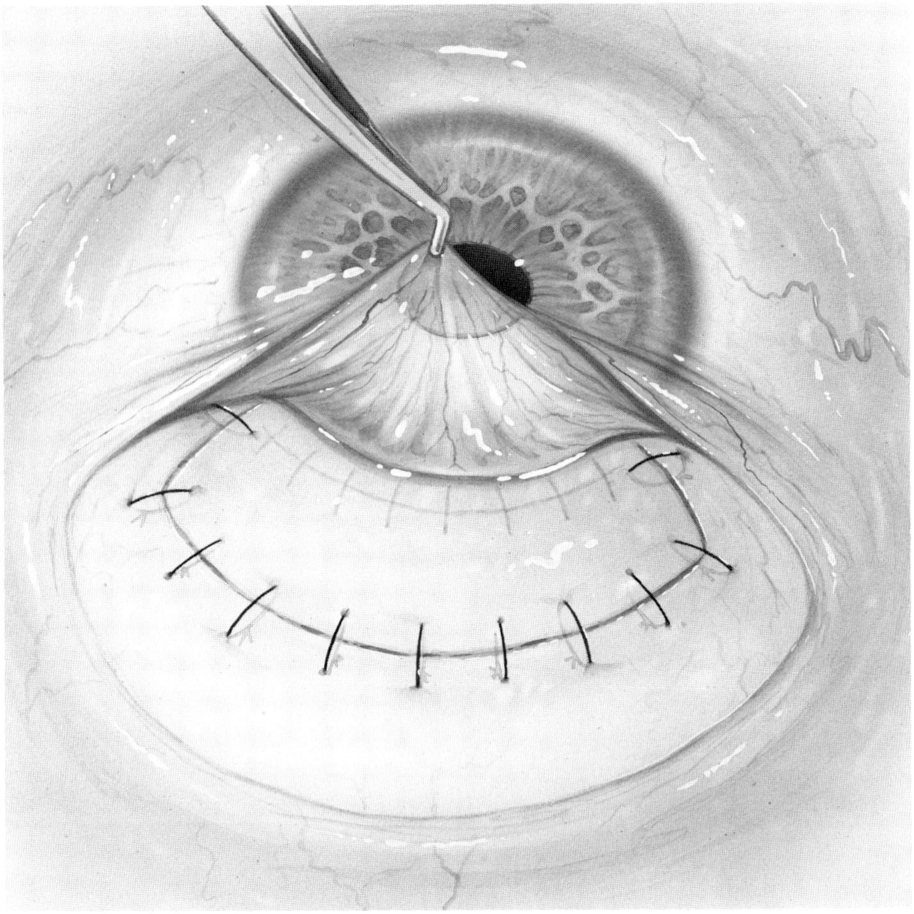

11

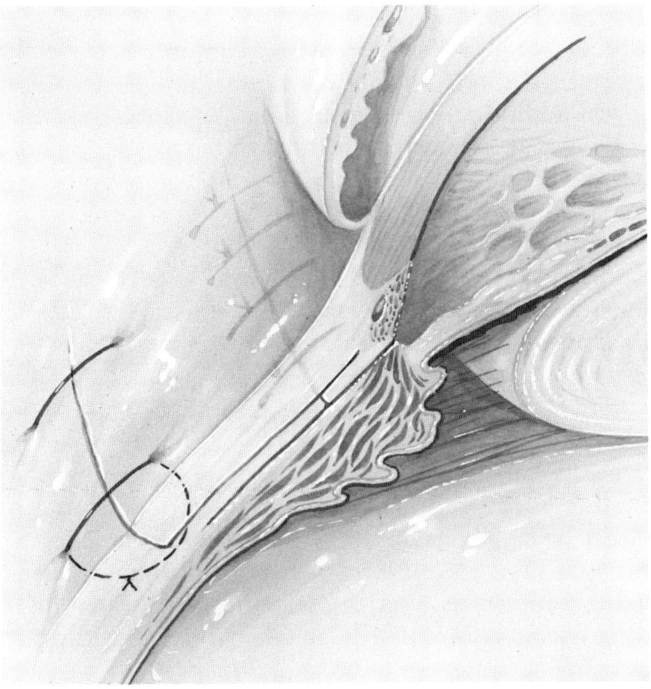

3.**10** and **11** The scleral lamellar window is closed.

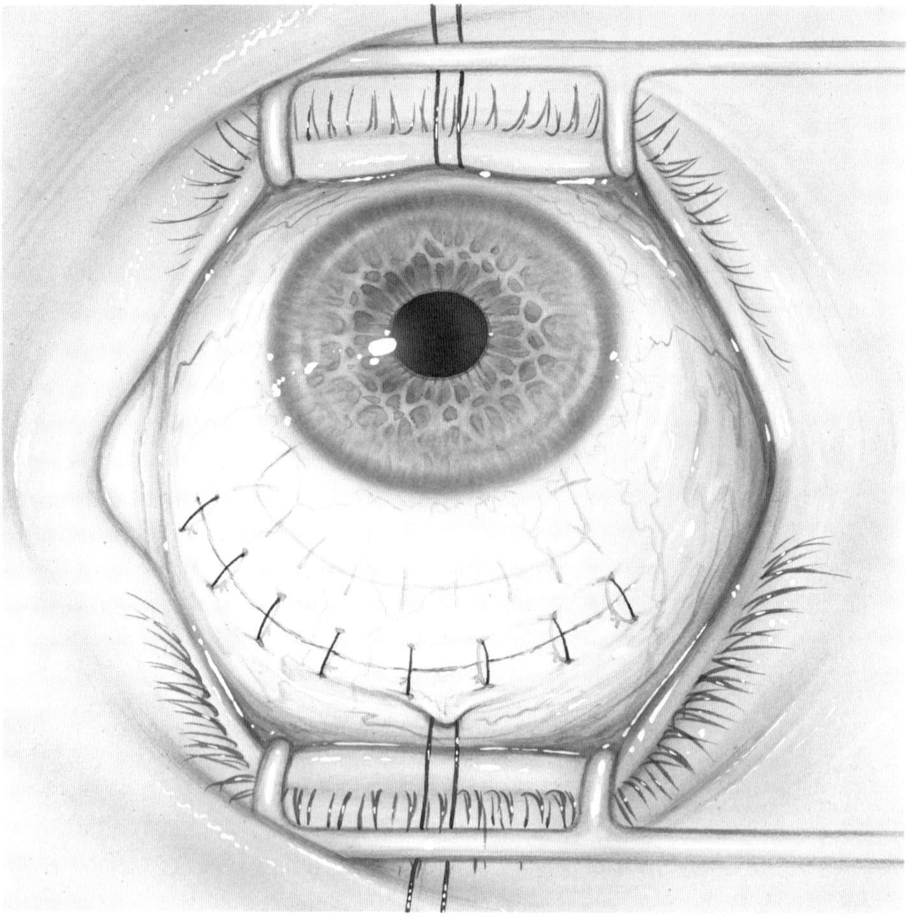

3.**12** The conjunctiva overlying the sclera is sutured.

Intraoperative Complications

Surprisingly, after bipolar cautery of the ciliary muscle, *hemorrhage* has not been a problem in our experience (despite initial misgivings). Anterior *synechiae* can be avoided be careful apposition of the anterior portion of the ciliary muscle to the sclera immediately behind the scleral spur.

If the cyclodialysis exceeds 90–120° a peripheral iridotomy is recommended to avoid a pupillary block.

Direct *contact with the lens* can be avoided by pushing it back by injection of air and/or hyaluronic acid into the anterior chamber.

Vitreous prolapse is commonly associated with traumatic cyclodialysis following contusion. Usually, it does not extend into the scleral surgical wound. Circumscribed focal vitreous prolapses at the pupillary margin are not surgically treated.

Admonitions and Suggestions

Watertight wound closure is mandatory with both the ciliary muscle and the scleral sutures.

In extensive cyclodialysis of more than 150° it can be extremely difficult to determine the real extent of the traumatic cyclodialysis by preoperative gonioscopy. The marked hypotony leads to deformation of the globe by the gonioscope, and corneal folds prevent good visualization of the angle.

If ocular hypotony persists in spite of a correctly performed direct cyclopexy, repeat gonioscopy may reveal additional areas of traumatic cyclodialysis that could not be detected at the initial preoperative examination. In this case a repeat direct cyclopexy of the remaining areas of cyclodialysis must be performed; this poses no special problems.

Originally, bovine fibrinogen was used to achieve fibrous connection between ciliary muscle and sclera; I am now convinced that this is unnecessary.

Simultaneous Intraocular Procedures

If the lens is opaque, extracapsular or intracapsular cataract surgery can be performed at the same time as direct cyclopexy via a transcorneal approach. If extracapsular surgery is feasible, posterior chamber lens implantation can be performed with intracapsular fit. If there is traumatic retinal detachment it can be rectified at the same session – after direct cyclopexy.

Postoperative Management and Complications

Cyclopegic medication and local corticosteroids are necessary postoperatively.

Often, in the first few days postoperatively, there may be an excessive but temporary *increase in pressure* which cannot be controlled with medication. It is remarkable that the patients sometimes complain of symptoms as in acute glaucoma, in spite of the fact that the pressure may only be in the range between 20 and 30 mm Hg! Occasionally, normalization of pressure may be delayed for several weeks. In our series of 30 eyes treated in this manner, there have so far been no persistent cases of secondary open-angle glaucoma.

In the normotensive eye a careful examination of the fundus periphery is not so difficult. If postcontusional peripheral *retinal tears* are found, retinopexy must be performed.

Regular pressure checkups are of course necessary to rule out late-onset secondary open *angle glaucoma* due to contusion. We advise our patients to see an ophthalmologist once a year.

Results

Direct cyclopexy achieved a reapposition of the ciliary muscle to the scleral spur without ensuing secondary angle-closure glaucoma in the 30 eyes of our series. The functional improvement depended on the extent of additional damage to the macular area and optic nerve: irreversible retinal folds and intraretinal edema sometimes delayed improvement in visual function for three to nine months.

Alternatives

Argon laser photocoagulation of the cleft can be successful in some instances if the extent of the cyclodialysis is very small. In our experience it is inadequate for closure of cyclodialysis clefts extending over more than 30°.

Bibliography

[1] Best, W., Hartwig, H.: Traumatic cyclodialysis and its treatment. *Klin. Mbl. Augenheilk.* 170: 917–922, 1977.

[2] Harbin, T. S.: Treatment of cyclodialysis clefts with argon laser photocoagulation. *Ophthalmology* 89: 1082–1083, 1982.

[3] Mackensen, G., Custodis, M.: Contribution to the surgical treatment of ocular hypotony after cyclodialysis. *Klin. Mbl. Augenheilk.* 161: 10–16, 1972

[4] Maumenee, A. E., Stark, W. J.: Management of persistent hypotony after planned or inadvertent cyclodialysis. *Amer. J. Ophthalmol.* 71: 320–327, 1971.

[5] Naumann, G. O. H., Völcker, H. E.: Direct cyclopexy in the treatment of the persistent hypotony syndrome due to traumatic cyclodialysis. *Klin. Mbl. Augenheilk.* 179: 266–270, 1981.

[6] Naumann, G. O. H., Völcker, H. E.: Direct cyclopexy for persisting hypotony. In: *Current Management in Ophthalmology,* ed. Koch, D. D., Parke, D. W., Paton, D. Churchill Livingstone, Edinburgh, 1983, pages 143–150.

Block Excision for Tumors of the Anterior Uvea

Surgical Principles

Malignant melanomas of the uvea are notorious for their tendency to invade the sclera. Malignant melanomas of the choroid appear to be treated most satisfactorily with ruthenium or other radioactive scleral applicators – if enucleation can be avoided. However, malignant tumors of the anterior uvea are not susceptible to this radiation therapy. If not more than 150° of the circumference of the ciliary body and/or iris root and chamber angle are involved, local tumor excision is possible. In 90 % of eyes containing malignant melanomas of the uvea, serial sections show scleral invasion. The extent of the scleral invasion cannot normally be detected clinically (particularly if the tumor is small or nonpigmented). Total resection can, therefore, only be achieved by the removal of *all* sclera and/or cornea adjacent to the tumor, together with the neighboring retinal, vitreous, and lens tissue. The resulting defect is then covered with a tectonic corneal or corneoscleral graft.

Preparation for Surgery

Before surgery a general medical checkup is advisable, to rule out metastases.

If the malignant melanoma extends posteriorly beyond the ora serrata, chorioretinal scarring must be induced posterior to the tumor by laser photocoagulation and/or cryocoagulation to prevent postoperative retinal detachment.

To inhibit the tumor's potential for metastasization, preoperative radiation with 30 Gy in 10 doses of 3 Gy each is advised. Higher doses of preoperative radiation should *not* be given, to avoid complications of radiation arteriopathy of the ciliary vessels (see below).

Conjunctival bacterial cultures are prepared, as in direct cyclopexy.

As a rule general anesthesia is necessary, and controlled arterial hypotension is desirable at the time of the actual tumor removal to minimize hemorrhage from the dissected uveal vessels. The pupil is kept miotic, particularly if the clear lens is to be preserved.

Instruments

A standard keratoplasty instrument tray is required. Large-diameter corneal trephines are needed, permitting microscopic observation and control of the cutting edge during the procedure. Thus, trephines up to 18 mm in diameter are required, i.e., beyond the range customary in standard keratoplasty.

A Flieringa ring is mandatory to prevent collapse of the globe. In special circumstances, modified Flieringa rings may be used.

Bipolar cautery is essential to stop bleeding from cut uveal vessels.

Healon is helpful to prevent collapse of the globe and to reduce hemorrhage from small uveal vessels.

Surgical Technique

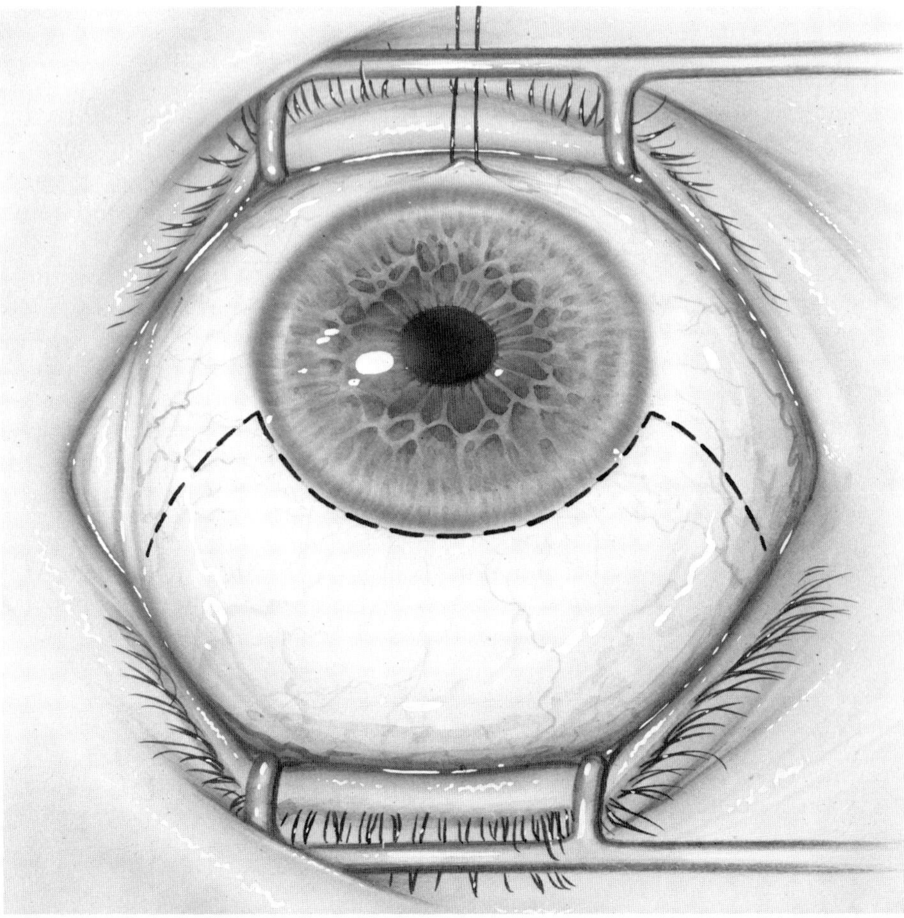

3.**13** Usually, a wide canthotomy is performed to facilitate access to the equatorial and posterior surfaces of the globe. An extensive fornix-based flap is created with radial incisions. Direct sutures are placed through the extraocular muscles.

14

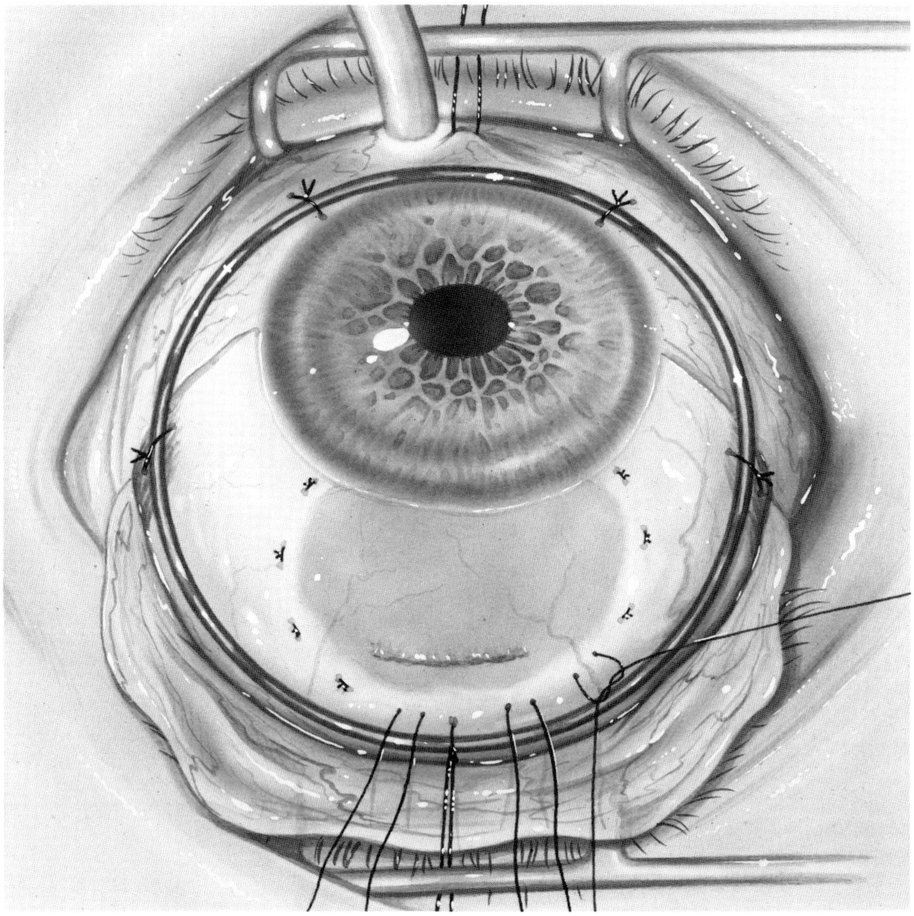

3.**14** The Flieringa ring is secured over the sclera to surround the extent of the lesion. The rectus muscle attached to the sclera overlying the tumor is separated. The edge of the tumor is marked by 8-0 or 10-0 interrupted nylon sutures or episcleral cautery.

3.**15** Diaphanoscopy with intensive fiber optic illumination is used to outline the margins of the tumor.

15

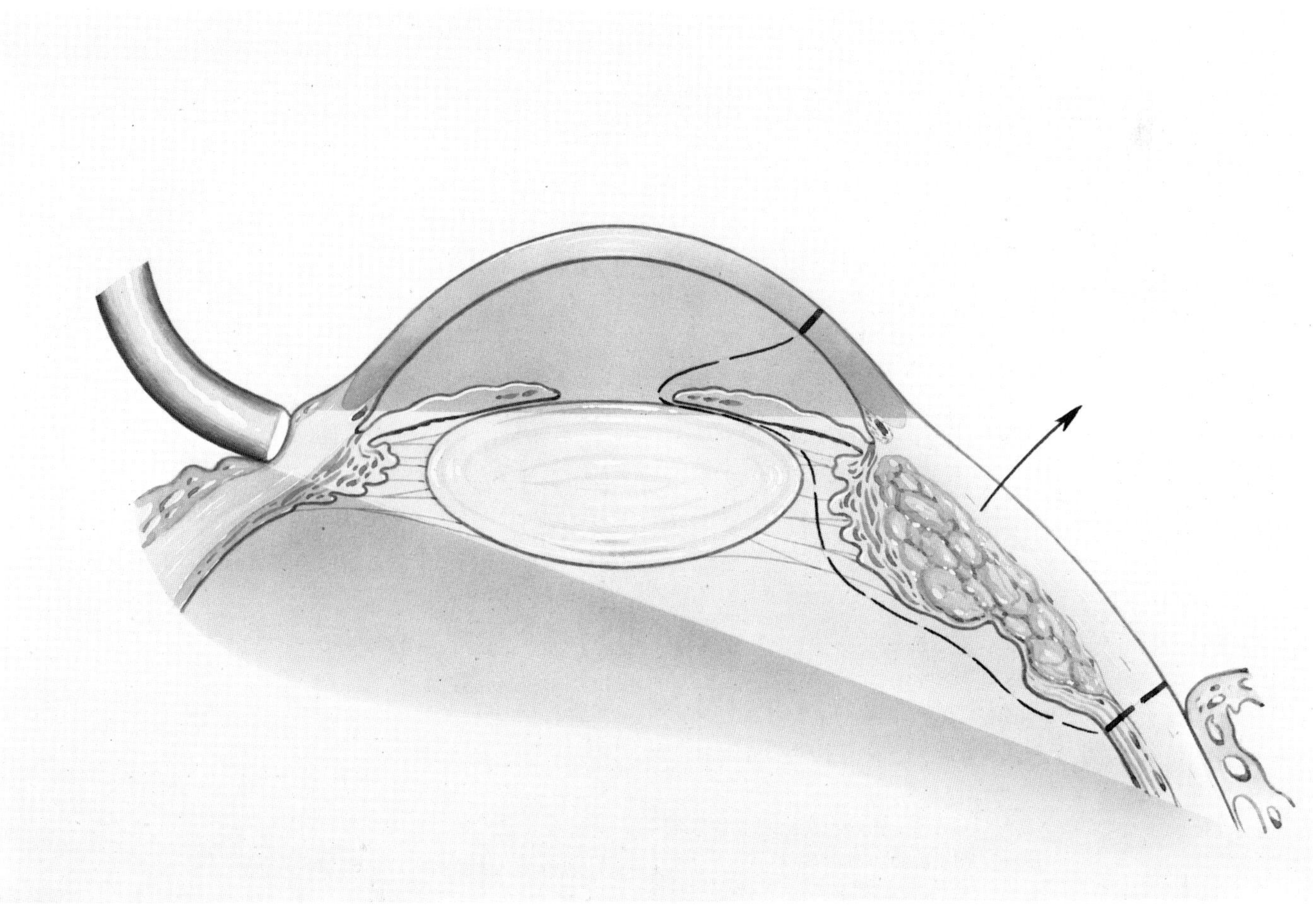

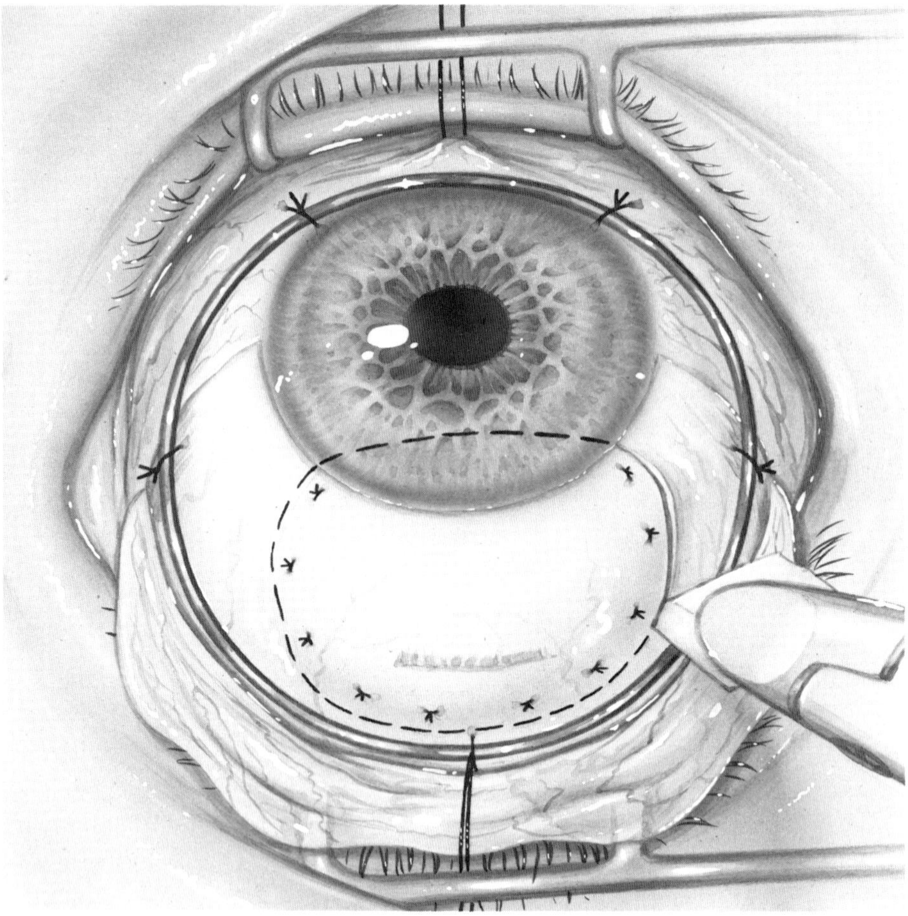

3.**16** An incision is made beyond the markings delineating the tumor, initially only in the superficial layers. Transcorneal paracenteses into the anterior chamber beyond the tumor edge facilitate reformation of the anterior chamber at the end of the procedure.

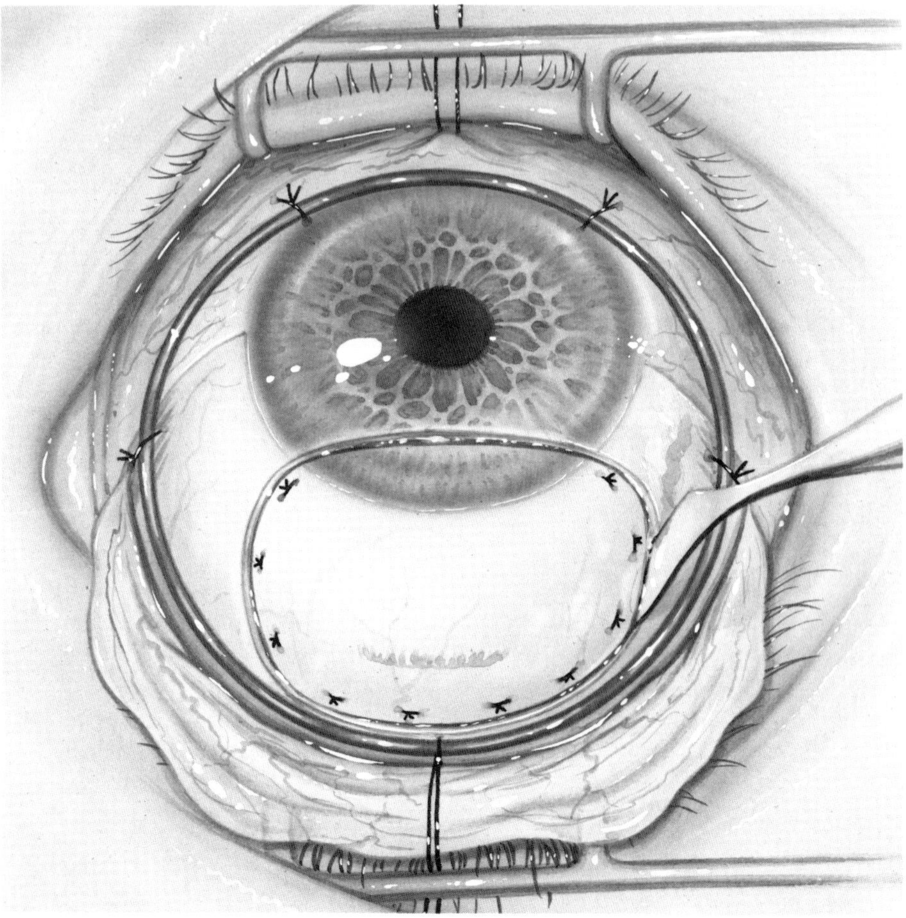

3.**17** The superficial incision is deepened into the sclera and cornea. Intensive diathermy is applied to coagulate the deep scleral and underlying uveal vessels.

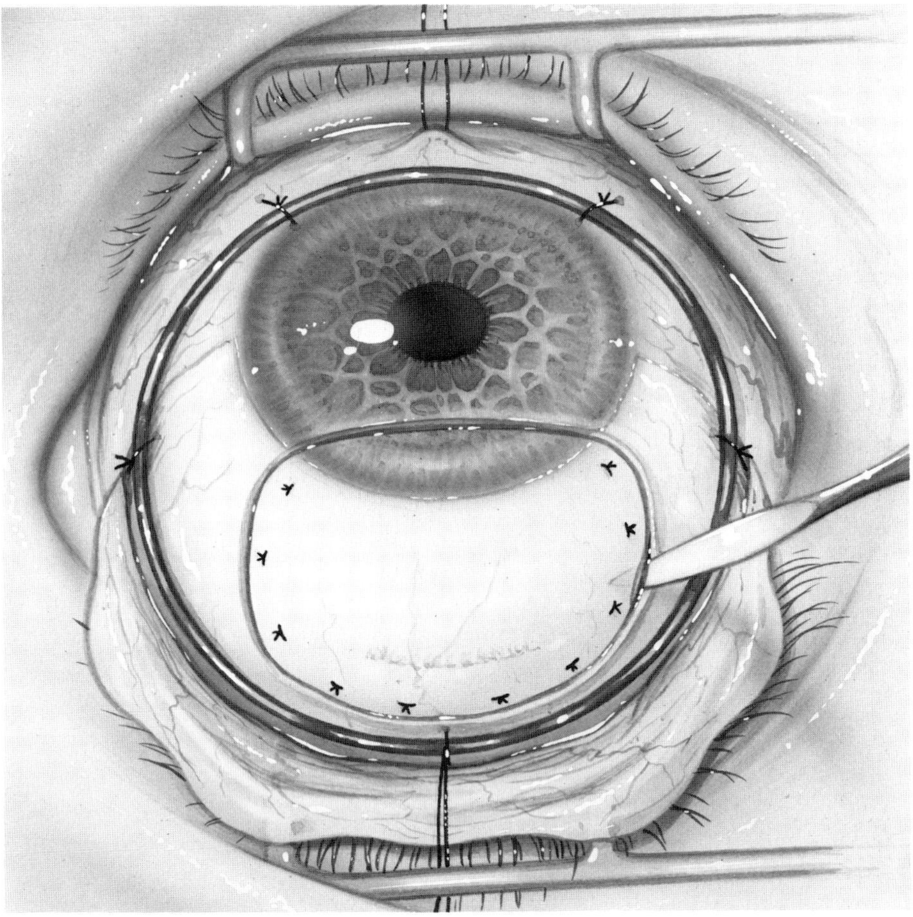

3.**18** A deep posterior sclerotomy is performed to open the posterior chamber.

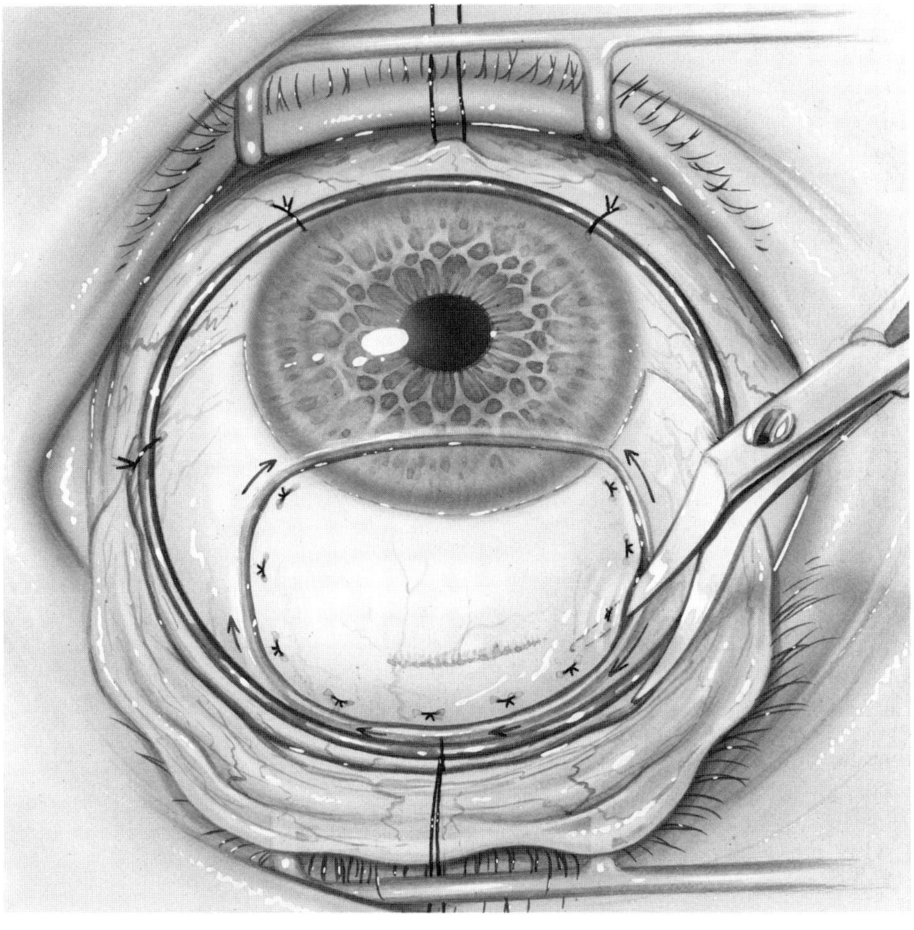

3.**19** Angled scissors (e.g., Troutman) are used to dissect the sclera, ciliary body and/or choroid, including the retina and vitreous.

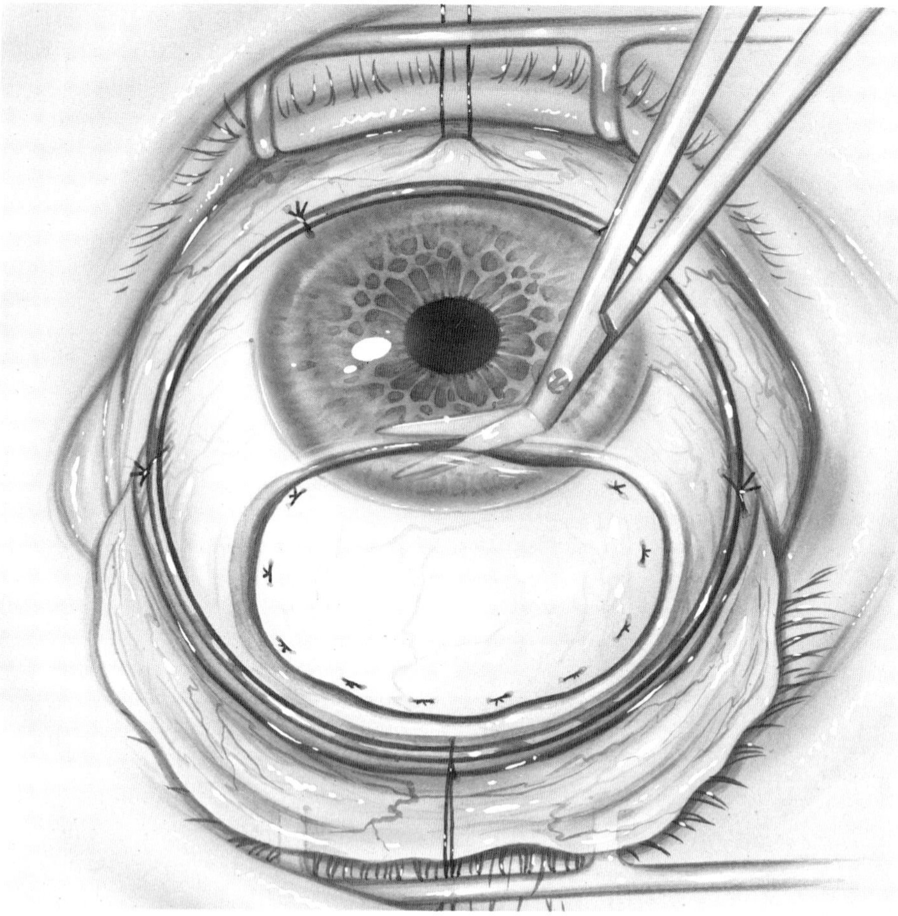

3.**20** Dissection continues through the pars plicata and the corneal segment.

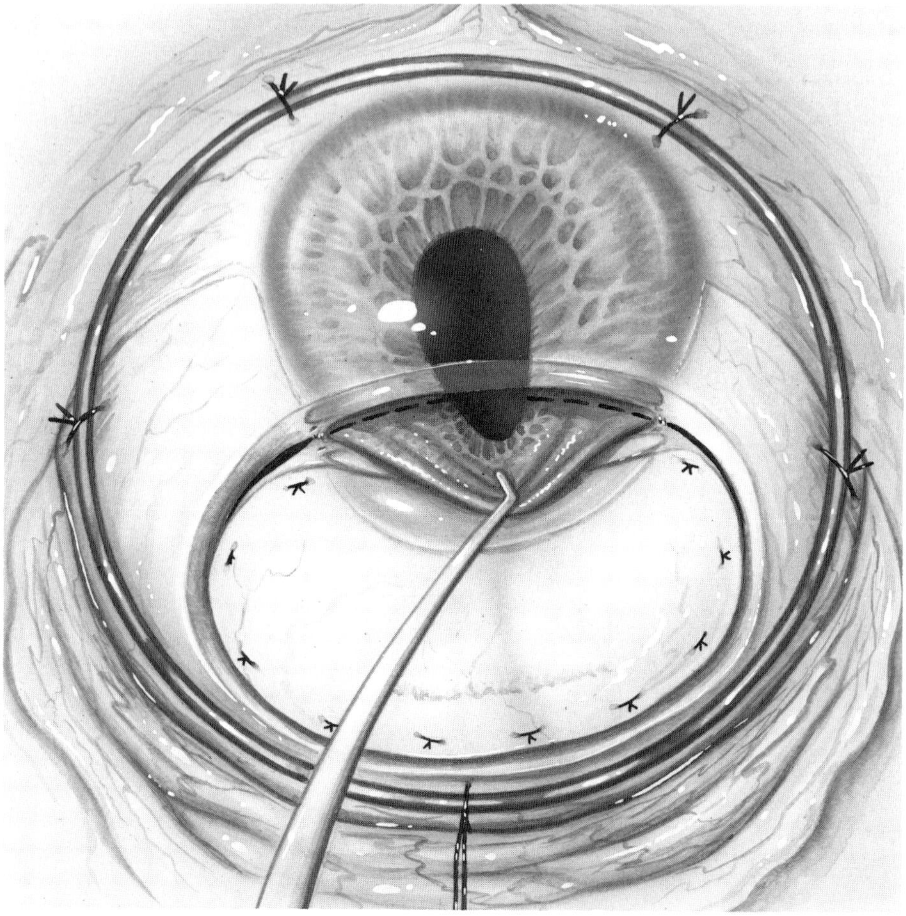

3.**21** A sector iridectomy is performed adjacent to the anterior edge of the tumor.

22

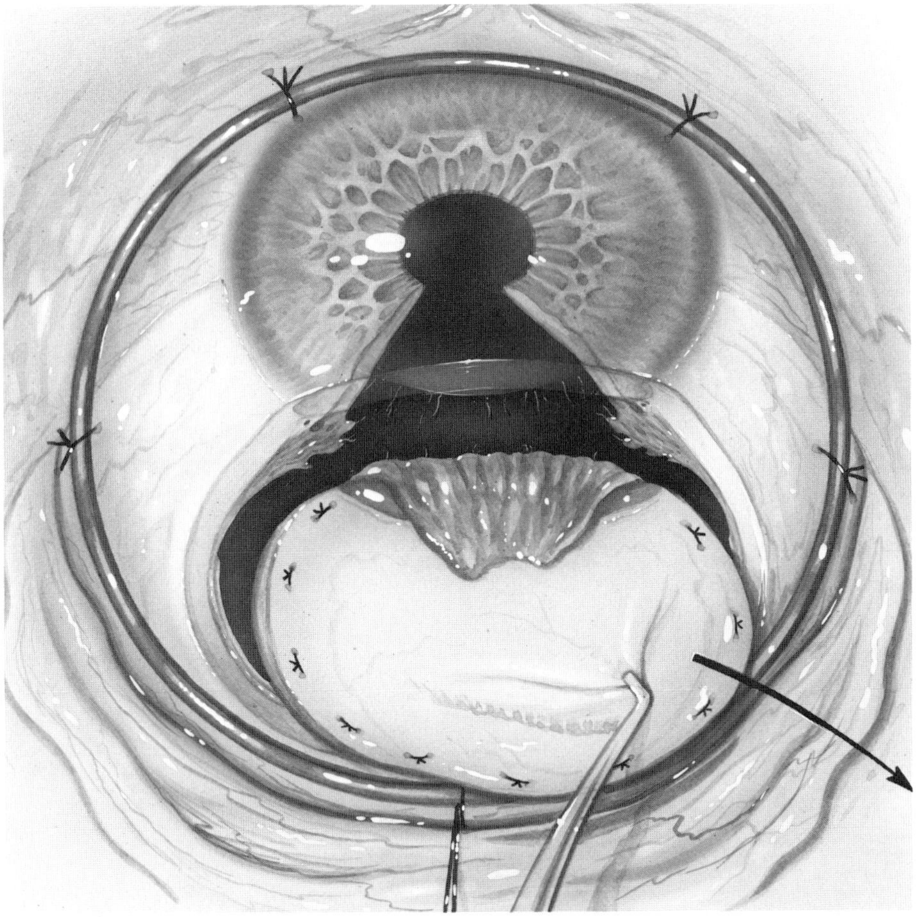

3.**22** The entire tumor, including the adjacent cornea, sclera, retina, vitreous, and iris, is mobilized *en bloc*.

3.**23** Direct bipolar cautery is applied particularly to the dissected vessels of the major arterial circle of the iris and the long ciliary arteries. The lens is removed if the block excision exceeds 120° of the circumference or if the lens is excessively cataractous.

23

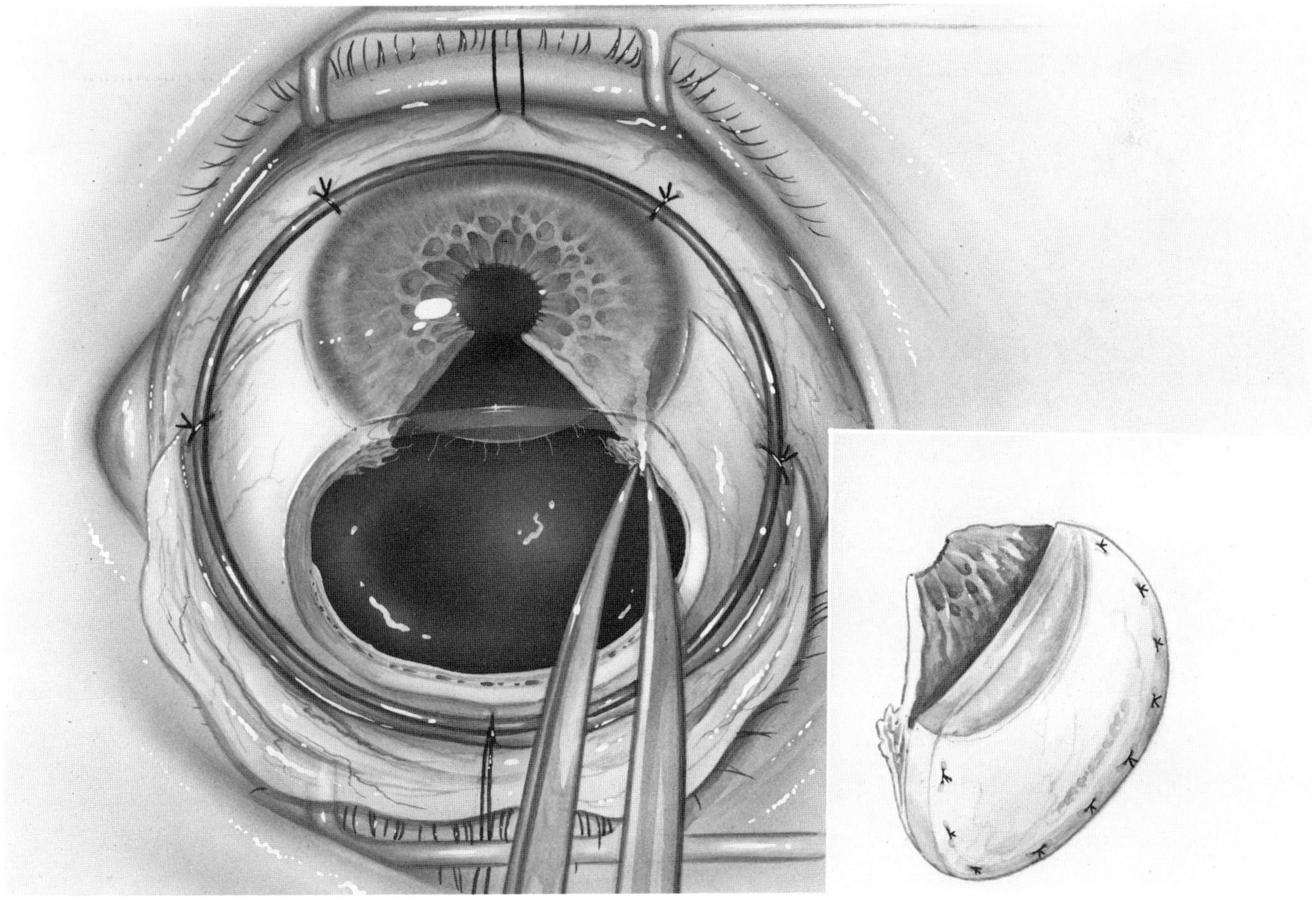

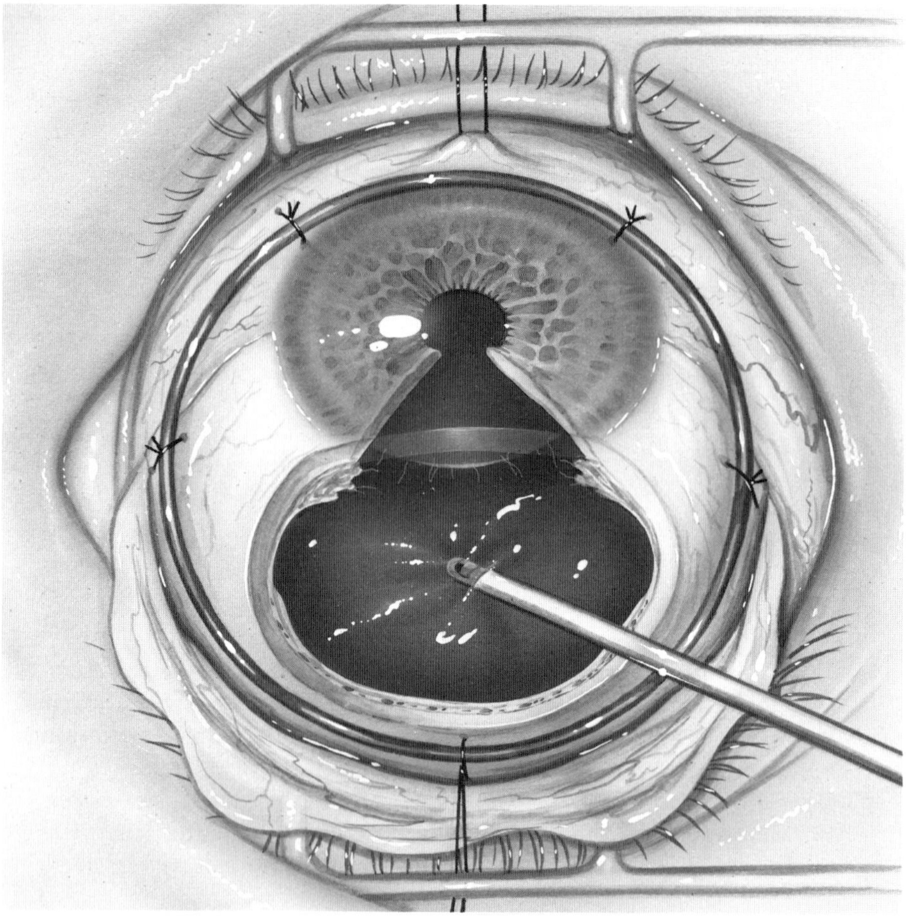

3.**24** Anterior vitrectomy is performed by the sponge or suction-cutting technique.

25

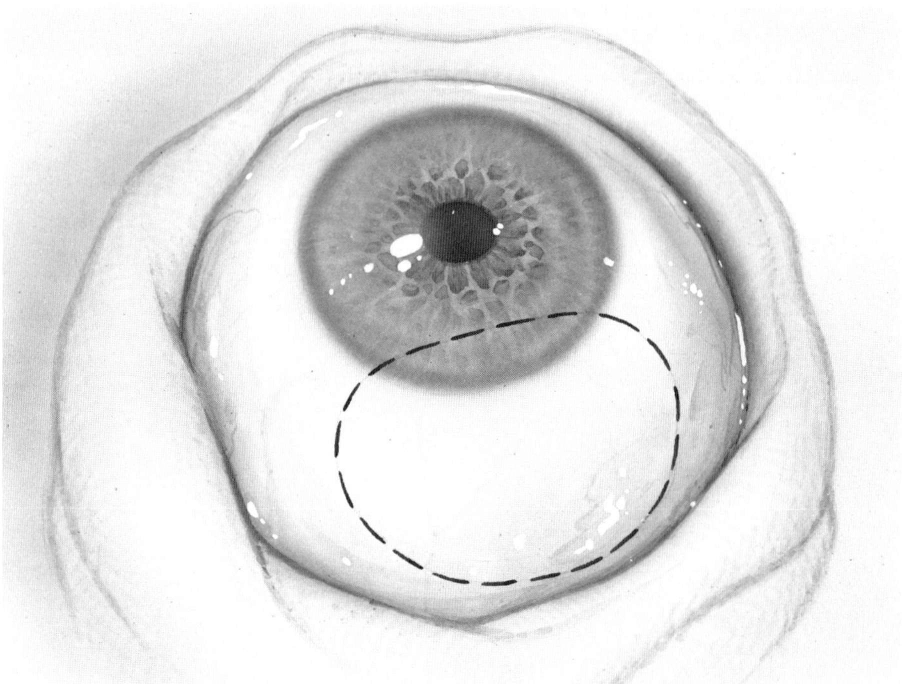

3.**25** and **26** A corresponding corneoscleral transplant is obtained from a donor eye. The diameter of the transplant should be 0.5–1 mm larger than that of the block excision. If the excision is not round, the shape of the transplant should be fashioned with plastic tissue (e.g., from the tissue margins covering the surgical area).

26

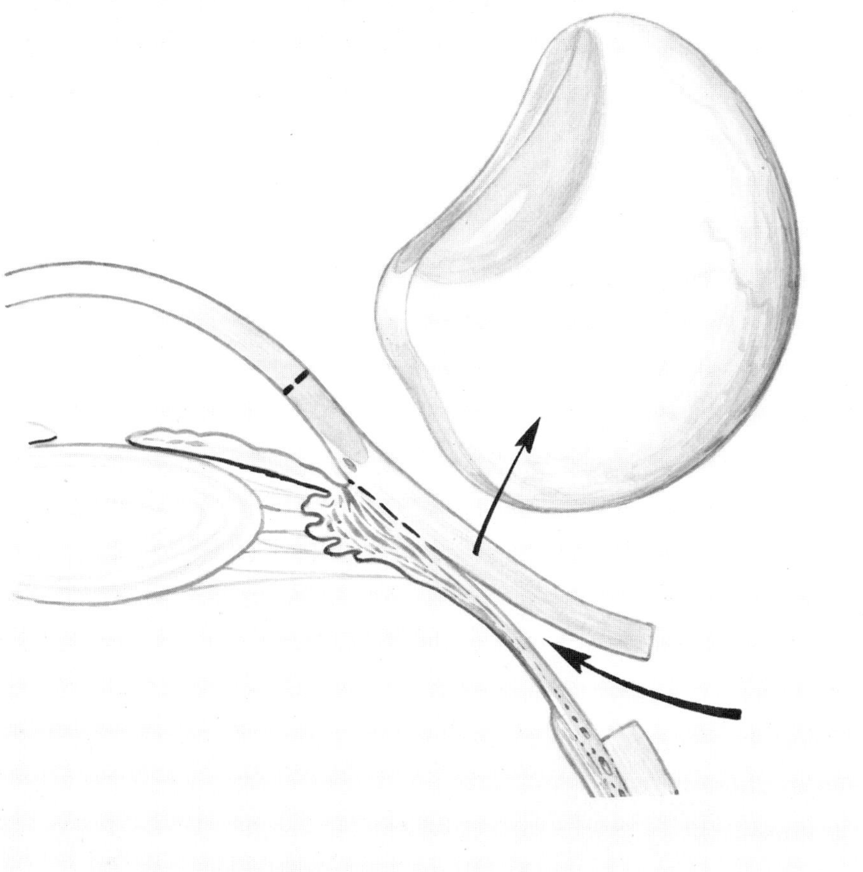

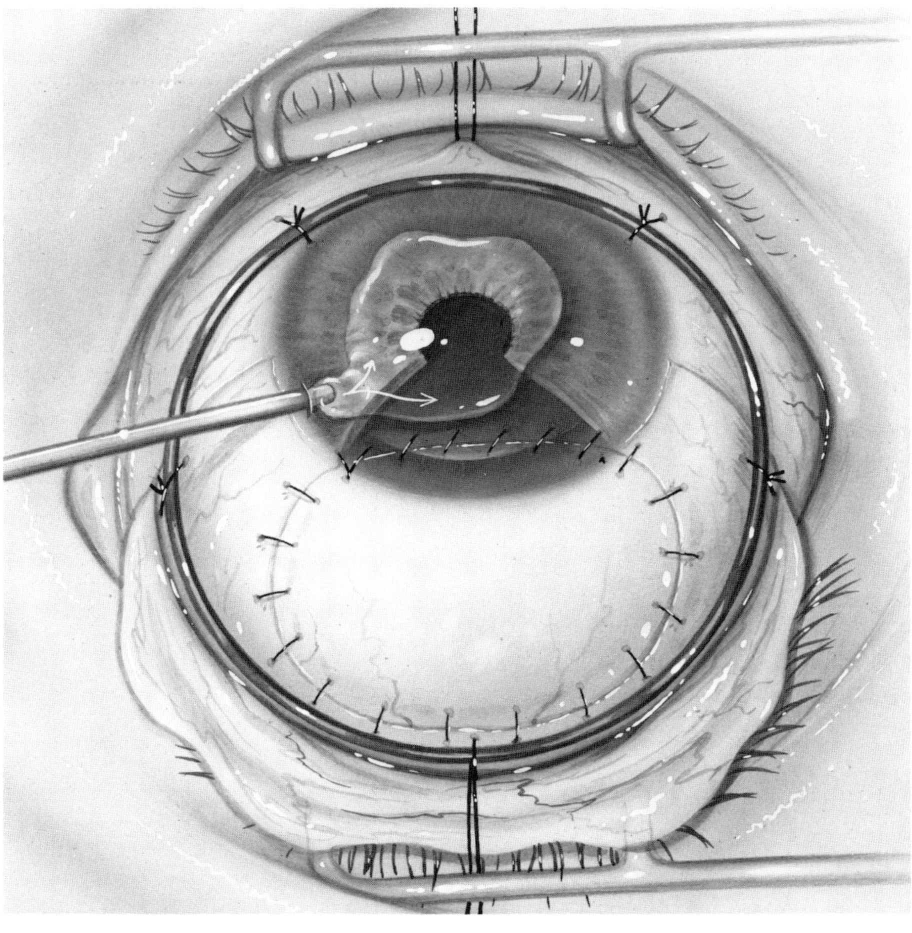

3.**27** The corneoscleral transplant is inserted and fixed in the area of the sclera with interrupted sutures or 8-0 or 10-0 nylon running sutures. A 10-0 nylon running suture is placed in the area of the cornea. Healon, Ringer's solution and/or air is injected to reform the anterior chamber via the preplaced transcorneal paracentesis stab incisions.

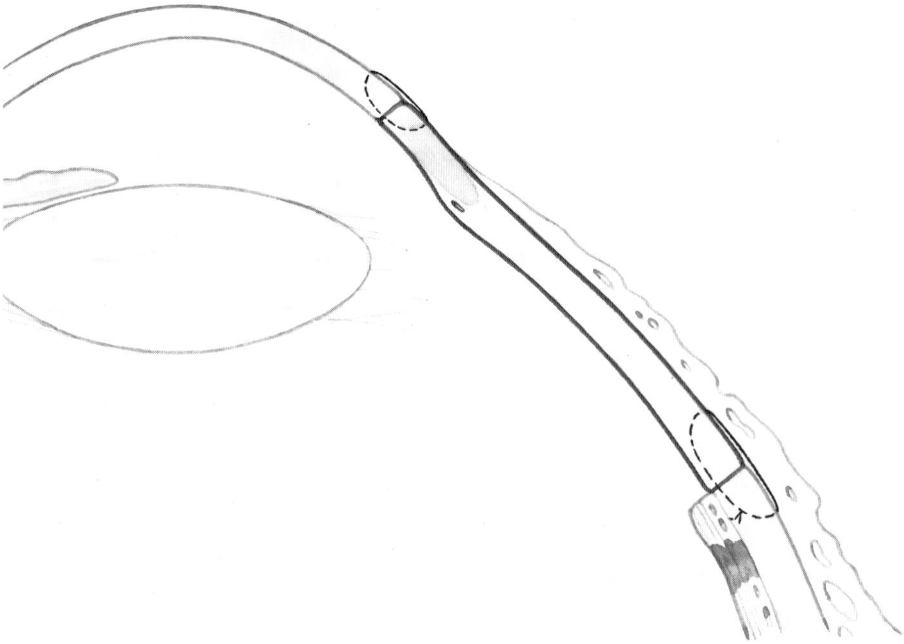

3.**28** The disinserted rectus muscle is reaffixed to the transplant.

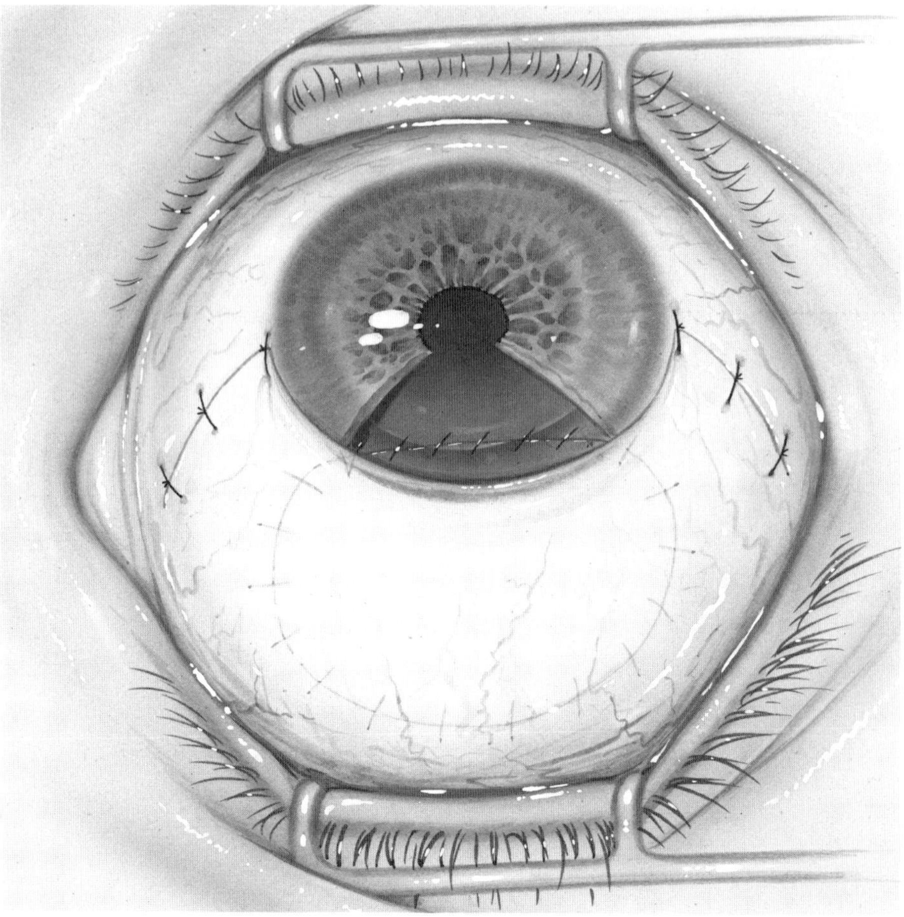

3.**29** The adjacent conjunctiva is mobilized and the conjunctival defect closed.

Modifications

A simple sector iridectomy is only justified for those circumscribed iris tumors that do not encroach on the structures of the angle. The iridectomy can be avoided in tumors of the posterior ciliary body and anterior choroid not involving the pars plicata. I believe, however, that most tumors of the choroid and posterior pars plana are better treated with episcleral ruthenium applicators. In large block excisions, removal of the lens is advisable, because often a cataract develops postoperatively, even if the lens is not injured during the procedure. Preoperative retinopexy is unnecessary in anterior ciliary body tumors.

Intraoperative Complications

This rather extensive procedure, in which often more than one-third of the anterior segment is removed, always involves a number of complications.

Intraoperative *hemorrhage* cannot be completely avoided, in spite of the use of controlled arterial hypotension and bipolar cautery. It usually clears from the anterior chamber without difficulty. Vitreous hemorrhages take some time to clear: if necessary, pars plana vitrectomy can be performed.

Vitreous loss is usually extensive in all tumors extending to the pars plana of the ciliary body. Careful anterior vitrectomy by sponge or instrument is necessary.

Damage to the lens equator sometimes occurs during the cutting procedure. Larger tumors indent the lens equator more than can be appreciated preoperatively. In case of doubt the lens should be removed, because otherwise a cataract will develop, requiring an additional surgical procedure.

Deformation of the wound margins after block excision: careful application of a standard or modified Flieringa ring and injection of Healon reduce this problem.

Misalignment of the corneoscleral tectonic graft can be corrected after placing the preliminary interruped sutures and injection of Healon and air into the globe.

Postoperative Management and Complications

As this procedure involves an extensive opening of the eye, we recommend antibiotics systemically for two days and systemic corticosteroids in decreasing doses for at least one week. Thereafter high doses of local corticosteroids are recommended, tapering off over one year.

The patient should be examined weekly by an ophthalmologist for six weeks, and with decreasing frequency thereafter.

Removal of the running corneal sutures is performed after 12 months or later.

In roughly 100 block excisions for tumors of the anterior uvea and epithelial ingrowth, ranging from 7 mm in diameter to 18 × 14 mm, we have experienced the following postoperative complications.

Hemorrhage can occur on the first day or, more often, five to seven days after surgery. Anterior chamber hemorrhage clears up within a short time, while vitreous hemorrhage may take several weeks or months to be resorbed.

Retinal detachment does not occur, we have found, if proper retinopexy is performed preoperatively. However, in two patients we saw retinal detachment originating from a preoperatively undetected retinal defect remote from the tumor.

Due to the intraocular hemorrhage a transient rise in *intraocular pressure* can develop; this must be treated with the usual local and general measures. Ocular hypotony can occur if more than 150° of the pars plicata is removed. Therefore, I do not recommend this when the tumor involves more than 180° of the pars plicata. In four early cases in our series of block excisions we attempted to remove more than 180° of the circumference of the pars plicata. Phthisis bulbi developed in these four eyes.

With a few exceptions, *immunologic graft reaction* develops weeks or months after grafting, giving rise to the picture of a more or less pronounced anterior uveitis. Corticosteroid therapy is indicated as a countermeasure. The graft reaction stops as soon as the corneoscleral graft is vascularized and scarred. In some patients, surprisingly, the large eccentric graft remains clear indefinitely in its corneal aspect.

Local tumor recurrence: In two patients with malignant epithelioid melanomas of the anterior uvea, we have seen local recurrences remote from the original iris tumor. Block excision is definitely contraindicated if more than the circumscribed nodular tumor area involves the angle structures. This may be difficult to detect in the initial phase, with individual cell-seeding into the anterior chamber from the loose surface of the tumor. Particularly careful follow-up is indicated in patients with malignant melanomas containing epithelioid cells.

If postoperative *glaucoma* occurs in spite of an open angle, one should be very suspicious of an early seeding of tumor cells into the trabecular meshwork.

General metastases: Of more than 50 patients who have undergone block excision for malignant melanomas of the anterior uvea, four died two to four years after surgery.

Block excisions extending over more than 120° of the circumference are frequently followed by postoperative *cataract.* This is particularly true where there is an impression mark of the tumor on the lens. If marked tumor indentation is present, we recommend simultaneous intracapsular removal of the lens during the procedure. If one chooses not to remove the lens and a cataract develops, it can usually be removed by standard intracapsular or extracapsular techniques. However, I am hesitant about recommending lens implantation in such eyes.

Admonitions and Suggestions

Examination of the peripheral fundus must be performed with extreme care, not only in the vicinity of the tumor. All retinal defects should be closed by cryocoagulation or laser coagulation *before* block excision. Otherwise, retinal detachment may develop, originating in these areas in consequence of the anterior vitrectromy which is usually necessary.

Preoperative retinopexy is very important. If extensive collateral retinal detachment or retinal detachment at the ora inferiorly is present, block excision is not advisable.

Preoperative radiation should be given in doses not exceeding, 3 Gy, otherwise the danger of radiation vasopathy can diminish an excellent postoperative result. We have seen this two years after postoperative radiation with 20 Gy in only two doses.

Results

We have performed this procedure in more than 50 patients with tumors of the anterior uvea, over one-third also involving the anterior choroid. The results were certainly not worse than after enucleation (Table 1).

Table 1. Summary of 36 eyes with tumors of the anterior uvea treated by block excision (1981).

Diagnosis	malignant	28
	benign	8
Location:	ciliary body (iris)	21
	choroid (ciliary body)	15
Diameters:	5.5 mm –	
	18 × 15 mm –	
	20 × 12 mm	
Distance behind limbus:	3–18 mm	
Enucleations:		4
Tumor deaths (after 3 and 4 years)		2
Visual results:	0.3–1.0	14
	0.01–0.1	16
	infants	1
	light projection	1

Bibliography

Naumann, G. O. H.: Blockexzision intraokularer Prozesse, I. Tumoren der vorderen Uvea. *Klin. Mbl. Augenheilk.* 166: 436–448, 1975.

Naumann, G. O. H.: Block excision of tumors of the ciliary body and choroid, in Intraocular Tumors, ed. P. K. Lommatzsch and F. C. Blodi, *Fortschritte der Onkologie* Vol. 9. Akademie Verlag, Berlin 1983.

Naumann, G. O. H., Apple, D. J., von Domarus, D., Hinzpeter, E. N., Ruprecht, K. W., Völcker, H. E., Naumann, L. R.: *Pathology of the Eye.* Springer, New York, 1986.

Naumann, G. O. H., Hadlock, I.: *Zur Technik der Zyklektomie* (film shown at the 72nd Annual Congress of the *Deutsche Ophthalmologische Gesellschaft, 1972).* Ber. *Dtsch. Ophthal. Ges.* 72: 481–484, 1974.

Naumann, G. O. H., Völcker, H. E., Gäckle, H. E.: The block excision of malignant melanomas of the ciliary body and the peripheral choroid. *Docum. Ophth.* 50: 43–48, 1980.

Weidle, E. G., Völcker, H. E., Naumann, G. O. H.: Epitheleinwachsung in das vordere Augensegment an der Universitäts-Augenklinik Tübingen (1975–1978), in *Wundheilung des Auges und ihre Komplikationen.* Bergmann, Munich 1980, pages 141–145.

Block Excision of Cystic and Diffuse Epithelial Ingrowth

Surgical Principles

Both cystic and diffuse epithelial ingrowths practically always cover the anterior surface of the ciliary body in the chamber angle region. (Only the rare isolated cysts of the iris stroma sparing the angle can be removed completely by simple sector iridectomy.)

All epithelial ingrowth involving the angle requires removal of the adjacent structures of the iris, cornea, and pars plicata of the ciliary body. Otherwise recurrences originate from residual islands of the cystic or diffuse epithelial ingrowth always persisting in the eye after simple iridectomy.

This cannot be cured by resecting only the areas of cornea in contact with the epithelial ingrowth. As the fragile epithelial cyst or the diffuse epithelial ingrowth, sometimes consisting of only one to three cell layers, cannot be separated from the adjacent tissues, these have to be removed also. In other words, they serve as a mold for the delicate epithelial structures, assuring complete removal.

Preparation for Surgery

Preoperative radiation is *not* prescribed. Preoperative chorioretinal cryopexy is not usually necessary, because only in exceptional circumstances does epithelial ingrowth extend posteriorly beyond the pars plicata. Otherwise, the preparations for surgery are the same as for tumors (see foregoing section).

Preoperative Medication and Anesthesia

See "Block Excision for Tumors" above.

Instruments

See "Block Excision for Tumors" above.

Surgical Technique

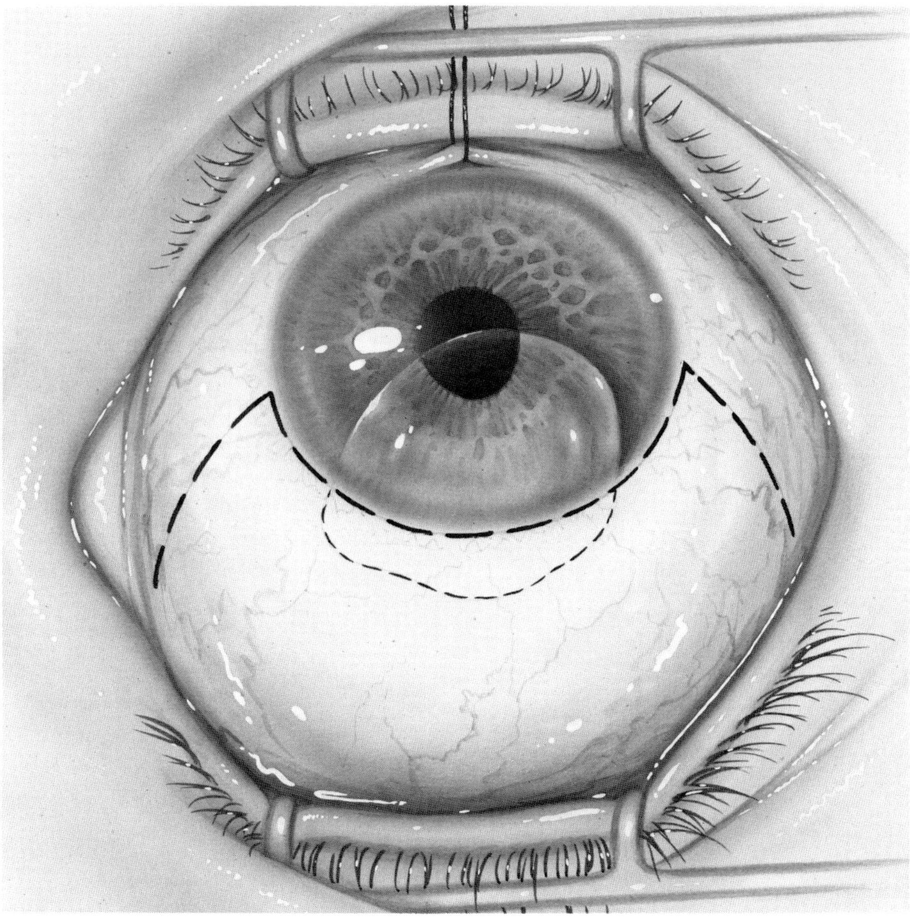

3.**30** An extensive fornix-based conjunctival flap is created with radial incisions at the margins. The opposing rectus muscles are held with direct traction sutures.

31

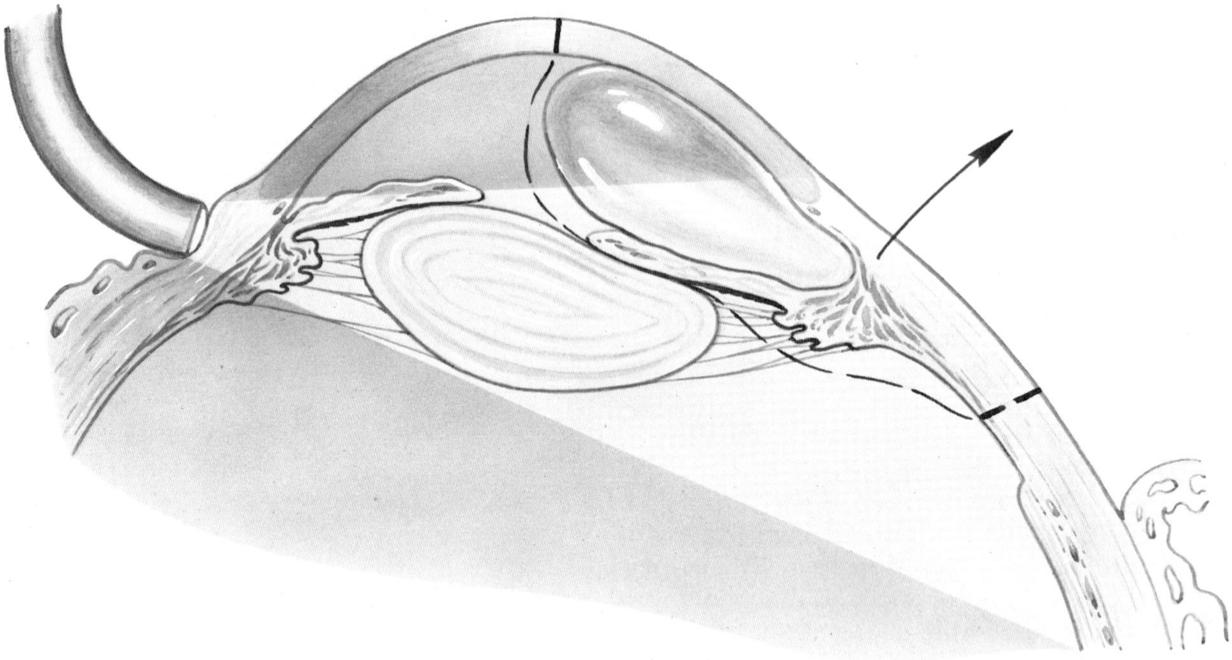

32

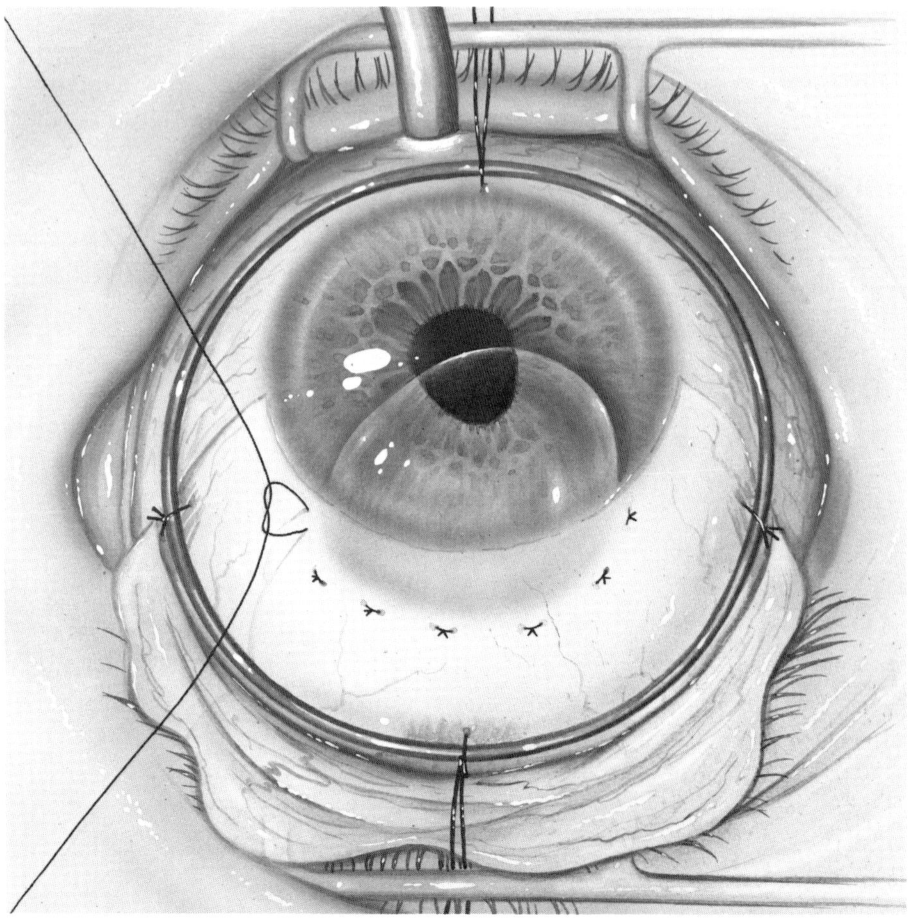

3.**31** The extent of the ingrowth is visualized via intensive fiber optic transillumination. This is particularly easy with cystic epithelial ingrowth.

3.**32** The margin of the lesion is delineated with simple interrupted sutures or coagulation marks. A Flieringa ring is fixed episclerally to surround the lesion.
Note: Simultaneous drainage of the cyst by a trans-corneoscleral paracentesis, and healon-injection into the anterior chamber reduces the size of the intact cyst. The extent of removal of cornea and pars plicata thus is minimized!

33

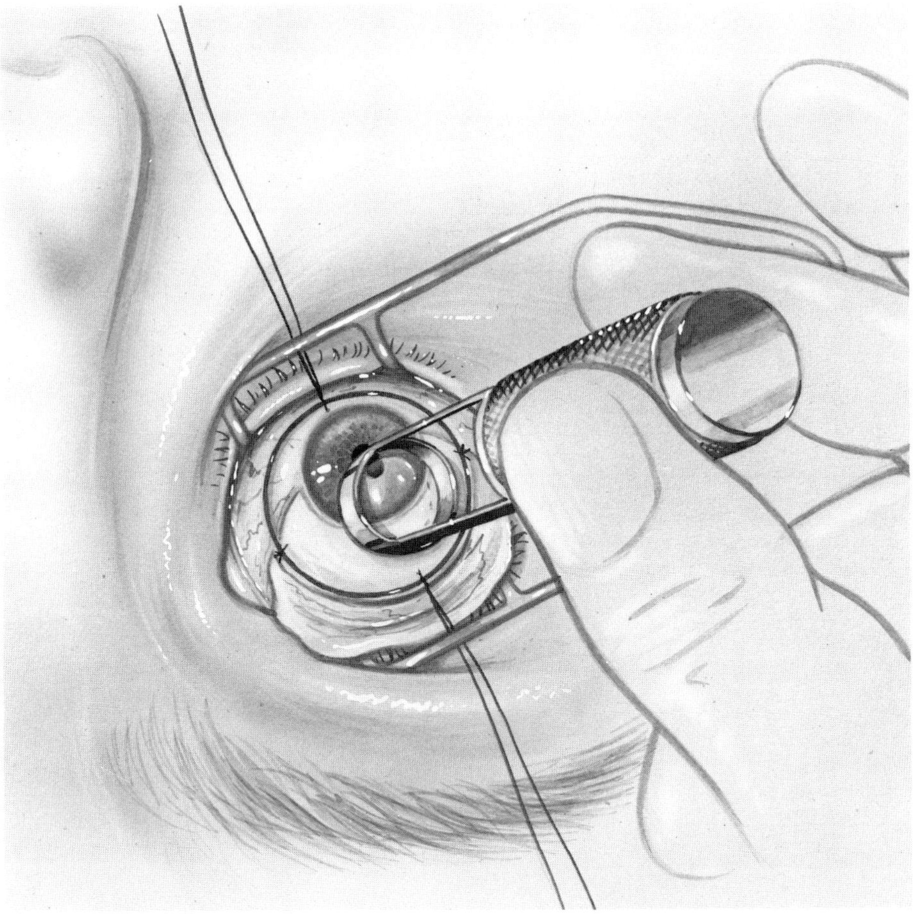

3.**33** A trephine of appropriate diameter is positioned over the lesion. The trephine must be open to permit microscopic observation and control of the cutting process.

3.**34** A superficial incision is made in the sclera and cornea adjacent to the cyst. Intensive diathermy is applied via a coagulation knife to the deeper scleral layers and the adjacent ciliary body tissue. A posterior sclerotomy is performed and the sclera and adjacent ciliary body and iris are dissected with scissors. A sector iridectomy is performed as in removal of tumors of the anterior uvea. The intact cyst or the diffuse ingrowth together with the adjacent tissues involved is removed *en bloc.*

34

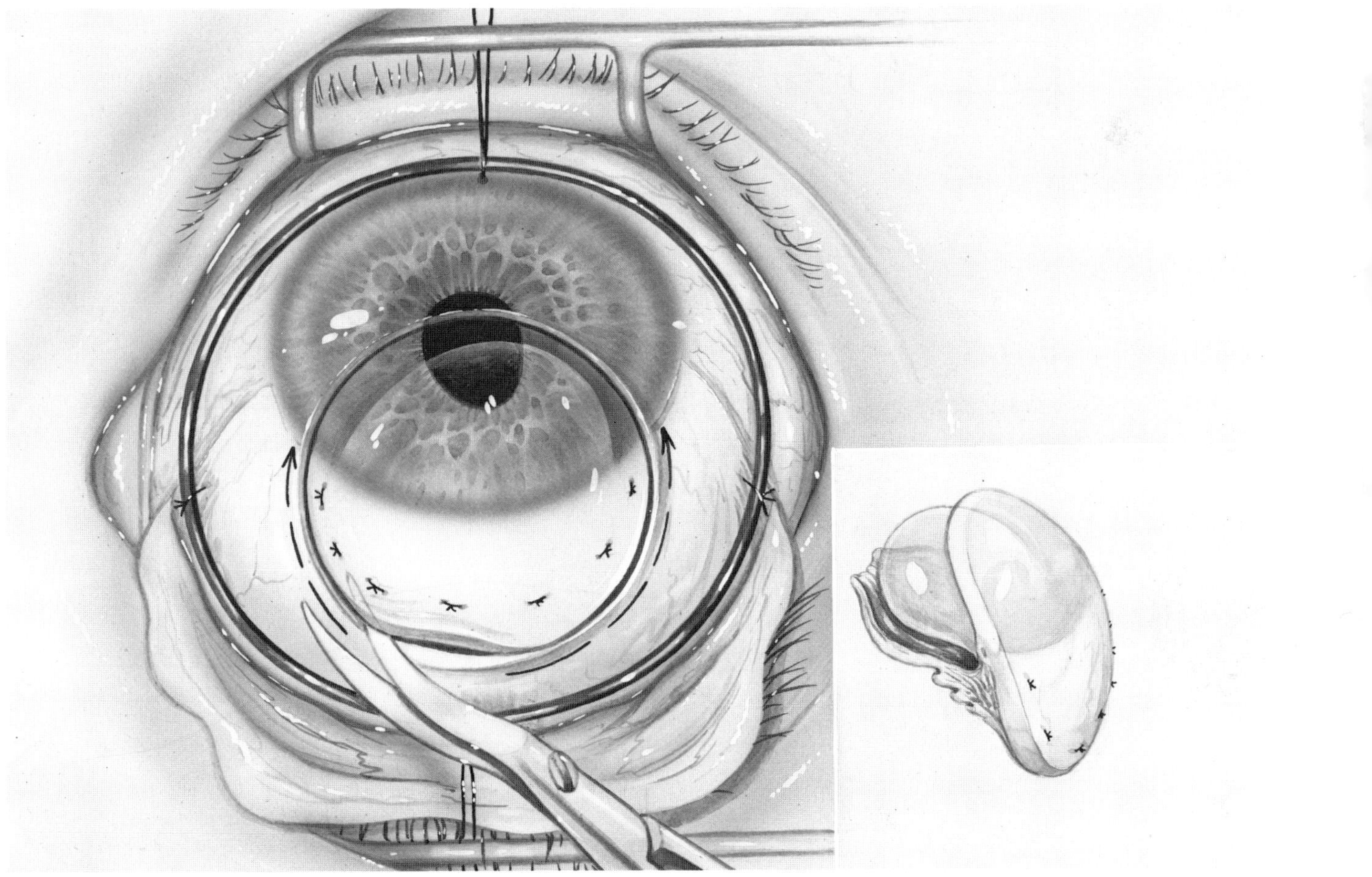

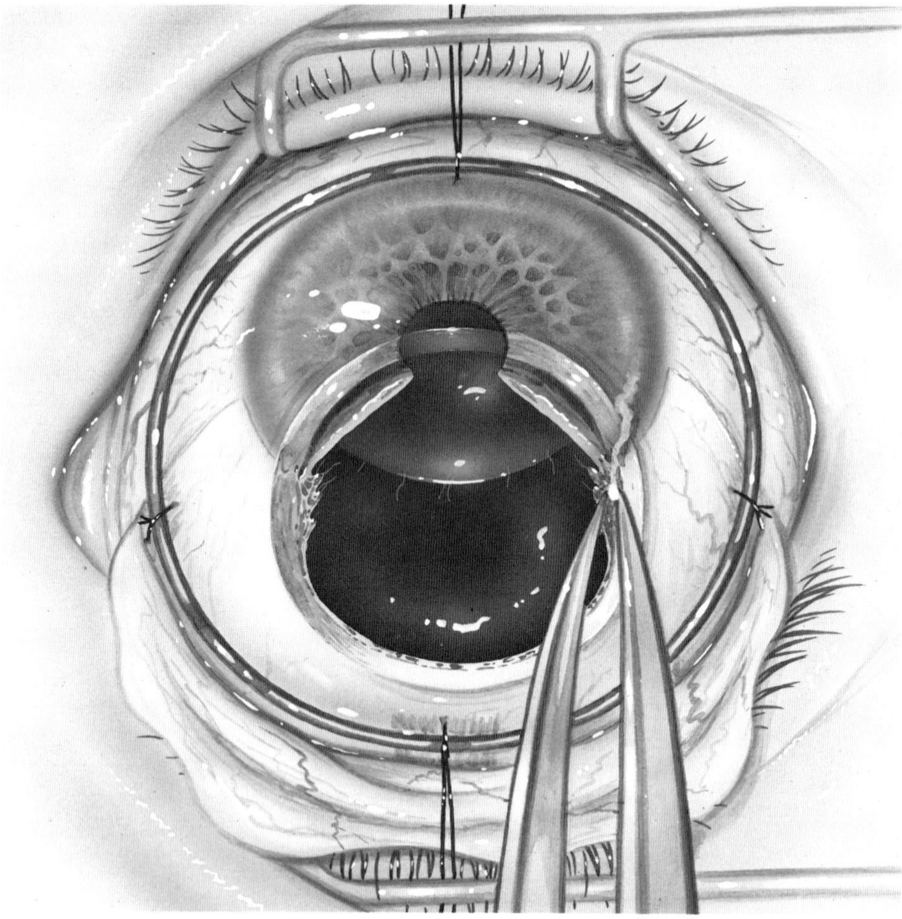

3.**35** Bipolar cautery of the major ciliary arteries and veins is done if necessary. An anterior vitrectomy is performed.

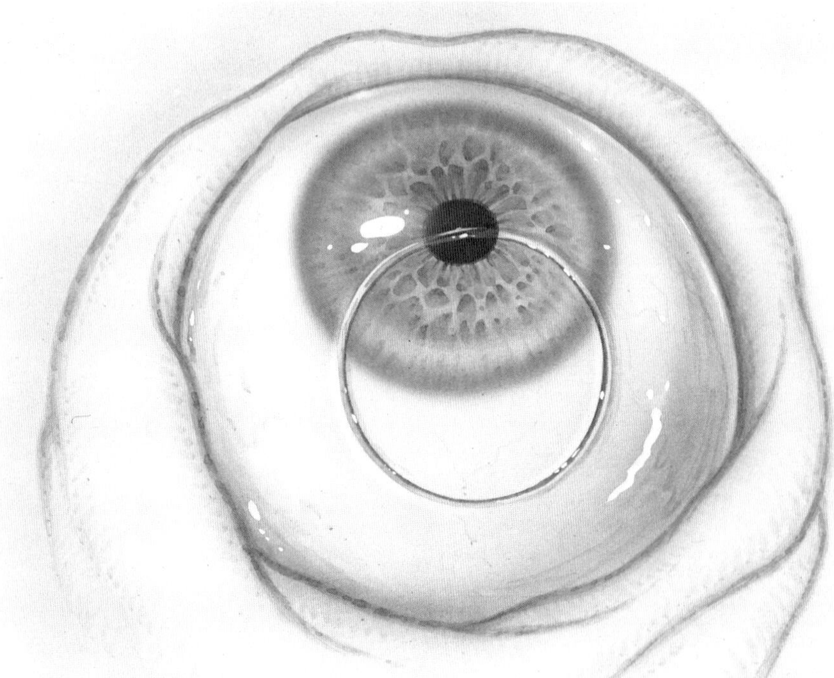

3.**36** The defect in the ocular wall is covered with a tectonic corneal or corneoscleral transplant graft of analogous shape and extent.

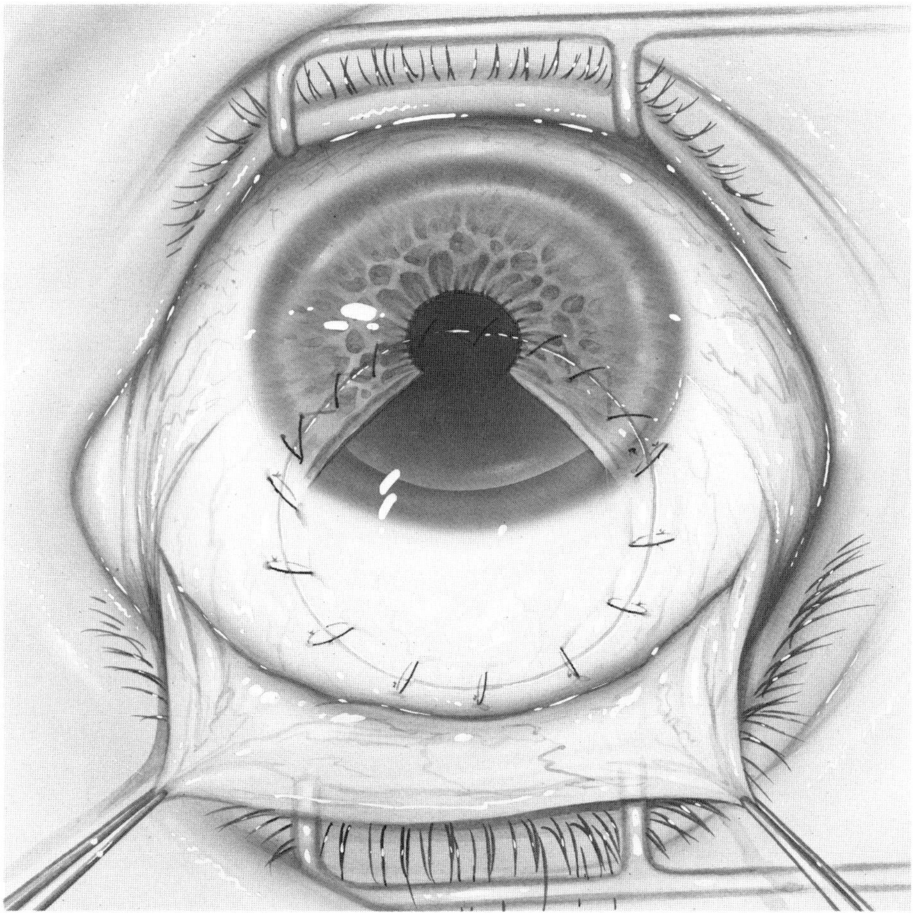

3.**37** Running sutures are used at the corneal edge of the wound, interrupted sutures at the scleral edge.

Modifications

A simple sector iridectomy will cure an epithelial ingrowth only if the lesion is confined to the iris and does not involve the angle structures. If the ingrowth does involve the angle structures, a simple iridectomy will convert a cystic ingrowth into a diffuse epithelial one and thus make matters worse.

Epithelial ingrowths involving more than 150–180° of the circumference cannot be cured by block excision (see fig. 3.32): in our experience the eye will become atrophic. In these situations we attempt to remove the epithelial ingrowth by closed anterior vitrectomy, trying to remove the epithelial structures together with the adjacent iris. Afterward we inject air into the anterior chamber and attempt to destroy the epithelium by cryocoagulation. This procedure has not been very effective: a recurrence has always occurred in the five eyes treated in this fashion.

Intraoperative Complications

Since preoperative radiation is not performed, intraoperative *hemorrhage* is less pronounced than with tumors. *Vitreous loss* occurs if the original trauma involved the vitreous surface.

The other complications associated with block excision of tumors are also encountered here.

Admonitions and Suggestions

If a cystic epithelial ingrowth involves the anterior chamber to such an extent that a block excision would involve more than 150° of the pars plicata, the following maneuver with Healon may be helpful.

A stab incision is made through the cornea or corneoscleral region into the lumen of the cystic epithelial ingrowth and fluid is aspirated. This usually causes the cyst to shrink somewhat. Through a preplaced transcorneal stab incision opposite the root of the cystic epithelial ingrowth, Healon is injected into the anterior chamber, thus compressing the cyst wall to a size that can be completely removed by our standard block excision technique.

As with tumors, the examination of the peripheral retinal fundus is important to rule out any retinal defects – particularly if vitreous loss is encountered.

Postoperative Management and Complications

If complete removal of the diffuse epithelial ingrowth is achieved, any pre-existing secondary open-angle *glaucoma* will clear up. Secondary angle-closure glaucomas require conventional therapy or direct pars plicata diathermy (see below).

Otherwise postoperative management and postoperative complications are similar to those for tumors, but usually to a lesser degree.

Results

We have performed more than 40 block excisions for cystic and diffuse epithelial ingrowth. If the ingrowth does not extend over more than 150° of the circumference, complete removal can be achieved with satisfactory anatomical and functional results.

Bibliography

[1] Naumann, G. O. H.: Blockexzision intraokularer Prozesse, I. Tumoren der vorderen Uvea. *Klin. Mbl. Augenheilk.* 166: 436–448, 1975

[2] Naumann, G. O. H. and H. E. Völcker: Blockexzision intraokularer Prozesse. II. Epitheleinwachsung in den vorderen Augenabschnitten. *Klin. Mbl. Augenheilk.* 166: 448–457, 1975.

[3] Naumann, G. O. H. and D. J. Apple with contributions by D. von Domarus, E. N. Hinzpeter, R. M. Manthey, L. R. Naumann, K. W. Ruprecht, H. E. Völcker: *Pathology of the Eye*, Springer Verlag New York-Berlin-Heidelberg-Tokyo, 1986

[4] Weidle, E. G., H. E. Völcker, G. O. H. Naumann: Epitheleinwachsung in das vordere Augensegment an der Universitäts-Augenklinik Tübingen (1975–1978) in: G. O. H. Naumann und B. Gloor (ed.) „*Wundheilung des Auges und ihre Komplikationen*", p. 141–145 Bergmann Verlag, München, 1980

Direct Pars Plicata Diathermy

Surgical Principles

The pars plicata of the ciliary body is coagulated by diathermy over 90–120° of its circumference in order to reduce aqueous secretion. This is never the first choice of surgical therapy.

It is a helpful approach to those secondary glaucomas without rubeosis iridis which are resistant to standard medical or surgical therapy, e.g., secondary open-angle glaucomas in aphakic patients after intracapsular cataract extraction or after extracapsular cataract extraction with a defect in the posterior lens capsule when there is no response to medication, laser trabeculoplasty, and/or glaucoma filtering procedures. Another main indication is complete and irreversible secondary angle-closure glaucoma after delayed therapy for pupillary block angle-closure glaucoma.

Preparation for Surgery

The procedure is only indicated if standard medical and surgical therapy (including laser trabeculoplasty) has failed. On the day before surgery a conjunctival swab and bacterial cultures are performed. Only if there is bacterial growth local antibiotics are given.

Preoperative Medication and Anesthesia

Local and systemic prostaglandin inhibitors are given to reduce the "paracentesis effects". Local anesthesia is generally sufficient, as the globe is not opened.

Instruments

In addition to the standard instrument tray for lamellar keratoplasty, a diathermy apparatus with an electrolysis needle 1–1 mm long is needed.

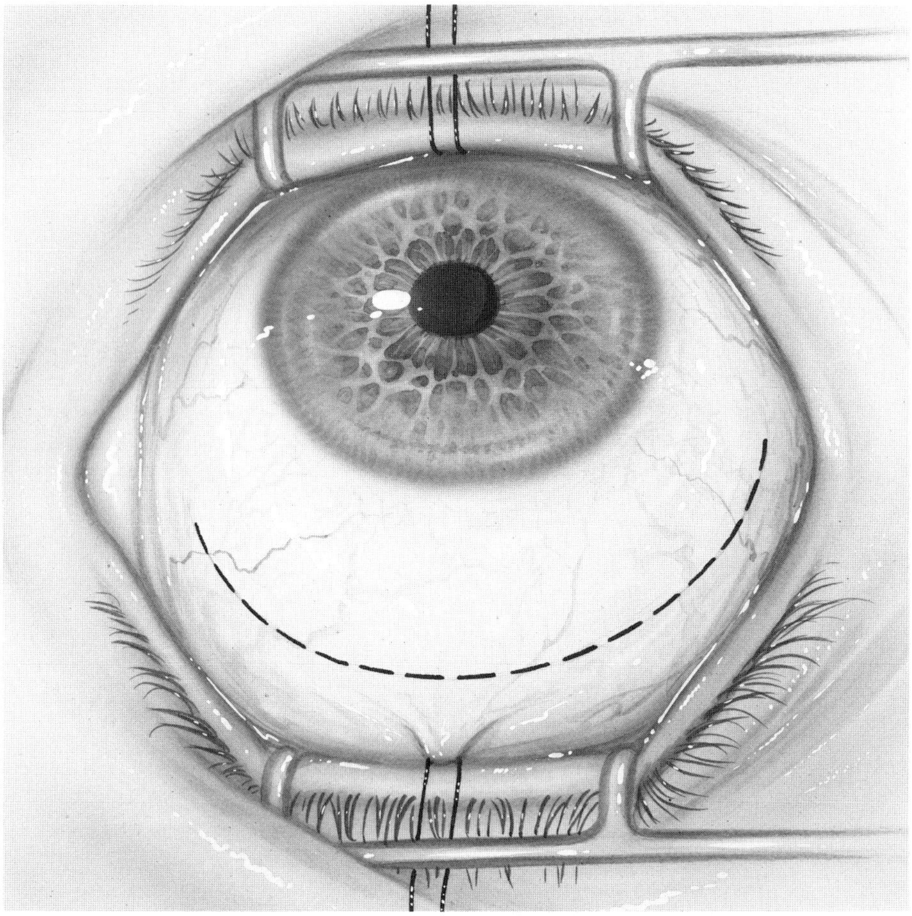

Surgical Technique

3.**38** A wide limbus-based conjunctival flap is created over 120–150°.

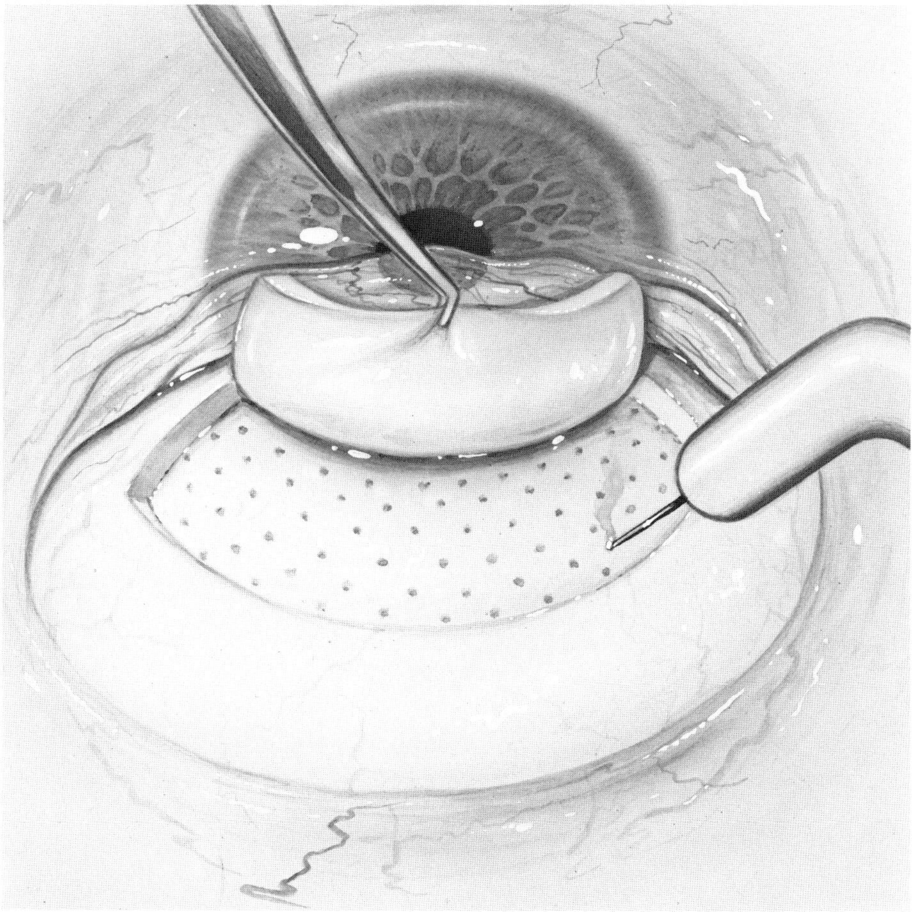

3.**39** A very thick limbus-based scleral flap 4 mm wide is prepared, involving 90–120° of the circumference. An effort is made to leave only very few layers of the basal sclera, so that the ciliary muscle can be seen through these remaining deep scleral layers.

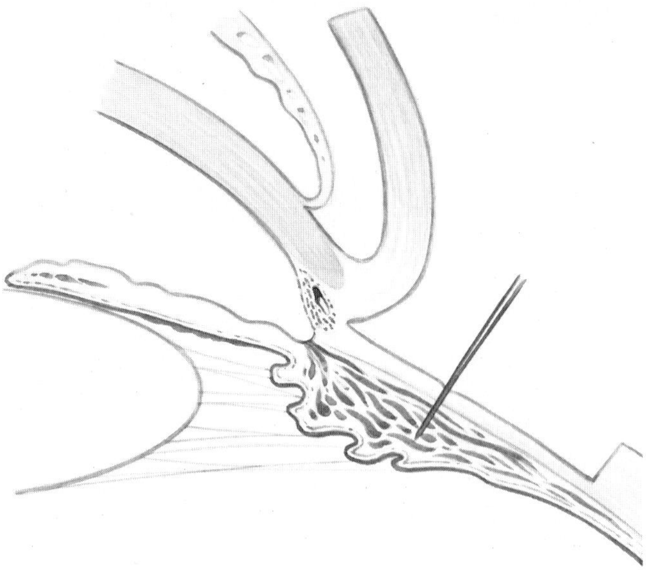

3.**40** The diathermy applications are performed by inserting the diathermy needle 2 mm behind the scleral spur and about 1–2 mm through the sclera. In aphakic eyes longer needles are used. In phakic eyes care must be taken not to injure the lens. Intensive diathermy applications are performed to achieve destruction of the treated sector of the pars plicata of the ciliary body.

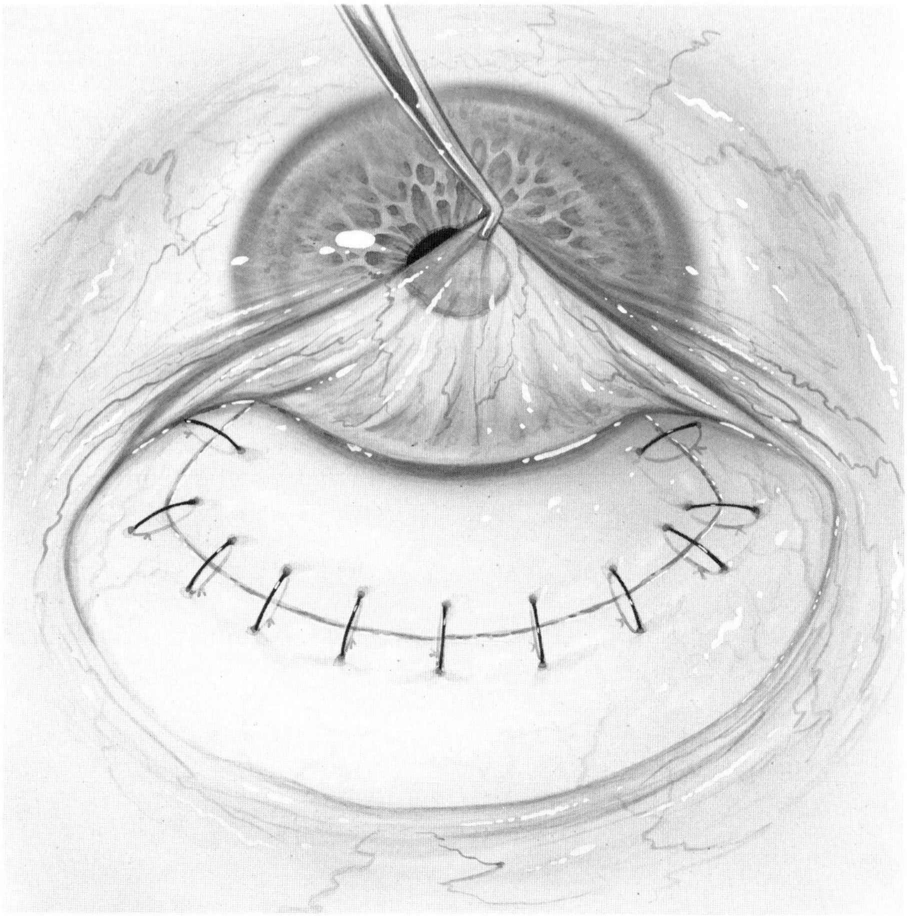

3.**41** The scleral flap is then closed with interrupted sutures of 10-0 or 8-0 nylon.

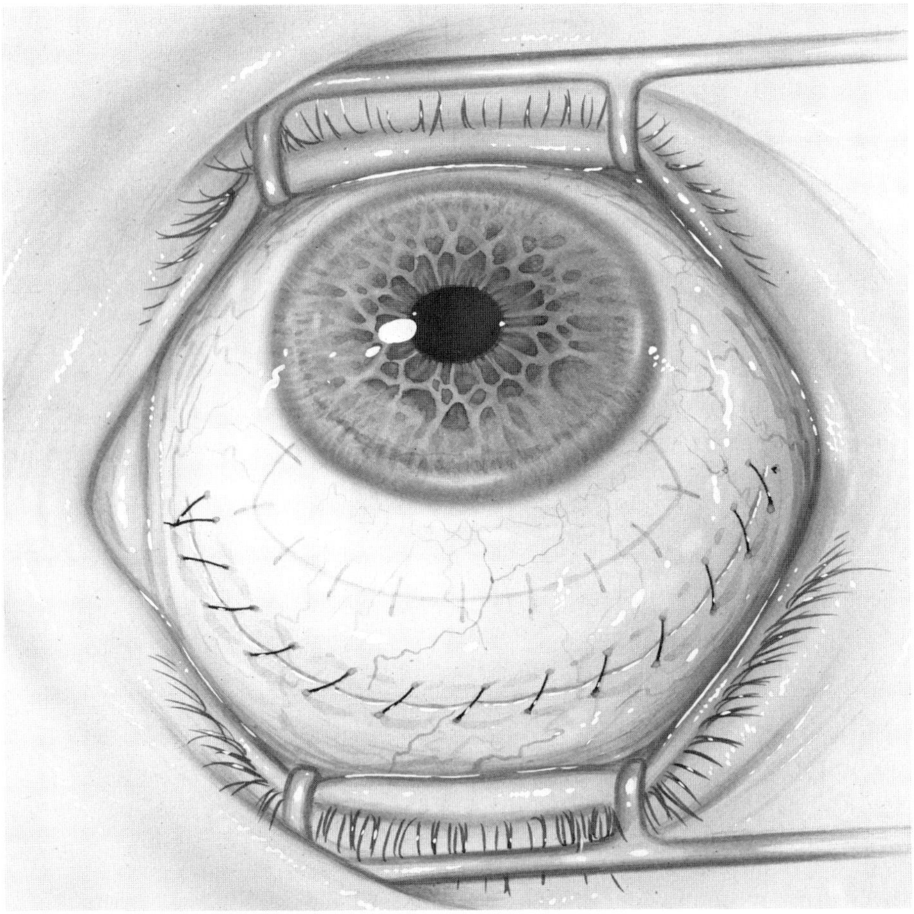

3.**42** The conjunctival flap covers the entire area of the procedure.

Modifications

In our experience, cryocoagulation often fails to produce a lasting effect (see below). Diathermy through all the layers of the sclera leads to necrosis of the entire eye wall and to staphyloma, so we do not use it.

Intraoperative Complications

Transscleral loss of aqueous: If the needle passes through the basal layer of the sclera and the ciliary body into the posterior chamber, aqueous may be lost. This is not of any significance. Care must be taken to achieve a watertight closure of the scleral and conjunctival wound.

Vitreous losses through needle punctures: If the scleral window is placed too far posteriorly, vitreous may be incarcerated by the diathermy needle. Additional needle applications must be placed more anteriorly.

Admonitions and Suggestions

The lamellar scleral flap should be as thick as possible, assuring sufficient viable scleral tissue to cover the area of intensive diathermy coagulation. Otherwise, late scleral staphyloma may develop. As the diathermy applications destroy most of the deep scleral layers, watertight closure of the scleral and conjunctival wound is mandatory.

Postoperative Management and Complications

Postnecrotic anterior uveitis. As a significant part of the pars plicata of the ciliary body is destroyed, there is always a marked inflammatory reaction immediately after surgery. This can be reduced by preoperative medication with prostaglandin inhibitors (see above) and treated by local and if necessary systemic corticosteroids. Some *hemorrhage* occurs in the first few postoperative days or after an interval of five to seven days, when spontaneous postoperative intravascular thrombolysis occurs.

Postoperative cataract. Care must be taken not to injure the lens equator; cataracts will then seldom appear. However, over the course of months and years, these eyes usually develop a nuclear cataract much earlier than other eyes.

Results

Intraocular pressure is lowered to some extent in practically all eyes. Depending on the degree of involvement of the chamber angle, this implies regulation of pressure with or without additional medication. If pressure is not satisfactorily regulated even with medication, the procedure can be repeated at another site. Additional cryocoagulation may be necessary to achieve a balance between inflow and outflow of aqueous and compensation of pressure.

Pars Plicata Excision and Reconstruction of the Anterior Segment

Surgical Principles

This is an extreme and exceptional approach to aphakic eyes with massive glaucoma in relatively young patients. It is only indicated in "hopeless" secondary angle-closure glaucoma without rubeosis iridis. Most of the conditions in this category follow serious complications after anterior segment surgery or long-delayed wound closure after neglected trauma. Most of these eyes have an extremely shallow anterior chamber or none at all ("athalamia"). This is the "last resort" surgical procedure for otherwise "lost" eyes.

Preparation for Surgery

An extensive preoperative work-up including A and B ultrasonography, electroretinography, and VEP is indicated to rule out contraindicative pathology of the posterior segment. In posttraumatic eyes, X-ray studies should be done to rule out foreign bodies. Local and systemic prostaglandin inhibitors are given to reduce the "paracentesis effect". Otherwise preparations are the same as for all intraocular surgery.

Preoperative Medication and Anesthesia

The procedure should be performed under general anesthesia, including controlled arterial hypotension. Patients in the older age groups are not usually suitable for this type of surgery.

Instruments

The same instruments are required as for block excision of tumors.

Surgical Technique

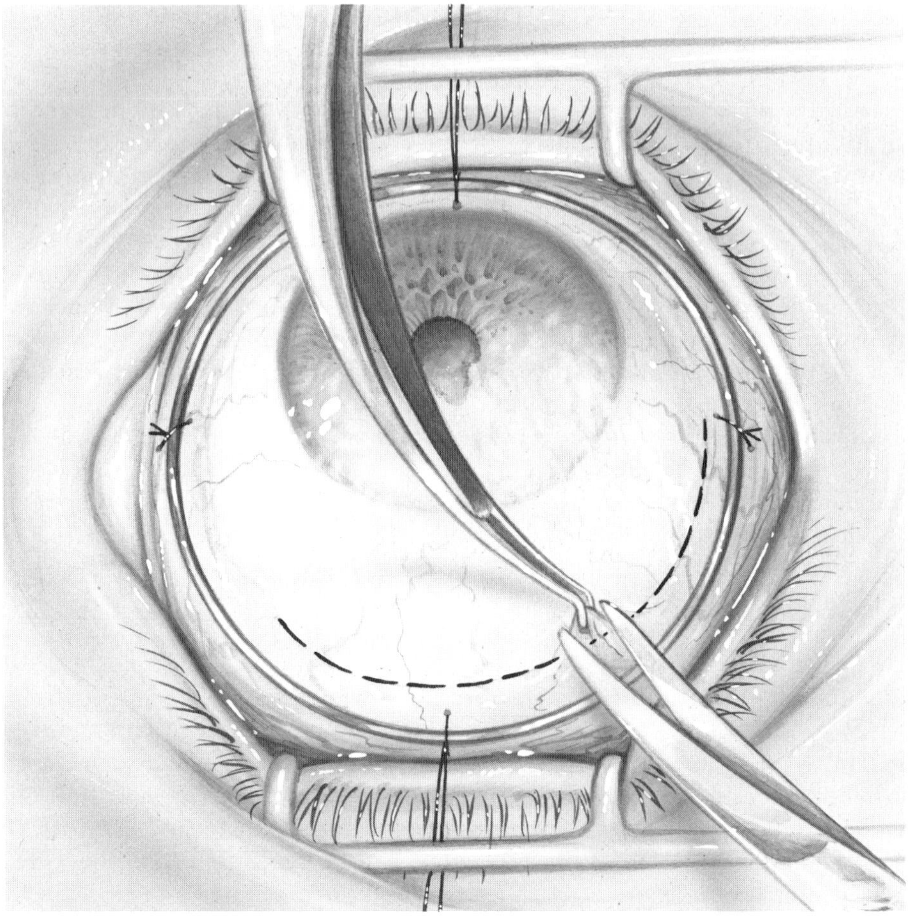

3.**43** An extensive limbus-based conjunctival flap is created. A Flieringa ring is applied to prevent collapse of the globe.

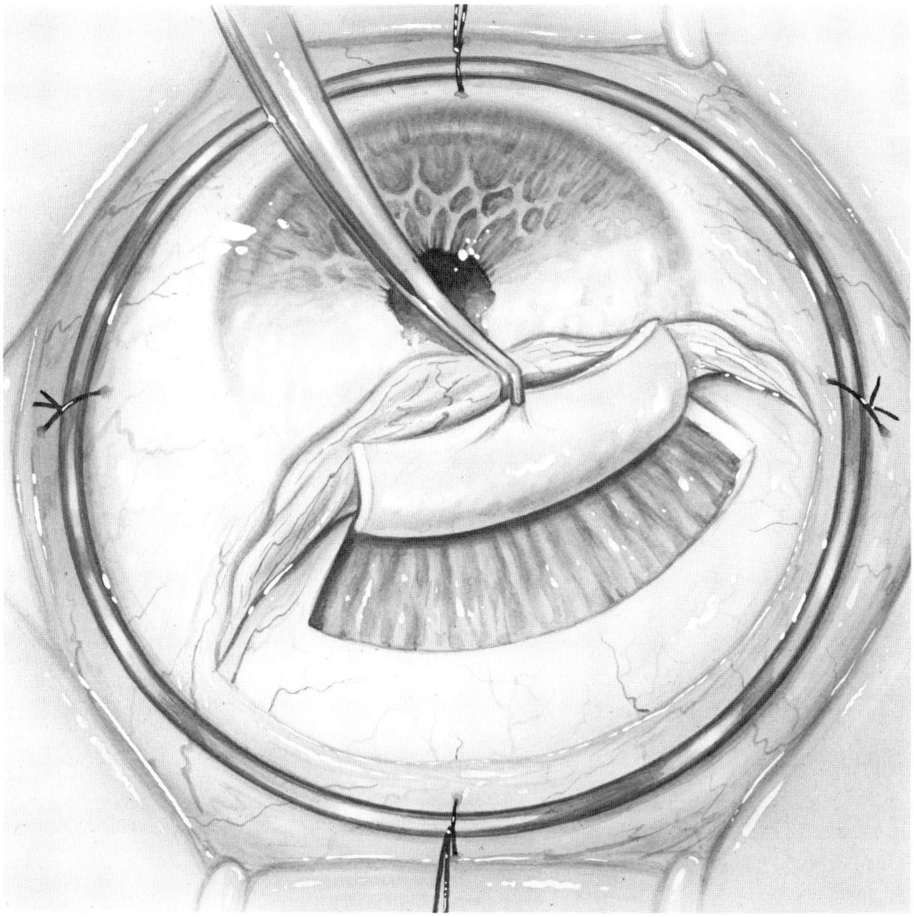

3.**44** A 4 mm broad limbus-based scleral flap including *all* layers of the sclera is prepared over 90–120°. The ciliary muscle is thus exposed in this area.

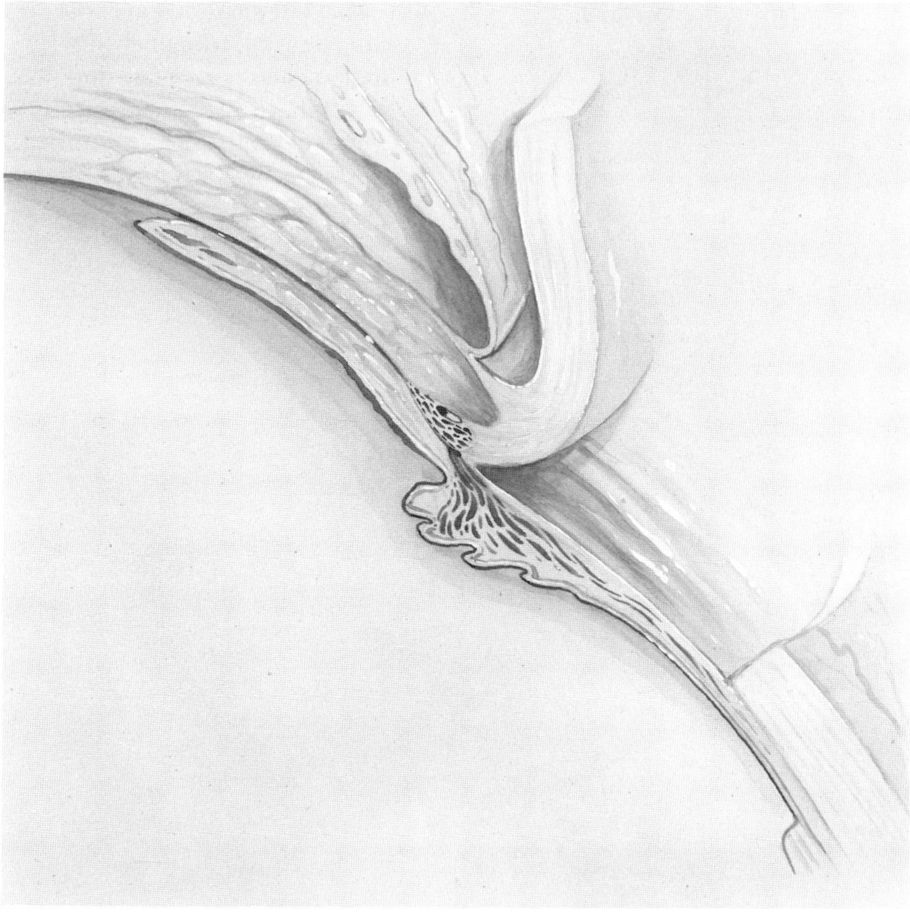

3.**45** It is surprising how easily the sclera can be separated from the ciliary muscle by *blunt* dissection up to the scleral spur. Only a few emissary vessels and nerve bridges (Axenfeld) have to be cut with scissors.

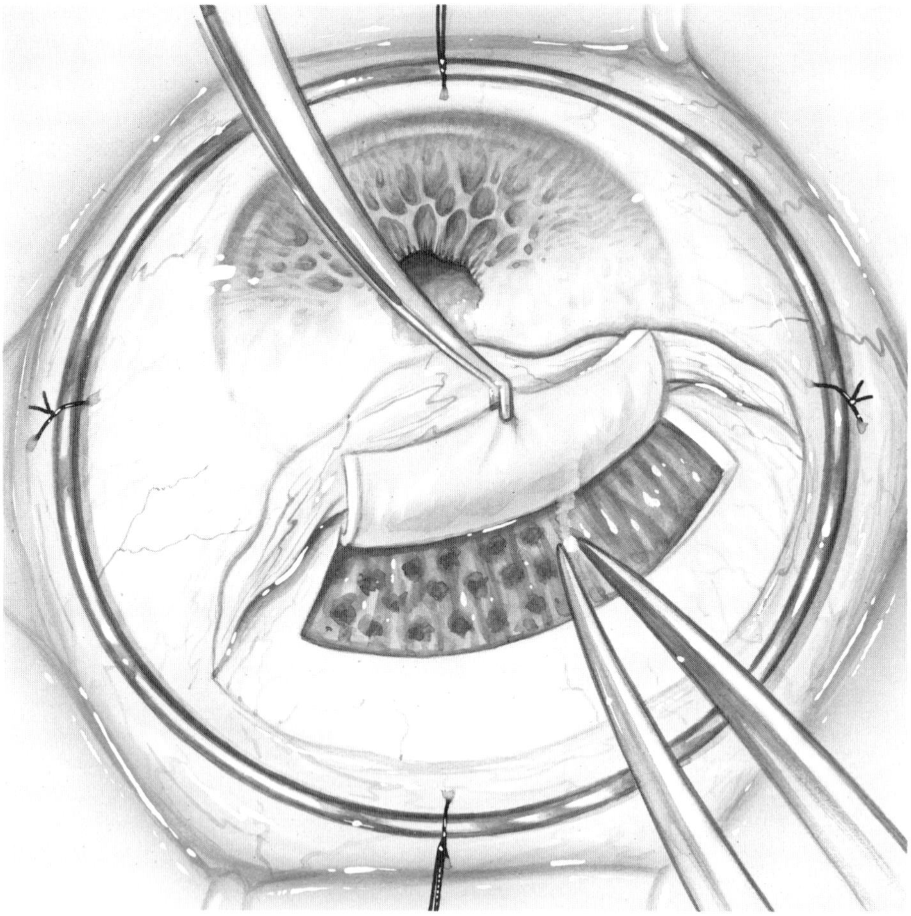

3.**46** Intensive bipolar cautery of the ciliary muscle is performed to prevent hemorrhage after excision of the tissue.

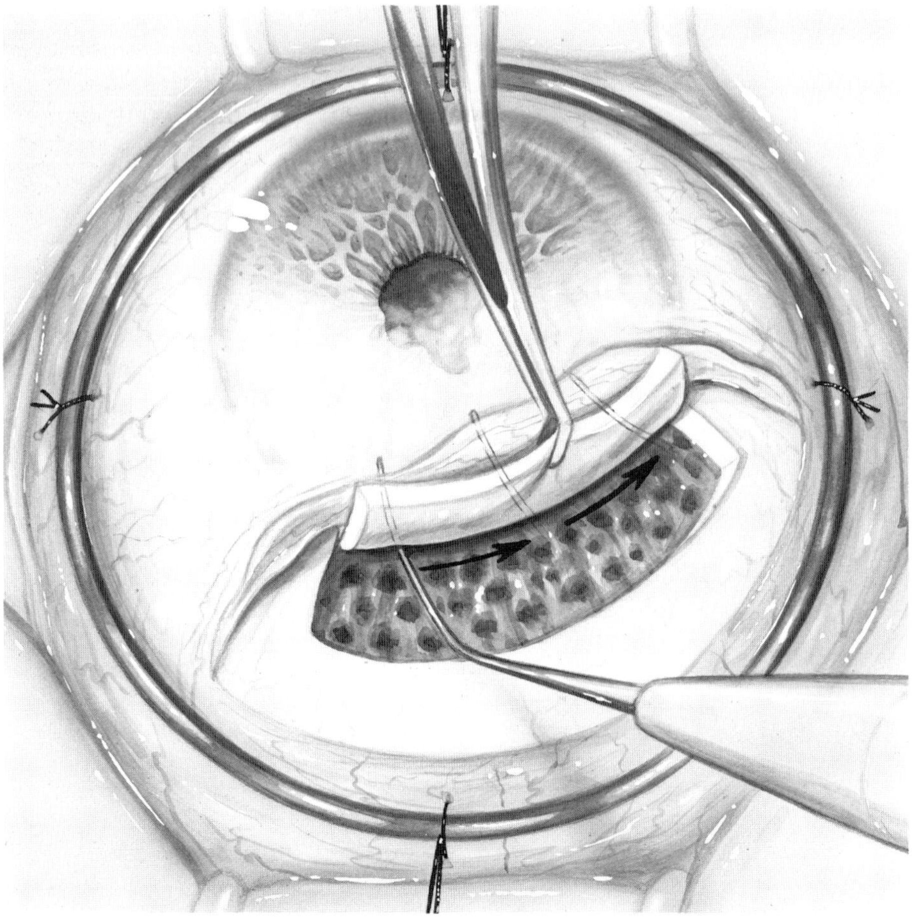

3.**47** The disinsertion of the ciliary muscle from the scleral spur must be performed initially with a sharp instrument such as a hockey knife. An iris spatula or a trabeculotomy probe can then be inserted and the ciliary muscle separated bluntly from the scleral spur.

48

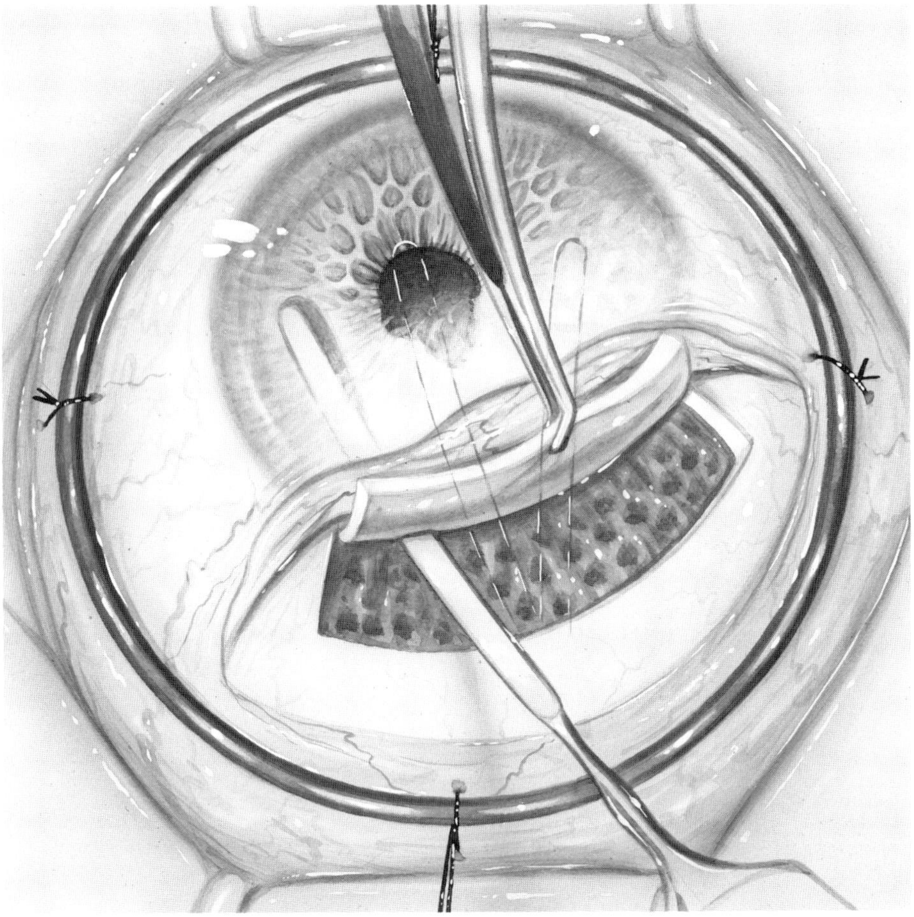

49

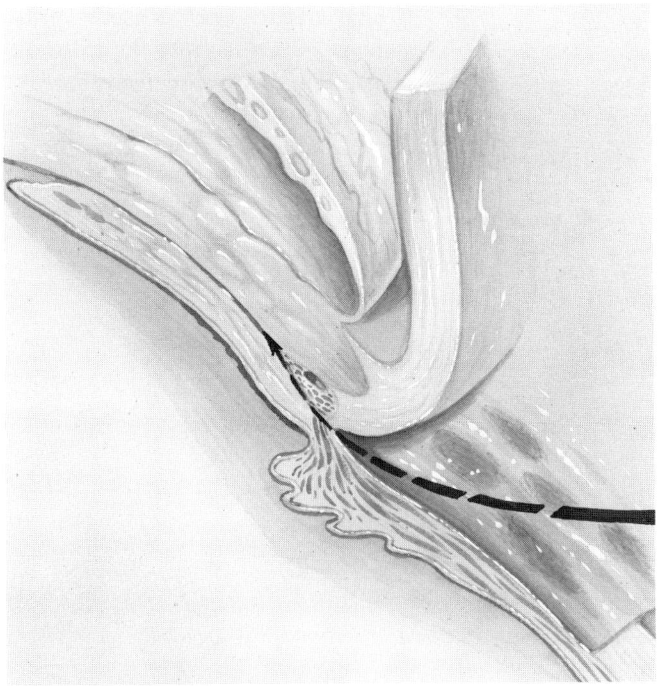

3.**48** and **49** An iris spatula is inserted between Descemet's membrane and the more or less extensively adherent iris and scar tissue. This is bluntly separated as much as possible through an initially performed trans-scleral paracentesis.

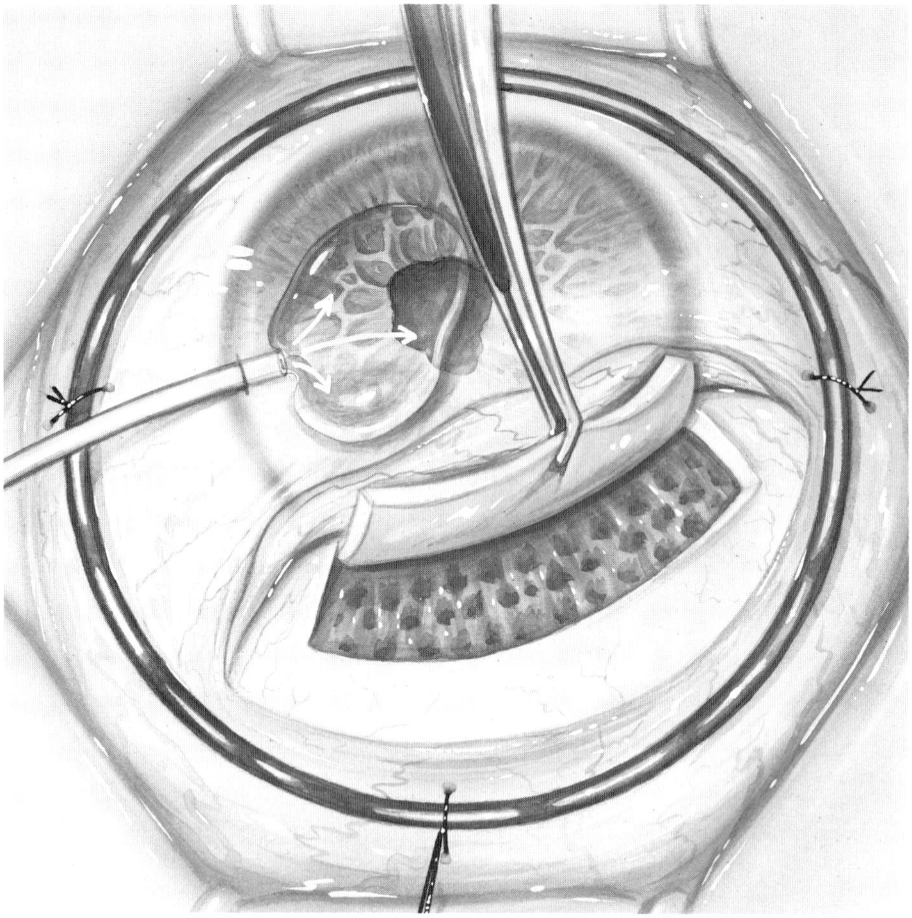

3.**50** Healon is injected into the anterior chamber to separate the scar tissue and iris from the cornea in the area of the adherent leucoma and also to reduce hemorrhage from these scars.

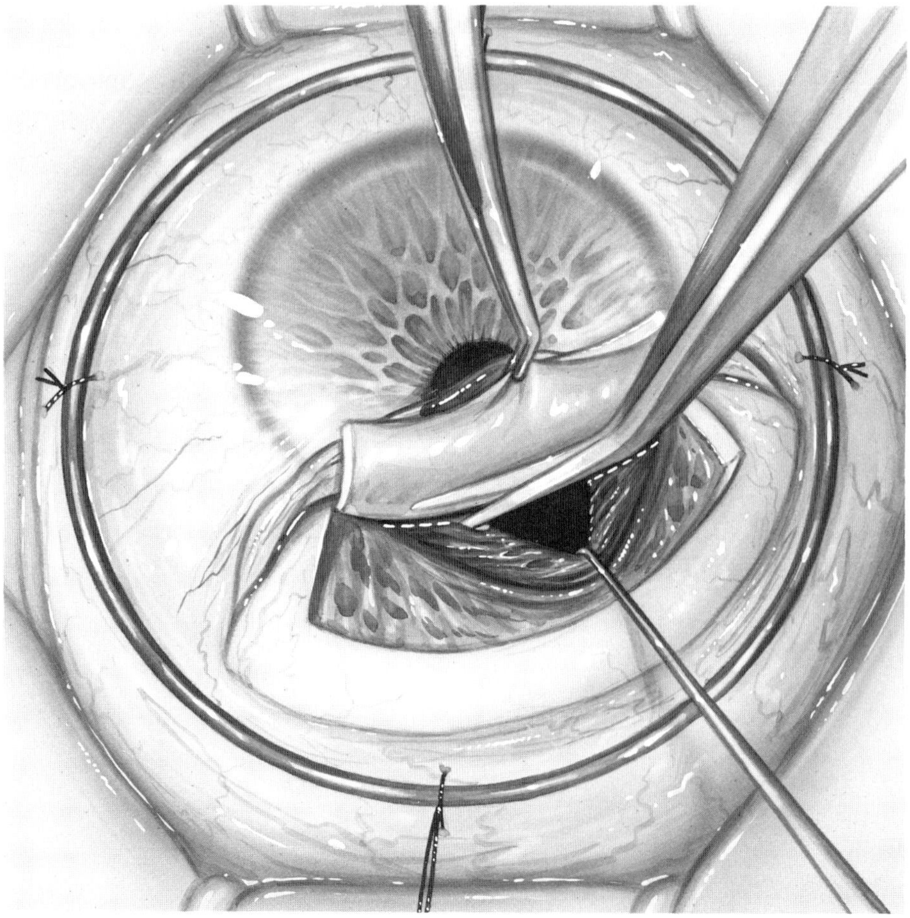

3.**51** An iris hook is used to pull the pupillary iris into the wound so that a sector iridectomy can be performed.

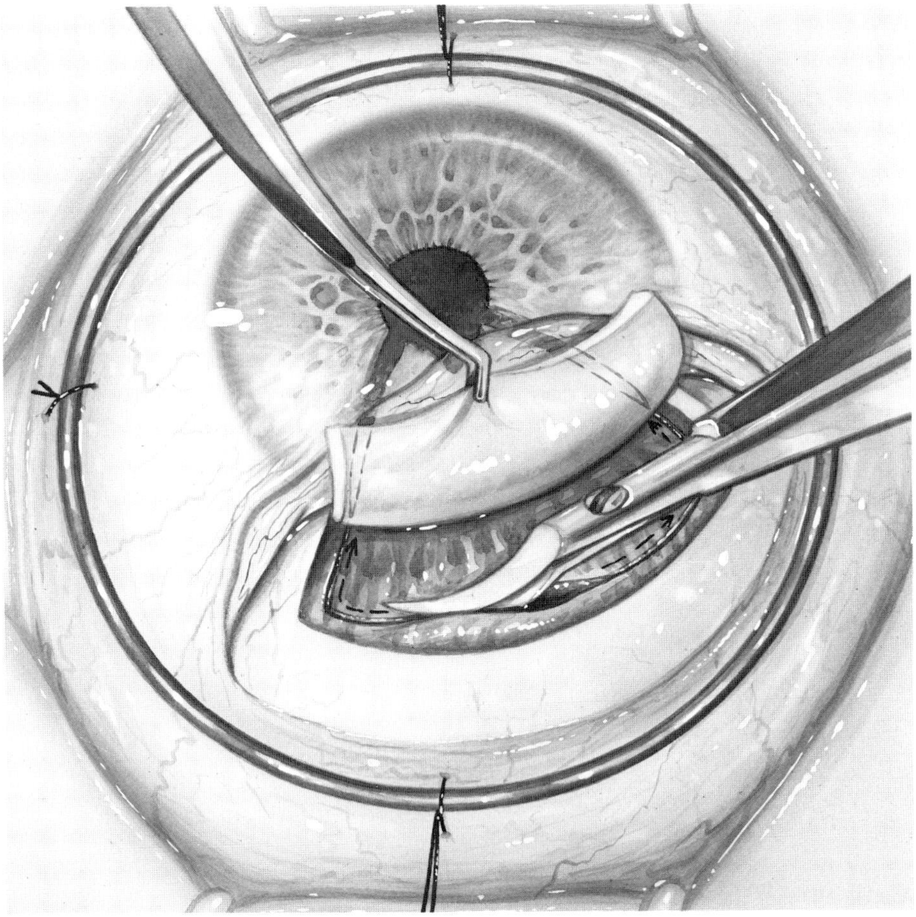

3.**52** The pars plicata is then excised in the area of the scleral window.

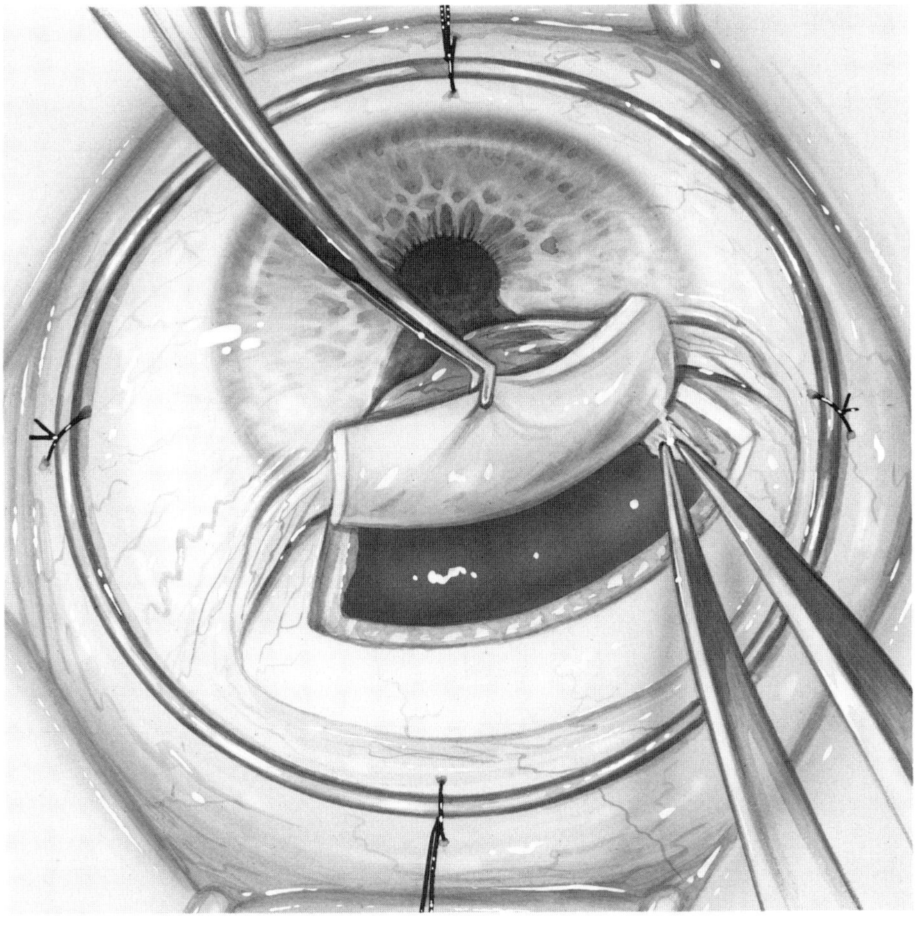

3.**53** Direct bipolar cautery stops the bleeding just as after block excision for tumors or epithelial ingrowth.

54

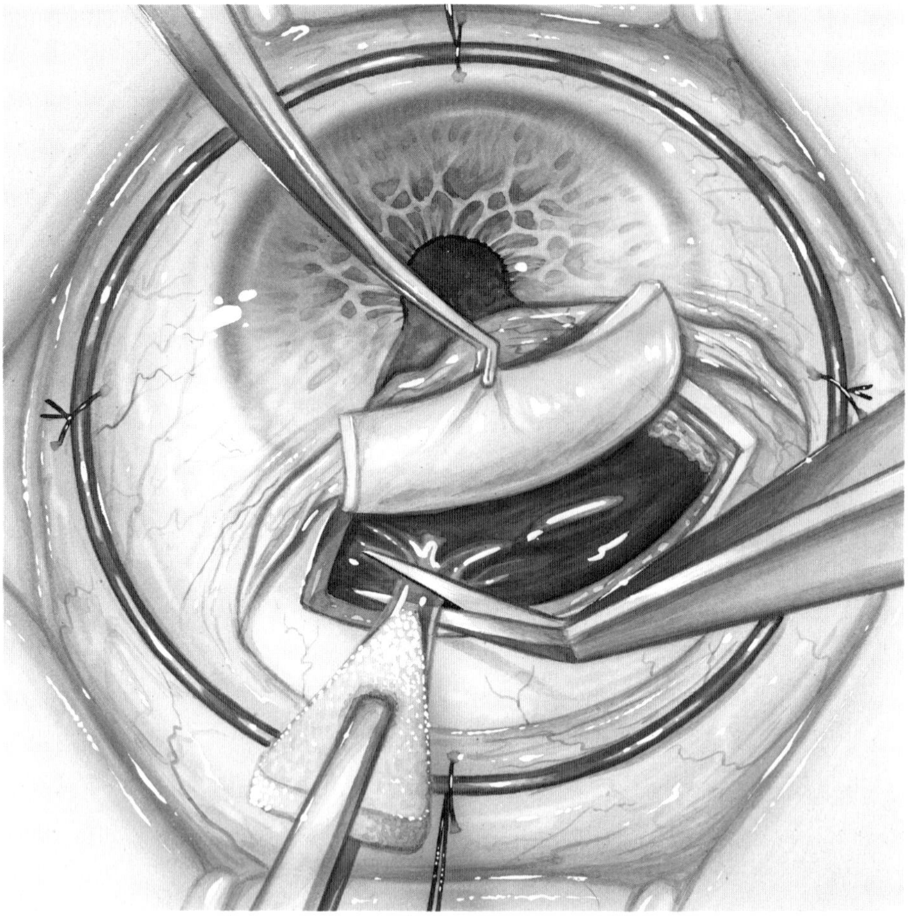

55

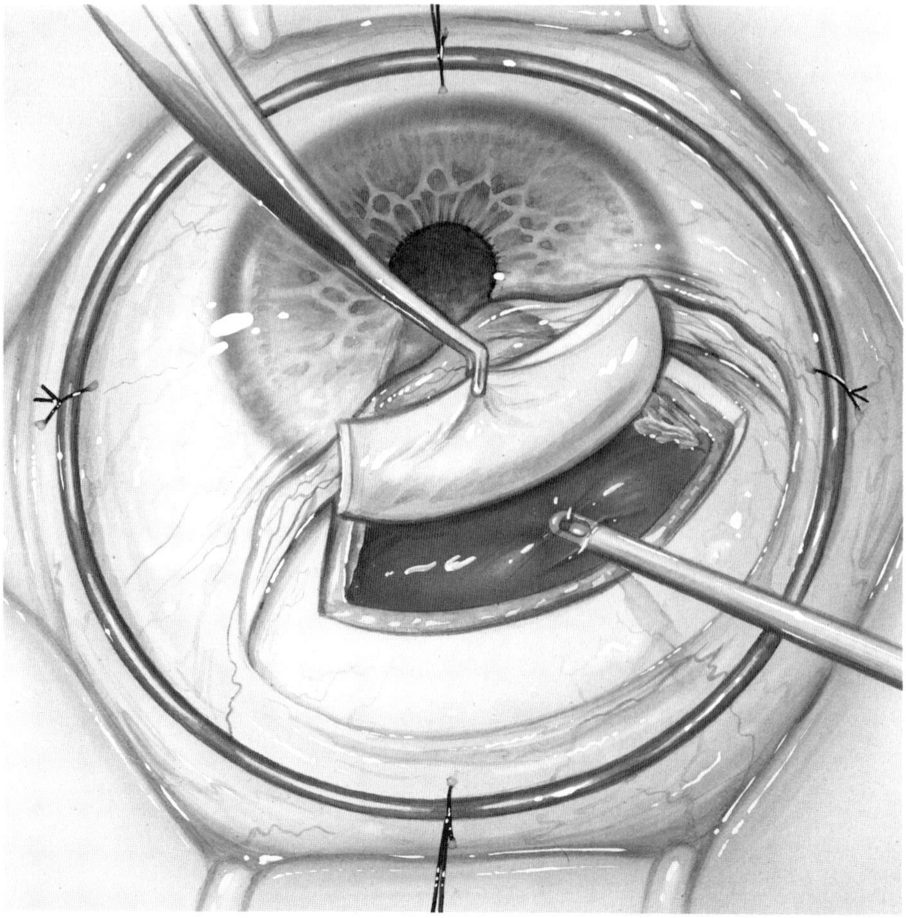

3.**54** and **55** Anterior vitrectomy is done either by sponge or by cutting/aspiration instruments. Healon is again injected into the anterior chamber after the scleral flap has been fixed to the sclera with interrupted sutures.

56

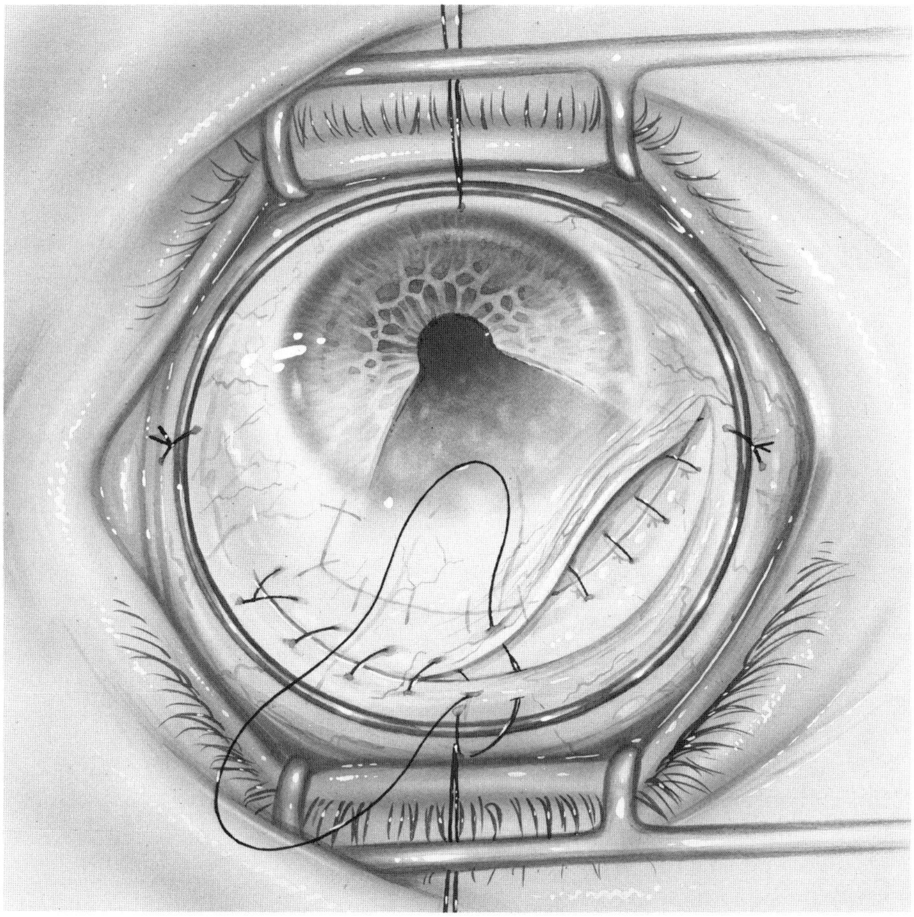

57

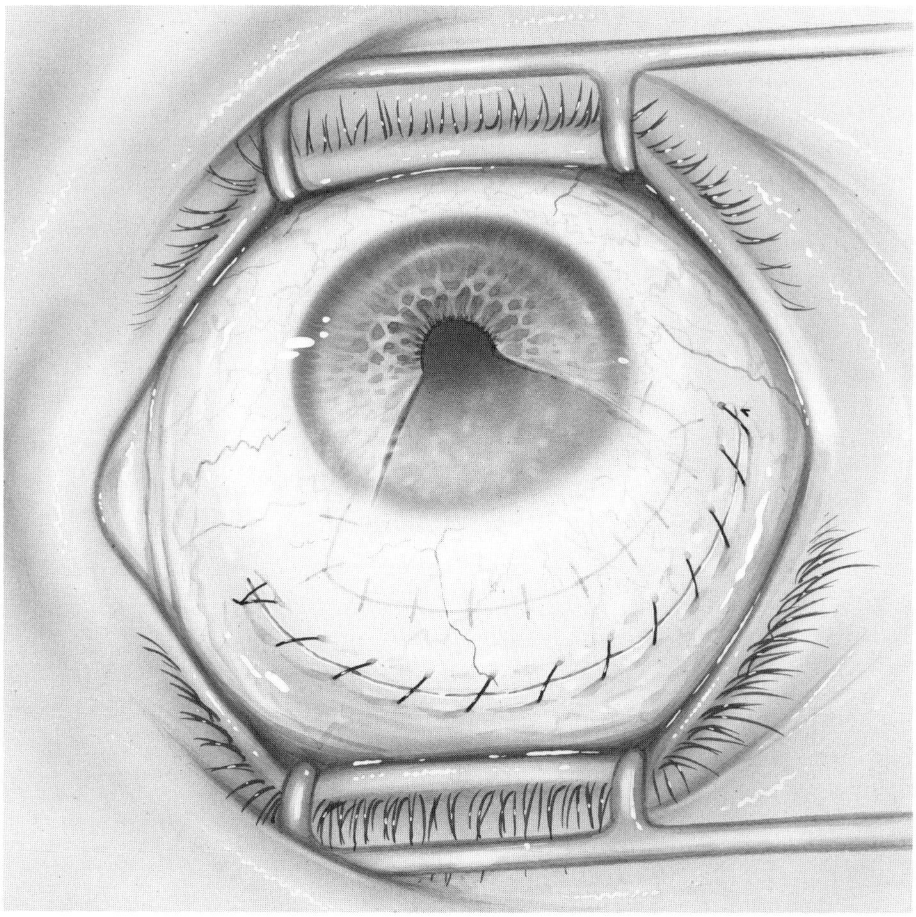

3.**56** and **57** The scleral and conjunctival flaps are closed.

Modifications

The procedure described is an "ultima ratio" attempt to preserve an otherwise lost eye with intractable secondary angle-closure glaucoma with athalamia. Therefore, it is indicated only where all other forms of medical or surgical therapy have failed. The prognosis for a successful Molteno implant may be improved.

Intraoperative Complications

Hemorrhage. As the anterior uveal vessels are cut and extensive scarring of the anterior segment is excised or bluntly dissected, hemorrhage usually occurs. It can be reduced by a combination of short-term controlled arterial hypotension, bipolar cautery, and injection of Healon to reduce hemorrhage from capillary vessels.

Vitreous loss. Vitreous is usually incarcerated into the anterior uveal scar tissue together with variable amounts of lens tissue. Therefore, the procedure always involves an anterior vitrectomy by sponge or instrument.

Corneal endothelial decompensation. In these eyes the corneal endothelium has always been damaged by the preceding surgical or accidental trauma, leading to bullous keratopathy. In view of the extent of the procedure we do not recommend the performance of a penetrating keratoplasty at the same time. Rather, we advise the patient that a penetrating corneal graft will be necessary at a later date to clear the optic axis.

Retinal detachment. In view of the vitreous incarceration in the anterior uveal scar, traction on the peripheral retina is common. Therefore, particular care must be taken not to injure any retinal traction folds. If the retina is cut, an encircling retinal detachment procedure is necessary.

Persistent secondary angle-closure glaucoma. As in these eyes practically the entire circumference of the angle is usually closed by the peripheral anterior synechiae, obstruction of outflow will persist. If this is not balanced by a reduction of inflow via excision of the pars plicata, additonal antiglaucoma medication and, if necessary, cryocoagulation are indicated, or a Molteno implant may be considered.

Admonitions and Suggestions

Any attempts to "free the angle" by separation of very peripheral anterior synechiae are useless. They may also lead to rather extensive hemorrhage, which may be difficult to control.

When stripping anterior synechiae away from Descemet's membrane, it is always difficult to find the right plane of separation of the synechiae from the membrane. However, care should be taken not to separate Descemet's membrane from the stroma.

Postoperative Management and Complications

Hemorrhage may recur immediately after surgery or after 5 to 7 days; it usually clears spontaneously.

Secondary glaucoma often persists as a problem in view of the preoperatively existing angle closure – despite pars plicata excision. If medical therapy fails to control pressure, a Molteno implant may be considered.

After intraocular pressure has been brought under control, a penetrating keratoplasty is indicated to clarify the *optic axis.*

Results

Our experience so far covers about 40 eyes. In about 50 percent of these hopelessly scarred eyes the intraocular pressure was compensated. The preconditions for a later penetrating keratoplasty are improved.

Transconjunctival and Transscleral Cryocoagulation of the Ciliary Body

Surgical Principles

Cryocoagulation of the pars plicata of the ciliary body usually has only a temporary effect in reducing intraocular pressure. It is indicated if standard antiglaucoma therapy has failed or cannot be performed. Our indications are mainly painful and secondary glaucoma *with rubeosis iridis* if the eye is blind and the patient rejects enucleation. It is also indicated in seeing eyes with secondary glaucoma with rubeosis iridis and in those aphakic eyes where conventional antiglaucoma therpay cannot be performed.

Preparation for Surgery

Bacterial cultures of the conjunctiva are not necessary, as the eye is not opened.

Preoperative Medication and Anesthesia

Carbonic anhydrase inhibitors, beta-blockers, and epinephrine derivatives are given about 60 minutes before surgery to reduce elevation of intraocular pressure. Local and systemic prostaglandin inhibitors are given to reduce the postoperative reaction to the pars plicata necrosis.

Instruments

Cryocoagulation apparatus is required which is capable of generating −70° to −80 °C.

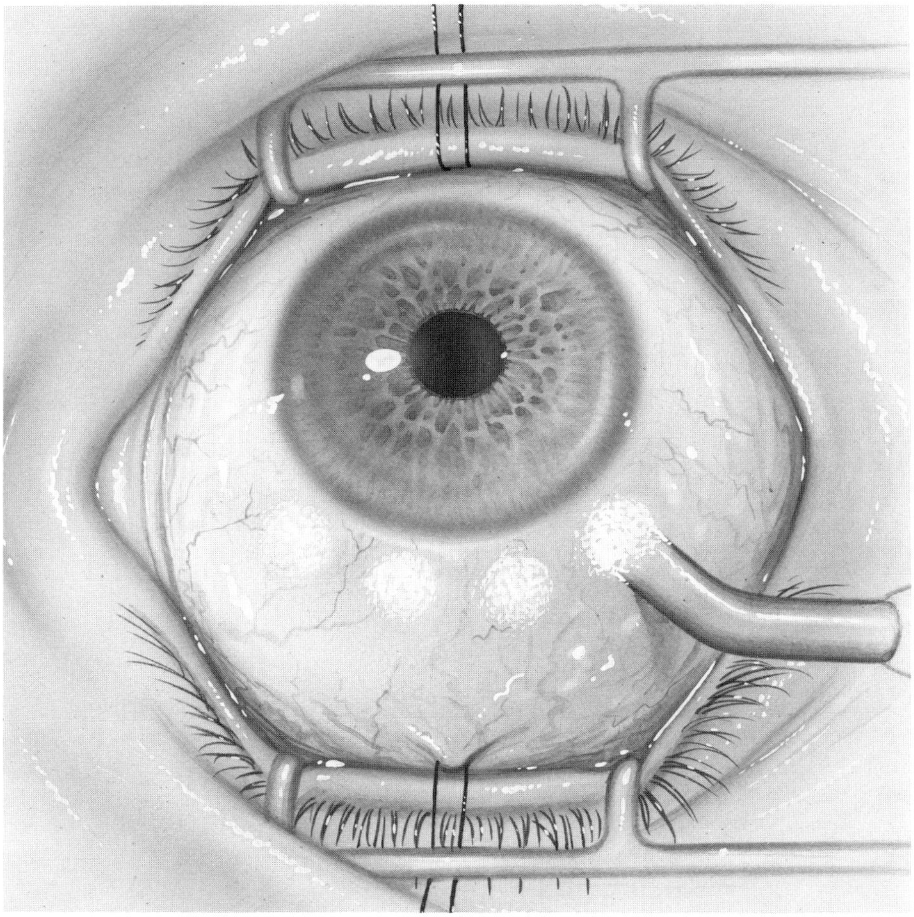

Surgical Technique

3.58 The globe is rotated with a squint hook and the conjunctival surface dried with standard swabs. The cryoprobe is applied about 3–4 mm behind the limbus for 45 seconds at −70° to −80 °C. The cryo effect is then thawed and the application repeated in the same manner. Altogether a minimum of six freeze-and-thaw cycles are done.

Intraoperative Complications

In spite of retrobulbar local anesthesia, the patient often complains of pain due to an acute rise in *intraocular pressure*. For this reason the patient should be given carbonic anhydrase inhibitors and beta-blocking agents one hour before the procedure.

If the cryoprobe is turned during freezing, vessels may be fractured at the edge, leading to *hemorrhage*. Care must be taken not to rotate the cryoprobe.

Admonitions and Suggestions

Care should be taken not to apply the cryoprobe through the peripheral retina, as excessive cryo application may lead to retinal defects.

Postoperative Management and Complications

An *inflammatory reaction* may be quite marked due to the tissue destruction. Therefore, preoperative therapy with prostaglandin inhibitors is important.

It is impossible to determine whether postoperative *hemorrhage* stems from the area of necrosis or from preexisting rubeosis iridis.

Results

The reduction in intraocular pressure after cryocoagulation is usually only temporary. The patient should know this before the procedure is performed.

4

Lens

Jörg Draeger, Jared M. Emery, Klaus Heilmann,
Stephen H. Johnson, Douglas D. Koch, Richard P. Kratz

Intracapsular Cataract Extraction

Klaus Heilmann

Surgical Principles

Essentially, this operation consists in total removal of the opaque lens in order to restore clear optic conditions.

Until artificial lens implantation was reintroduced, intracapsular cataract extraction (ICCE) was the classic procedure for cataract and is still regarded as such by many authors today. When there are no complications, the disadvantages of extracapsular extraction (ECCE) are avoided, i.e., lens remnants in the capsule and the development of new fiber bundles from the capsular epithelium. The continuing development of laser technology bears witness to the fact that these problems still play a part in ECCE, despite advances in surgical technique. The great advantage of ICCE lies in the fact that – provided there are no other pathologic changes – optimal vision can be restored. Manually, the procedure can be more difficult than ECCE, and the intraoperative and postoperative complications it entrains may be more severe.

The advances made in the safety of ICCE and the improvements in the results obtained have been due to the introduction of new methods of preparing the patient, microsurgical instruments, magnifying visual aids, and modern suture techniques and suture materials. Prior to the discovery of enzymatic zonulolysis and the introduction of phakoerysis and cryoextraction a certain degree of maturity of the cataract was desirable, in order to minimize the resistance of the zonula during extraction. Since the aids mentioned above have been available the primary criterion has been the extent to which the lens-related visual disturbance handicaps the patient in his everyday life.

Advanced age is not a contraindication for cataract surgery. Retinal detachment, absence of retinal function, and optic nerve atrophy have to be ruled out, i.e., it must be established prior to surgery that restoration of vision or a meaningful improvement in vision is likely.

Preparation for Surgery

Customary preparation for an intraocular operation.

Preoperative Medication and Anesthesia

Local antibacterial treatment of both eyes for one week. In cases of doubt a conjunctival smear should be made and bacteriologically tested.

Instillation of a short-acting mydriatic 45, 30, and 15 minutes before commencement of surgery.

In principle ICCE can be performed under local anesthesia. However, this author generally opts for tracheal intubation, the premedication for this being at the anesthetist's discretion, in particular taking the (in most cases advanced) age of the patient into account. As an anesthetic we prefer Fluothane, because it enables anesthesia to be deepened quickly, while the patient still wakes up rapidly and in a calm state. Postoperative nausea and vomiting are very rare. Fluothane also causes a great drop in IOP, which is desirable for ICCE.

We use mannitol to immobilize the vitreous by dehydration. Thirty minutes before the operation 250 ml of the 20 % solution are infused. Carefully applied manual pressure on the eye can also be extremely effective.

Instruments

The usual microsurgical instruments for intraocular surgery are used.

1

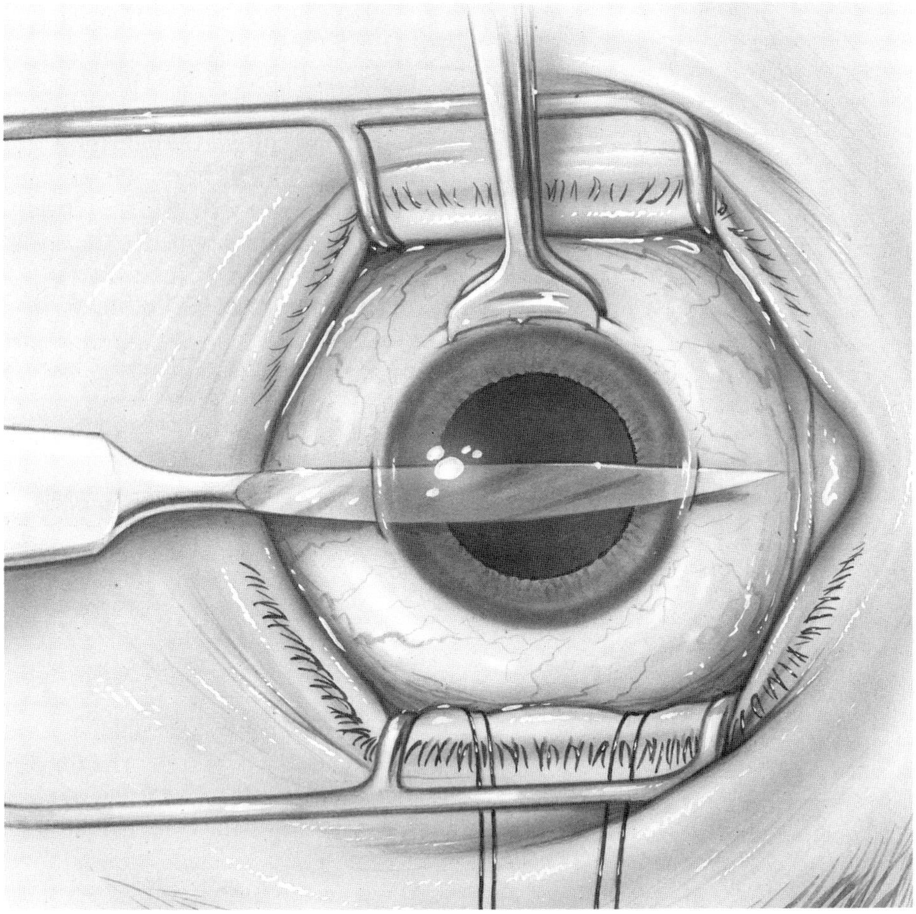

2

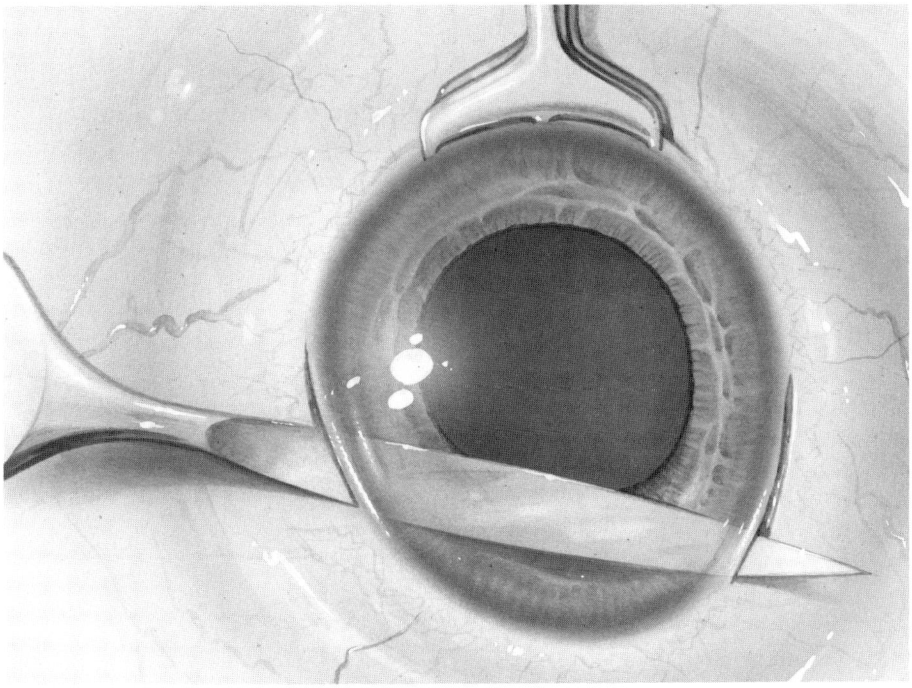

Surgical Technique

(The description is for surgery on the left eye.)

4.1 A holding suture is applied through the insertion of the superior rectus muscle at 12 o'clock, approximately 8 mm behind the limbus. The Colibri lid retractor (J. I. Barraquer) is then inserted; it is placed under the upper lid first, and then under the lower lid, without compressing the spring. Subsequently the surgical field is flushed.

The globe is grasped firmly at 6 o'clock with fixation forceps and pulled gently downward. Using the tip of the Graefe knife, the conjunctiva is perforated at 3 o'clock 1,5 mm from the limbus and pushed forward toward the limbus. The anterior chamber is punctured about 0.5 mm outside the limbus. The blade of the knife must be parallel to the iris with the cutting edge directed upward. The knife is now pushed through the anterior chamber. The knife tip reemerges from the bulb 0.5 mm outside the limbus and from the conjunctiva 3 mm from the limbus.

4.2 After withdrawal of the blade the knife is moved gradually forward and upward (clockwise) on the withdrawal side and subsequently upward on the side where it was inserted (counterclockwise), simultaneously withdrawing it.

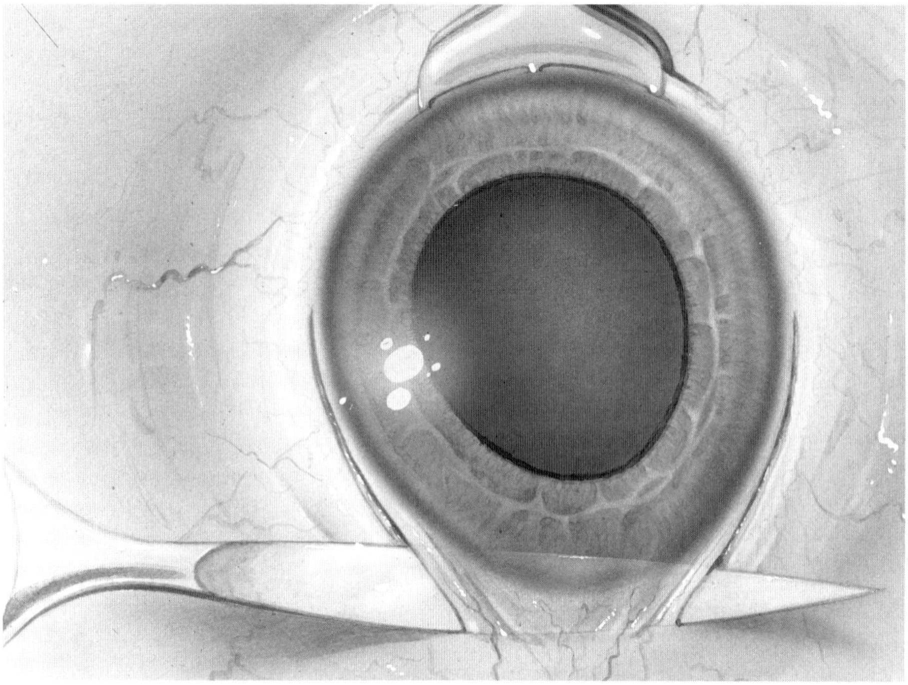

4.3 With this second movement the sclerocorneal incision should be completed, and the conjunctival flap completed with the same or the next incision. While cutting, care must be taken to insure that no pressure whatsoever is applied to the globe and that the incision is 0.5 mm outside the limbus at all points.

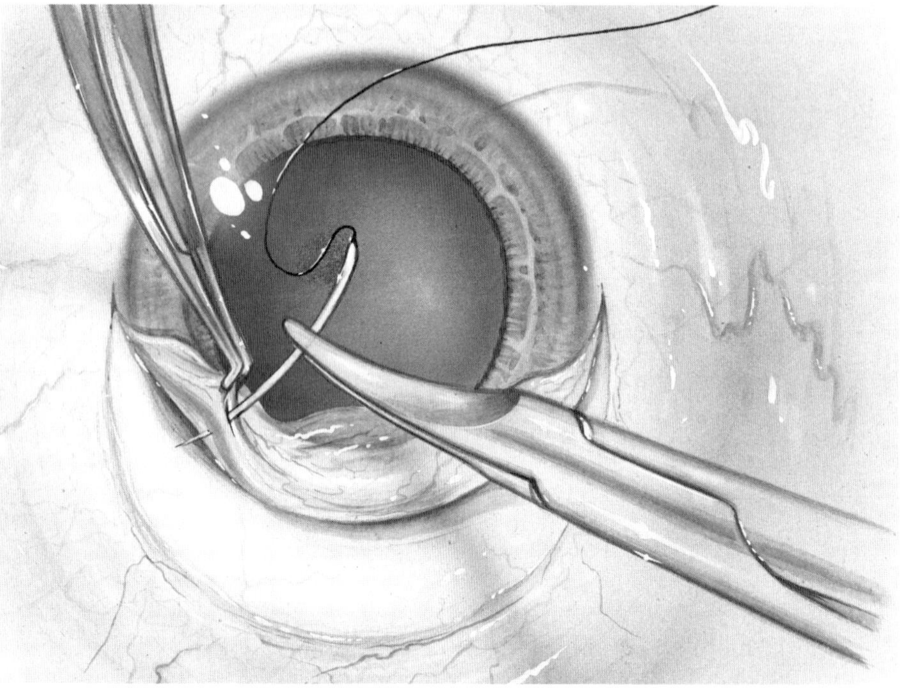

4.4 The conjunctival flap is folded back over the cornea and the border of the corneal wound grasped with the Colibri forceps. The needle with the welded-in Vicryl suture (9-0 monofilament Vicryl) is taken up with the short Barraquer needle holder and inserted into the cornea adjacent to the forceps, 0.5 mm from the border of the wound and in front of the beginning of the corneal flap.

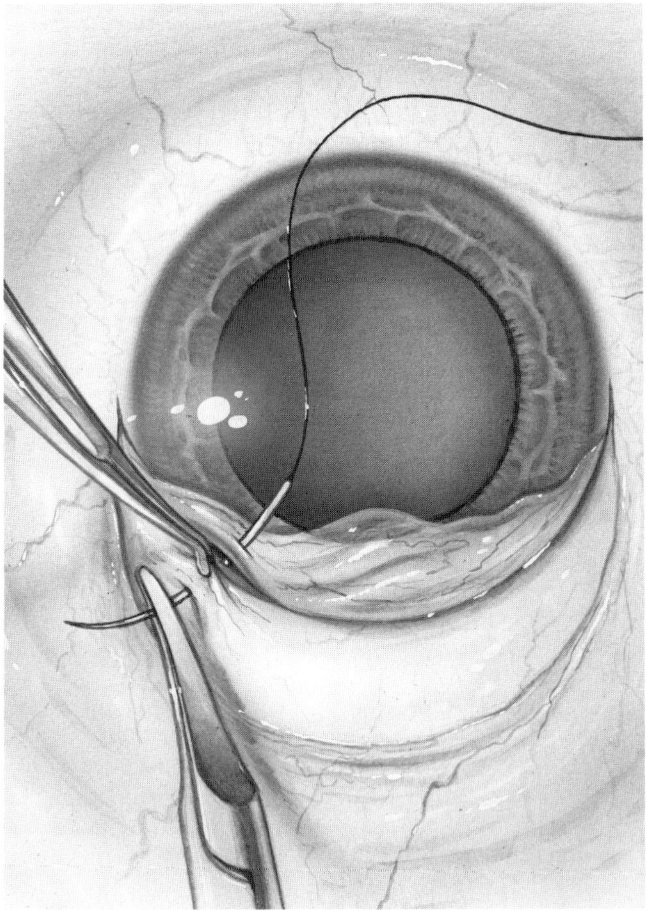

4.5 When the tip appears in the wound the corneal border of the wound is released and its scleral border is grasped. The needle then penetrates the scleral edge of the wound from inside, so that each suture bite is made with a single movement. If the suture has been placed correctly no wrinkling of the cornea should occur.

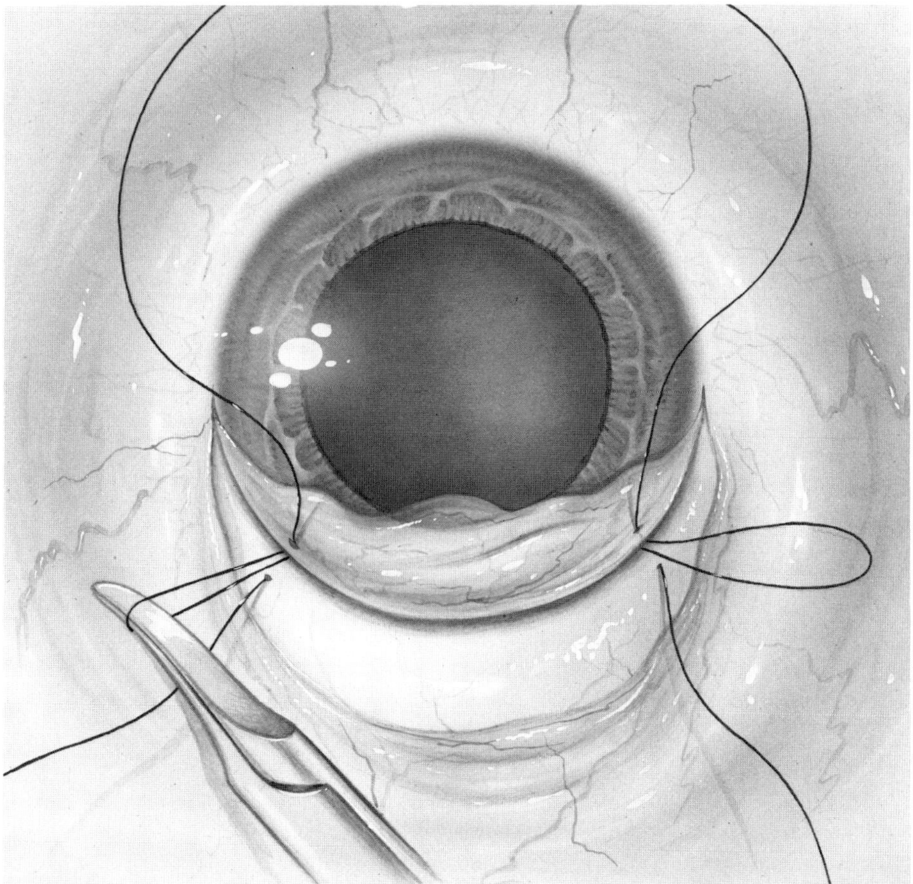

4.6 After laying two sutures forward, at 2 and 10 o'clock, the sutures are positioned, by pulling them out and looping them, so that they represent no obstruction during the rest of the operation.

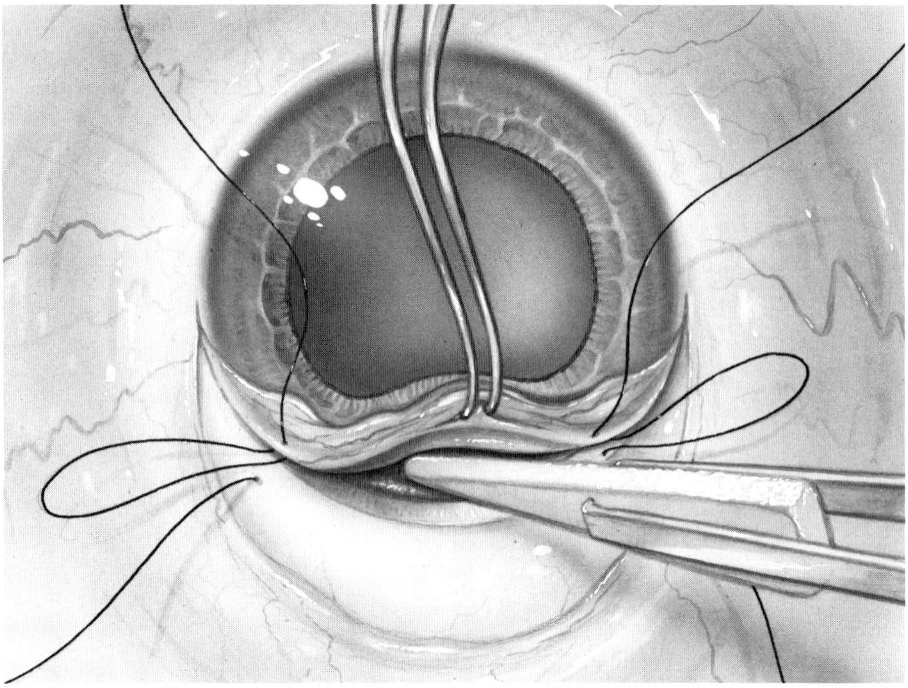

4.7 Using the iris forceps, the anterior chamber is opened at 12 o'clock (left hand) and the iris, slightly wrinkled by mydriasis, is gently pushed downward with a wedge-shaped sponge (right hand).

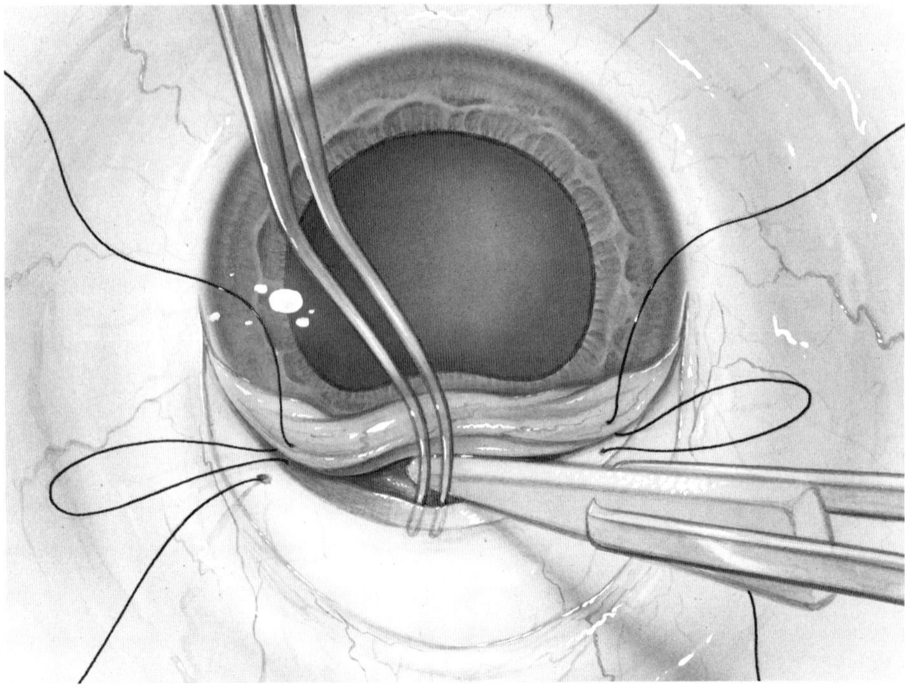

4.8 With the wedge-shaped sponge (right hand) the anterior chamber is held slightly open; now the base of the iris can be observed directly. Using the forceps, the iris is grasped, lifted slightly, and pulled out.

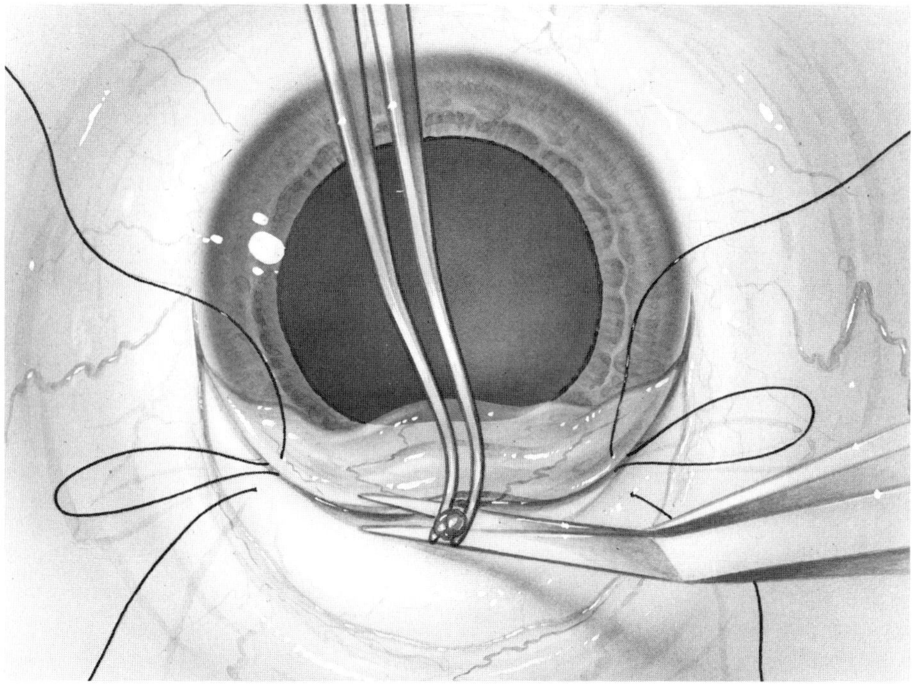

4.**9** The sponge is removed. The cornea falls back so that the forceps is now only holding the tip of the iris which has been pulled out. This is cut off with the De Wecker scissors. This technique results in a small, very regular basal iridectomy.

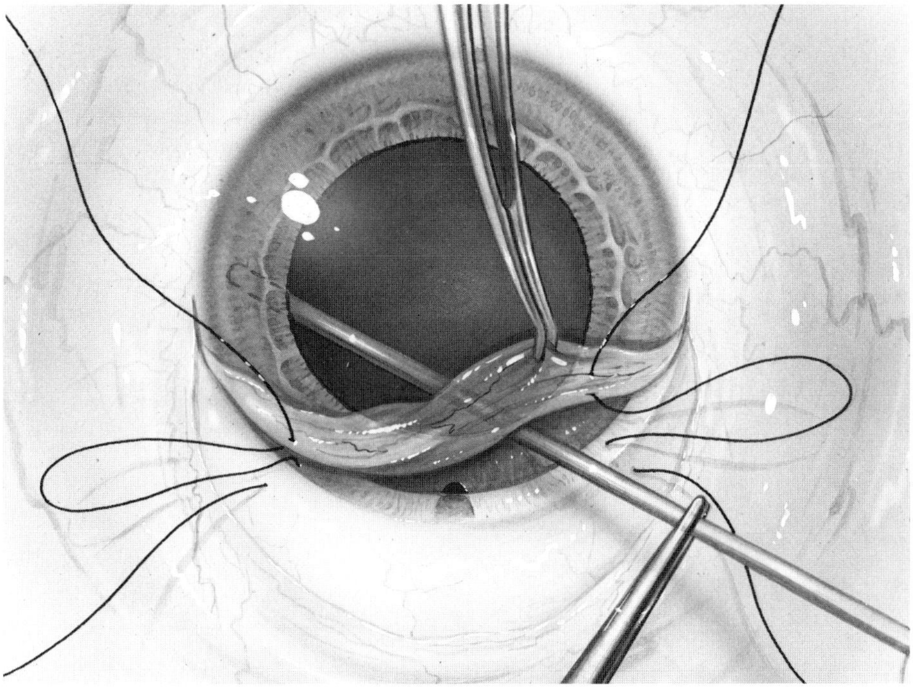

4.**10** The anterior chamber is flushed with balanced salt solution so that it is free of blood prior to performing the enzymatic zonulolysis. Any coagulated blood can be removed with the sponge. Alpha-chymotrypsin (1 mg dissolved in balanced salt solution) must be instilled into the posterior chamber very carefully and accurately. To insure that the cannula is guided correctly it is advisable to hold and guide it with forceps. The posterior surface of the iris should hardly be touched during the flushing procedure, and for this reason the lens is depressed slightly. For zonulolysis in the two lower quadrants this author instills the enzyme behind the pupillary margin, in the two upper quadrants carefully through the iridectomy. While the enzyme is taking effect (two to three minutes) the anterior chamber is again flushed with balanced salt solution, and preparations are made for cryoextraction.

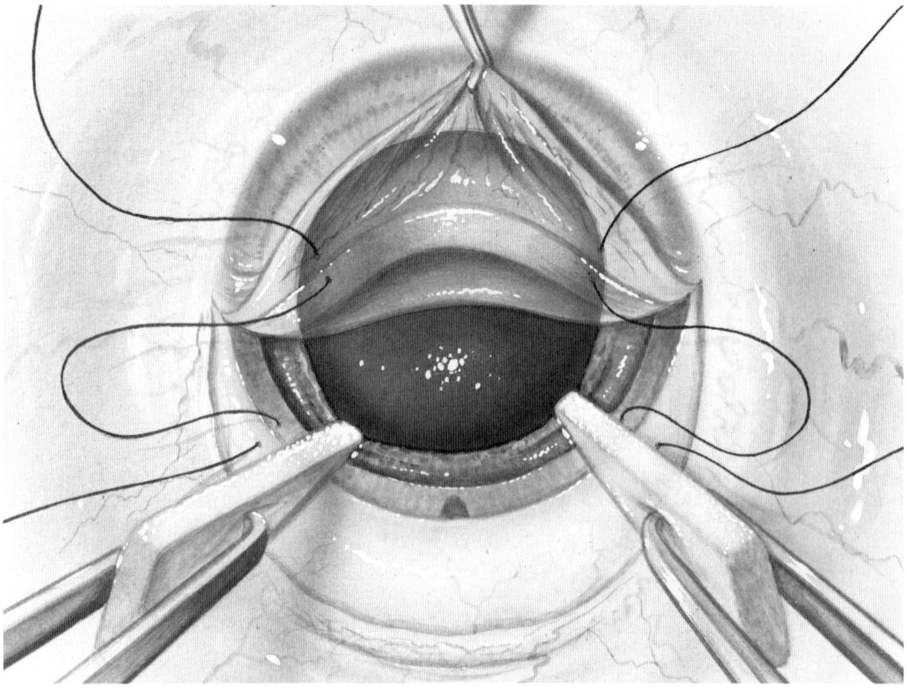

4.11 The assistant unfolds the cornea by taking hold of the conjunctiva with forceps, and if necessary stroking the iris upward a little at 2 o'clock. If necessary the surgeon dries the lens surface with a wedge-shaped sponge and pulls the iris gently upward at 11 o'clock with a dry sponge.

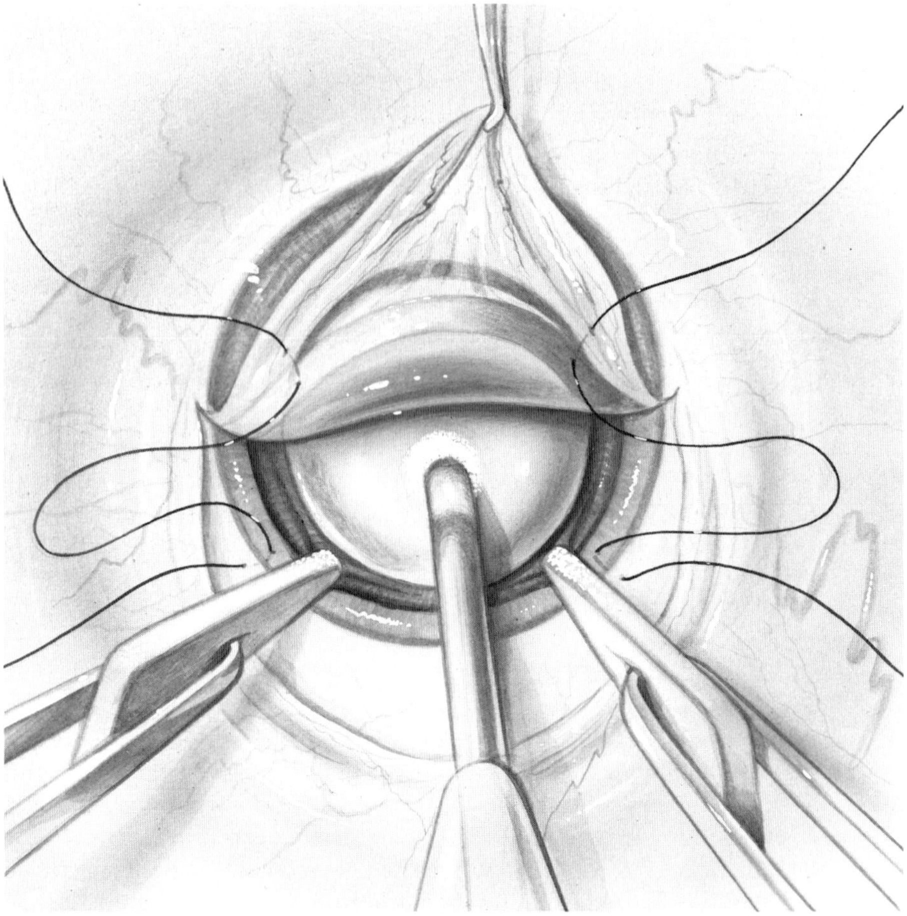

4.12 The cryoextractor is placed on the anterior surface of the lens capsule and the freezing procedure initiated with the foot switch. It is advisable to wait five to ten seconds before starting the extraction procedure and to make sure that the extractor is not touching the corneal endothelium, or that iris tissue has not been frozen.

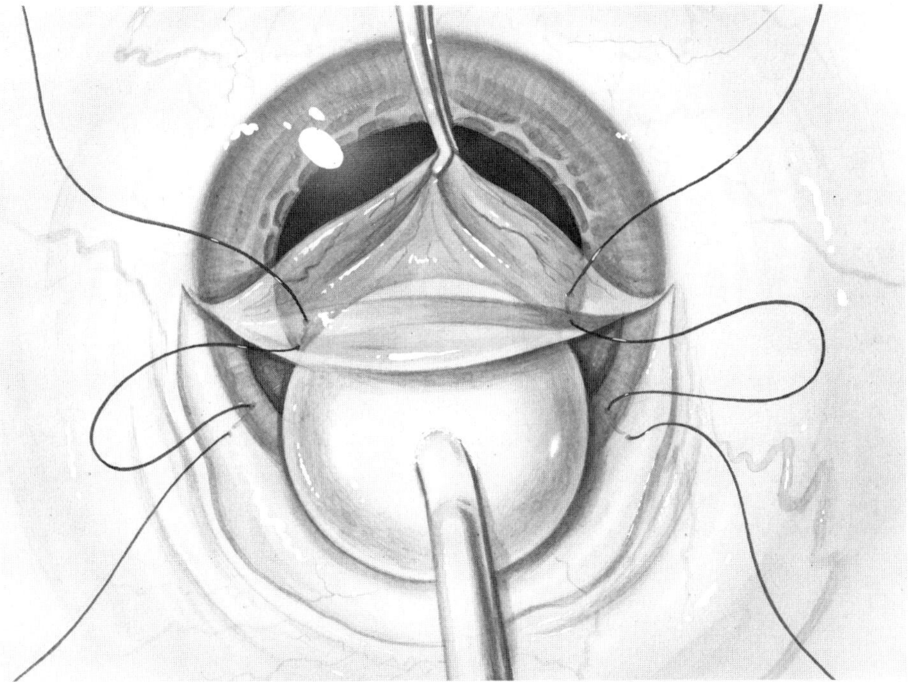

4.**13** The extraction procedure is begun by rotating the lens slightly to detach it completely from zonular fibers, and then turning and lifting it. As soon as the upper margin of the lens becomes visible the traction on the cornea can be relaxed, so that when extraction is completed it falls back into its original position.

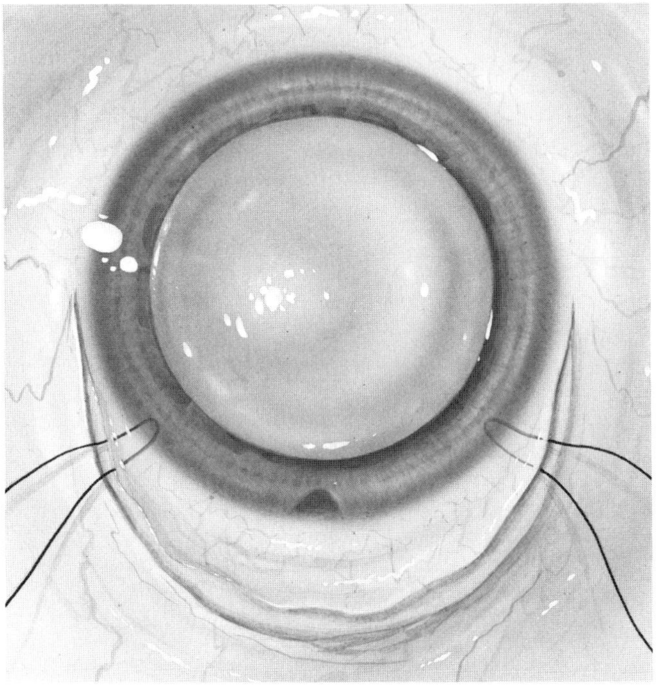

4.**14** Gentle immobilization of the vitreous is achieved by laying the lens on the surface of the cornea and ending the cryo procedure. The suture threads laid forward are tautened and prepared for knotting. If the vitreous is still, acetylcholine can be instilled into the sclerocorneal wound opening to constrict the pupil.

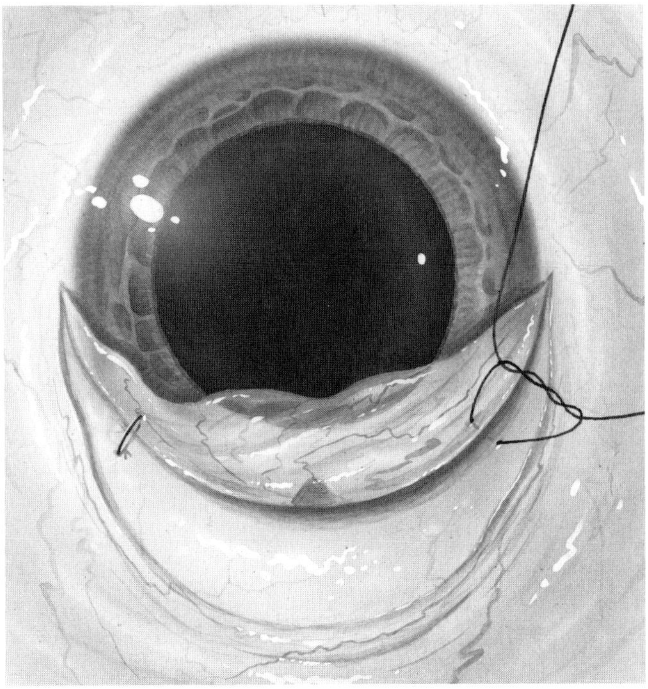

4.**15** The sutures which were laid forward are knotted and additional acetylcholine is administered to the wound.

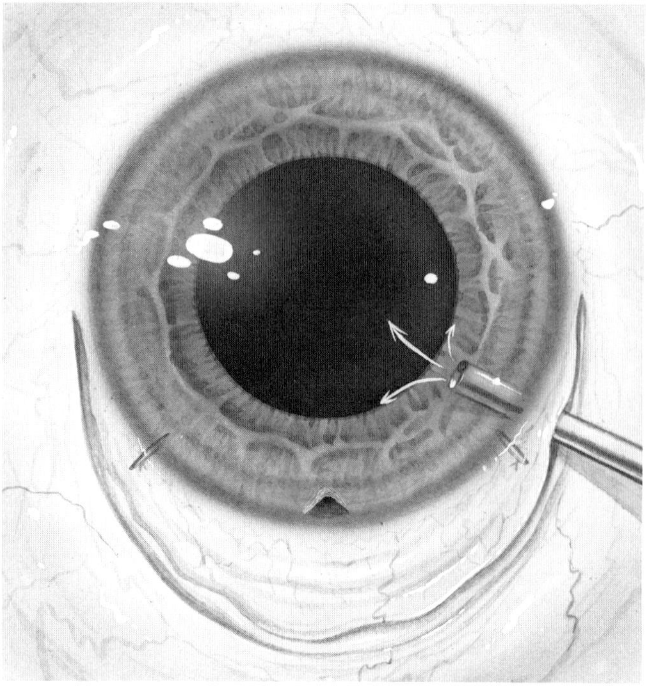

4.**16** The instillation of acetylcholine into the anterior chamber usually produces a rapid and extensive miosis. Additional sclerocorneal sutures are placed and knotted, always with the objective of achieving watertight wound closure.

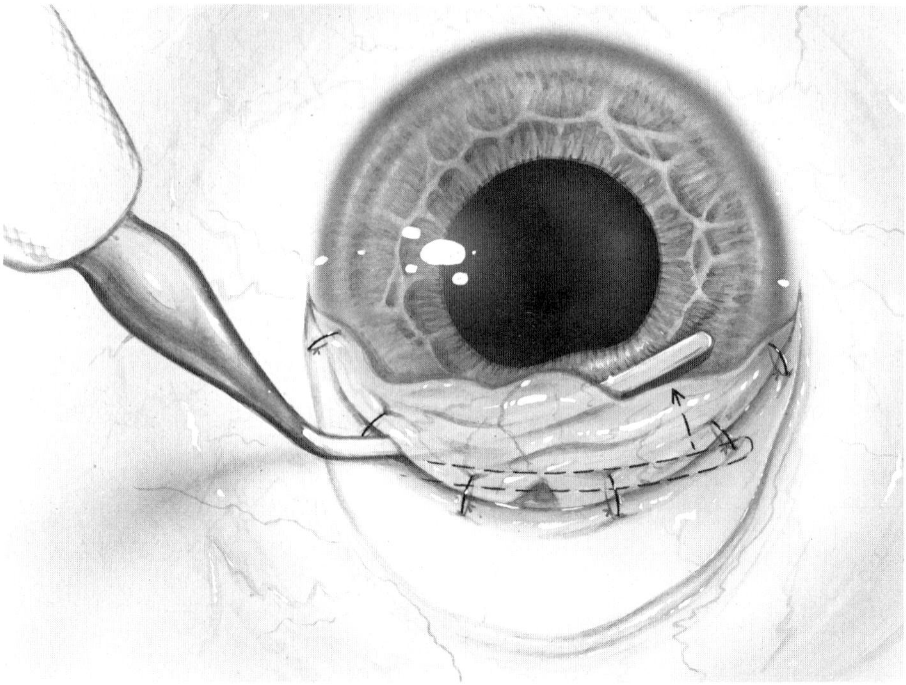

4.**17** If there is any iris caught in the wound or miosis is insufficient, the iris can be returned carefully to its original position using the Castroviejo spatula by stroking lightly over its surface and on the inner surface of the incision wound.

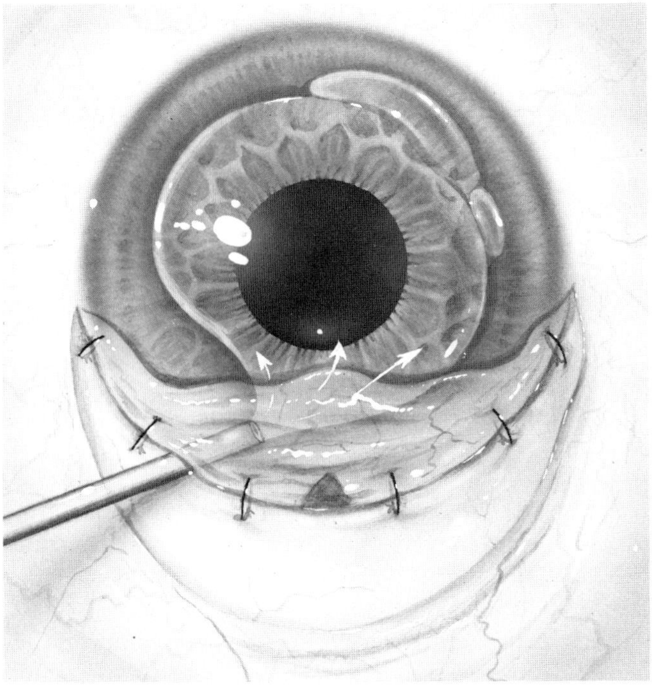

4.18 Insufflation of the anterior chamber has proved extremely efficacious, especially for pushing back the vitreous and restoring the configuration of the globe. If the air bubble becomes shallower and continues to spread at the end of the operation it is a sign that the incision wound is not watertight.
Some authors substitute balanced salt solution for the air at the end of the procedure.

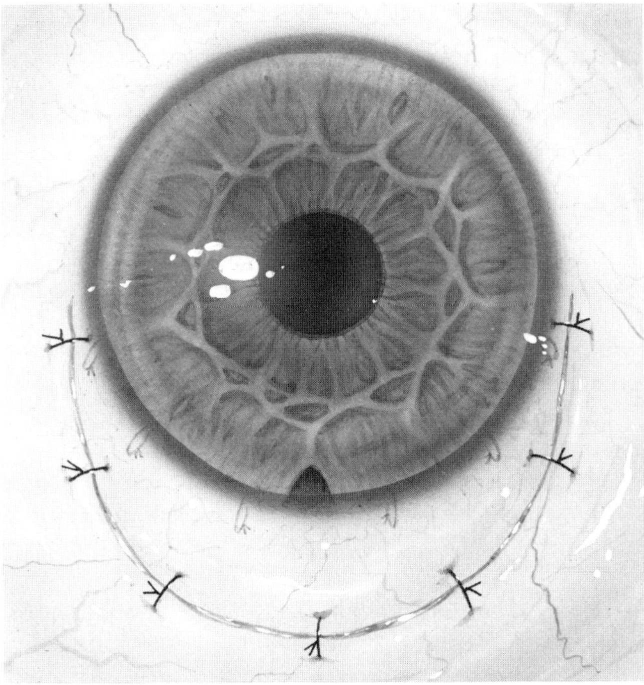

4.19 The conjunctival flap is smoothed back over the sclera, and the conjunctival wound is closed with interrupted sutures of 7-0 silk.
At the end of surgery the sclerocorneal wound should be closed watertight; the anterior chamber should have been restored with air or fluid, and the pupil should be round and centric.

Complications

Cataract incision: If the globe is poorly fixed the incision will be irregular and jagged, even with a knife which cuts well. The holding suture is necessary, because it limits movement of the globe and prevents the upward and downward deviation which is normal under anesthetic.

This author prefers a sclerocorneal incision. If the points at which the cataract knife is inserted and withdrawn are too close to the limbus, the conjunctiva may be severed at the limbus: as a result, a part of the incision would subsequently be devoid of the corresponding conjunctival cover. If the points of insertion and removal are too far inside the sclera severe bleeding may occur, the ciliary body may be exposed, and the ciliary border of the iris may be damaged. If the knife is not kept parallel to the iris when it is inserted, either a very large intracorneal incision area or a damaged iris will be the result.

If the wrong pressure is applied to the knife and fixation forceps, or if the knife is tilted, aqueous humor will drain off prematurely and the iris will fall in front of the knife blade. It is advisable to withdraw the knife with a slight downward rotation and to complete the incision with scissors. If the knife has already been pushed beyond the pupillary margin the iris will merely be grazed, or a more or less extensive, irregular peripheral iridectomy will be the consequence. It is wrong to try to extend the incision directly upward; a sawing action is essential.

If the knife is inadvertently introduced into the anterior chamber with the cutting edge downward, it must be removed completely. Injuries to the lens with the cataract knife are extremely rare.

Iris: Operations on the iris performed in combination with cataract surgery are intended primarily to prevent pupillary block. In most cases a small basal peripheral iridectomy is fully sufficient. If the central portion of the iris is grasped, as is possible when the pupil is greatly dilated, the result will be an iridectomy which is either larger than intended or close to the sphincter.

When attempting to achieve the smallest possible basal iridectomy, it may happen that only the iris stroma will be severed while the pigment epithelium remains intact. In this eventuality the pigment epithelium can be perforated by stretching it with the wedge-shaped sponge.

If the ciliary body is injured during the iridectomy, severe bleeding may result. This can be avoided by performing the iridectomy 0.5 mm basally in front of the ciliary border of the iris.

If the zonular and/or the vitreous limiting membrane are grasped together with the iris, the vitreous may be lost.

Enzymatic zonulolysis: If the iris is inadvertently touched quite forcefully with the cannula while flushing with alpha-chymotrypsin, atrophic areas will result and pigment will be dispersed.

As soon as the lens is freed from the zonula, it starts to protrude. If unskilfully manipulated it could be dislocated posteriorly. For this reason the lens must be depressed with great care when instilling alpha-chymotrypsin.

Lens extraction: In all cases with complications, inadequate dilatation of the pupil and a cataract incision which is too short are disadvantages.

Spontaneous protrusion of the lens is extremely rare under general anesthetic. In cases of intumescent cataract the capsule is very brittle and tears very easily. The freezing procedure has to be prolonged; occasionally it is completely impossible. In such cases removal with capsule forceps and/or an Arlt loop is indicated.

In certain cases the vitreous body follows the lens out of the eye without the limiting membrane being torn. While the lens is suspended on the cryoextractor the assistant can facilitate detachment from the vitreous by flushing the lens with alpha-chymotrypsin from below.

If the vitreous protrudes following extraction, patience is required. It is important initially to avoid miosis, because this causes vitreous to be caught in the pupil, assuming a mushroom shape, and the limiting membrane of the vitreous may tear. For this reason the two sutures laid forward are knotted first. An effective way of forcing the vitreous body back out of the anterior chamber is to introduce air carefully into the latter. As soon as this has been done the pupil can be contracted with acetylcholine. Care must be taken to insure that no air finds its way behind the pupillary margin and into the posterior chamber.

During extraction the limiting membrane of the vitreous may be ruptured. In this eventuality an anterior vitrectomy must be performed following extraction, and vitreous carefully removed from the anterior chamber and the wound.

Loss of vitreous usually occurs when IOP has been insufficiently lowered preoperatively, or due to deficient surgical technique. General anesthesia and hyperosmotic infusion represent the best prophylaxis for vitreous loss.

Postoperative Management

After the operation antibiotic and miotic drops are administered; some authors prefer to apply the same drugs in the form of ointment. If an intraocular lens was implanted following extraction, dexamethasone is injected subconjunctivally. The eye is dressed and additionally protected with a metal patch.

For the following few days the patient is positioned with his/her head raised slightly so that the air bubble displaces the iris away from the incision area.

The dressing is changed for the first time 24 hours after surgery. Subsequently the patient is remobilized. A dressing is worn for one week; antibiotic and, if necessary, substances acting on the pupil are administered daily. The conjunctival sutures are removed one week postoperatively. Dexamethasone and chloramphenicol drops are then given in combination for a further two weeks.

Most postoperative complications which occur after cataract surgery are attributable to inadequate wound closure, blockage of the aqueous circulation, or pinching of the vitreous body.

Bibliography

[1] Barraquer, J., Troutman, R. C., Rutllàn, J.: *Die Chirurgie des vorderen Augenabschnittes, Bd. I.* Enke, Stuttgart 1965.

[2] Fasanella, R. M.: *Komplikationen in der Augenchirurgie und ihre Behandlung.* Enke, Stuttgart 1968.

Intracapsular Cataract Extraction with Iris-Supported Posterior Chamber Lens Implantation

Klaus Heilmann

The surgical principle of this procedure, preparation for surgery, preoperative medication and anesthesia, and instruments are as described under "Intracapsular Cataract Extraction," page 4.2.

Surgical Technique

(The description is for an operation on the left eye.)

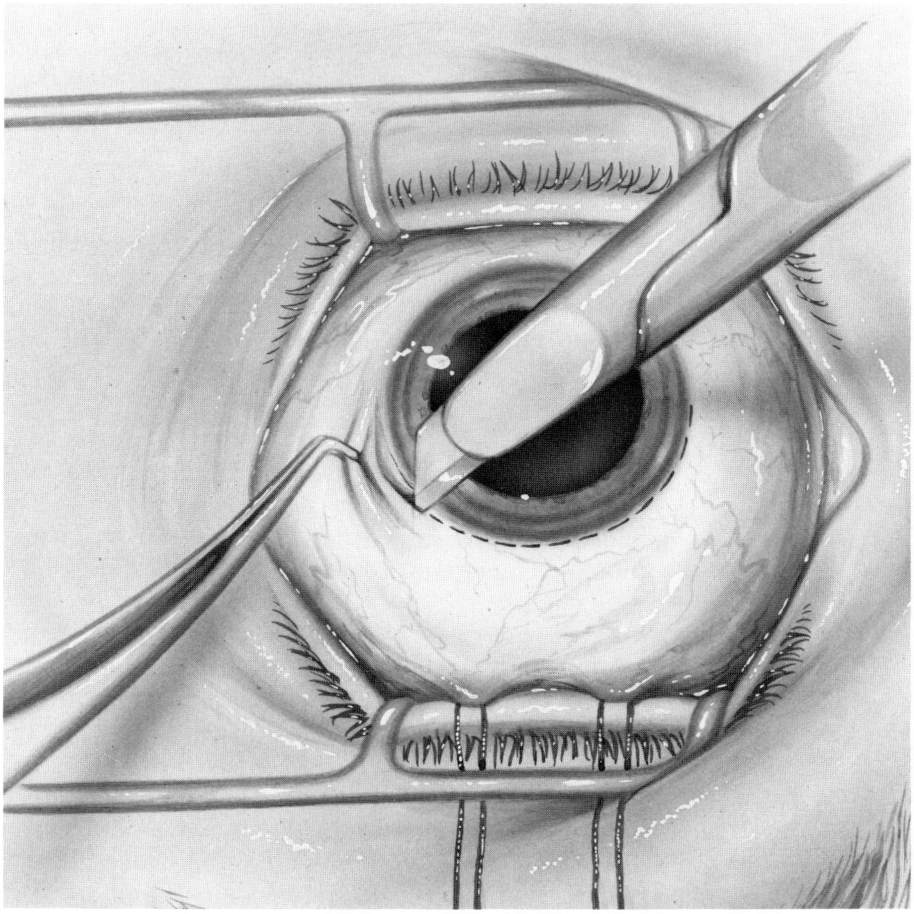

4.20 After placing the holding suture through the superior rectus muscle and inserting the Colibri lid retractor, the conjunctiva is grasped at 3 o'clock with the fixation forceps. Slight tension is applied with them while cutting along the cornea with the razor blade knife, keeping as close to the cornea as possible. If this is done correctly bleeding should be minimal.

21

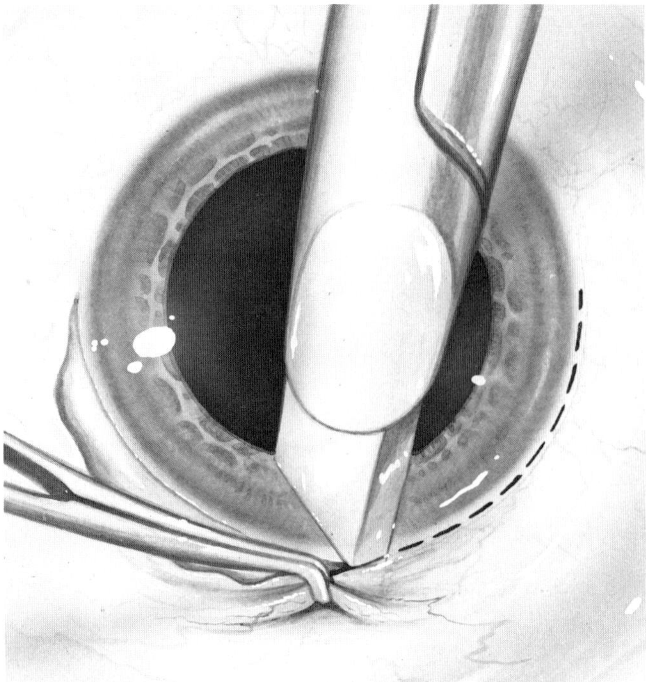

22

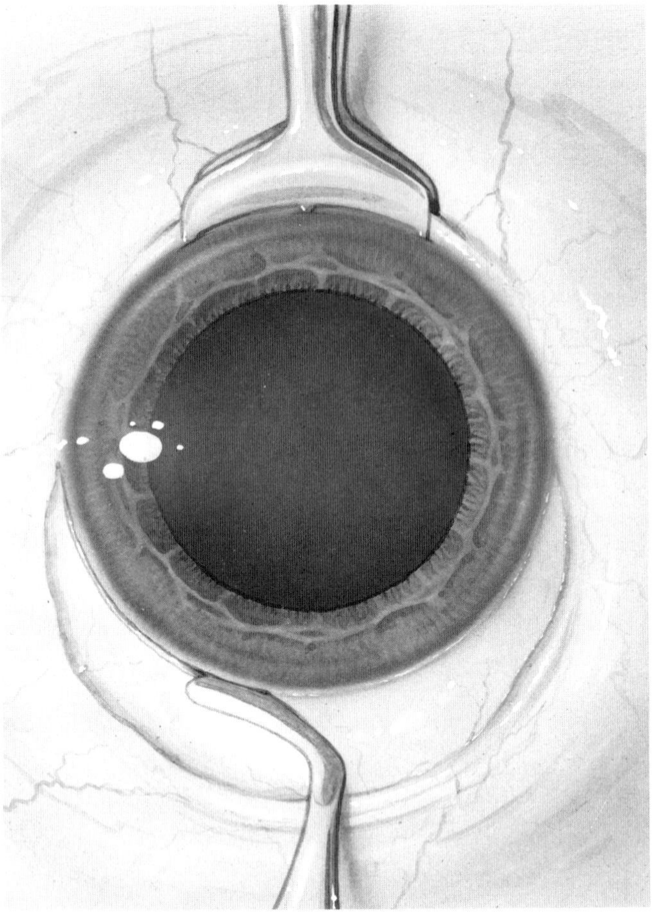

23

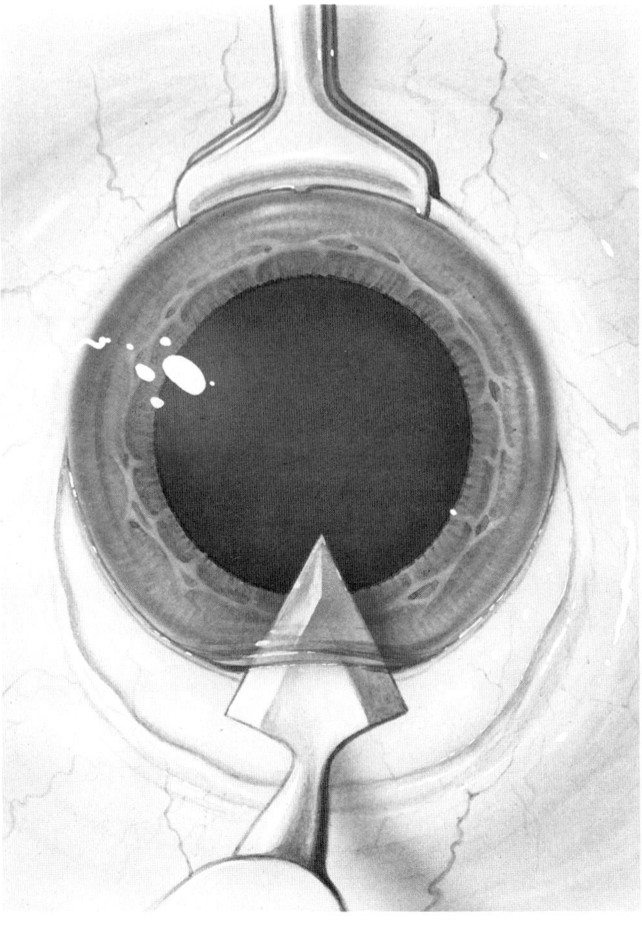

4.**21** The conjunctiva will automatically retract from the limbus. Any bleeding is stopped with a thermocautery or, better still, with bipolar forceps. If the conjunctival flap still interferes in the region of the incision, the margin is undermined and the conjunctiva is pushed farther back.

4.**22** Cutting a shallow groove with the hockey knife facilitates the subsequent corneoscleral incision. The blades of the scissors will slide along this groove as though of their own accord.

4.**23** The globe is grasped at 6 o'clock with Barraquer fixation forceps and pulled downward a little. Next a curved lancet (12×12 mm) is introduced into the anterior chamber at 12 o'clock, 0.5 mm outside the limbus. The blade must be held almost perpendicular to the corneal surface (radial to the midpoint of the eye). After inserting it into the anterior chamber one changes direction immediately, now guiding the blade parallel to the iris; injury to the iris and the lens is thus avoided. After creating a paracentesis some 3 mm wide the lancet is slowly withdrawn from the anterior chamber. There will be some seepage of aqueous.

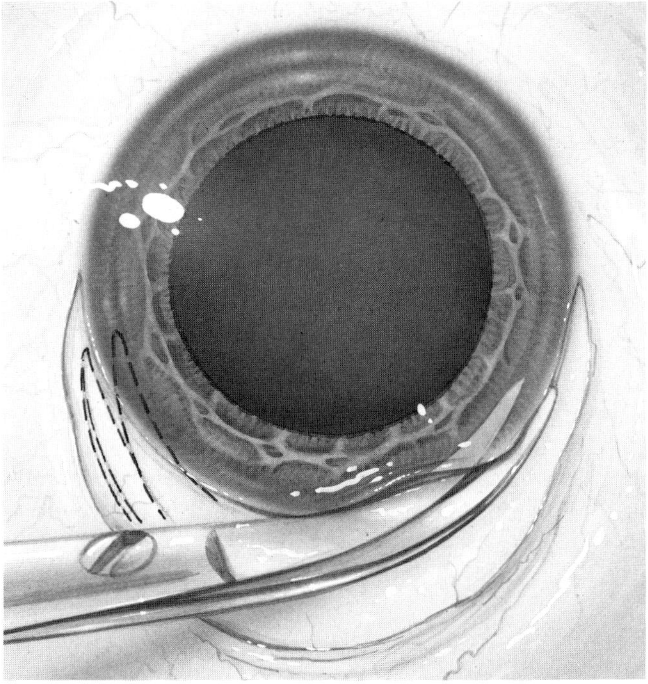

4.**24** Curved eye scissors are introduced into the opening thus created, and the incision is extended, first toward 9 o'clock and then toward 3 o'clock. Care must be taken to ensure that neither iris tissue nor conjunctiva are caught between the blades of the scissors. Cutting is continuous, i.e., the inner blade of the scissors does not leave the anterior chamber, so that an almost completely unserrated cut results.

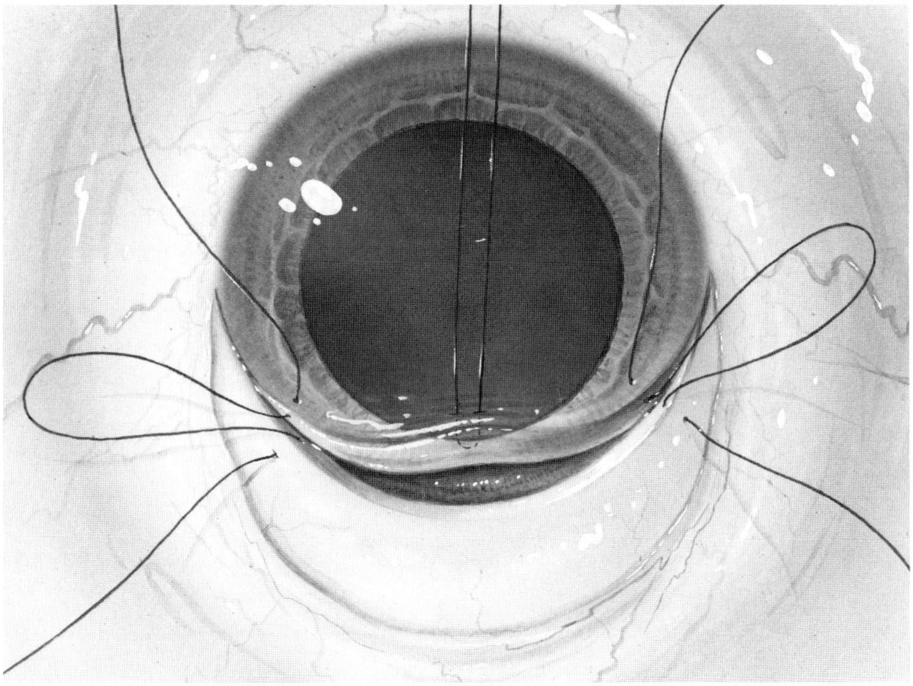

4.**25** Two corneoscleral sutures (monofilament 9-0 Vicryl) are placed at 2 and 10 o'clock. A similar suture is placed at 12 o'clock for raising the cornea. For the following steps in the procedure see Figs. 4.7 to 4.13, pages 4.6 to 4.9.

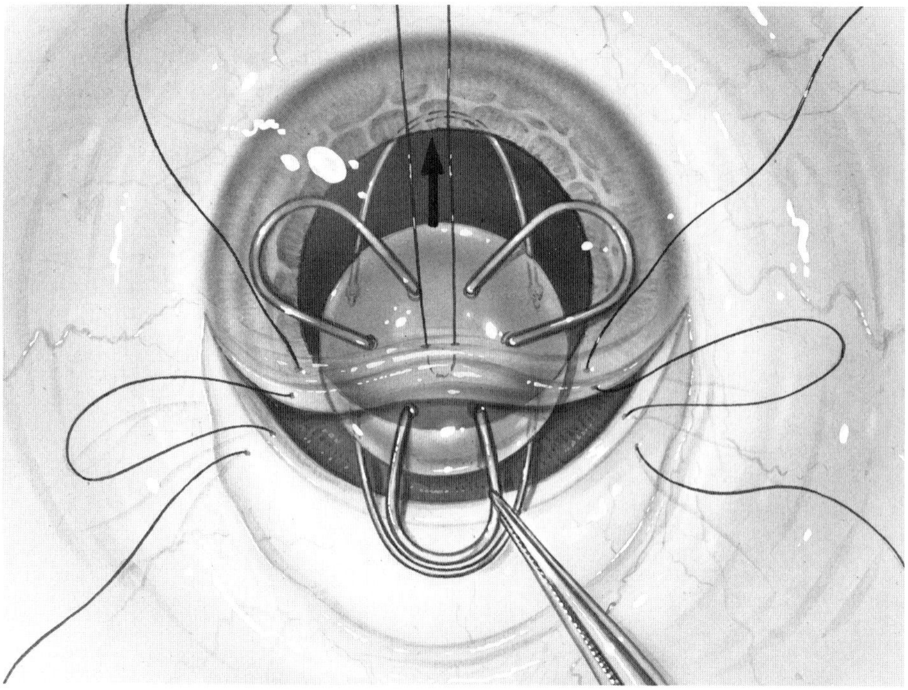

4.26 The cornea is raised very gently on the holding suture. The lens (Severin iris clip lens) is grasped with forceps at the edge of the top anterior haptic and – without touching the corneal endothelium – introduced into the anterior chamber in such a way that its lower posterior haptic slides under the pupillary margin at 6 o'clock. Care must be taken to ensure that the two lower anterior haptics of the lens simultaneously come to rest over the iris. (In most cases the corneal endothelium is not at risk; coating the anterior surface of the implant with a viscous substance ensures that the endothelium will be protected in all cases.)

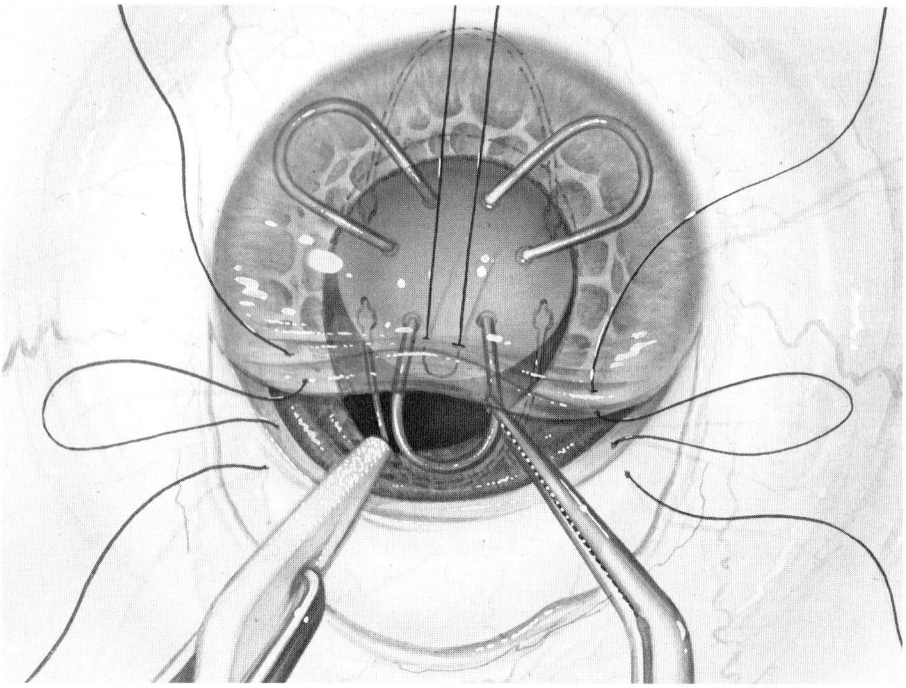

4.27 When it is certain that the haptics are positioned as described above, the body of the lens is carefully pushed down until its upper edge extends beyond the pupillary margin. The iris is pulled up slightly using a wedge-shaped sponge and the lens lowered somewhat, until the pupillary margin can slip between the upper posterior and anterior lens haptics.

28

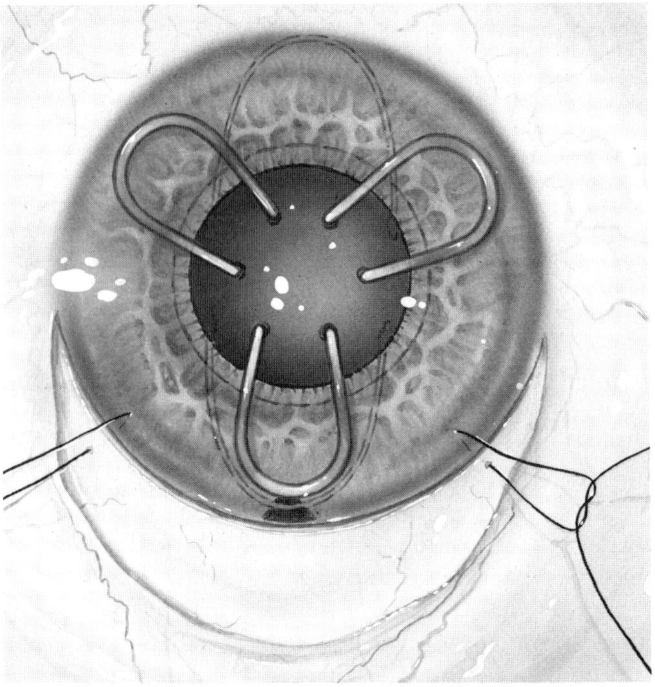

30

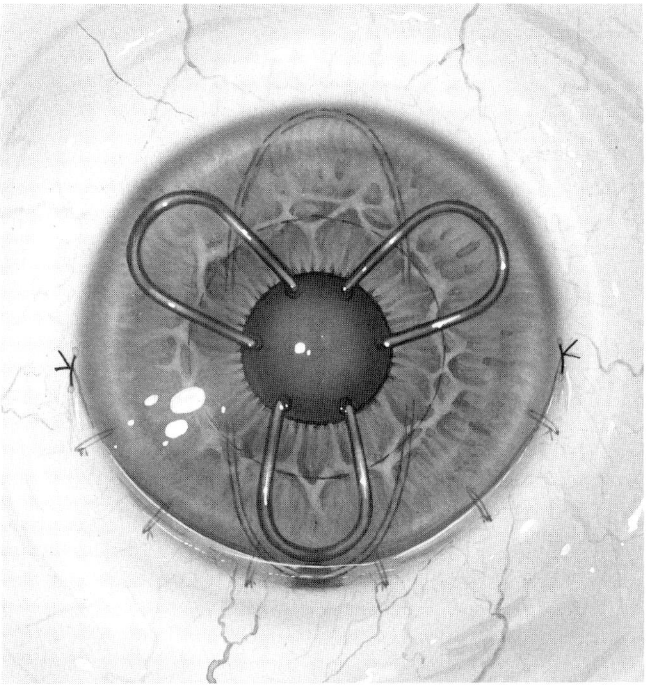

29

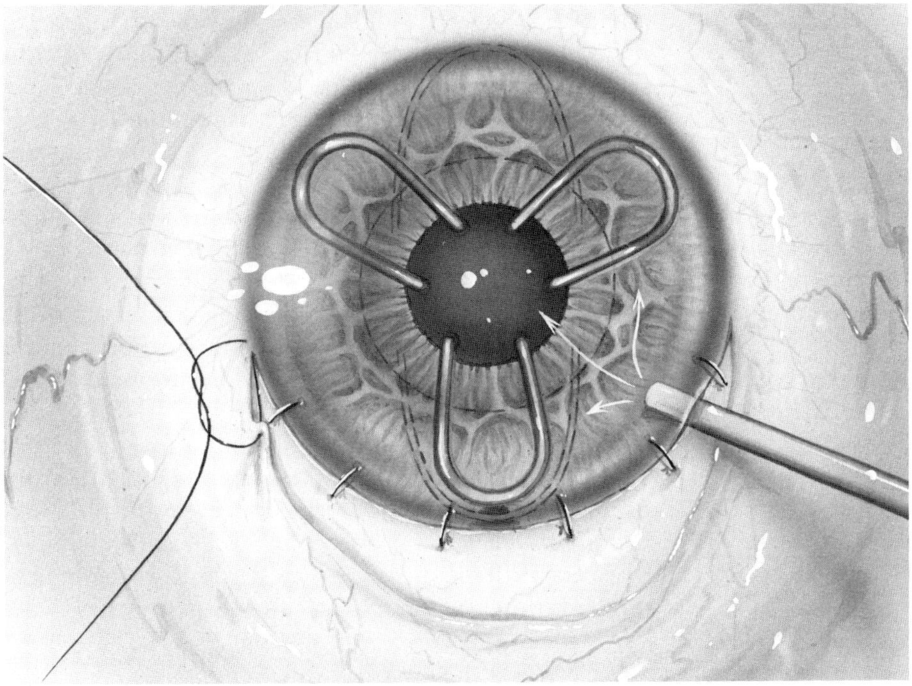

4.**28** The pupil is contracted immediately with acetylcholine, and the anterior chamber is flushed several times with balanced salt solution. The sutures placed in preparation are knotted, the holding suture is removed, and additional sutures are placed and knotted.

4.**29** More acetylcholine is instilled, and subsequently air. This must be done with great care to prevent air entering the posterior chamber and changing the position of the lens.

The conjunctiva is spread apronlike over the sclerocorneal wound and closed with two single 7-0 silk sutures.

4.**30** At the end of the procedure the wound should be closed and watertight, the pupil moderately dilated to contracted, and the lens centric.

Complications

If the vitreous bulges after the intracapsular cataract extraction, and the limiting membrane of the vitreous threatens to tear, either the lens implantation must be forgone or an attempt must be made to cause the vitreous to recede by filling the anterior chamber with a viscous substance such as sodium hyaluronate (Healon) or methylcellulose.

Correct positioning of the lens is facilitated, and dislocation into the vitreous cavity avoided, if the pupil is contracted with acetylcholine before implantation. Instillation of a viscous substance into the eye separates the anterior hyaloid membrane from the posterior surface of the iris, thus facilitating insertion of the lens implant and reducing mechanical damage of the vitreous. Miotic medication is continued after implanting the lens. Fixation of the lens on the iris is not practised by this author. Lens dislocation in the first few postoperative days or later is a very rare occurrence.

Postoperative Management

Postoperative management is as described for intracapsular cataract extraction, page 4.12.

Results

With careful microsurgical technique this procedure, which technically is not altogether simple, produces good visual results. The criticism of the procedure voiced by many authors is based less on the operation itself than on the possible surgical complications.

If no adhesion occurs between the pupillary margin and the lens, some pupillary "play" remains due to the lightness of the lens. In very elderly patients, provided no macular complications arise, very good central visual acuity can be achieved.

Bibliography

[1] Rosen, E. S.: IOL implantation with special reference to intra-capsular cataract extraction. *Cataract*: 20–30, April 1984

[2] Severin, S. L.: The Severin posterior chamber lens. In: Rosen, E. S., Haining, W. M., Arnott, E. J. (eds.): *Intraocular Lens Implantation*. Mosby, St. Louis 1983, pages 327–334.

Anterior Chamber Intraocular Lens Implantation

Douglas D. Koch

Surgical Principles

Anterior chamber lens implantation is currently the second most frequently utilized form of pseudophakic correction;[1] it is indicated in older patients who strongly desire pseudophakic correction and whose zonular-capsular support is deficient or absent, thereby precluding posterior chamber lens implantation. Potentially suitable eyes, therefore, are those that have undergone intracapsular cataract extraction or have weak zonules or large posterior capsule openings (exceeding 6 mm).

A wide variety of anterior chamber lenses are available for implantation. Selection of a particular lens type is probably less critical than is proper determination of lens size, proper lens positioning in the anterior chamber angle, and proper management of the vitreous. There are few definitive data available to guide the surgeon in selecting a particular anterior chamber lens design. This author prefers a flexible lens that has a minimal area of contact with the anterior chamber angle. Rigid lenses are difficult to size appropriately and can cause marked tenderness to touch and distortion of the iris and pupil. These problems are partially alleviated with more flexible lenses, although careful lens sizing must still be performed intraoperatively. Lenses with a broad arc of chamber angle contact may be less desirable because they can be associated with the formation of broad peripheral anterior synechiae.

In this chapter, secondary implantation of the UV 11 H Stableflex lens, manufactured by Optical Radiation Corporation, is described. The principles and techniques of lens insertion are essentially identical, irrespective of the specific lens design and of whether the implantation is primary or secondary.

Preparation for Surgery

The preoperative routine is as for extracapsular cataract extraction.

Preoperative Medication and Anesthesia

Local anesthesia is employed as described in the section on extracapsular cataract extraction. It is helpful to constrict the pupil prior to implanting the lens. If this is a secondary implantation and a vitrectomy is not anticipated, 2% pilocarpine drops are given 30 minutes preoperatively.

Instruments

A standard cataract and intraocular lens instrument tray is required. Optional extras are: sodium hyaluronate; Thorpe gonioprism or other surgical goniolens; automated vitrector if anterior vitrectomy is planned.

Surgical Technique

31

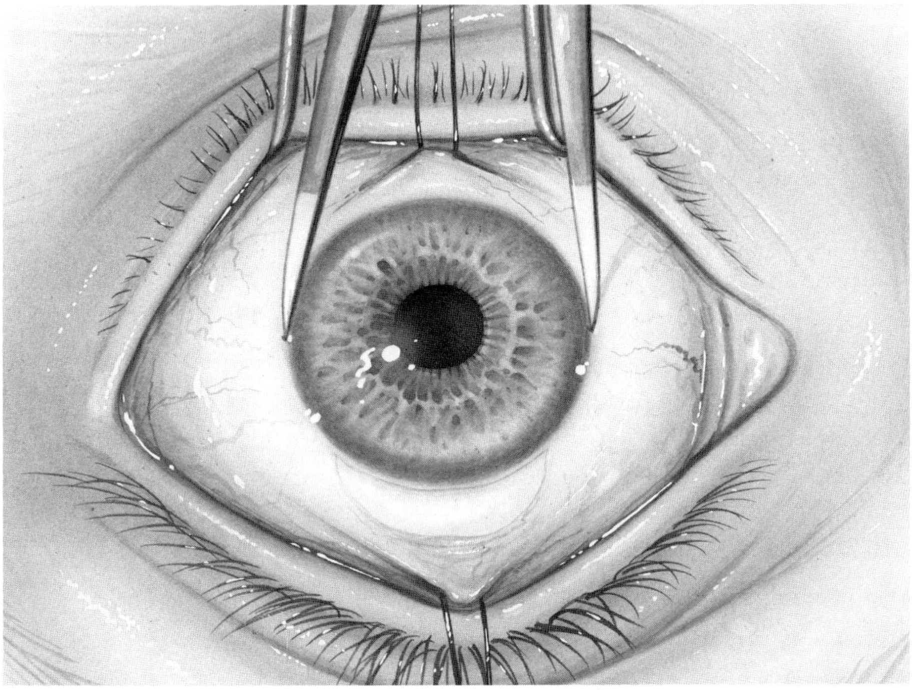

32

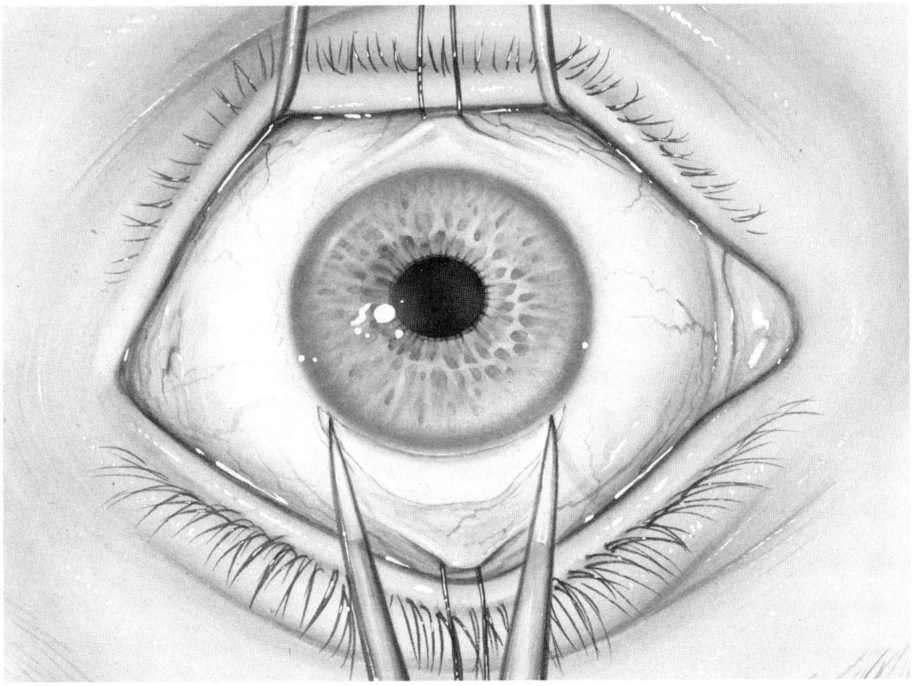

4.31 The calipers are used to measure the corneal diameter—the so-called "white-to-white" distance. The white-to-white measurement plus one provides a rough estimate of the anterior chamber diameter, but it is only an estimate and should not be the major criterion for determining the lens size.

4.32 The length of the incision is determined by the diameter of the intraocular lens optic and should exceed the optic size by 1 mm. This is marked with calipers. The incision can be made superiorly or temporally. If preexisting astigmatism exceeds 2 D, a scleral flap is formed along the steep or flat meridian; this flap is recessed or resected, respectively, under intraoperative keratometric control.

It is helpful to leave at least a 1 mm internal scleral lip between the iris and the incision; this provides room for haptic implantation without haptic contact with the wound or sutures. Therefore, entry into the anterior chamber should be made relatively anteriorly. If a superior incision is planned, the incision and anterior chamber entry can be made in the mid- or anterior limbus while still preserving an adequate scleral lip. The temporal limbus is narrower and more posteriorly located. A limbal incision temporally should therefore be shelved anteriorly to avoid anterior chamber entry near the iris root; a clear corneal incision temporally facilitates preservation of an adequate scleral lip.

33

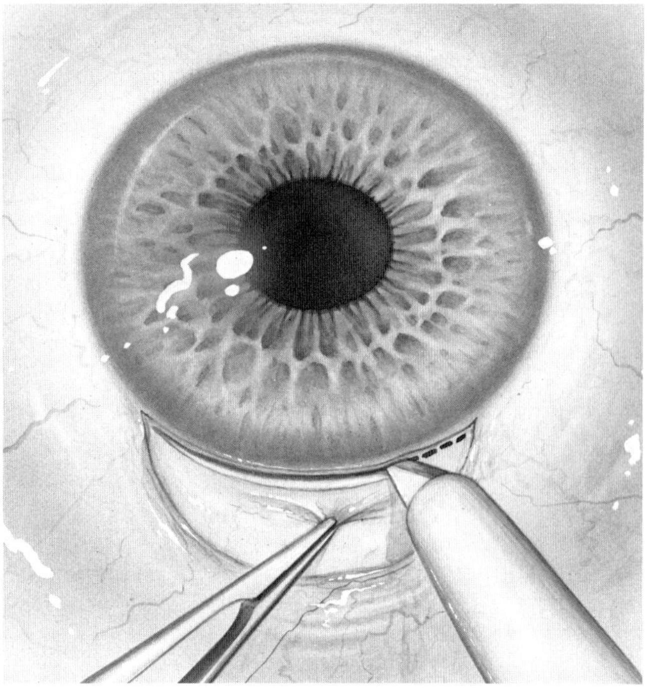

34

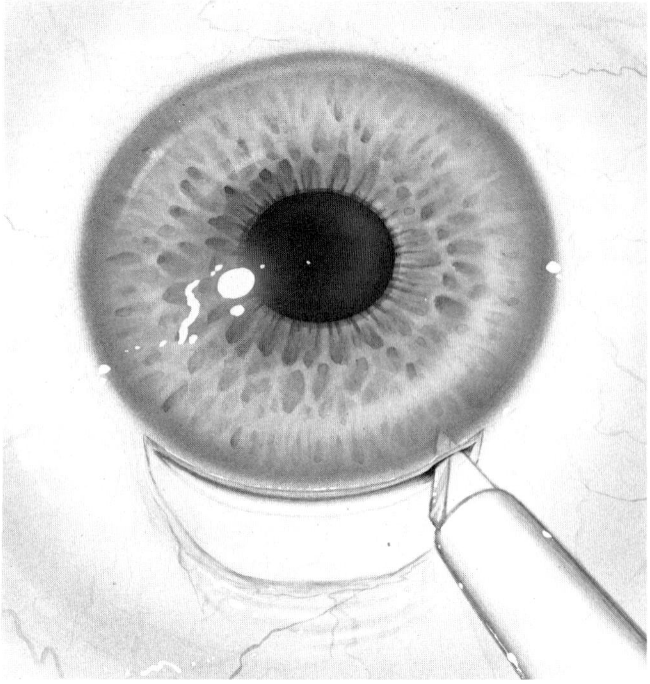

35

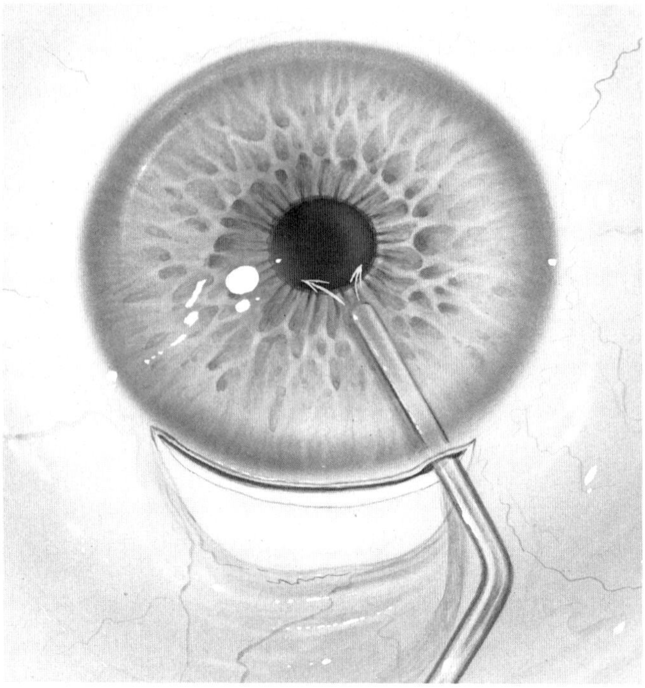

4.**33** A vertical groove is made with a microsurgical steel knife.

4.**34** A stab incision is made into the anterior chamber. If an anterior vitrectomy is planned, it should be performed at this stage of the operation. This procedure is described in the section on corneoscleral lacerations.

4.**35** Acetylcholine is injected to constrict the pupil.

36

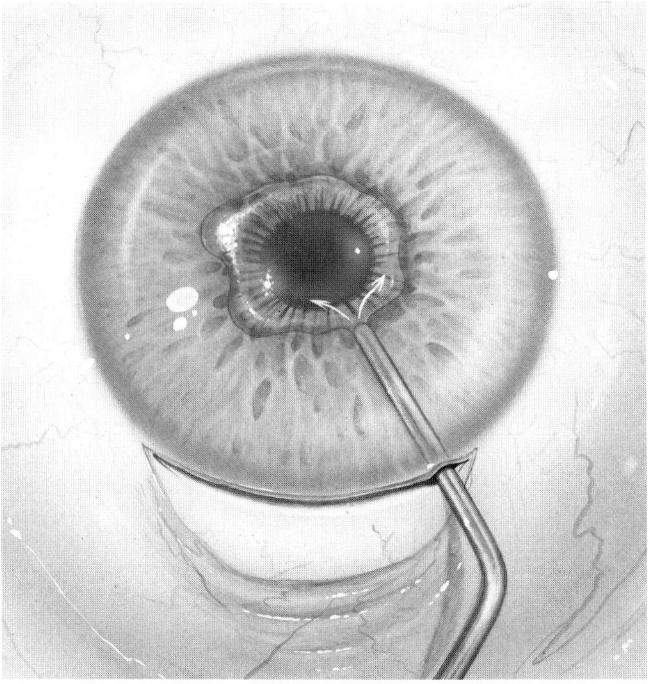

38

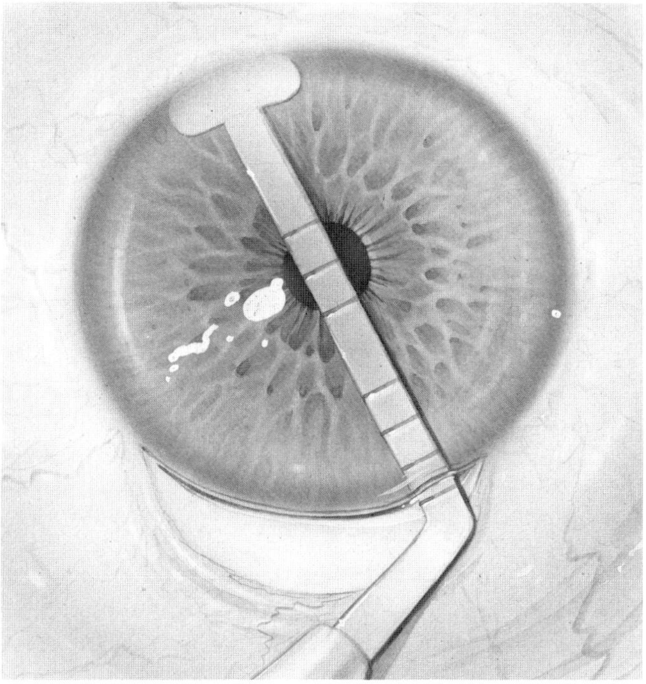

37

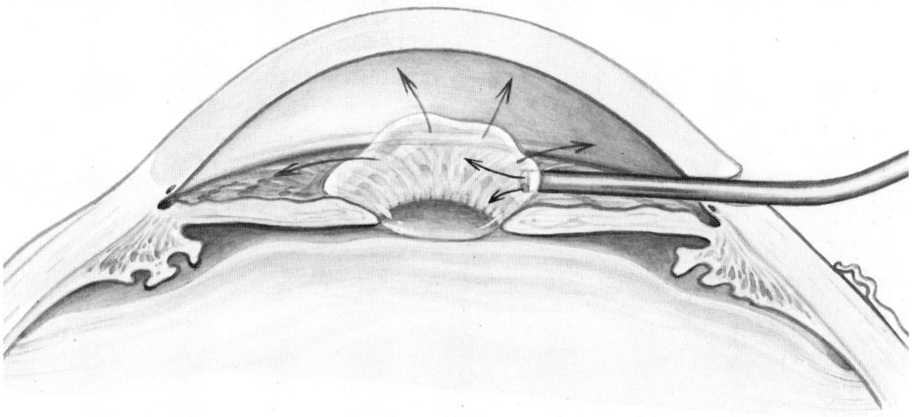

4.**36** and **37** The anterior chamber is filled with sodium hyaluronate or air. The injection is first made over the pupil in order to mechanically block anterior movement of the vitreous.

4.**38** The Tennant or Kelman anterior chamber gauge can be used to measure the anterior chamber diameter. These instruments provide a better estimate of anterior chamber diameter than does the white-to-white measurement. However, the ultimate determinant of the appropriate lens size is the adequacy of lens fit after insertion.

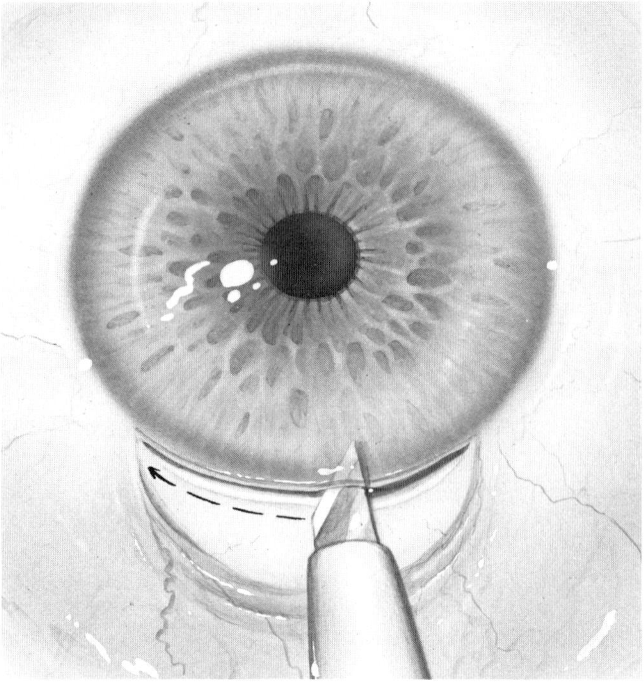

4.39 The wound is enlarged to 7 mm with the microsurgical knife.

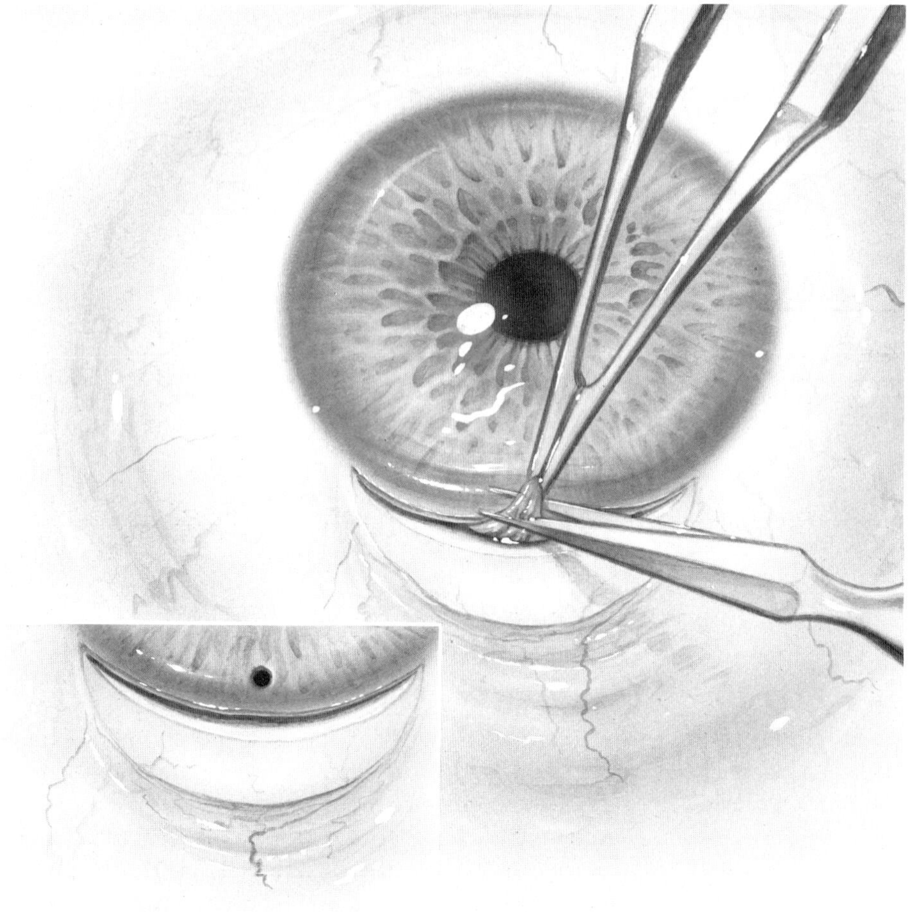

4.40 An iridectomy is made if one is not already present; it should be placed in the mid-periphery, approximately 2 mm from the iris root. An iridectomy reduces the risk of pupillary block by the vitreous or lens optic; however, pupillary block can still occur if the lens haptic or vitreous occludes the iridectomy.

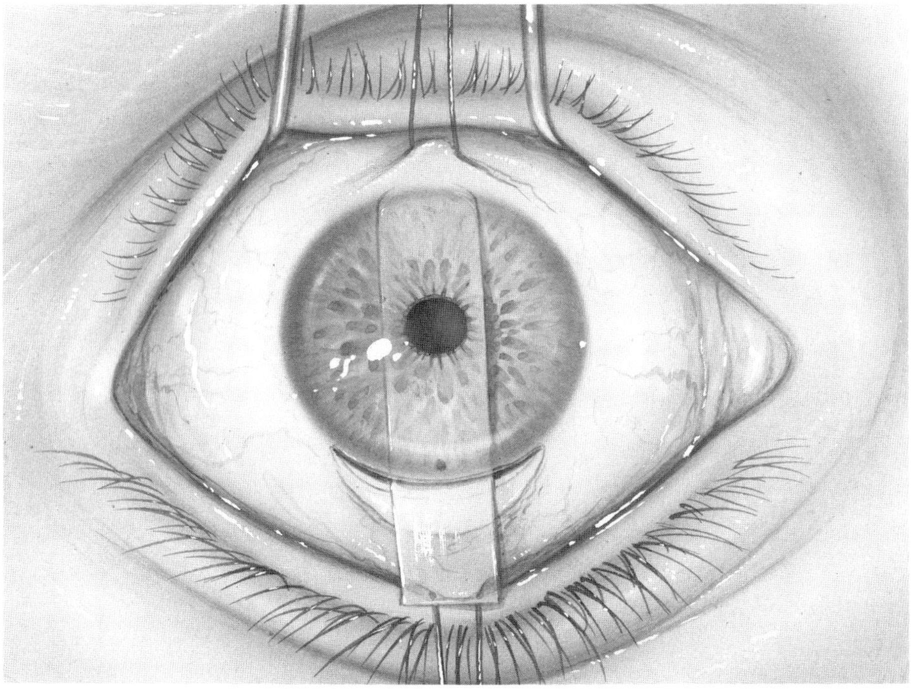

4.41 A Sheets glide is made using a Sheets glide cutter or utility scissors. The glide is inserted across the anterior chamber and positioned securely in the opposite anterior chamber angle. The glide helps to prevent iris tuck by the haptics as they are passed over the iris.

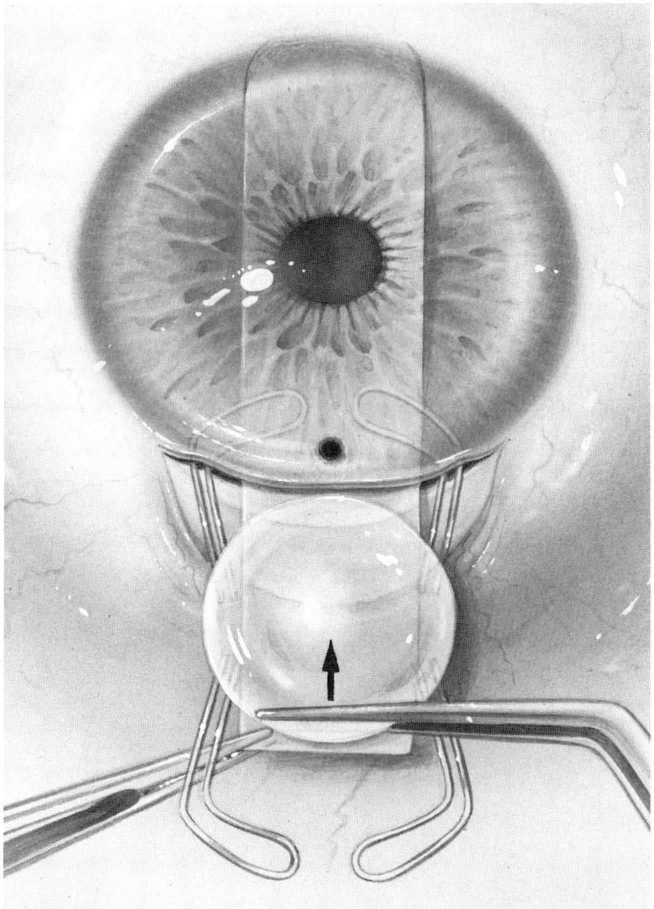

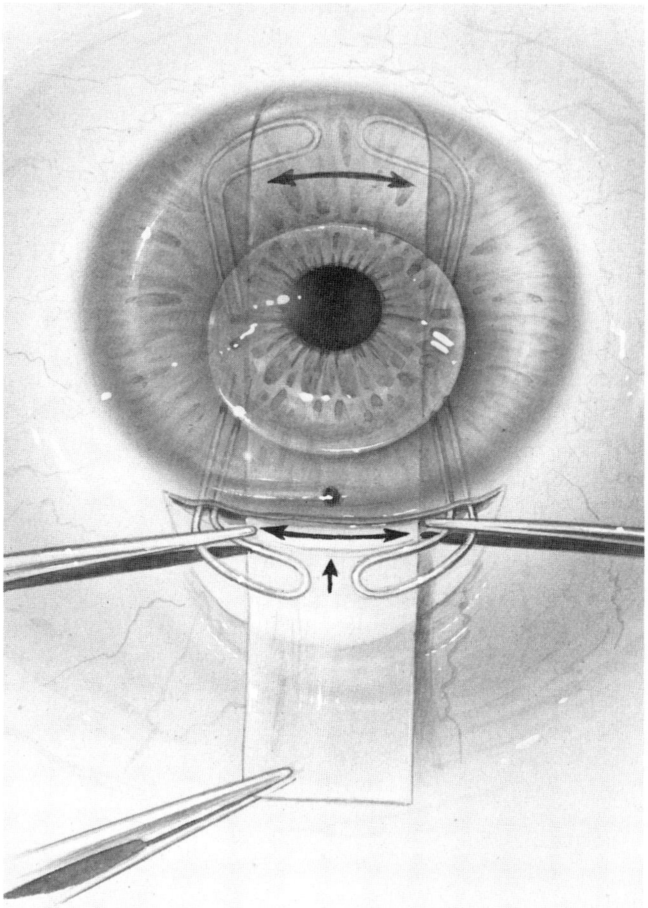

4.42 The optic is grasped with smooth forceps during the initial phases of lens implantation, and its inferior edge is tilted down to avoid Descemet's membrane and to prevent the inferior haptics from touching the corneal endothelium.

4.43 A pendulum movement is used while sliding the lower haptics into the inferior anterior chamber angle. The continuous back-and-forth motion disengages the iris if it gets caught on the haptics, thereby avoiding iris tuck. This maneuver is especially helpful if a Sheets glide is not employed. With the lower haptics in position in the inferior angle, the upper haptics of a correctly sized lens should extend onto the sclera 0.5–1.5 mm, depending upon the position of the incision.

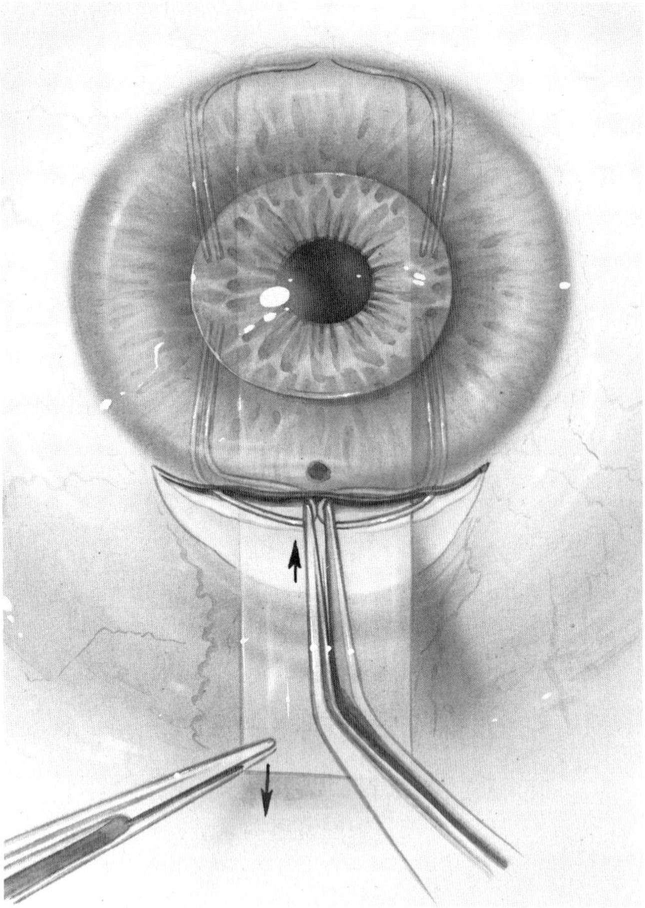

4.44 In inserting the upper lens haptics of this flexible lens, it is helpful, but not necessary, to retract the sclera with 0.12 mm forceps. (With rigid lenses, retraction of the posterior wound edge is recommended to avoid inferior angle or iris injury.) Both upper loops are grasped with smooth forceps. The loops are flexed inferiorly and directed posteriorly into the anterior chamber angle.

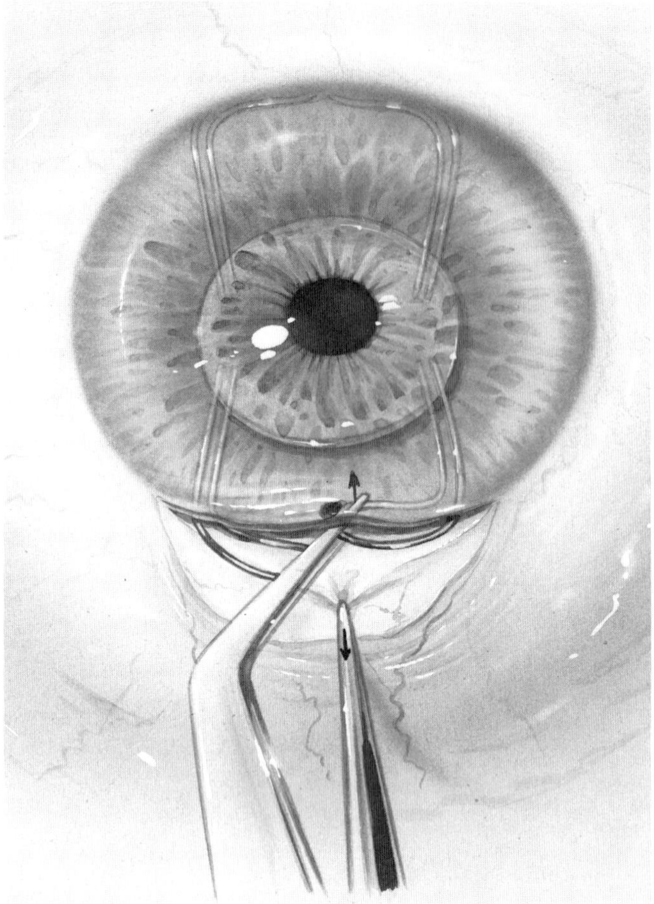

4.45 An alternative method is to insert each upper loop separately. This is facilitated by grasping the inner portion of the loop; if the outer portion is grasped, the forceps mechanically interferes with loop placement into the angle recess.

The accuracy of lens size can be assessed by gently pushing on the sclera overlying the superior haptics. The lens should flex slightly but not move freely. Similarly, the Sinskey hook can be inserted, and lateral pressure can be applied at the junction of the haptic and optic. Again, slight resistance to movement should be encountered. Signs of excessive lens size are excessive resistance to lens movement, gaping of the wound, and ovaling of the pupil in the absence of iris tuck.

46

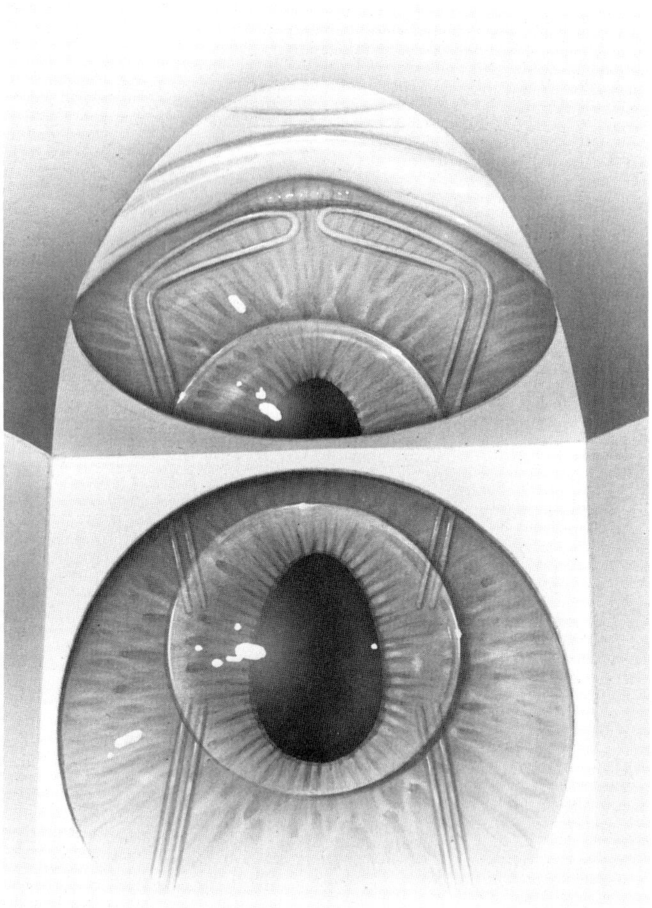

47

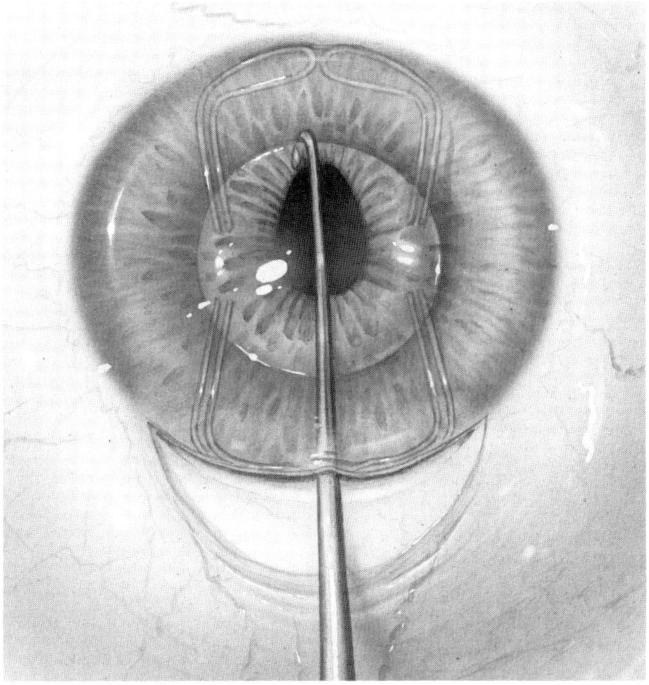

4.**46** Gonioscopy can be performed to ensure that there is no iris tuck superiorly or inferiorly. The pupil is usually oval if iris tuck is present; however, this is not an infallible sign because the pupil can be round when iris tuck is present, and the pupil can be oval when no iris tuck exists (especially after an iris tuck has been released). In this drawing, inferior iris tuck is illustrated.

48

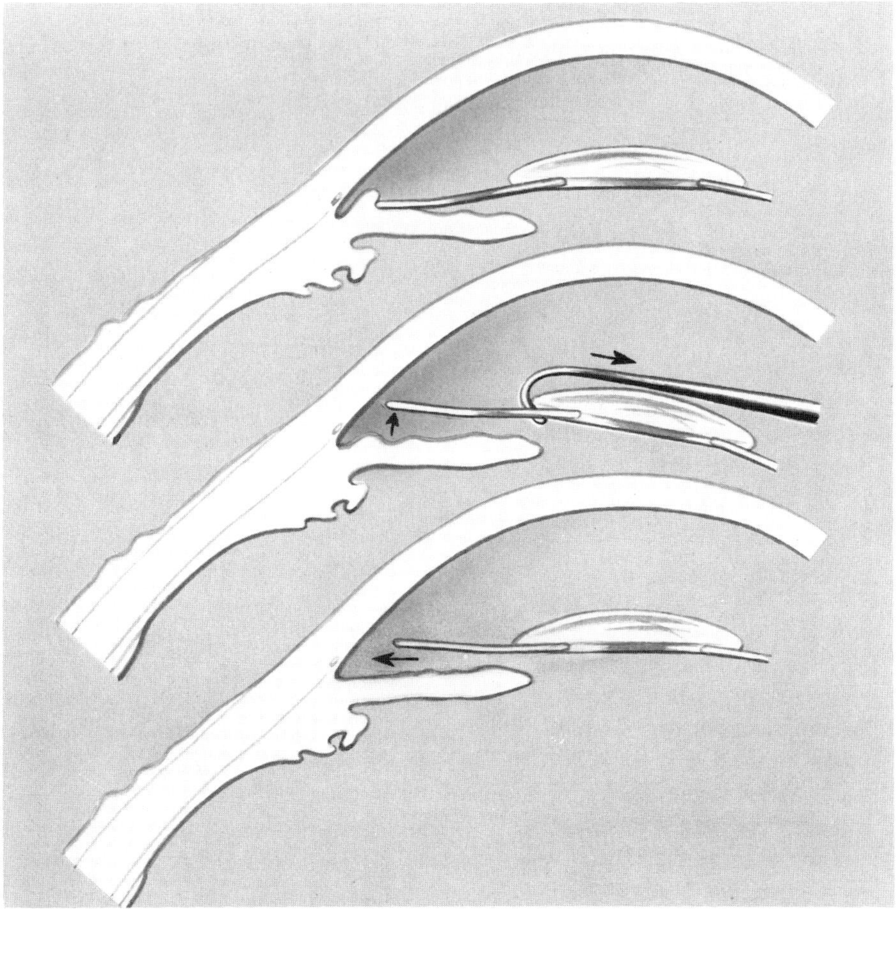

4.**47** and **48** Iris tuck can be relieved by retracting the lens from the area of the tuck using a microsurgical hook. The lens is then slightly elevated and allowed to glide back into the angle. This can be done safely and atraumatically if anterior chamber depth is maintained with sodium hyaluronate or air.

A superior tuck is readily released by pushing the optic inferiorly while elevating it slightly. The upper haptic is then allowed to slide back into the angle while the elevation is maintained.

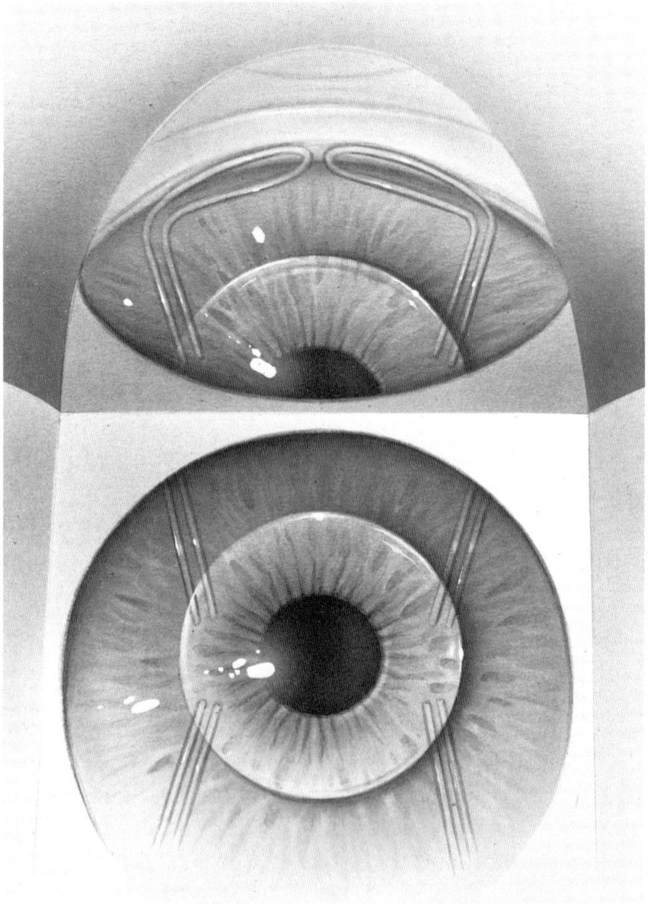

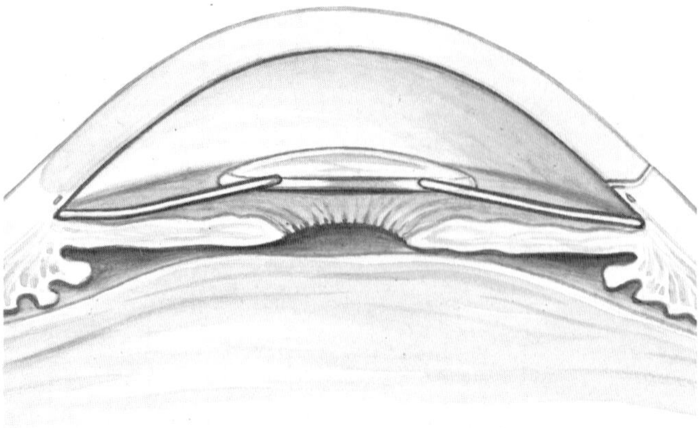

4.49 and **50** The lens loops are in the proper position in the anterior chamber angle, without iris tuck.

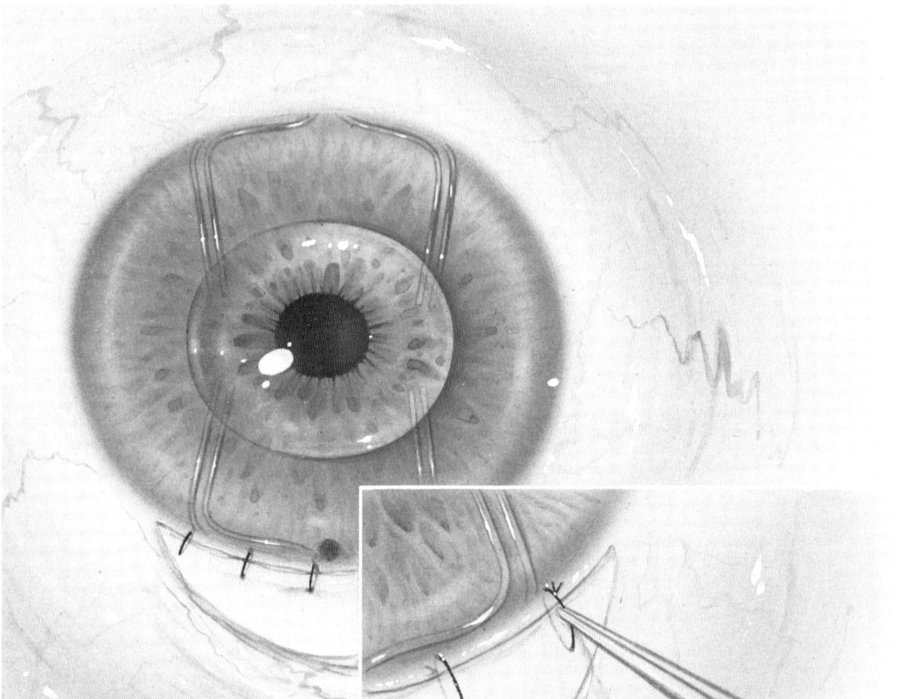

4.51 The wound is sutured with interrupted sutures. The knots are buried.

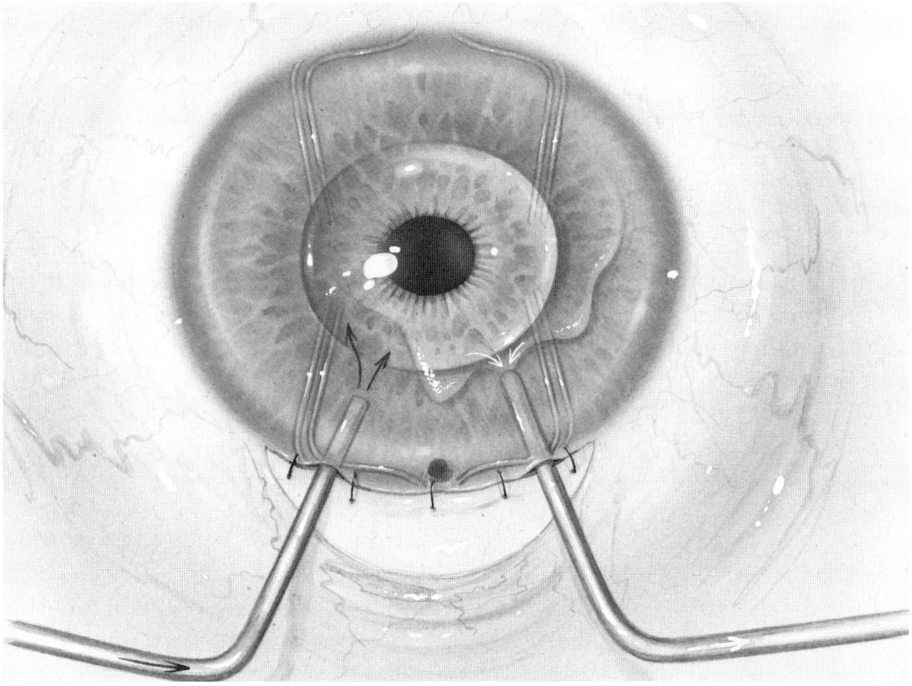

4.52 The sodium hyaluronate or air is aspirated. To maintain adequate anterior chamber depth, it is helpful to have the assistant inject balanced salt solution while the surgeon aspirates the sodium hyaluronate or air. The hyaluronate is easily aspirated using a 27-gauge cannula on a 3 ml plastic syringe containing balanced salt solution.

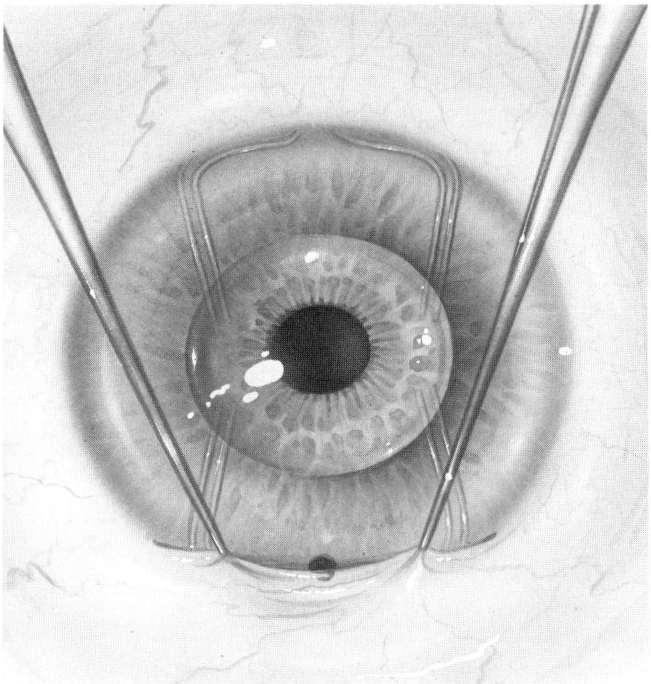

4.53 The wound is checked to ensure that it is sufficiently water-tight. If a conjunctival flap was made, the conjunctiva is manually retracted over the wound. Suturing of the conjunctival flap is not necessary. The eye is dressed with a combination antibiotic and corticosteroid ointment. Eserine ointment is instilled to maintain pupillary constriction, which protects against pupillary capture of the lens optic.

Complications

Wound: It is important to examine the wound carefully following lens implantation to ensure that a portion of the superior haptic is not entrapped in the incision; this can escape detection unless the wound is meticulously inspected.

Cornea: Direct lens contact with the corneal endothelium can occur if anterior chamber depth is inadequate or if the inferior haptics are directed anteriorly during lens insertion. Sodium hyaluronate is preferable to air in avoiding these problems. It affords greater visibility and predictability; an air bubble can suddenly escape if there is significant vitreous pressure or wound gape during insertion.

Iridectomy: Lens haptics positioned near a peripheral iridectomy can migrate posteriorly through it. It is therefore advisable to position the lens such that none of its haptics overlie or are adjacent to a peripheral iridectomy. Despite this precaution, the lens, especially when undersized, can rotate such that the haptic enters the iridectomy; this problem is less common with flexible lenses, and it rarely if ever occurs when the iridectomy is mid-peripheral.

Vitreous: Vitreous present in the anterior chamber during lens implantation predisposes to an increased incidence of postoperative complications. If the vitreous is not removed, it becomes entrapped in the haptics or in the wound. This results in chronic vitreous traction, which in turn can cause chronic iridocyclitis, cystoid macular edema, retinal detachment, and the vitreous wick syndrome. Typically, in these instances, vitreous presents to the wound immediately after the anterior chamber is entered.

If vitreous is present in the anterior chamber, an anterior vitrectomy is usually required to avoid vitreous entrapment in the wound or haptics. Unfortunately, in the author's experience, performing an anterior vitrectomy at the time of secondary implantation increases the incidence of postoperative retinal detachment. In a series of 35 secondary anterior chamber lens implants (follow-up ≥ 1 year), postoperative retinal detachment occurred in two of 15 (13 %) patients who underwent vitrectomy.[2] None of the 20 non-vitrectomized patients developed this complication. These risks must be weighed before proceeding with secondary implantation; pre- and postoperative follow-up must include careful peripheral retinal examinations.

Occasionally, vitreous in the anterior chamber can be mechanically pushed back through the pupil, especially if the vitreous face is intact. Following a small stab incision, air is immediately injected into the anterior chamber to force the vitreous back through the pupil. The air is then replaced with sodium hyaluronate, which is first placed over the pupil and then into the inferior angle until the entire anterior chamber is filled. In this fashion, vitreous removal and adherence to the intraocular lens can sometimes be avoided.

If vitreous presents to the wound after the lens has been implanted, management depends on the amount of vitreous present. A small vitreous strand can usually be swept away from the wound with an iris spatula after wound closure. Slightly greater amounts of vitreous loss can often be managed by performing a minimal vitrectomy using microsurgical sponges. Extensive vitreous loss is best managed by automated anterior vitrectomy. It is usually easier to remove the implant first and then reinsert it when the surgeon is assured that no vitreous remains in the anterior chamber.

Admonitions and Suggestions

Meticulous preoperative examination is essential for patients being considered for secondary anterior chamber lens implantation. Gonioscopy should be performed to ascertain if peripheral anterior synechiae are present and to examine any existing iridectomies. The lens haptics must not be inserted against peripheral anterior synechiae: this can lead to further synechia formation, migration of the endothelium onto the haptics and iris, and eventual corneal decompensation and glaucoma.[3]

The corneal endothelium should be carefully assessed preoperatively, especially in secondary implant patients. If possible, a quantitative measurement or estimate of endothelial cell density should be obtained. If specular micrography is not readily available, a sufficiently accurate estimate of endothelial cell density can usually be obtained with a semiquantitative device such as a reticle for the slit lamp ocular.[4]

There is a higher incidence of cystoid macular edema if the interval between intracapsular extraction and secondary lens implantation is less than one year;[5] therefore, it is prudent to wait at least one year following the original surgery. Fluorescein angiography is advisable in any patient whose history suggests that cystoid macular edema might be present. Secondary anterior chamber lens implantation can exacerbate pre-existing cystoid macular edema and is usually contraindicated in these patients.

Postoperative Management and Complications

The eye patch is removed on the morning following surgery. Prednisolone acetate drops are begun and continued for eight weeks following surgery.

Pupillary capture of the lens optic can occur in rare instances. This is managed by vigorously dilating the pupil while the patient is supine. Administration of oral osmotic agents such as glycerol can assist this process by reducing vitreous pressure. If the capture is successfully broken, miotic drops are begun and continued for several days. If the pupillary capture cannot be broken pharmacologically, then surgical intervention is preferable. Persistent pupillary capture can lead to chronic iridocyclitis.

Pupillary block glaucoma can occur despite a patent iridectomy. An iridectomy can be occluded by vitreous or by the haptic, as was noted above. Signs of pupillary block include elevated intraocular pressure, shallow anterior chamber, and convex bulging of the iris. If the lens optic is in contact with the iris over 360° around the pupil, it is likely that the lens itself is the cause of pupillary block. Pupillary block can usually be alleviated with an Nd: YAG or argon laser iridotomy. It is advisable to make several iridotomies, as they can easily become occluded. Surgical iridectomy is reserved for those instances in which laser iridotomy is unsuccessful or in which intimate contact of the iris and corneal endothelium precludes laser treatment.

A lens that is too small can change position or "propeller" post-operatively. Gross lens movements can be detected by having the patient assume a supine position. As the patient looks either up or down, the lens can be seen to move. Subtle lens movements can be detected at the slit lamp by having the patient look laterally and then rapidly refixate. It is extremely rare for a lens to achieve secure fixation if movement is present postoperatively. Chronic lens movement can lead to corneal endothelial decompensation and cystoid macular edema. The problem can be managed by replacing the lens with a larger lens or by suturing the haptic to the iris with a polypropylene suture.

An oversized lens can result in chronic eye pain and excessive tenderness to touch. One or more of the lens haptics can migrate from the chamber angle into the iris and ciliary body. Progressive ovaling of the pupil often occurs. Indications for lens removal or replacement include intolerable eye pain and chronic iridocyclitis accompanied by glaucoma or cystoid macular edema.

Results

In the United States Food and Drug Administration study, visual acuity of 20/40 or better was obtained by over 90 % of primary anterior chamber lens patients without pre-existing eye pathology (excluding cataract).[6] In evaluating the results of secondary anterior chamber implants, a key statistic is the percentage of patients that retain their best-corrected preoperative acuity. In two recent reports, less than 10 % of patients lost two or more lines of Snellen visual acuity.[7, 8] In this author's series, best corrected preoperative acuity was preserved in 92 % of cases.[2] The major causes of visual loss in these series have been cystoid macular edema and retinal detachment.

References

1 Stark, W. J., Terry, A. C., Worthen, D., Murray, G. C.: Update of intraocular lenses implanted in the United States. *Amer. J. Ophthalmol.* 98: 238–239, 1984.

2 Wong, S. K., Koch, D. D., Emery, J. M.: Secondary intraocular lens implantation. J. Cataract Refract. Surg. (in press).

3 Rowsey, J. J., Gaylor, J. R.: Intraocular lens disasters. *Ophthalmology* 87 (7): 646–664, 1980.

4 McIntyre, D. J.: Comparative endothelial biomicroscopy. *Amer. Intra-Ocular Implant Soc.* J. 5: 346–348, 1979.

5 Shammas, H. J. F., Milkie, C. F.: Cystoid macular edema following secondary lens implantation. *Amer. Intra-Ocular Implant Soc.* J. 7: 40–42, 1981.

6 Stark, W. J., Worthen, D. M., Holladay, J. T. et al.: The FDA Report on Intraocular Lenses. *Ophthalmology* 90: 311–317, 1983.

7 Kraff, M. C., Sanders, D. R., Lieberman, H. L., Kraff, J.: Secondary intraocular lens implantation. *Ophthalmology* 90: 324–326, 1983.

8 Lindstrom, R. L., Harris, W. S.: Secondary anterior chamber lens implantation. *CLAO J.* 10 (2): 133–136, 1984.

Extracapsular Cataract Extraction and Posterior Chamber Lens Implantation

Jared M. Emery and Douglas D. Koch

Surgical Principles

The aim of this surgical procedure is to remove the lens, including all cortical remnants, while leaving the zonules intact and the posterior lens capsule intact and clear. It is desirable to leave an ample, intact rim of anterior lens capsule as support for a posterior chamber lens to be held within the capsule bag. Alternatively, the posterior chamber lens may be placed outside the capsule bag so that the haptics make contact with the ciliary sulcus. Capsular bag implantation is discussed elsewhere in this chapter; sulcus implantation is described here.

Preparation for Surgery

Preparation of the patient for surgery is a highly personalized process that each ophthalmologist handles according to his own preferences, personality, and style. In-depth patient counseling by the physician and his aides will reduce the patient's anxiety by providing detailed information about what the problem is, and what the physician will do to solve the problem. This counseling should include information about experiences that the patient will have in the immediate preoperative, operative, and postoperative periods.

We prefer to do cataract/lens implant procedures on an outpatient basis. The patient is advised not to eat or drink after midnight the day before surgery, but routine medications are taken with a small amount of water in the morning as usual.

On the day before surgery, the patient receives an ocular and general physical examination. Routine preoperative photographs are taken, including a fullface view to document the position of the lids and a slitlamp view of the cataract. A-scan ultrasonography is used to determine the power of the lens to be implanted. Urinalysis is performed, and blood is tested for complete blood count, serum electrolytes, creatinine, and blood nitrogen. An electrocardiogram is obtained. Detailed consent forms are discussed and signed with the patient.

Preoperative Medication

Most of our patients have outpatient cataract surgery. The patient is given a 500 mg Diamox Sequel approximately 45 minutes to one hour before surgery. Good pupillary dilation is achieved with 1 % cyclopentolate hydrochloride and 10 % phenylephrine hydrochloride, one drop of each to the eye in question approximately 30 minutes before surgery.

Instruments

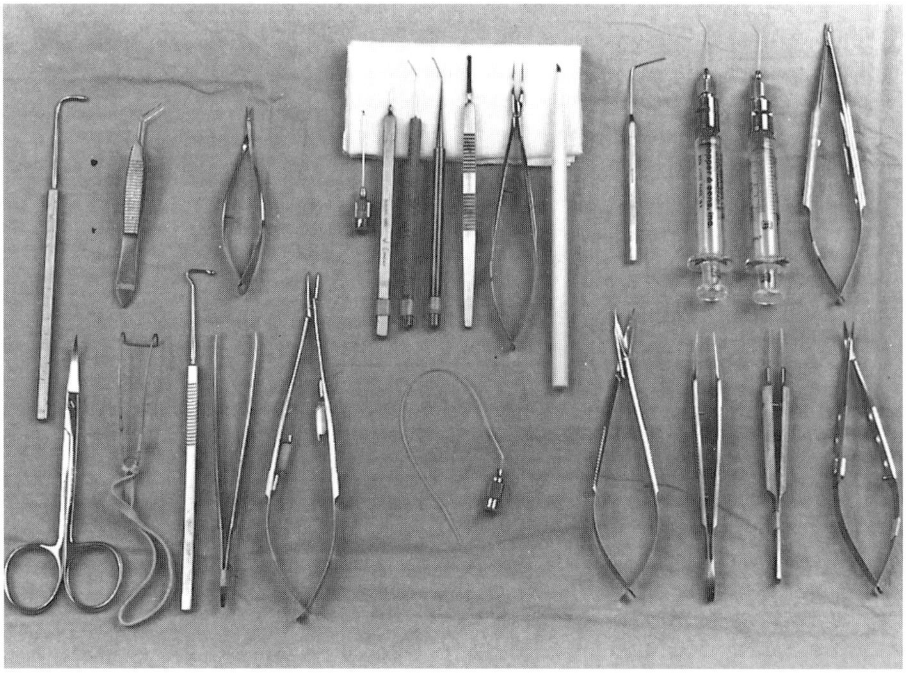

4.54 The instruments we prefer are shown arranged for surgery.[1] *Two row (left to right):* nucleus expressor, Bechert intraocular lens insertion forceps, Vannas capsulotomy scissors, Kelman irrigating cystotome, Jaffe modification of Sinskey hook, Bechert nucleus rotator, Tennant iris hook, Tooke knife, Maumenee cross-action forceps, Medical Workshop 30° Superblade, Barraquer iris spatula, syringe with Katena 30-gauge cannula for air injection, syringe with Katena 30-gauge cannula for balanced salt solution injection, McIntyre fishhook needle holder. *Bottom row (left to right):* utility scissors for cutting drape, Jaffe lid retractor, Jameson muscle hook, Kuhnt fixation forceps, Castroviejo needle holder (for rectus suture placement), anterior chamber maintainer (made by threading fragment of Guibor lacrimal cannicular tubing onto end of McIntyre 26-gauge cannula), sharp-pointed Westcott-type scissors, Castroviejo suturing forceps (0.12 mm teeth), Tennant tying forceps, Barraquer corneoscleral scissors.

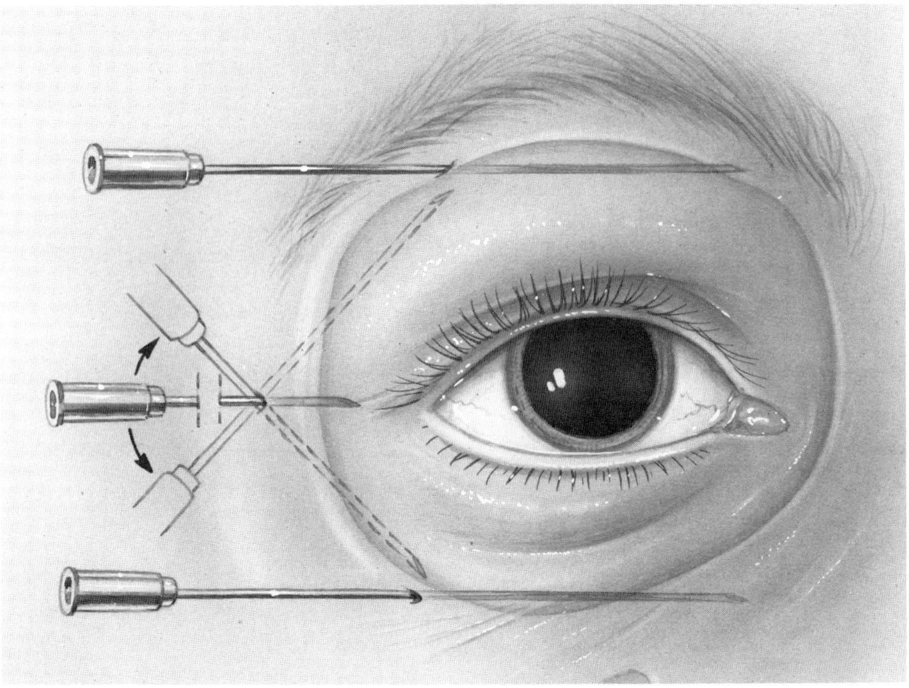

Surgical Technique

4.**55** Two to five milliliters of a 50-50 mixture of 0.5 % Marcaine and 2 % Xylocaine is injected as illustrated to achieve lid akinesia and analgesia.

56

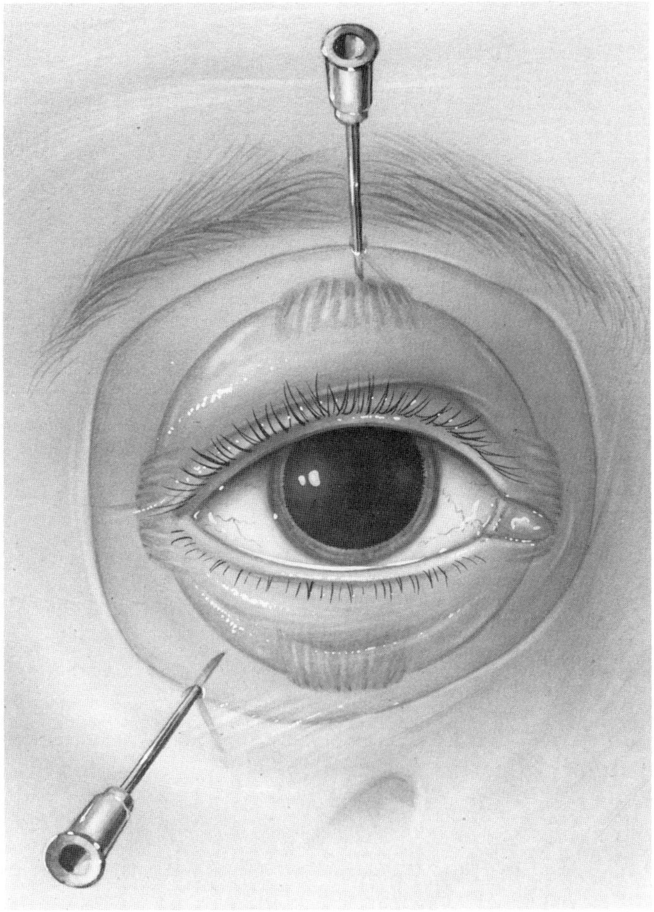

57

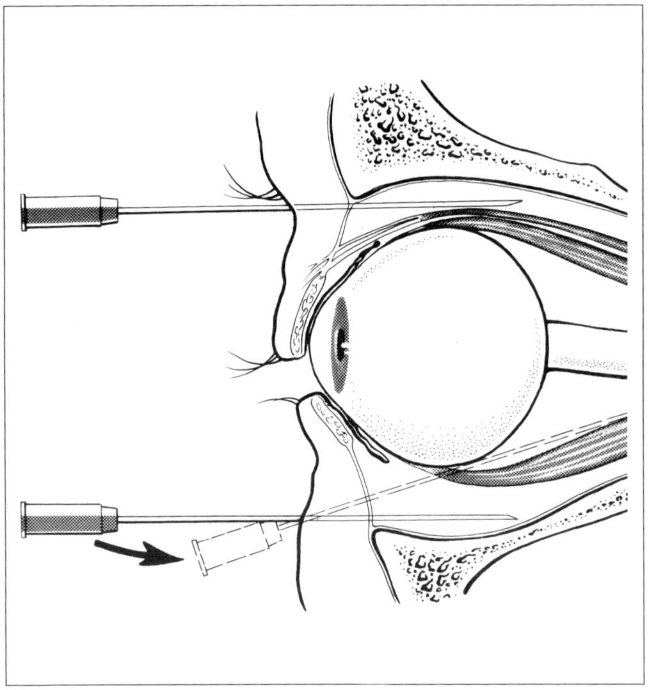

4.**56** and **57** 2.5 ml of 0.5 % Marcaine and 2.5 ml of 2 % Xylocaine are mixed in a 5 ml syringe. A disposable 23-gauge Atkinson[2]-type round-point needle is used to give the retrobulbar injection into the muscle cone in the inferior temporal quadrant while the ipsilateral eye remains in fixed gaze toward its upper nasal quadrant. 4 ml of the anesthetic solution is injected into the muscle cone. An additional 1 ml is injected near the roof of the orbit at about half the depth of the retrobulbar injection while the patient gazes downward. This superior injection insures good akinesia of the superior rectus and superior oblique muscles, as well as anesthesia in the region where the superior rectus muscle suture will be placed.

58

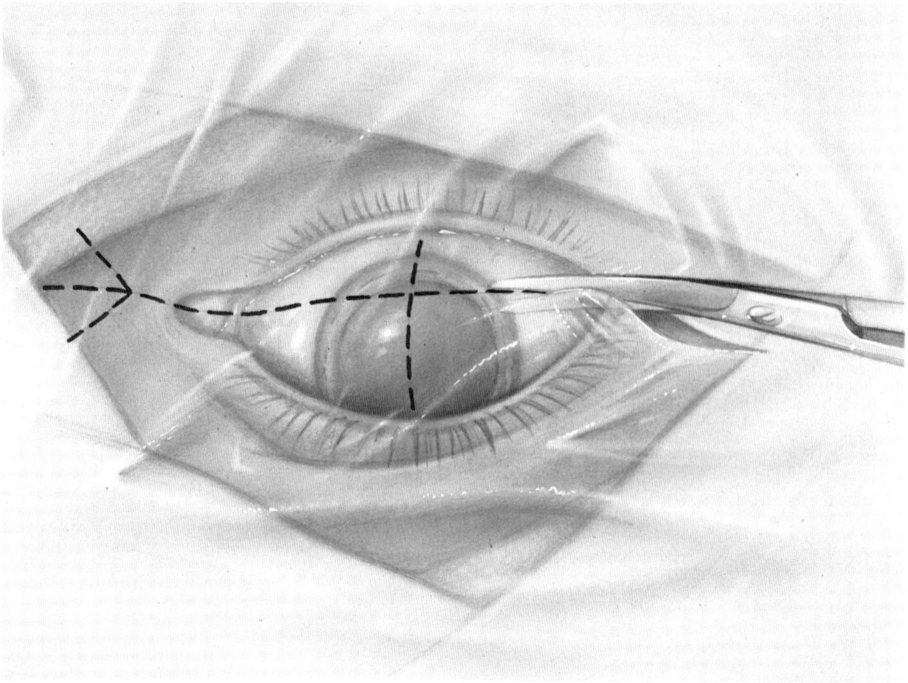

59

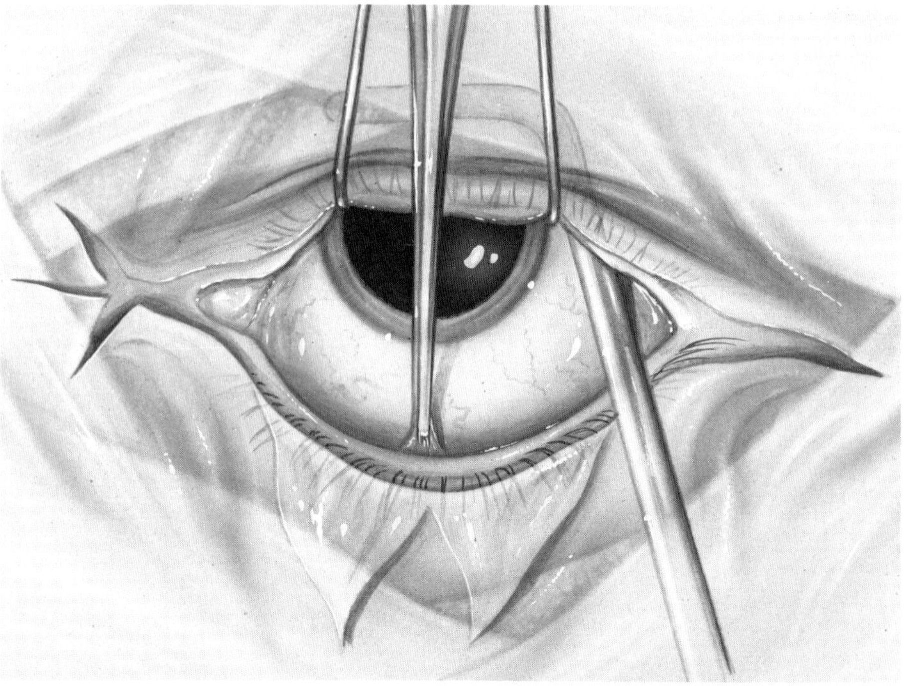

4.58 After cleansing of the periocular skin and lids, and irrigation of the cul-de-sacs with an antibiotic solution, the area is dried. Cellulose sponges are used to dry the lid margins to enhance adhesion of a plastic drape. After placing the usual cloth or paper disposable drapes so that only the eye and a small amount of skin adjacent to the lids are exposed, a large unperforated plastic drape (3 M) is applied to the opened lids. The adhesive material will not adhere to wet tissue, and therefore it does not adhere to the cornea or conjunctiva. The drape is cut as illustrated.

4.59 The eye is rotated downward with the muscle hook, while the superior rectus muscle is grasped at its insertion with Kuhnt forceps.

60

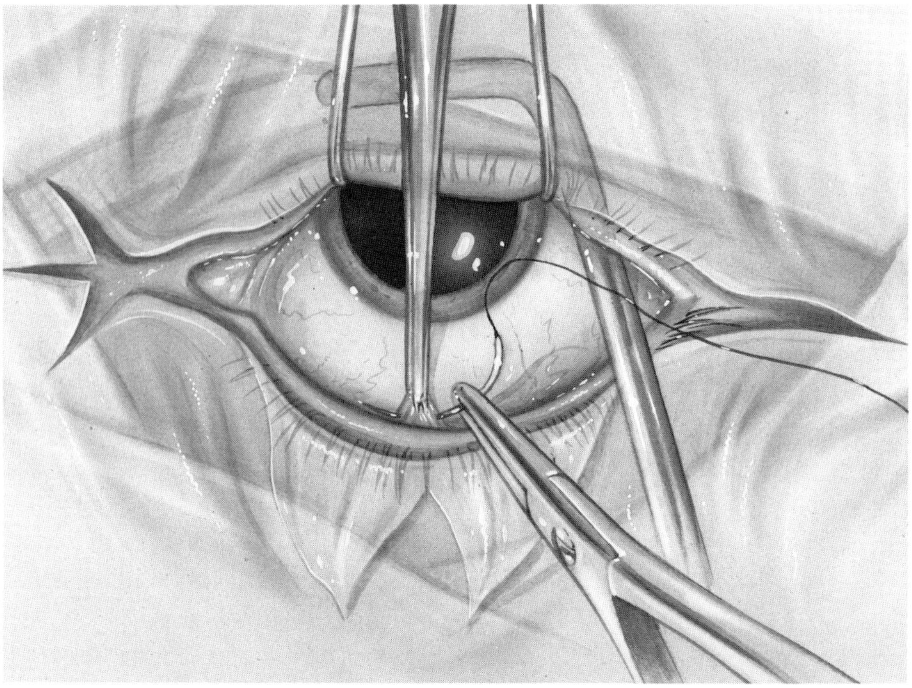

61

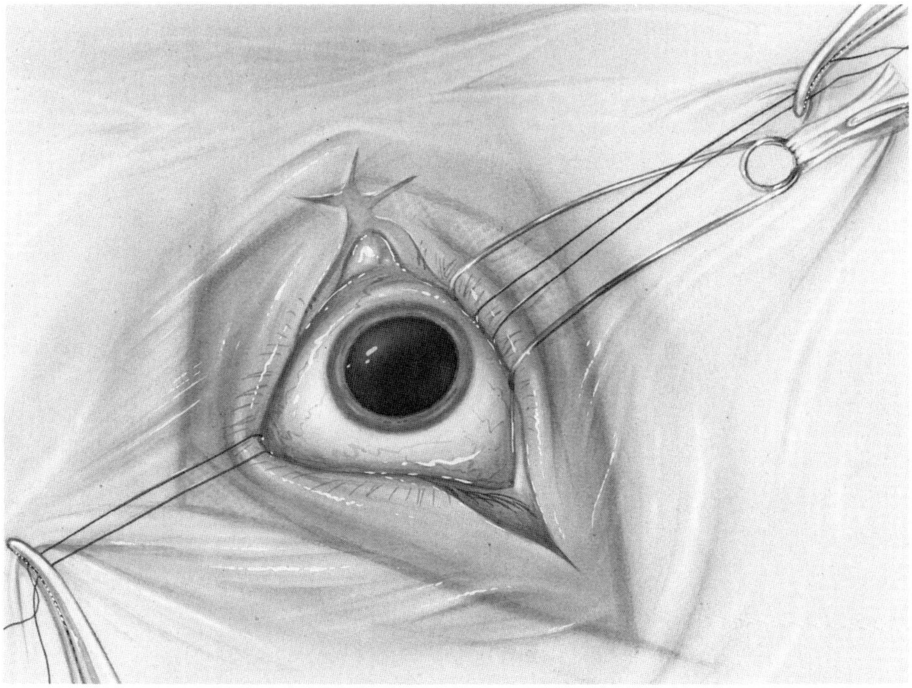

4.60 A 4-0 black silk suture is placed beneath the insertion of the superior rectus muscle. In a similar fashion, the muscle hook is placed in the superior cul-de-sac and used to rotate the globe upward while a 4-0 black silk suture is placed beneath the insertion of the inferior rectus muscle.

4.61 A Jaffe wire lid speculum is used to gently retract the lower lid. The speculum is attached via a rubber band to the drapes inferiorly, using a hemostat. The lid speculum holds the free edges of the adhesive drape tucked into the lower cul-de-sac in order to isolate the lashes outside the operating field. The adhesive drape flaps are tucked similarly into the superior cul-de-sac to isolate the superior lashes from the operating field, and the superior rectus bridle suture is retracted and clipped to the drapes superiorly with a hemostat, using the minimum amount of tension required to give good exposure to the operating site. The inferior rectus suture is then attached with light tension to the drapes inferiorly, using a hemostat.

62

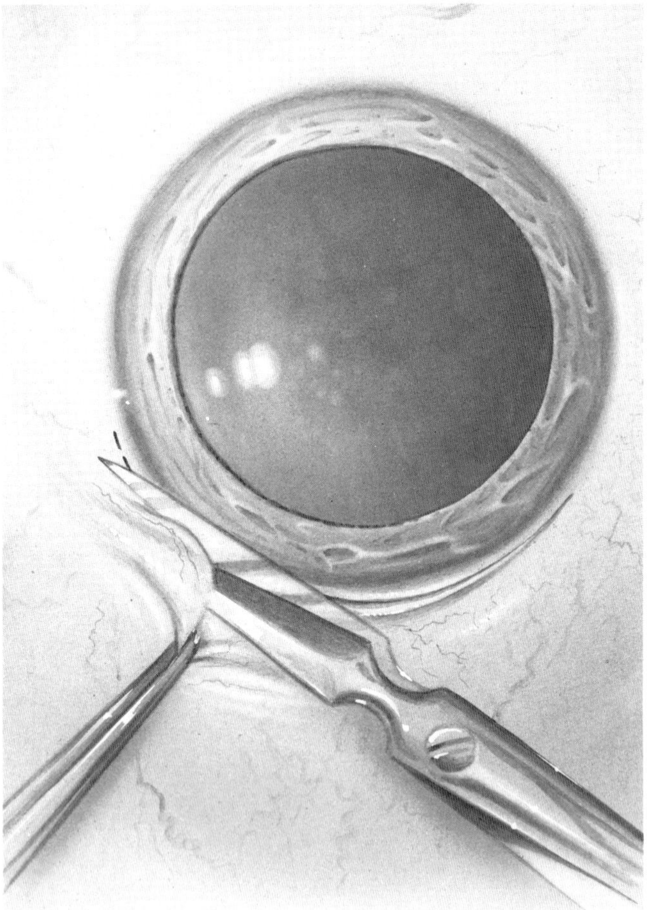

63

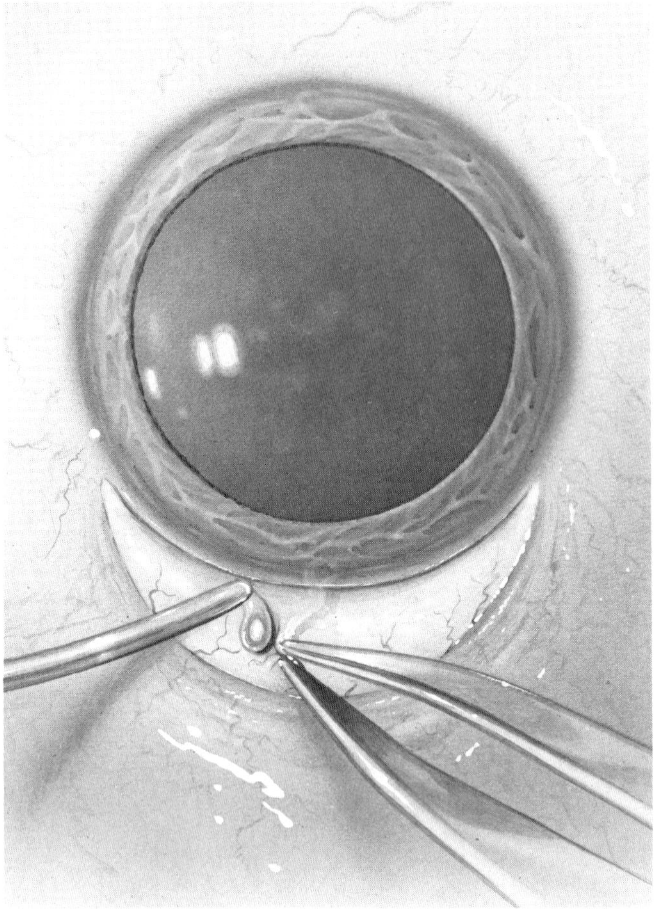

64

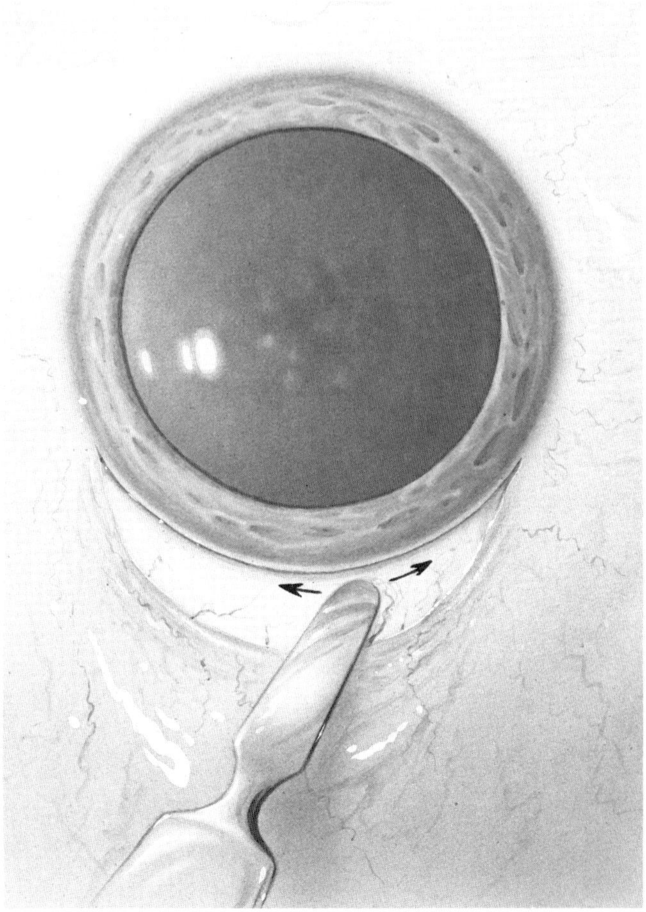

4.62 A 11–12 mm long fornix-based conjunctival flap is made straddling the 12 o'clock position.

4.63 Wet-field cautery is applied lightly just posterior to the limbus, obliterating all visible surface vessels.

4.64 The limbus is cleaned with a Tooke knife to clearly define limbal anatomy.

65

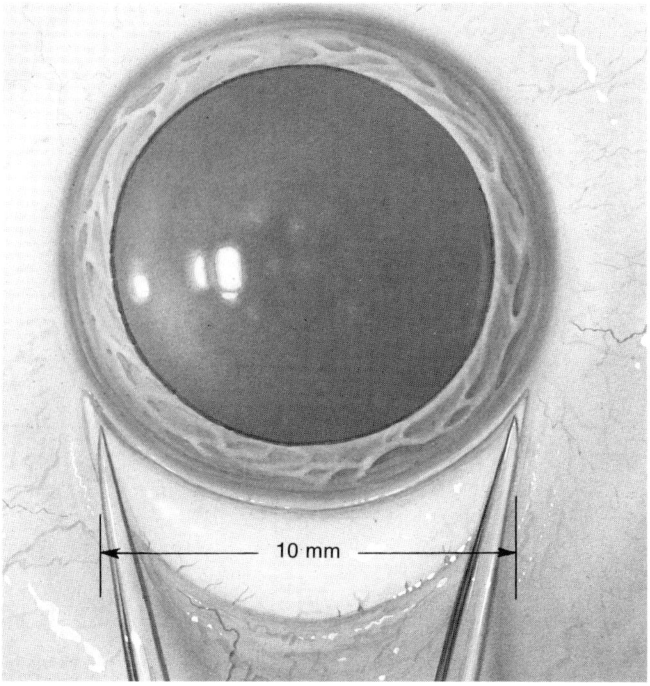

66

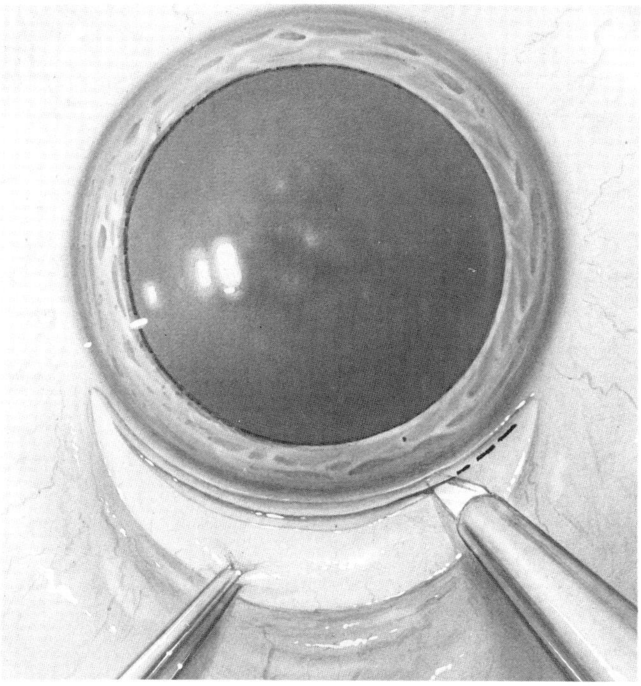

4.**65** A 10 mm chord length is measured with the caliper.

4.**66** A 30° disposable steel microblade is used to make a 10 mm partially penetrating incision. We make the groove at one of two locations: 1. mid-limbal, preferably at 70–80% depth; or 2. in the sclera, approximately 1–2 mm posterior to the anterior limbal border. The groove should be made with one pass and be as perpendicular as possible. If the posterior incision is used, shelve anteriorly after grooving to ensure that the wound entrance into the anterior chamber is relatively anterior.

67

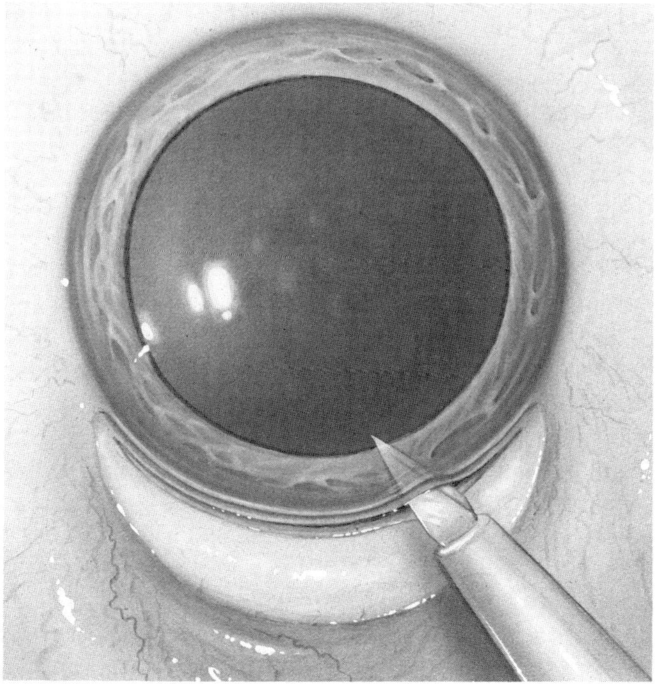

68

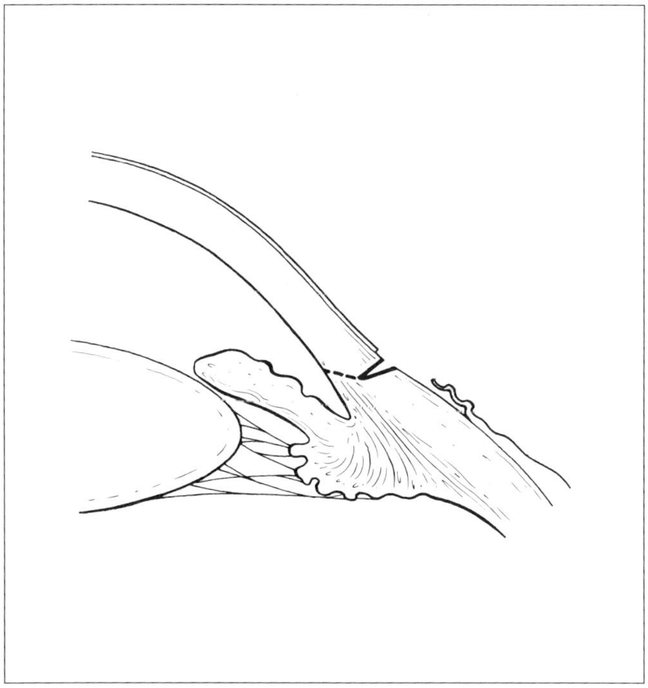

4.**67** and **68** The steel microblade penetrates the anterior chamber at approximately the 10–11 o'clock position, beginning at the base of the preplaced groove and cutting parallel to the iris plane. This incision is approximately 1.5–2.0 mm long.

69

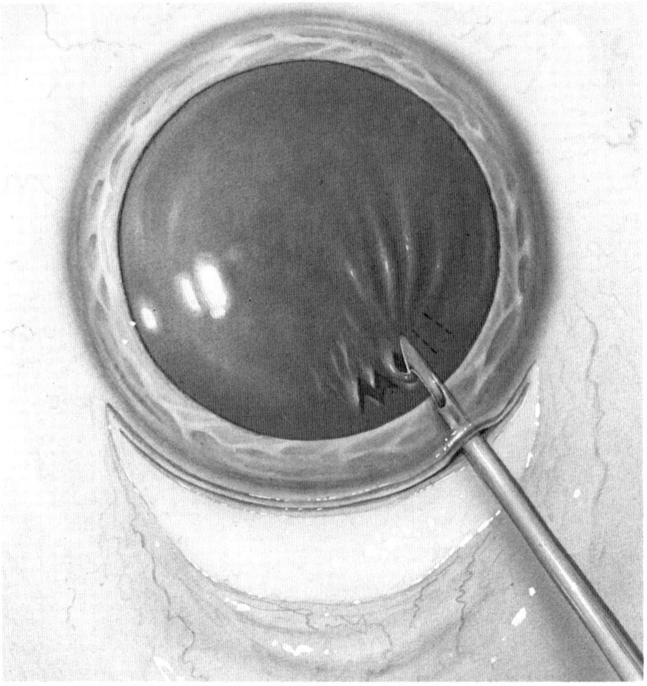

70

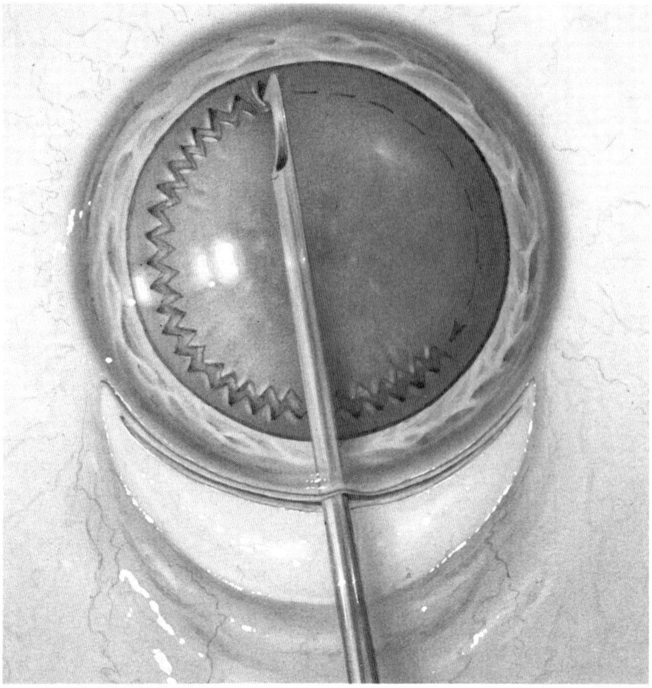

71

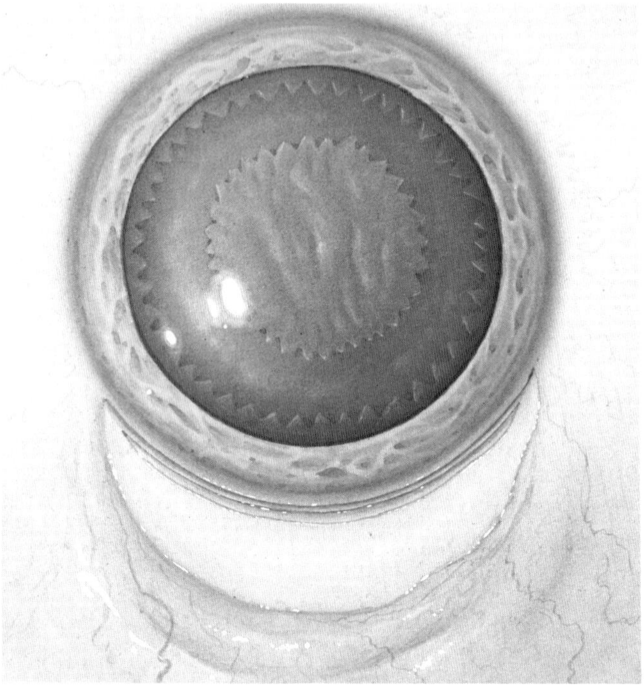

4.69 Sodium hyaluronate is injected into the anterior chamber, completely filling it so that the chamber is at normal or slightly distended depth. Illustrated here is a can-opener anterior capsulectomy using a Kelman cystotome. Initially, a sharp cystotome is used to create about three short tiny tears or punctures near the incision site. These initial tears are created by a movement of the tip of the sharp cystotome so as to puncture the capsule, and then to pull it slightly toward the incision site. Care is taken not to tear close to the zonules or the lens equator.

4.70 The cystotome cuts are continued with small tears each adjoining the previous cut, and each being made using a force vector toward the optic axis.

4.71 The Kelman cystotome capsulotomy is completed. Irrigation was not used here because sodium hyaluronate maintained the depth of the anterior chamber. In the absence of sodium hyaluronate, a constant infusion of balanced salt solution is required in order to maintain the depth of the chamber during the capsulotomy. Alternative methods that we like to use for anterior capsulectomy include: the technique as advocated by David J. McIntyre, using a 25-gauge disposable needle bent in such a way as to have a small microhook at its tip; and the Gills technique employing Stern-Gills scissors to create the entire capsulectomy or to cut the nasal and temporal portions of the flap after the superior and inferior portions have been cut with the bent 25-gauge needle. Prior to inserting the Stern-Gills scissors, the wound must be enlarged to its full extent as described subsequently. If capsular bag fixation is planned, be sure to leave the anterior capsular flaps sufficiently large to permit visualization for proper posterior chamber lens positioning.

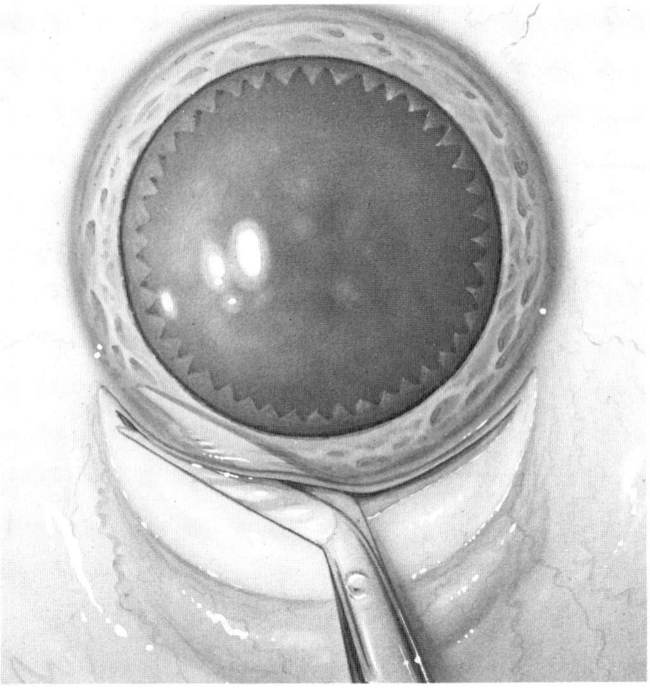

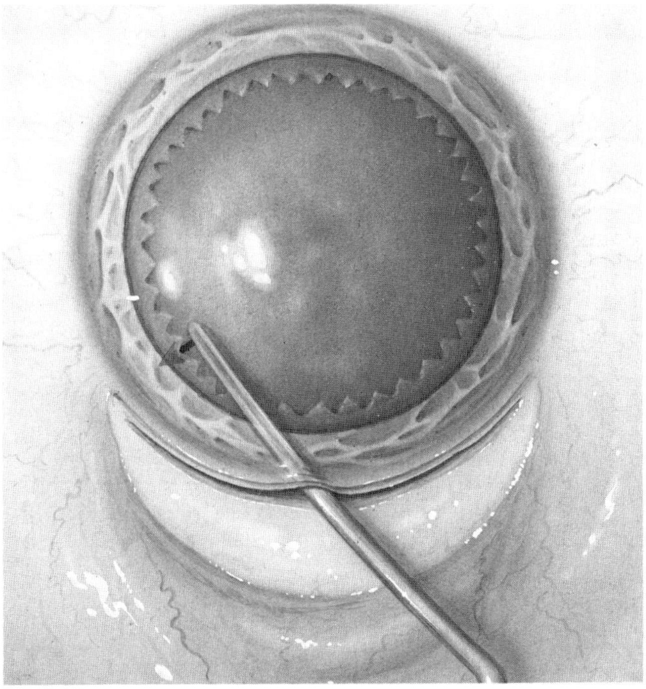

4.72 If sodium hyaluronate is not used, the incision may be completed using corneoscleral scissors as illustrated. Alternatively, sodium hyaluronate can be injected to deepen the anterior chamber adjacent to the wound to prepare for completion of the incision. The incision is then completed by cutting along the preplaced groove parallel to the iris plane using the microsurgical blade. To minimize trauma and stretching, the wound is not separated with forceps during this procedure. The incision is squared off so that it measures a full 10 mm at its internal aspect as well as at its external aspect. Though not illustrated here, at this time two interrupted 8-0 black silk sutures are placed for use as control sutures. These can be in different positions, depending on where the instruments for irrigation/aspiration will be inserted. It is important not to insert the irrigation/aspiration instrument through an excessively large opening, as this will facilitate iris prolapse. If irrigation/aspiration has to be done superiorly, then the sutures should be placed such that an approximately 2.5 mm opening is left superiorly. Another option is to place the sutures 2.5 mm from each end of the wound. Irrigation/aspiration can then be performed through these openings, thereby facilitating removal of the superior cortex. These sutures will not be tied until after the nucleus has been expressed.

4.73 The McIntyre 26-gauge cannula, attached to the Kelman-Cavitron irrigating cystotome handle or to a syringe filled with balanced salt solution, will be used to prepare the nucleus for expression. It is first used to loop the 8-0 black silk sutures around the margins of the groove. With irrigation flowing by gravity or by gentle injection through the syringe, the superior pole of the nucleus is brought anterior to the iris, as described by McIntyre.[3] The 26-gauge anterior chamber cannula is inserted into the anterior chamber at the 12 o'clock position. Its tip is passed under the margin of the anterior capsular leaflet at approximately the 2 o'clock position. The leaflet is retracted toward the lens equator with the capsule being stretched sufficiently to allow the nucleus equator to move anteriorly. Gentle irrigation is begun with a syringe, or is ongoing with gravity flow of irrigation using the Kelman-Cavitron handpiece. This creates a cleavage plane between the lens nucleus and the posterior capsule. The cleavage is assisted by moderate posterior pressure against the scleral wound lip while the instrument is held still parallel to the plane of the iris.

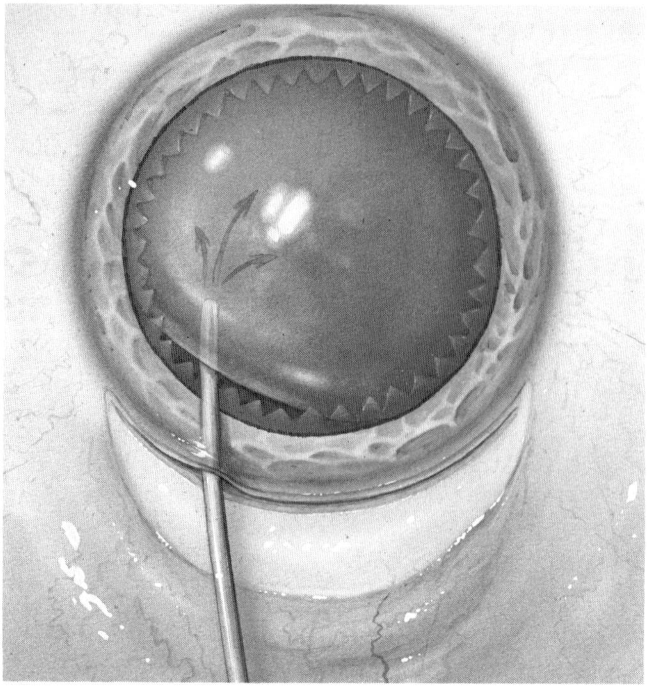

4.74 As the nucleus starts to move forward, the cannula rotates to the right beneath the equator of the lens, and the iris and superior anterior capsular flap are tucked under the equator of the nucleus.

75

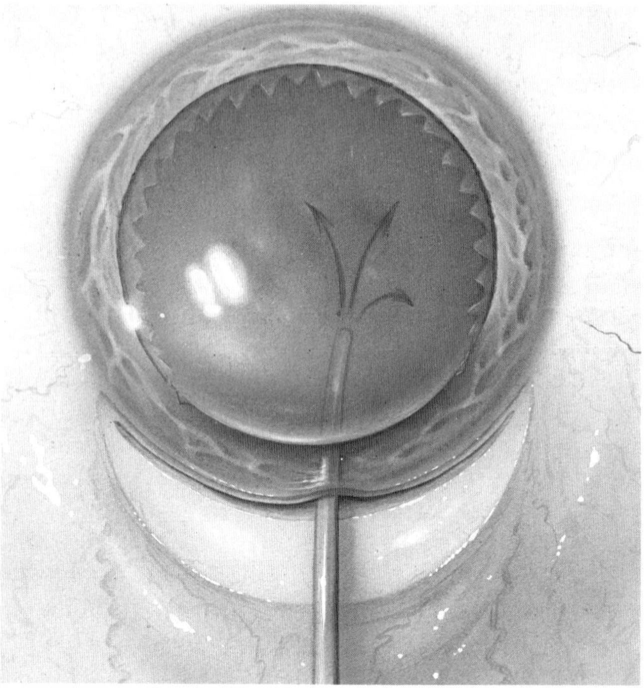

76

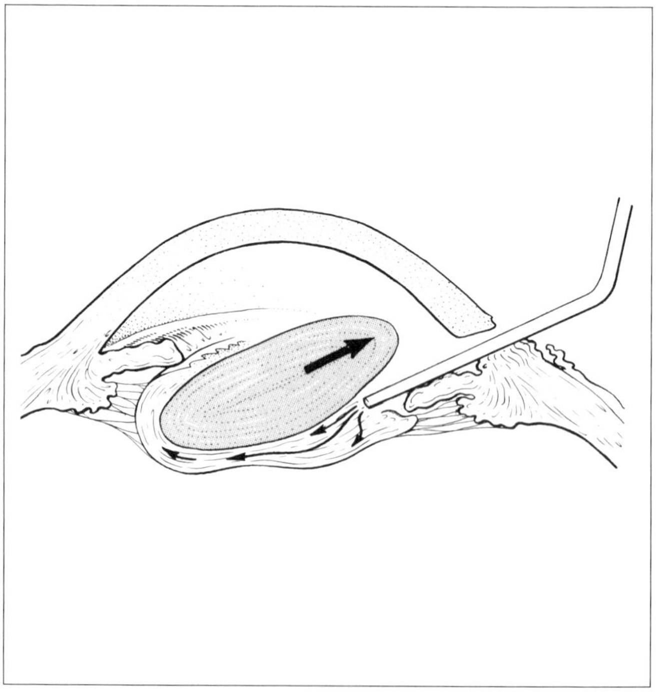

4.**75** and **76** Irrigation continues to cleave the nucleus away from the posterior capsule as the cannula is slid across to the right, bringing the superior equator of the nucleus anterior to the iris.

77

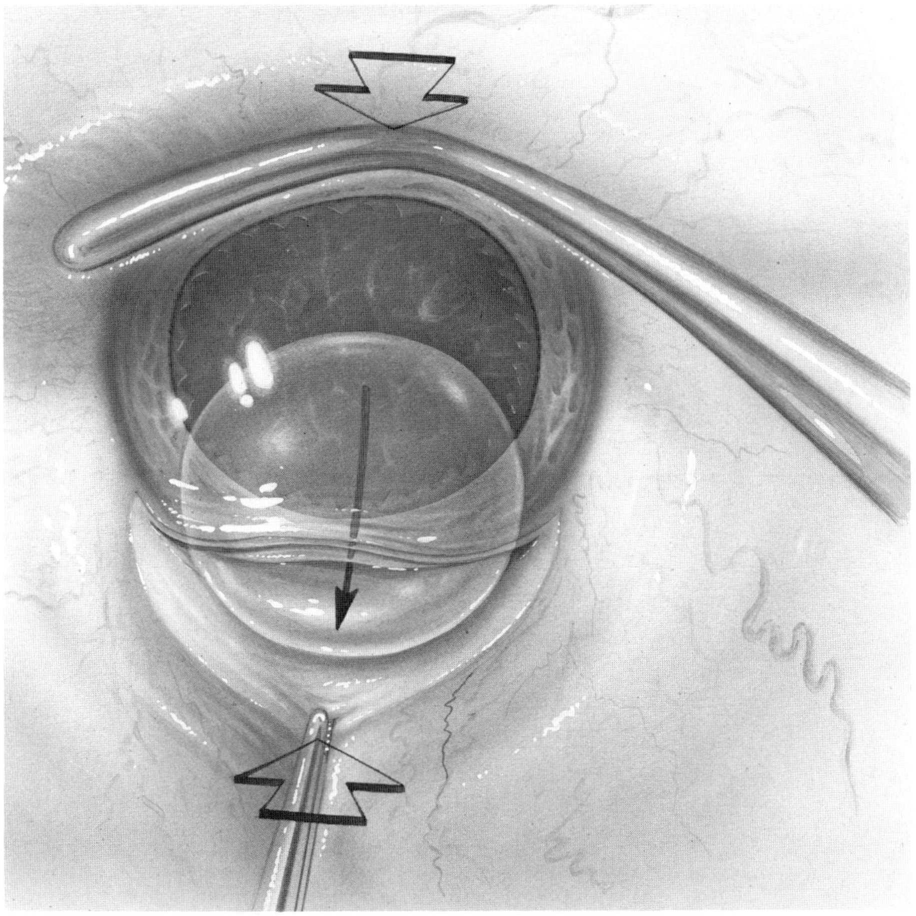

4.77 Bimanual expression technique. A small-toothed forceps is used to grasp the superior sclera 1–2 mm posterior to the incision site, and posterior pressure is applied, while simultaneously placing a lens expressor or muscle hook at the 6 o'clock position on peripheral cornea adjacent to the limbus. Gentle to moderate posterior force is alternated between the two instruments, causing the nucleus to gradually exit from the wound.

78

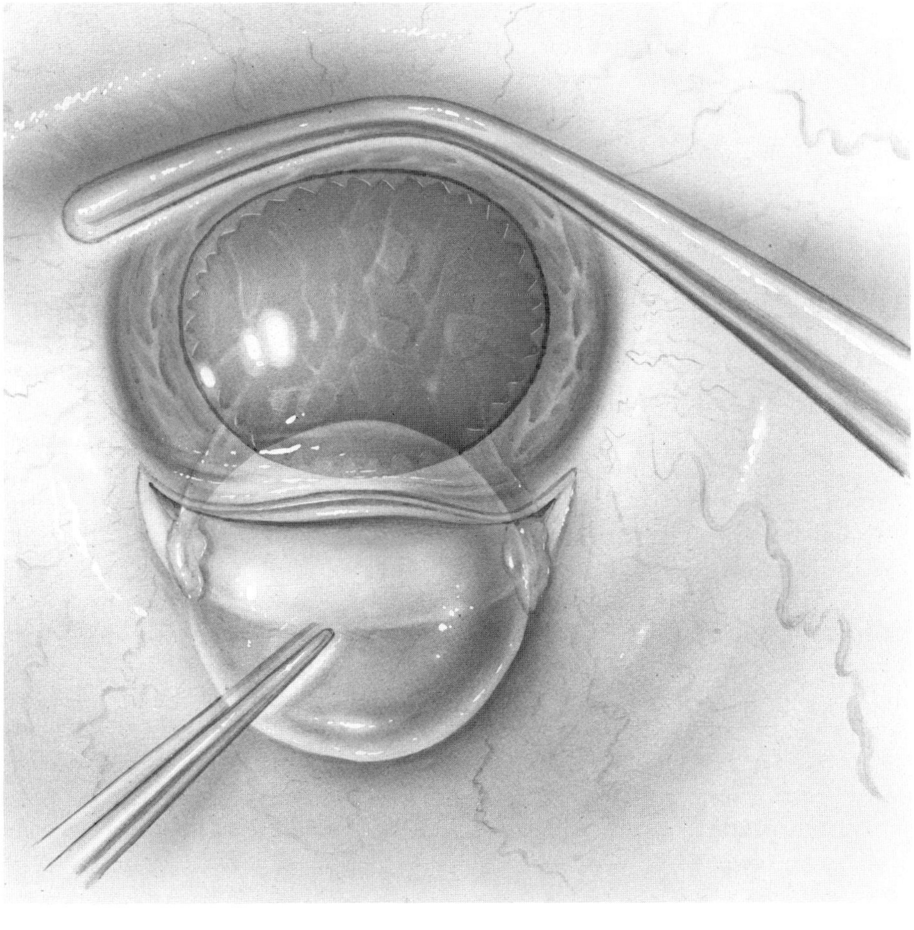

4.78 Completion of nuclear expression by the bimanual technique. Remember that, when using this technique, a baseline pressure is always maintained with the two instruments, while an additional increment of pressure is applied with the two instruments alternately. The nucleus extrudes slowly in most cases, and the surgeon should avoid the temptation to speed up the delivery by excessive application of pressure.

An alternative method for delivery of the nucleus involves the application of pressure solely at the superior location. We actually use this method about ninety percent of the time with good success, and use the bimanual technique only in those cases where the lens nucleus is not readily expressed by superior pressure alone. The superior pressure is applied by grasping the sclera 1–2 mm behind the posterior scleral lip and gaping the wound with pressure directed primarily posteriorly with a slight superior complement; or an irrigating lens loop may be used to depress the sclera 3 mm behind the wound.

79

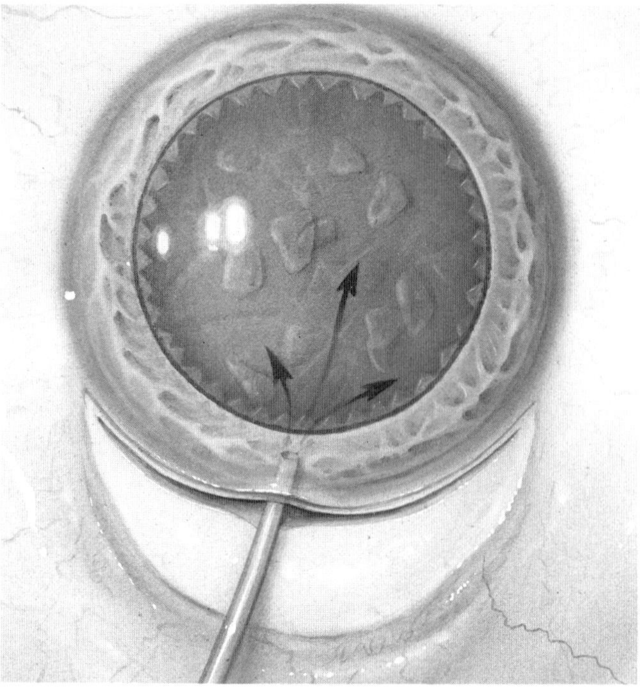

80

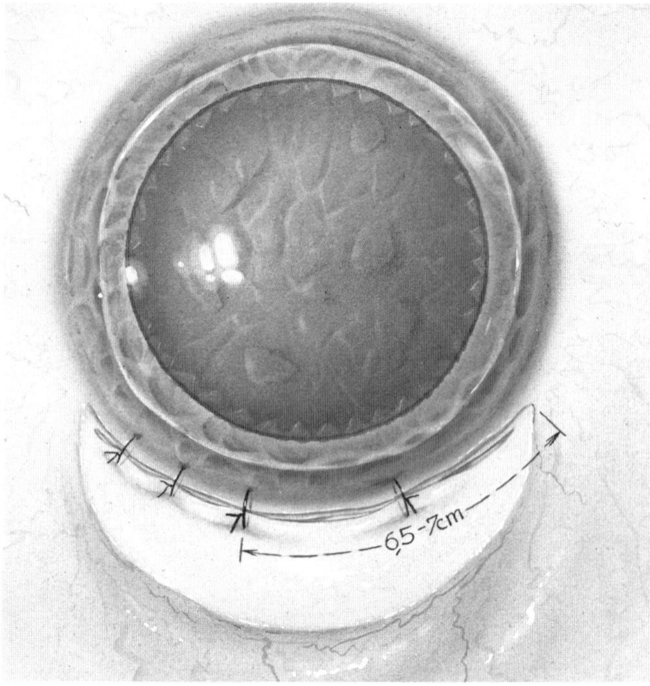

81

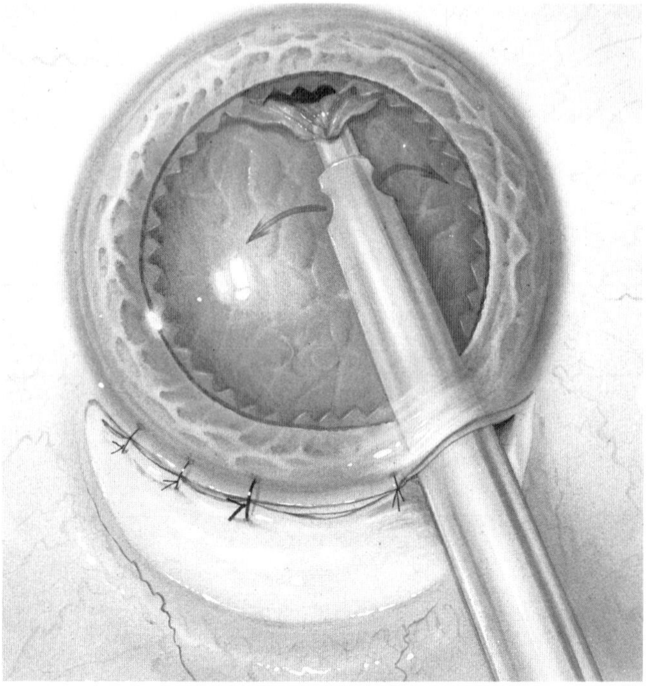

4.79 Loose cortex is irrigated away from the anterior chamber and from the wound margins, using balanced salt solution.

4.80 The preplaced 8-0 black silk sutures are tightened, tied and cut. Additional sutures may be placed as needed if the iris presents to the wound during subsequent removal of cortex.

4.81 Cortex removal may be accomplished using either the Kelman-Cavitron Phaco-Emulsifier aspirator system or a manual irrigation/aspiration system such as that devised and described by McIntyre.[4]

The basic principles of cortex removal are similar, whether the system is automated or manual.[5] One primary difference in our experience is that with the automated system the anterior chamber remains deeper, and therefore it might be somewhat easier and safer for the less experienced extracapsular surgeon than the manual technique, during which the anterior chamber tends to be more shallow and the maneuvers somewhat more difficult. The basic principles of the irrigation/aspiration process are as follows: When irrigating (but not aspirating), the instrument is inserted into the anterior chamber. For aspiration, the aspiration hole is aimed anteriorly and the tip of the instrument gently inserted beneath the iris and into the capsular fornix, while keeping as close as possible to the posterior capsule, thereby avoiding the possibility of aspirating the free anterior capsular flap. The point is to have the aspiration hole in contact with cortex in the capsular fornix so that when aspiration is initiated that cortex will occlude the aspiration opening selectively, thereby preventing the undesirable adherence of the tip to the anterior capsule. Once in position in the capsular fornix, aspiration is initiated and, after a second or so has been allowed for engagement of the cortical material, the tip is gently withdrawn into the pupillary space, where the aspiration port becomes visible to the surgeon.

82

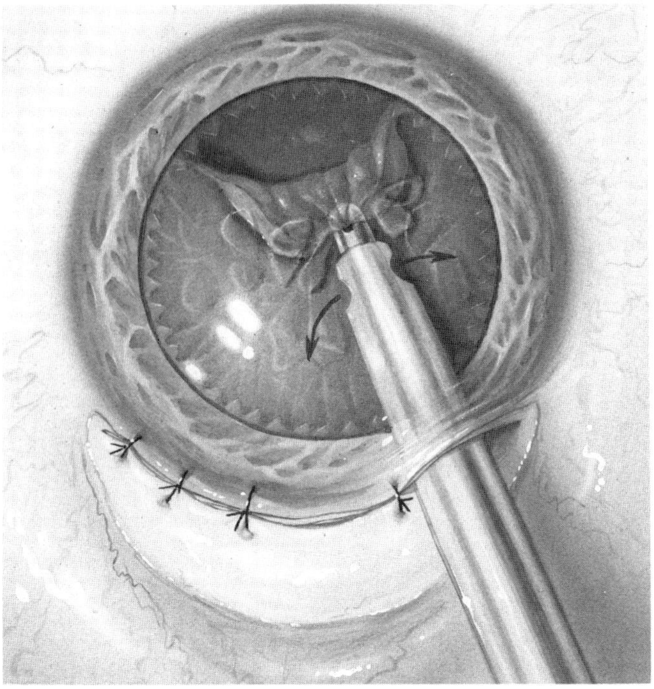

83

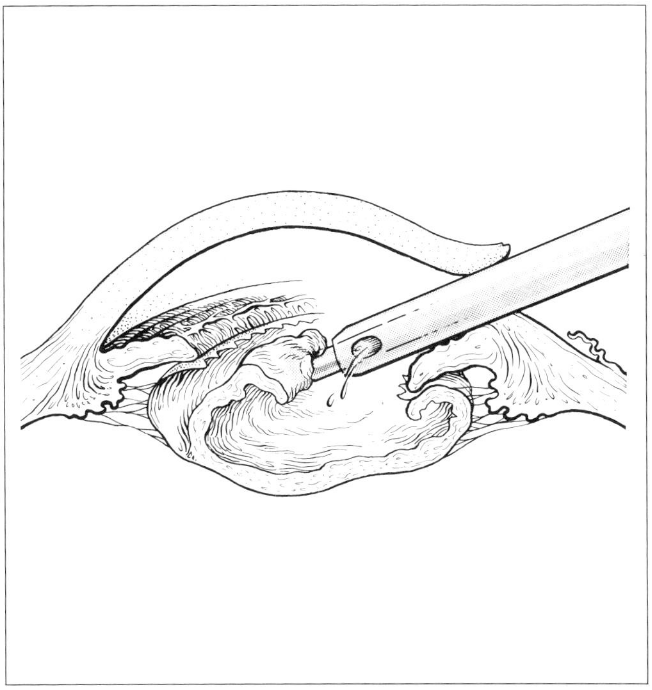

84

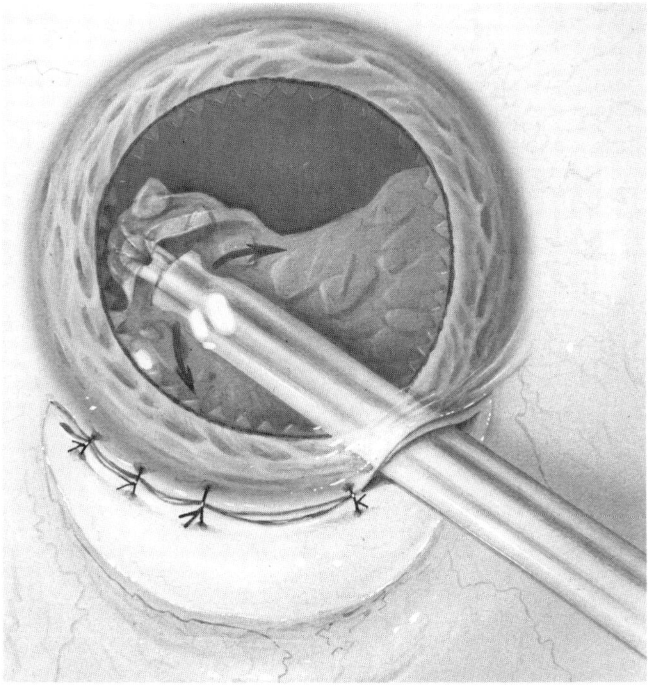

85

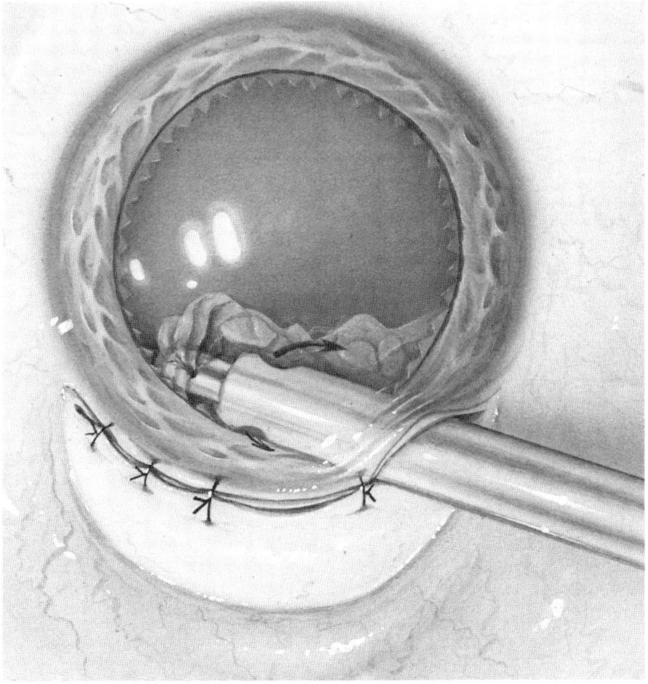

4.**82** and **83** The tip of the instrument is slowly brought into the center of the pupil, thereby stripping cortex away from the posterior capsule and simultaneously aspirating it.

4.**84** The cycle of placement of the tip into the capsular fornix, engagement of cortex, central stripping and aspiration is usually initiated at the 6 o'clock position, and then repeated systematically at the 5 o'clock, 4 o'clock and 3 o'clock positions.

4.**85** The process is continued at the 7 o'clock, 8 o'clock, and 9 o'clock positions, and then again at 2 o'clock and 1 o'clock until a patch of cortex remains immediately beneath the instrument adjacent to the site of entry into the anterior chamber.

86

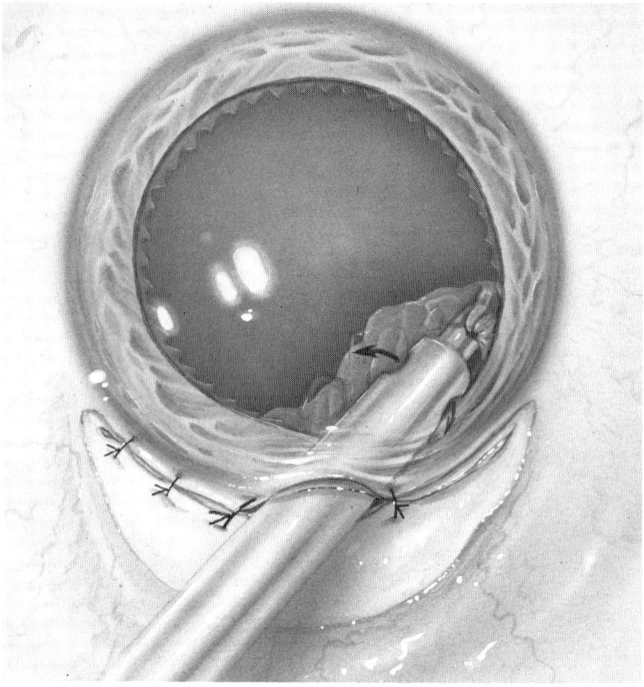

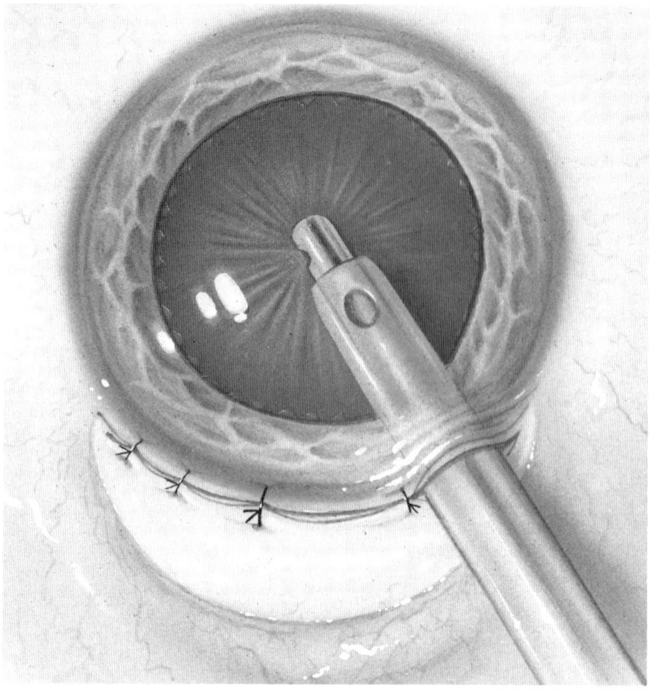

87

88

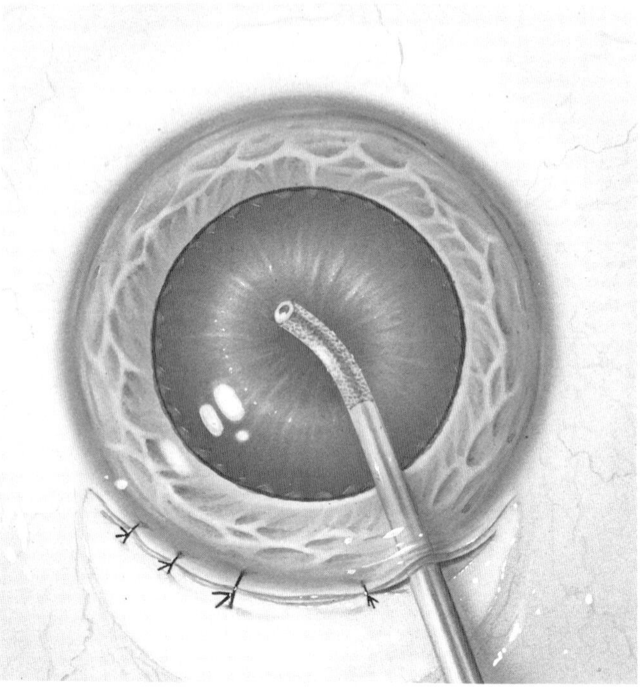

4.**86** The instrument is then inserted through a different location in the wound in order to obtain easier access to the cortical material remaining beneath the original entry site.

4.**87** The posterior capsule is cleaned by "vacuuming," using low aspiration pressure, with either the automated or manual aspiration instrument.

4.**88** Additional cleaning of the posterior capsule may be accomplished using a scrubbing action with the Kratz scratcher. With this instrument the anterior chamber is maintained by infusion of balanced salt solution by a gravity inflow, or by injecting with a syringe to which the instrument is attached.

We prefer to inject sodium hyaluronate in preparation for insertion of the lens implant. For this, a blunt 27-gauge injection cannula is attached to the syringe. The central anterior chamber is filled with hyaluronate, and then additional hyaluronate is injected beneath the residual anterior capsular flap in order to inflate the capsule for in-the-bag insertion (our current preference), or the injection may be placed in the posterior chamber between the iris and residual anterior capsule if one desires placement of the lens into the ciliary sulcus. It is best to avoid injecting hyaluronate beneath the iris adjacent to the wound, because this leads to iris prolapse.

Alternatively, the anterior chamber may be maintained using either air or balanced salt solution as illustrated here. The basic mechanics of insertion and placement of the lens are similar, regardless of whether one uses hyaluronate, air, or balanced salt solution. A disadvantage of air is that it tends to compress and obliterate the spaces of the posterior chamber, making it more difficult to place the lens implant accurately in the desired location, either in or out of the bag.

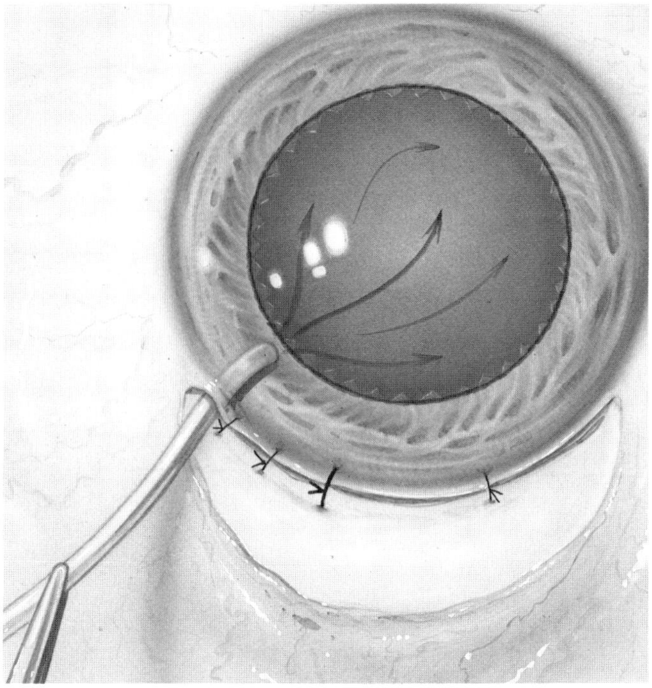

4.89 When maintaining the anterior chamber depth with balanced salt solution, permanent 10-0 nylon sutures are first placed in an interrupted fashion in the left-hand one-third of the incision site, if not already done before cortex removal. The residual 8-0 black silk sutures are still present at approximately the 11 and 1 o'clock positions. A small silicon (lacrimal) cannula attached to a source of balanced salt solution is threaded between the left-most suture and the edge of the wound. Fluid is injected into the anterior chamber as needed to maintain adequate anterior chamber depth for the subsequent maneuvers.

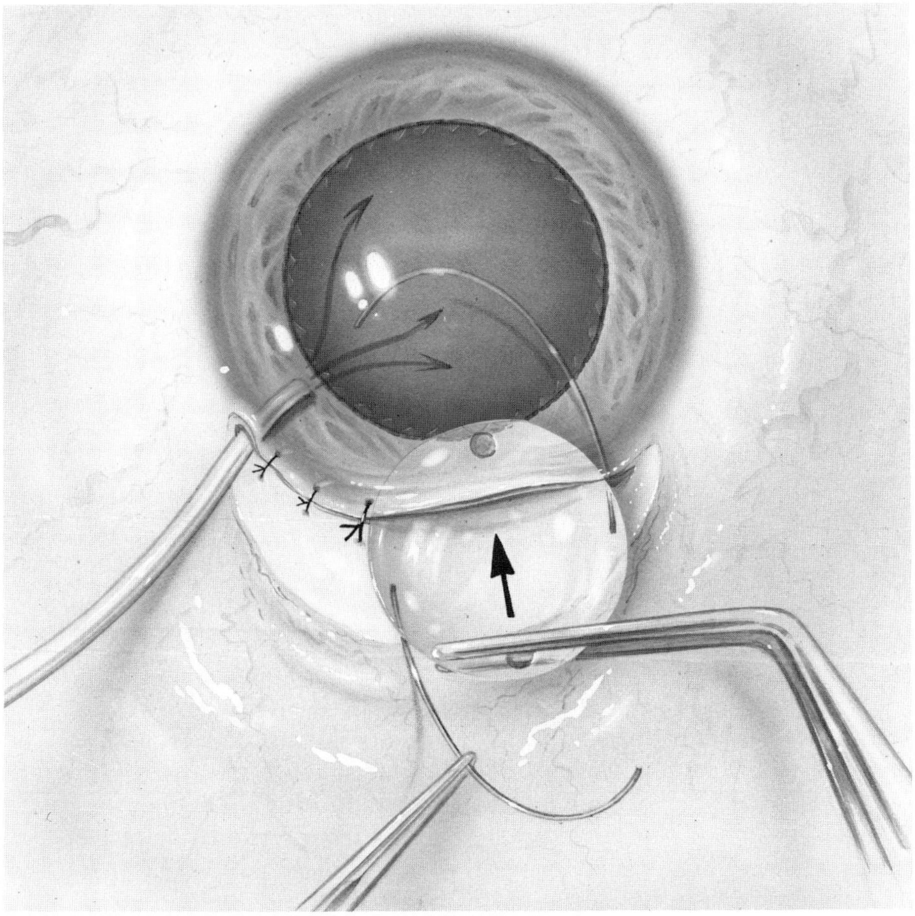

4.90 The 11 o'clock 8-0 black silk suture is removed, providing an adequate wound opening for passage of the lens implant into the eye. A Sinskey or Kratz type of posterior chamber intraocular lens as illustrated is our preference for ciliary sulcus placement, and a short C-loop design is our preference for capsular bag placement. We prefer an overall lens length of 14 mm and anterior angulation of the loops. The intraocular lens is held with the Bechert lens insertion forceps and inserted through the wound opening.

91

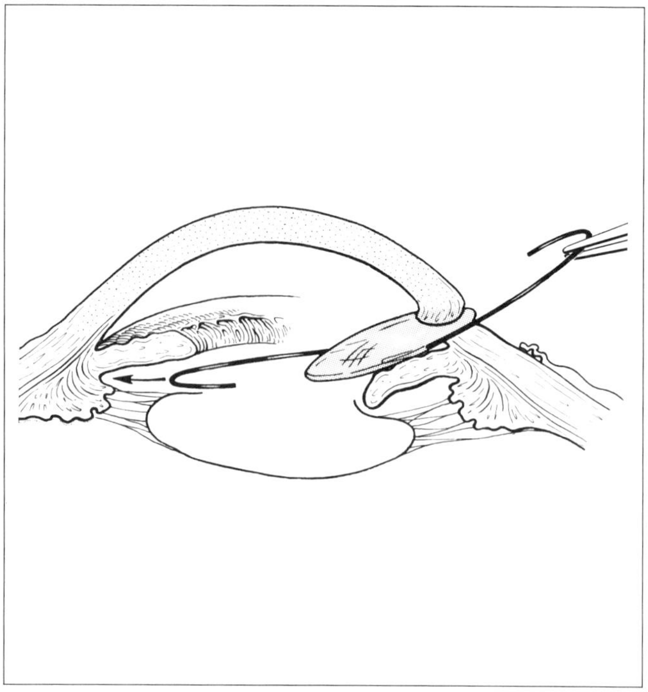

92

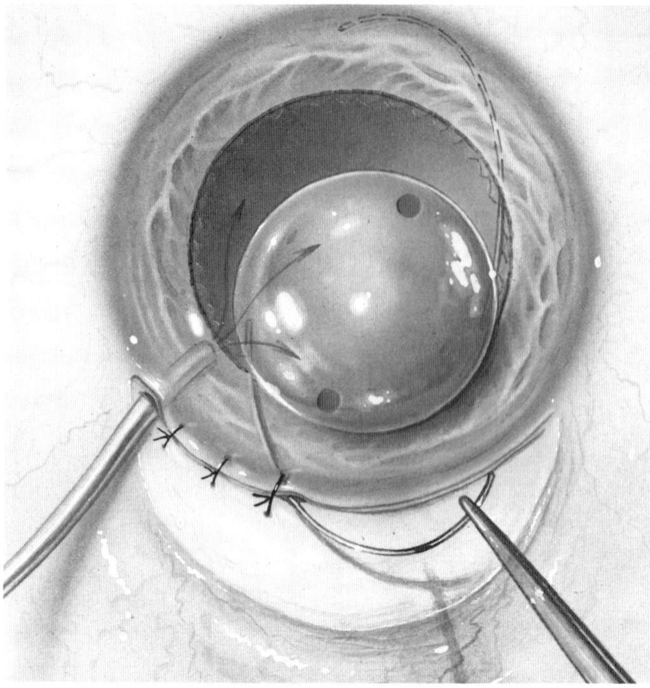

93

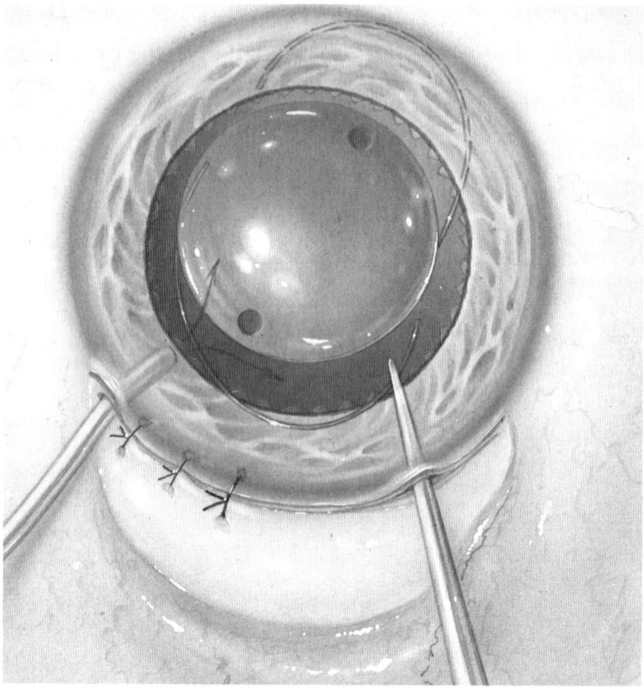

94

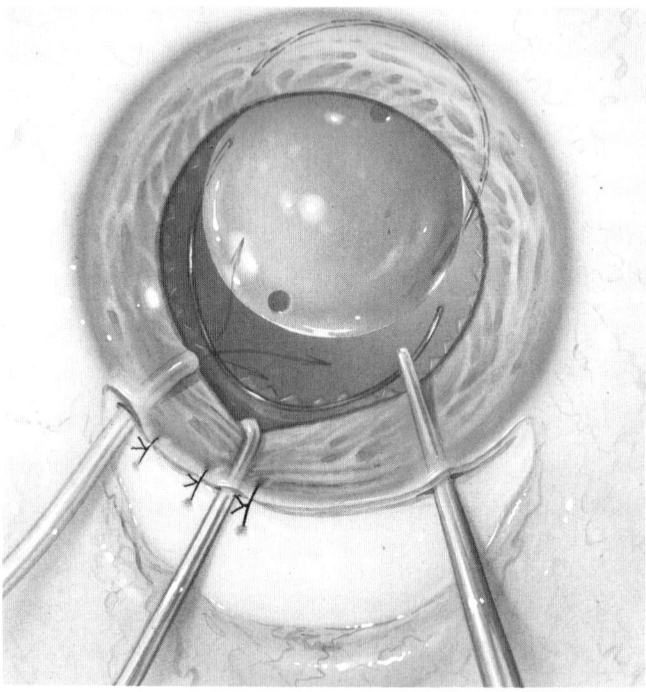

4.91 The inferior loop passes between the iris and the residual anterior capsular flap for ciliary sulcus placement.

4.92 The inferior loop of the lens is situated at approximately the 7:30 position. The superior loop is then grasped somewhat distal to its knee or apex and is passed into the anterior chamber while flexing the loop.

4.93 The knee of the superior loop is then positioned between the iris and the residual anterior capsular flap at approximately the 1:30 position. A slight counterclockwise rotation of the end of the forceps depresses the knee and allows it to readily pass beneath the iris and up into the region of the ciliary sulcus. The loop should be guided up under the iris and gently released to allow it to expand into the desired position. Note that the lens is partially rotated during the insertional maneuver. It is easier, because of mechanical advantage and better visualization, to insert the superior loop at the 1:30 position, rather than at the 12 o'clock position.

4.94 If the pupil is small or if the residual anterior capsular flap is not readily visible at the pupillary margin, a small iris hook may be used to retract the iris at the 1:30 position to permit better visualization and more accurate placement of the superior loop.

95

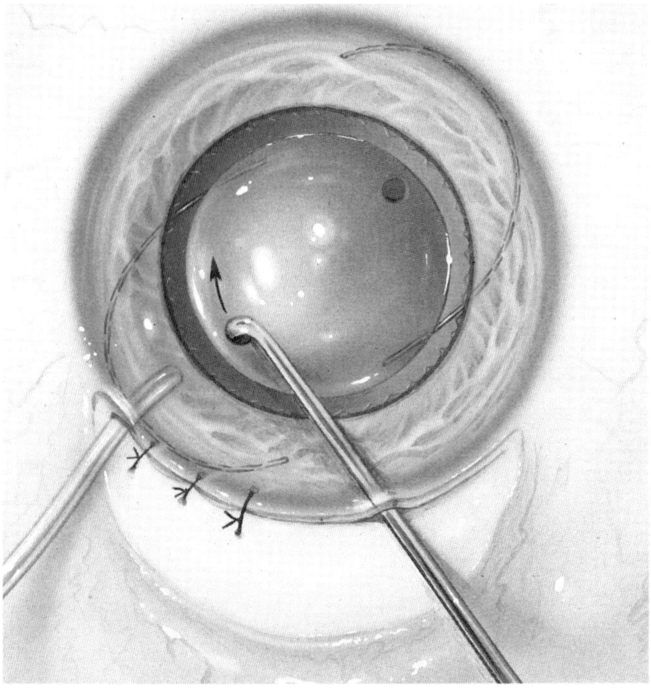

96

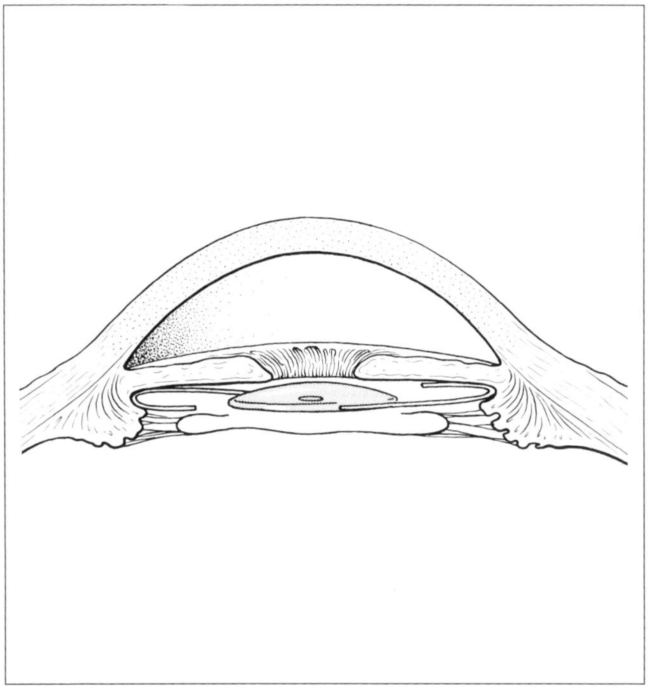

97

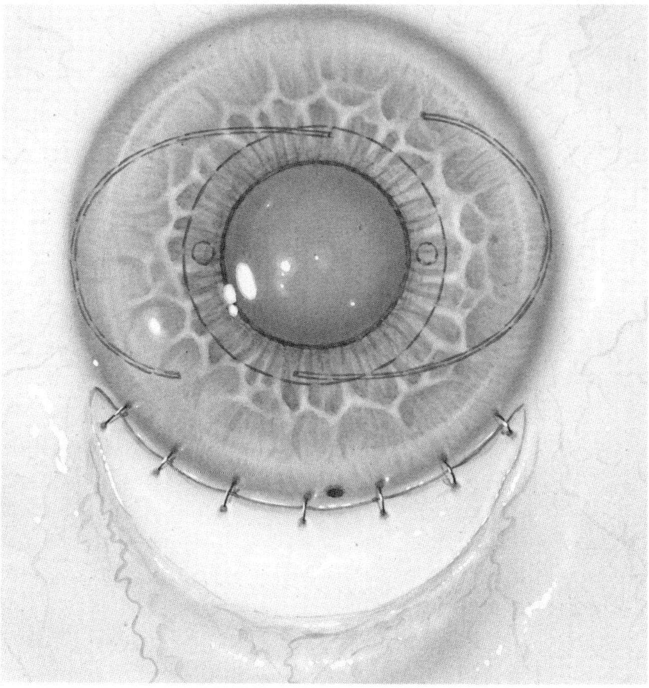

4.95 The lens is gently rotated slightly to ensure good centering. The surgeon should avoid excessive rotation, especially if the lens is placed in the capsular bag, since the rotation can cause a loop to slip out of the bag. Although we do not routinely employ a peripheral iridectomy, the surgeon may wish to place one at this time.

4.96 The posterior chamber intraocular lens is appropriately positioned in the ciliary sulcus.

4.97 The horizontal position is preferred for sulcus fixation. If the lens does not appropriately center in the horizontal location, continued rotation will usually result in better centering. The incision is closed with interrupted 10-0 nylon sutures. Before tying the last one or two 10-0 nylon sutures, we insert the irrigation/aspiration tip of the automated Kelman-Cavitron system with the aspiration port facing up to remove residual hyaluronate while irrigating with balanced salt solution. If the McIntyre instrument is used for hyaluronate removal, it is small enough to insert between adjacent sutures after closure is completed. Hyaluronate is readily aspirated from the posterior chamber and from beneath the intraocular lens as well as from the anterior chamber when the aspiration hole is moved in a circular fashion adjacent to the pupillary margin through 360°. (Another way to remove hyaluronate is to aspirate with a 27-gauge cannula attached to a 5 ml plastic syringe: move the aspiration hole in a circular fashion adjacent to the pupillary margin through 180°; refill the chamber with balanced salt solution and repeat aspiration on the opposite 180°; refill the chamber with balanced salt solution and aspirate residual hyaluronate from the central anterior chamber.) The lens implant usually remains in proper position, but if it becomes slightly displaced it is repositioned with a Sinskey hook after closure. The wound closure is completed with interrupted 10-0 nylon sutures. The residual 8-0 black silk suture is removed and replaced with a 10-0 nylon suture. We usually use approximately seven to eight sutures for closure of this 10 mm wound.

98

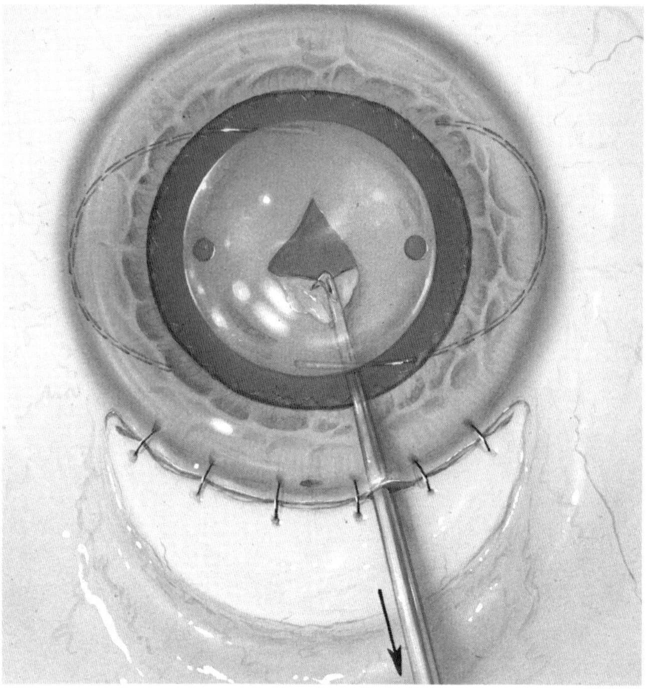

99

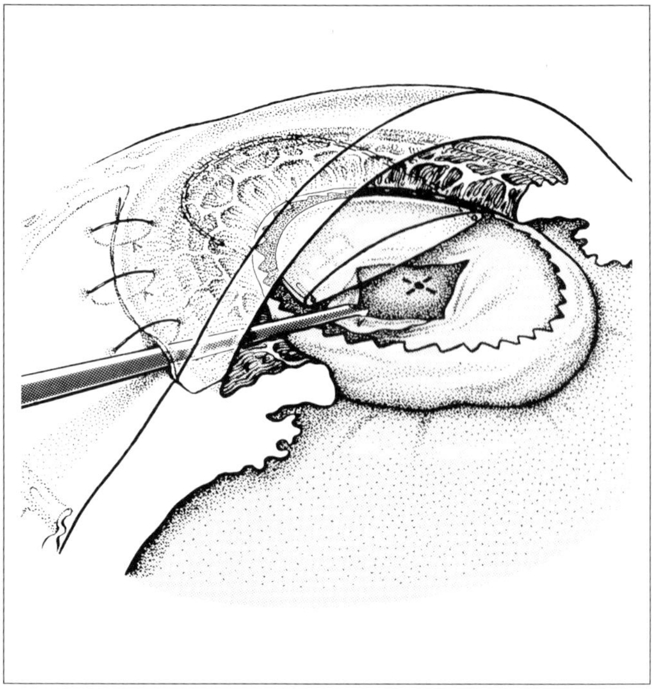

100

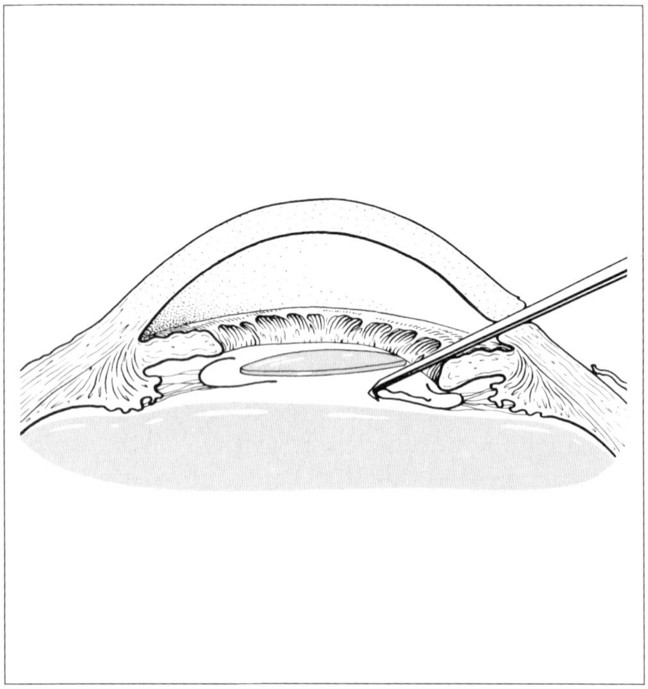

4.**98** to **100** We prefer to leave the posterior capsule intact whenever possible. We never open the capsule primarily unless there is a very significant opacification of the central posterior capsule due to residual fibrosis which cannot be removed, and even then in some of these cases we leave it intact and open the capsule with a YAG laser three months after the date of surgery. When this policy is followed, we believe that the incidence of cystoid macular edema is reduced and that the chances of vitreous incarceration between the posterior capsule and the lens are reduced.

Nevertheless, if there seems to be a pressing need for prompt restoration of vision, we will open an opacified posterior capsule primarily, as illustrated here. A 27-gauge disposable needle is fashioned with a small microhook at the tip. It is attached to a 5–10 ml syringe containing balanced salt solution. After complete closure of the incision, the needle is passed between two sutures into the anterior chamber, through the pupillary space, beneath the intraocular lens implant, and inferiorly to a position about 2 mm below the optic axis. Balanced salt solution in injected as needed in order to maintain the depth of the anterior chamber. Care is taken not to displace the intraocular lens from its desired position. The posterior capsule is engaged approximately 2 mm below the optic axis, and then a small tear is initiated by pulling superiorly. Once a small tear has begun, additional balanced salt solution is injected in order to allow fluid to pass through the hole and to push the vitreous face posteriorly to allow safer tearing of the posterior capsule. The posterior capsule tear is continued by tearing superiorly until an opening approximately 3 mm in diameter has been obtained. Continued injection of balanced salt solution keeps the vitreous face away from the microhook. Excessive manipulation is avoided in order to prevent rupture of the vitreous face. After completion of the tear in the posterior capsule, the microhook is turned to the side so that the flap is disengaged, and the hook is removed while injecting balanced salt solution to maintain the depth of the anterior chamber. The position of the lens is readjusted if necessary, but manipulation should be kept to a minimum after the capsulotomy.

101

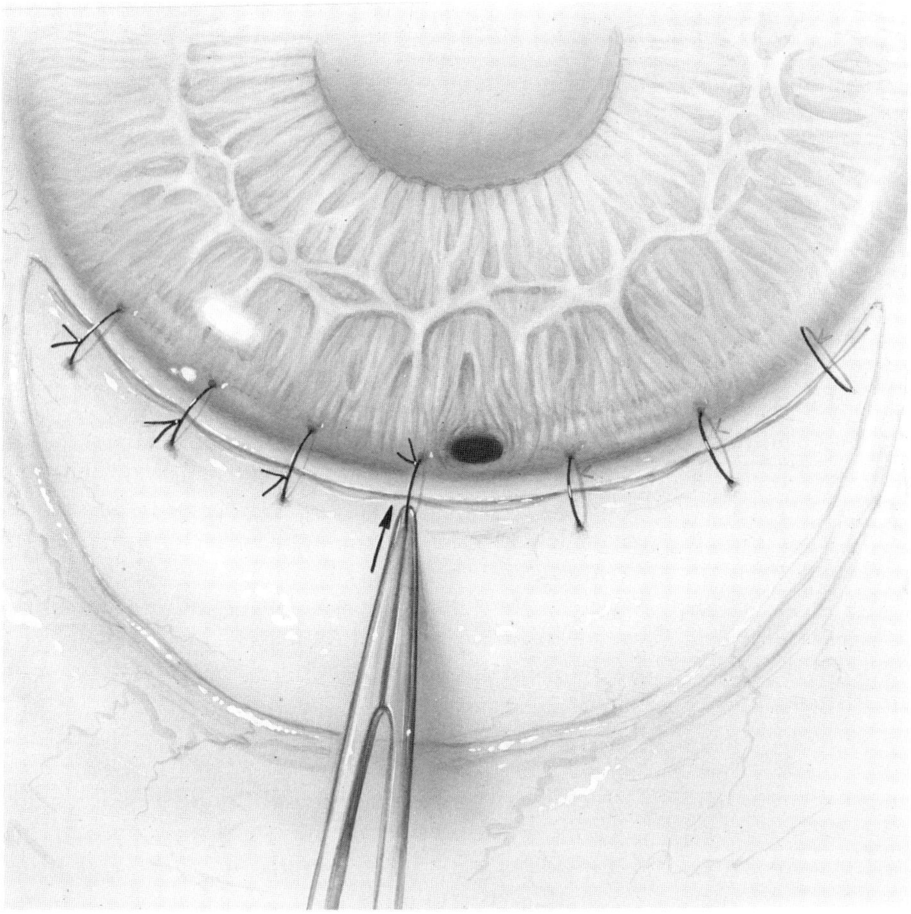

102

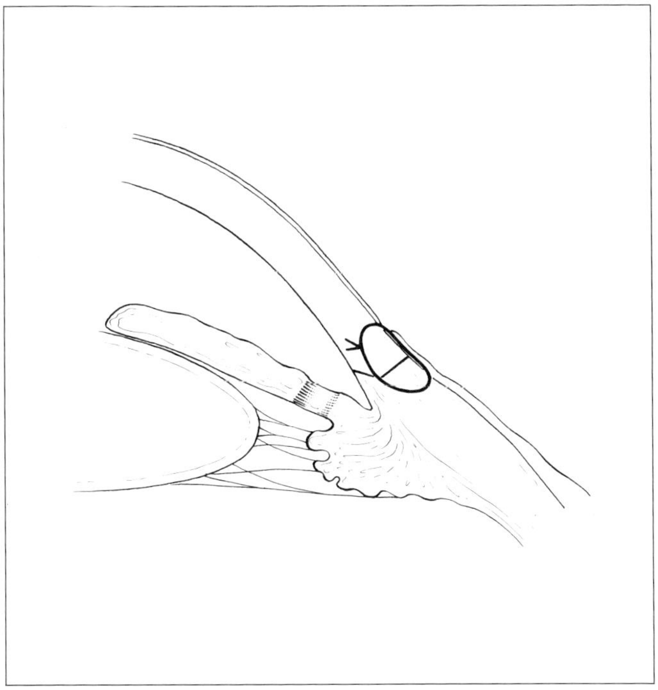

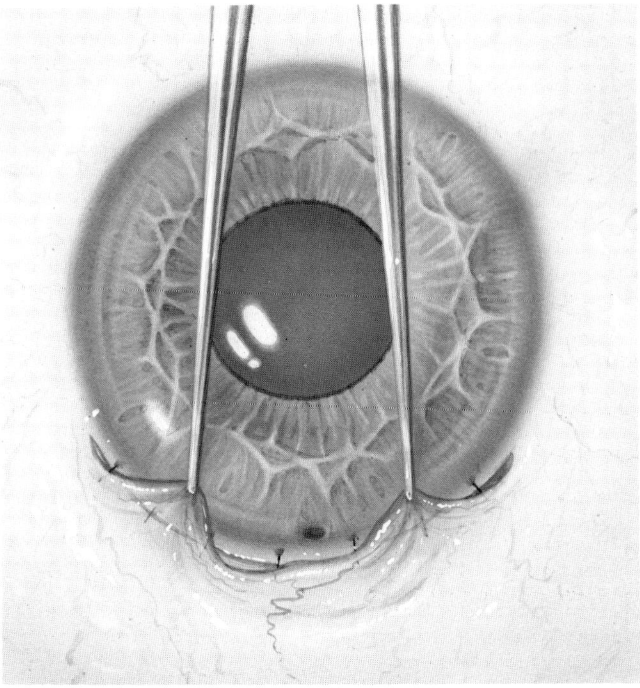

103

4.**101** and **102** After injection of acetylcholine hydrochloride to constrict the pupil and balanced salt solution to bring the eye to normal intraocular pressure, the wound is tested for watertightness. The wound, because of its clean two-plane incision, is watertight without excessive tightening of sutures, thereby minimizing astigmatism. The sutures are rotated to bury the knots in the corneal side of the incision.

4.**103** The conjunctiva is pulled back into its normal position for spontaneous reattachment. Suturing of the conjunctiva is unnecessary with this fornix-based flap.

Postoperative Management

We like to irrigate the eye with Neosporin solution, and then apply a small amount of topical eserine, 0.25 % ointment, followed by Neosporin or Maxitrol ointment. The eserine ointment pulls the pupil down so that it is small and central and thereby prevents iridocapsular adhesions that might cause an irregular pupil. We begin dilating with Mydriacyl 0.5 % q.i.d. on the day after surgery. The mydriatic is used primarily to move the pupil rather than to cause wide dilation, which again could result in an irregular pupil from synechia formation.

The intraocular pressure is measured on the morning following surgery. Pressure elevations above 40 mmHg can occur, especially if sodium hyaluronate was incompletely aspirated at the close of the surgery. Pressure elevations are managed with some combination of timolol, acetazolamide and, if necessary, oral glycerol.

Spectacles are prescribed six to eight weeks following surgery. Sutures can be removed selectively as noted below to minimize postoperative astigmatism. Approximately one diopter of with-the-rule astigmatism is desirable six weeks postoperatively; further regression towards sphericity will occur in subsequent months. One suture only is removed at each visit to avoid unwanted excessive shifts to against-the-rule astigmatism.

Timing of Suture Cutting

Postoperative Interval	*Astigmatism*
≤ 3 weeks	Never cut
4–5 weeks	≥ 5 D
≥ 6 weeks	≥ 2–5 D

References

[1] Emery, J. M., McIntyre, D. J.: *Extracapsular Cataract Surgery*. Mosby, St. Louis 1983.

[2] Atkinson, W. S.: *Anesthesia in Ophthalmology*, 2nd ed., Thomas, Springfield (Ill.) 1965, pages 64–76.

[3] Emery, J. M. McIntyre, D. J.: *Extracapsular Cataract Surgery*. Mosby, St. Louis 1983, Chs. 38–40.

[4] Emery, J. M., McIntyre, D. J.: *Extracapsular Cataract Surgery*. Mosby, St. Louis 1983, Ch. 11, pages 42–49.

[5] Emery, J. M., McIntyre, D. J.: *Extracapsular Cataract Surgery*. Mosby, St. Louis 1983, Ch. 28, pages 205–215.

Phacoemulsification with Posterior Chamber Intraocular Lens Implantation

Richard P. Kratz

Introduction

Phacoemulsification is a relatively new technique of planned extracapsular cataract extraction. It was first introduced at the American Academy of Ophthalmology in 1968 by Charles Kelman, M.D. The first classes were taught in 1971, and since then improved machines have been developed by Cavitron and other companies. Variations of the original Kelman technique have been devised, and one such variation is presented here.

Preparation for Surgery

Tetracaine drops are given, and the pupil is dilated with Cyclomydril and 1 % atropine, one drop of each. If this gives wide dilation in 20 minutes, no additional drops are used; if the pupil is still not widely dilated, the tetracaine is repeated, and one or two applications of 2.5 % phenylephrine are instilled. The Honan ballon is applied for 30 minutes at 30 mm Hg.

Instruments

Either the Cavitron Kelman Model 8000 or the United Surgical Systems Phacotron is used to emulsify the nucleus. Epinephrine 1:1000 (0.5 ml) is added to the 500 ml of balanced salt solution, making a dilution of 1:1,000,000.

Surgical Technique

104

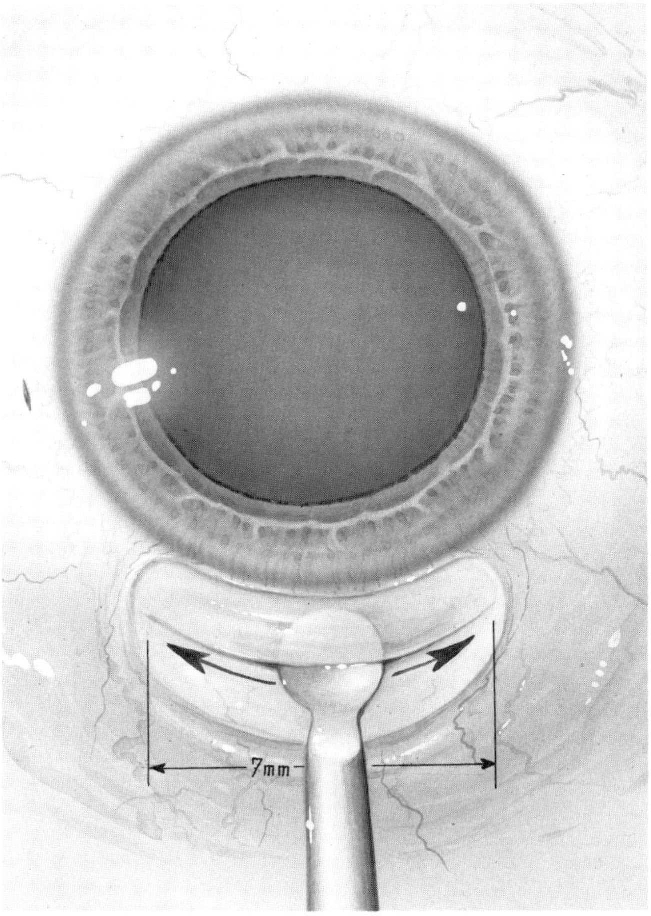

105

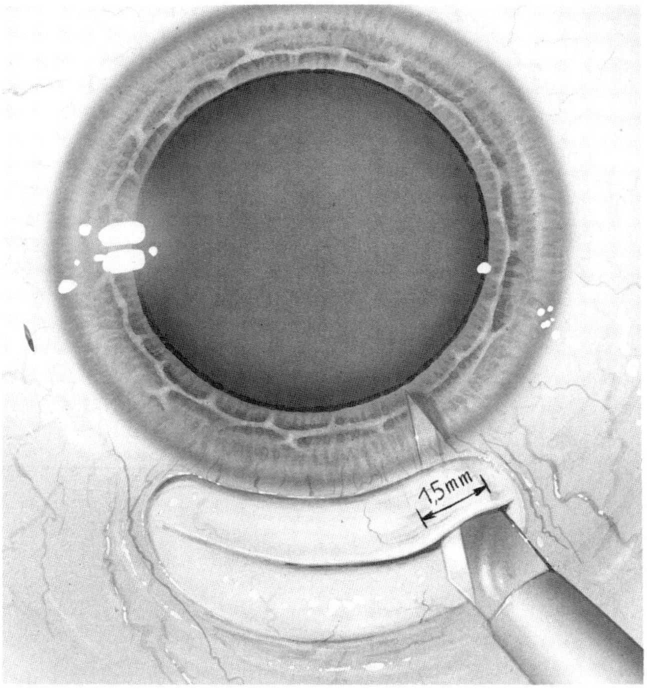

4.**104** A distance of 7 mm is measured at the limbus, and a 7 mm fornix-based conjunctival flap is prepared. A # 681.01 Grieshaber blade is used to incise the sclera to one-half of its thickness over the full 7 mm. This incision is placed 2 mm below the posterior edge of the limbus, or 3 mm below the anterior portion of the limbal arcade. A # 8121 Grieshaber blade is used to dissect forward into clear cornea. It is important to change the angle of the blade as it moves from side to side and as it changes from the scleral to the corneal radius of curvature.

4.**105** A 30° angled razor blade fragment is used to make a beveled 0.5 mm limbal puncture at 3 o'clock and to open 1.5 mm of the scleral pocket incision at 11 o'clock. The actual entry into the anterior chamber is at the anterior part of the limbal arcade, thus leaving a shelf in case an anterior chamber intraocular lens is needed.

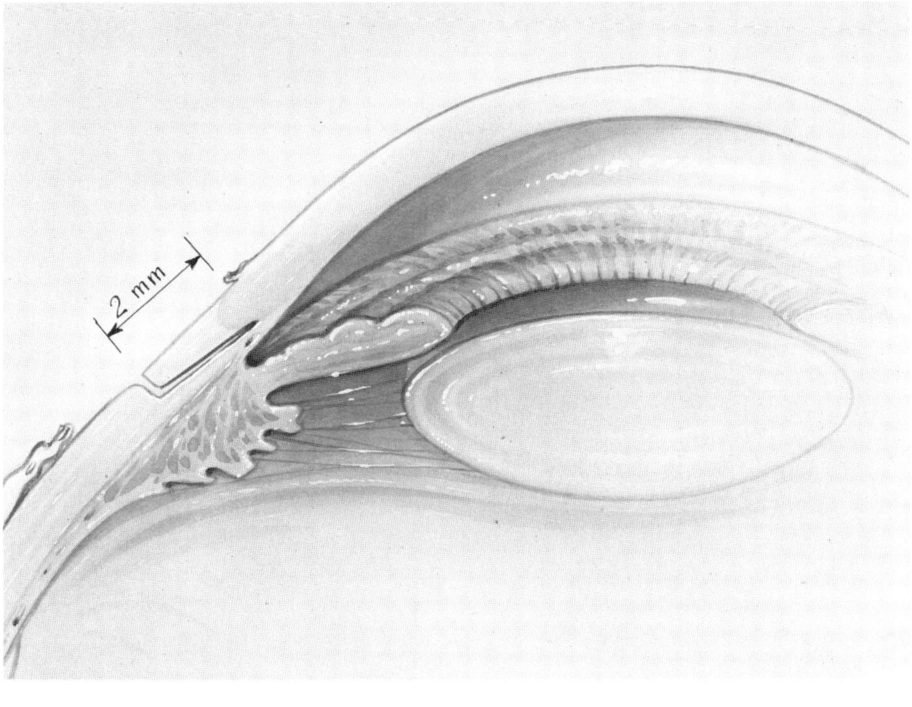

4.**106** The cross-section shows the depth and the angle of the incision into the sclera.

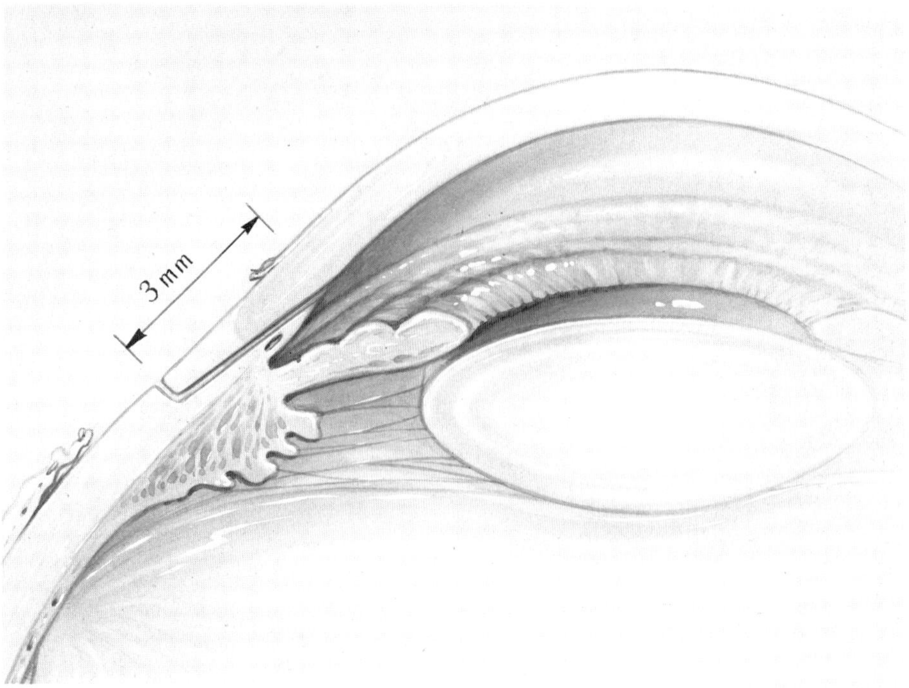

4.**107** The incision into the anterior chamber has been completed. Note that the entry is anterior to the trabecular meshwork rather than at the iris root. This gives a good scleral shelf in case an anterior chamber lens is used and avoids the bleeding and iris prolapse that occur if the incision enters at the iris root.

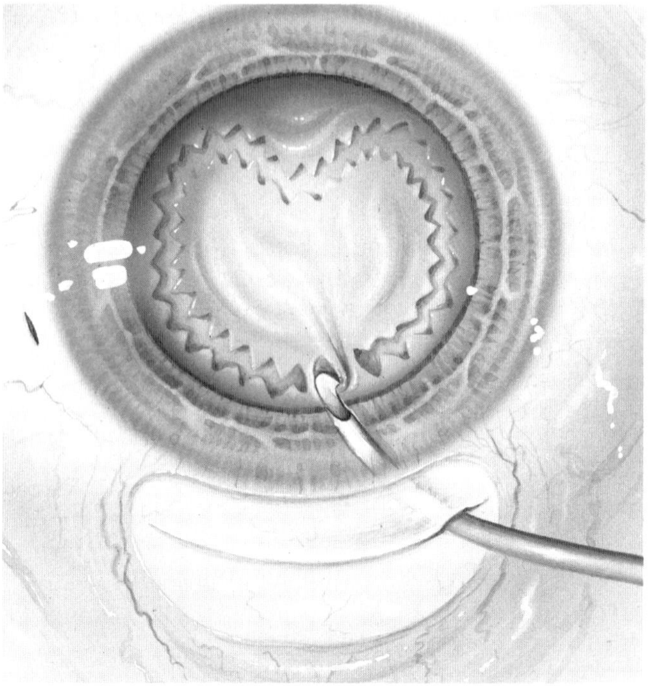

4.**108** A bent 25-gauge needle or a 23-gauge irrigating cystotome (Storz # E 0146) is used to do a can-opener-type anterior capsulotomy. The anterior chamber depth is maintained with balanced salt or Healon. The capsulotomy from 10 to 12 o'clock should be completed first, as it is difficult to get accurate cuts in this area if the capsule is not tight. The capsule should be removed as far into the periphery as possible in this area, as a large flap of anterior capsule makes it difficult to remove cortex here.

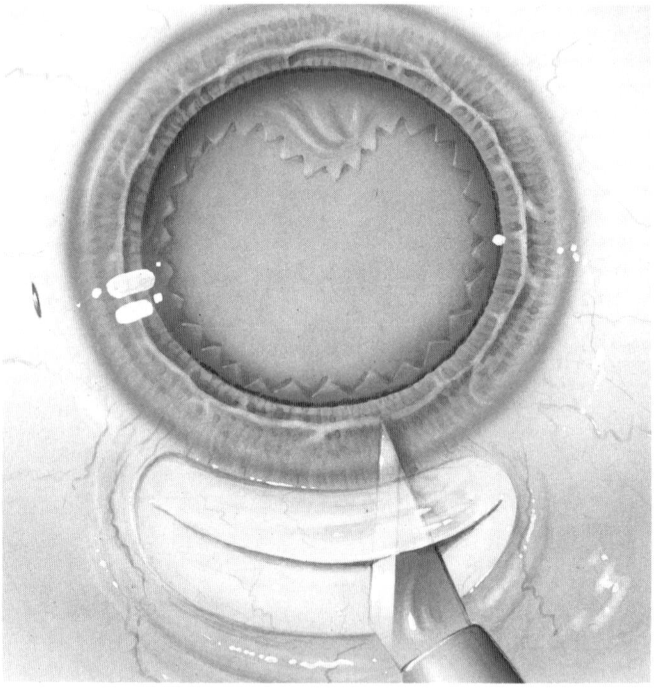

4.**109** The razor-blade is used to enlarge the scleral incision to 3 mm.

110

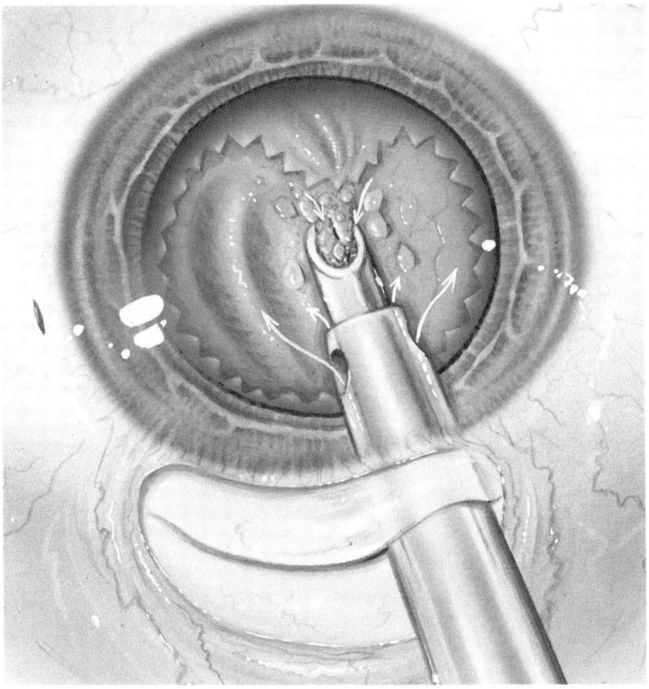

112

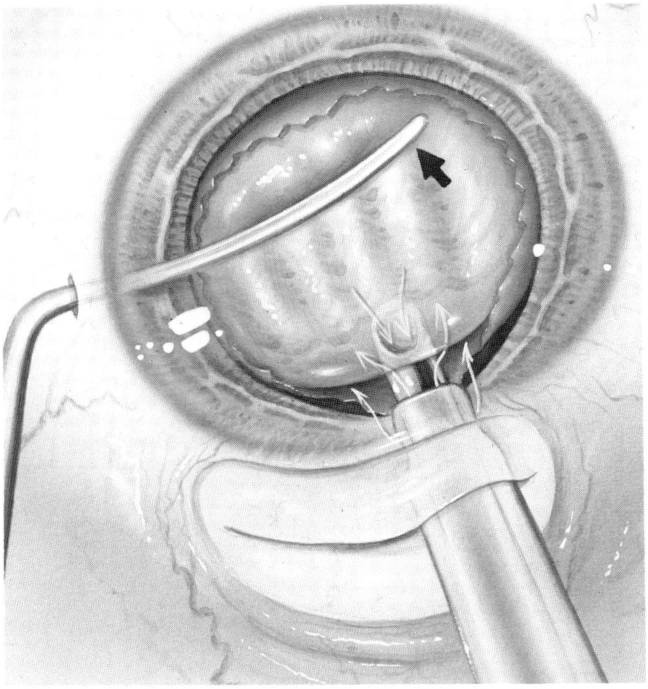

111

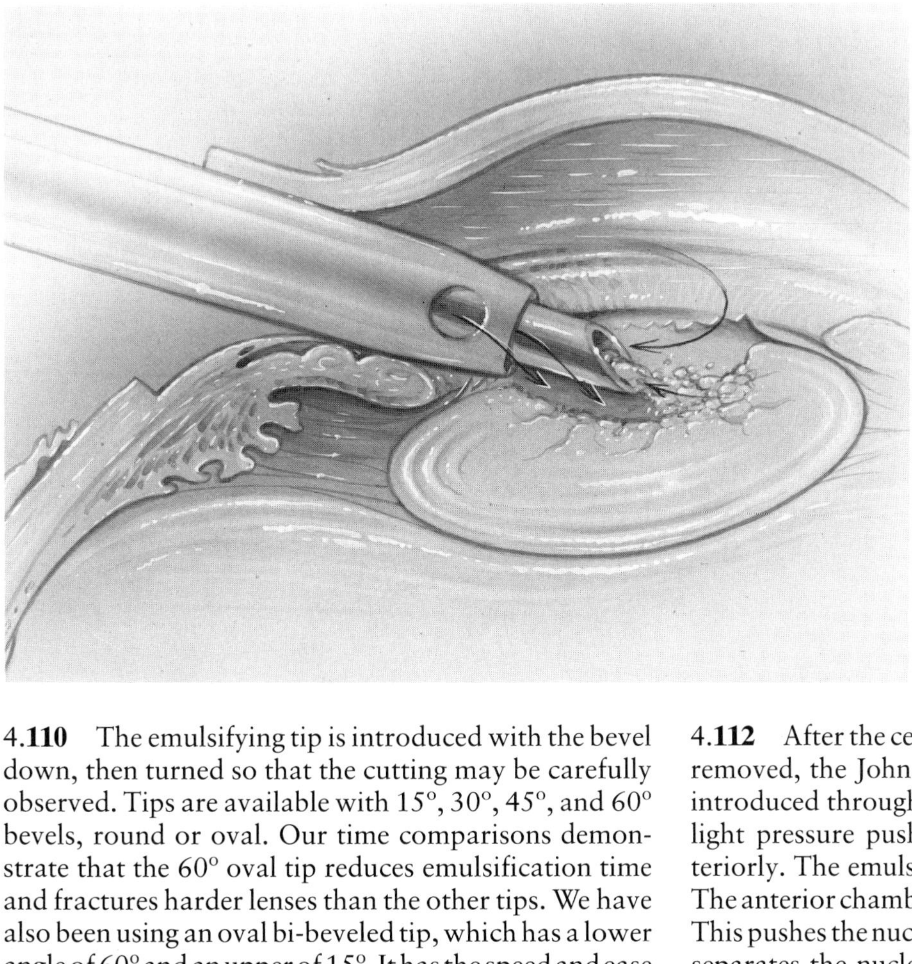

4.**111** Without subluxing the nucleus, the emulsification is carried out in the posterior chamber or at the plane of the iris. The emulsifier is held like a pool cue rather than a silver spoon. This gives greater side-to-side wrist action and permits the emulsifying tip to rest on the patient's brow. When the silver spoon grip is used, there is a tendency to lift up on the incision with the emulsifying tip. The pool cue grip allows the instrument to be steadied against the patient's forehead.

4.**110** The emulsifying tip is introduced with the bevel down, then turned so that the cutting may be carefully observed. Tips are available with 15°, 30°, 45°, and 60° bevels, round or oval. Our time comparisons demonstrate that the 60° oval tip reduces emulsification time and fractures harder lenses than the other tips. We have also been using an oval bi-beveled tip, which has a lower angle of 60° and an upper of 15°. It has the speed and ease of the 60° bevel and the aspirating power of the 15° bevel. The oval tips put more cutting surface on the nucleus with less stretch on the sclero-corneal incision.

4.**112** After the central portion of the nucleus has been removed, the Johnson spatula (Storz: special order) is introduced through the 3 o'clock limbal puncture, and light pressure pushes the nucleus inferiorly and posteriorly. The emulsifying tip is retracted to 11 o'clock. The anterior chamber is then allowed almost to collapse. This pushes the nucleus forward, and the emulsifying tip separates the nucleus from the cortex and flap of the anterior capsule. The flow of balanced salt is resumed.

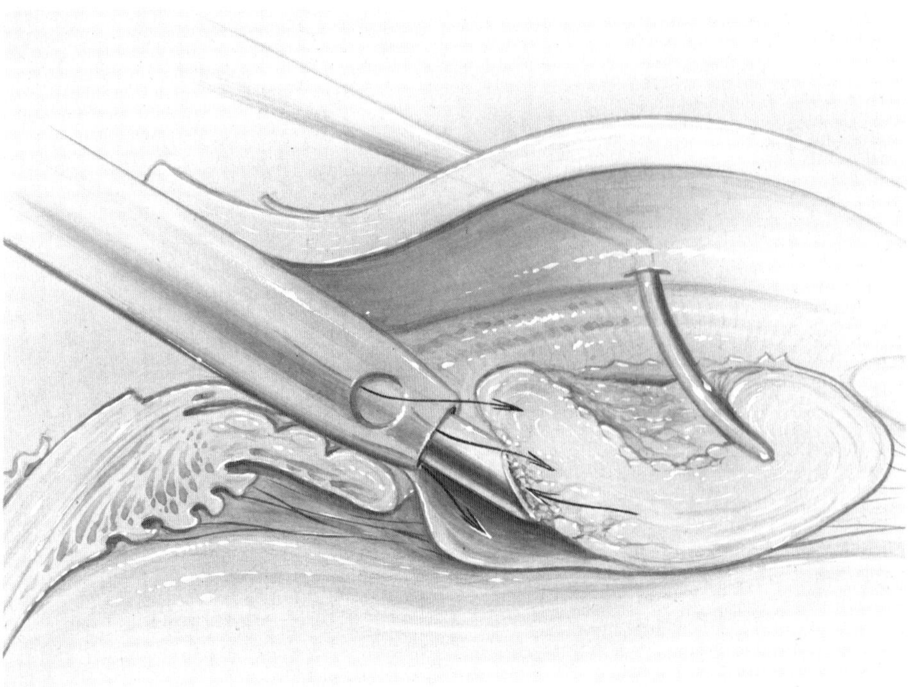

4.**113** The infusion of balanced salt easily separates the nucleus from the cortex with the aid of the spatula.

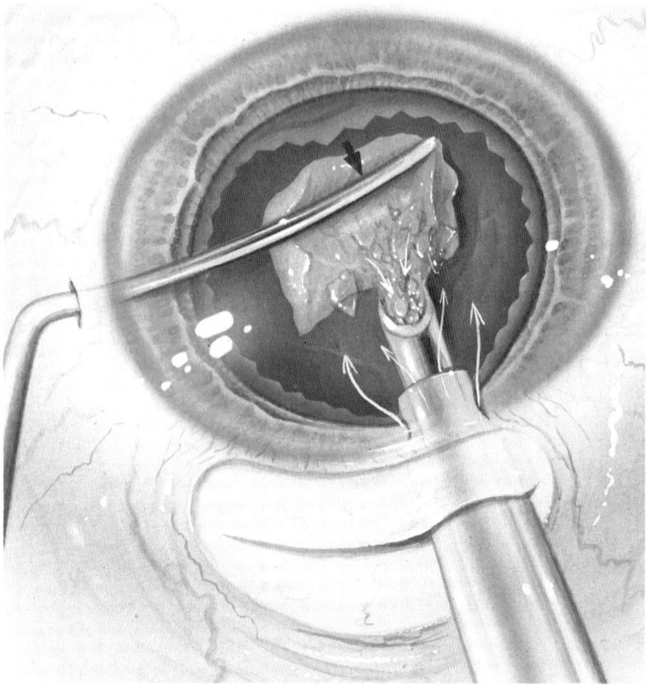

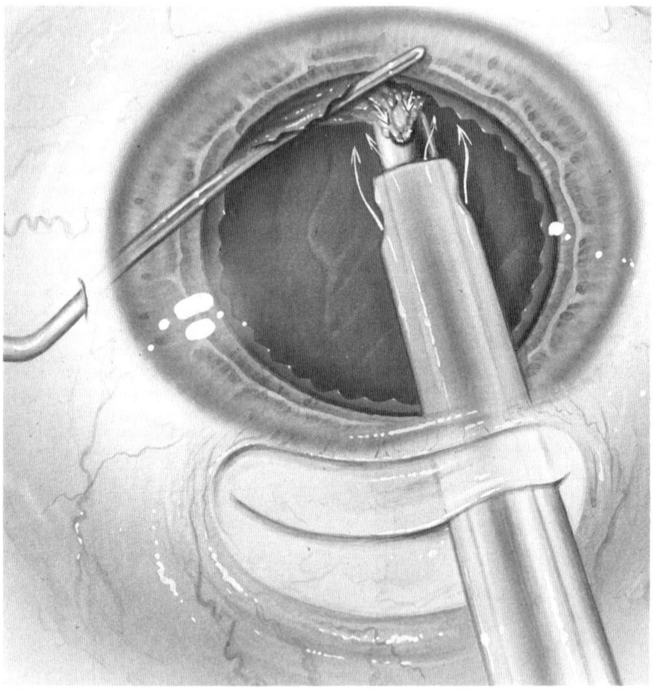

4.**114** The spatula is used to elevate, rotate, depress, or crush the nucleus. The spatula is also helpful to prevent contact of the nucleus with the endothelium and to prevent sharp edges of the nucleus from perforating the posterior capsule. Care should be taken not to touch the emulsifying tip while the power is on, as small flakes of metal will be left in the eye.

4.**115** When the emulsification has been completed, the 0.3 mm irrigating and aspirating tip is used to remove the cortical material. The spatula assists by retracting the iris or anterior capsule flap and by helping to steady the eye. The posterior capsule may be lightly cleansed with the 0.3 mm irrigating and aspirating tip under minimum vacuum. Polishing devices have been a disappointment, as the capsule will cloud anyway, and there is little advantage in risking premature rupture and vitreous loss. If a plaque is present, it is usually allowed to remain and then treated with the Nd: YAG laser in the postoperative period.

116

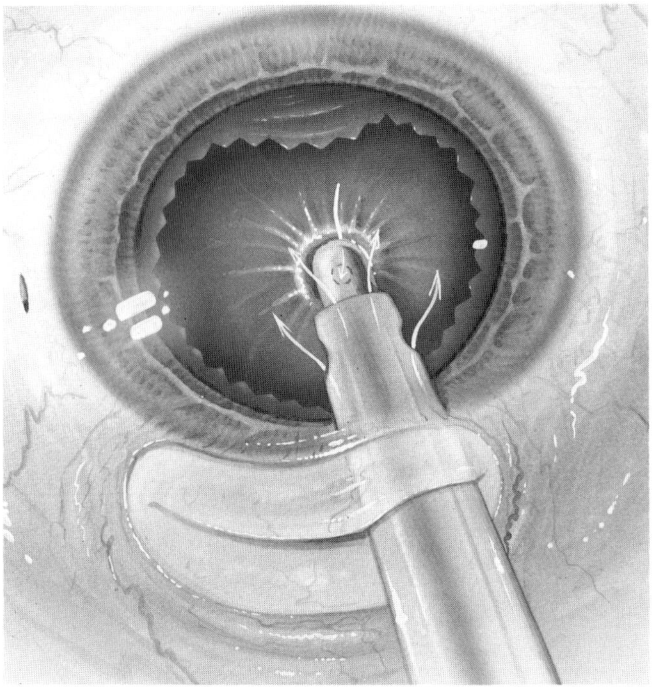

117

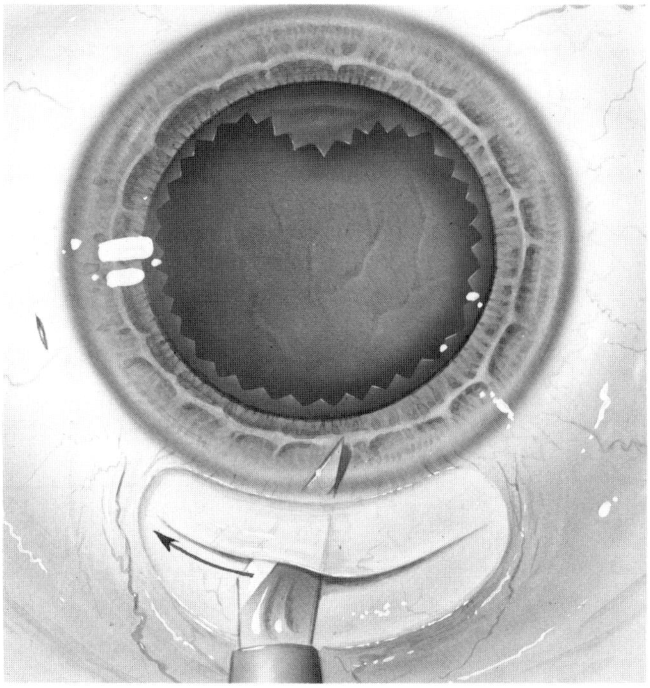

118

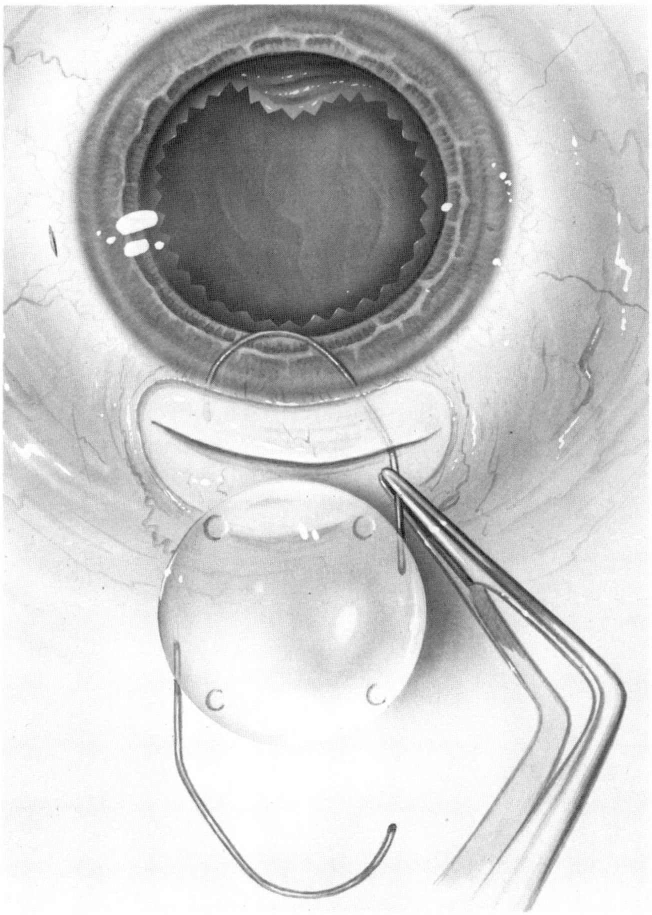

4.116 Occasionally, the posterior capsule is grasped by the irrigating and aspirating tip. This may be recognized when radial folds converge on the aspirating tip. Unless the capsule is promptly released, it may be torn, resulting in vitreous loss. The 0.3 mm tip is less apt to grab the capsule than the 0.5 mm or the 0.7 mm tip. We use a safety device consisting of a T-connector in the aspiration line. The T-connector has ten inches of silicone tubing and a 10 ml syringe partially filled with balanced salt. When the capsule is inadvertently gripped by the irrigating and aspirating tip, the flow is reversed through the aspirating port by simply infusing fluid from the syringe, which releases the capsule. The T-connector device may also be used to augment aspiration by increasing the vacuum after the cortex has been grasped. It is also used to deepen the chamber when the emulsifying tip is first introduced into the anterior chamber.

4.117 Healon is instilled into the anterior chamber, and the anterior capsule flaps are widely separated from the posterior capsule. Air or saline may be used, but visualization of the bag is more difficult with the former, and loss of the anterior chamber more common with the latter. The incision is enlarged to the full 7 mm with the razor-blade fragment.

4.118 The posterior chamber intraocular lens is inserted, using a Kratz forceps # 5848 (Katena). It is first grasped by the inferior haptic, as many of these loops have very low compression force, and grasping by the optic simply causes the loop to collapse rather than enter the eye.

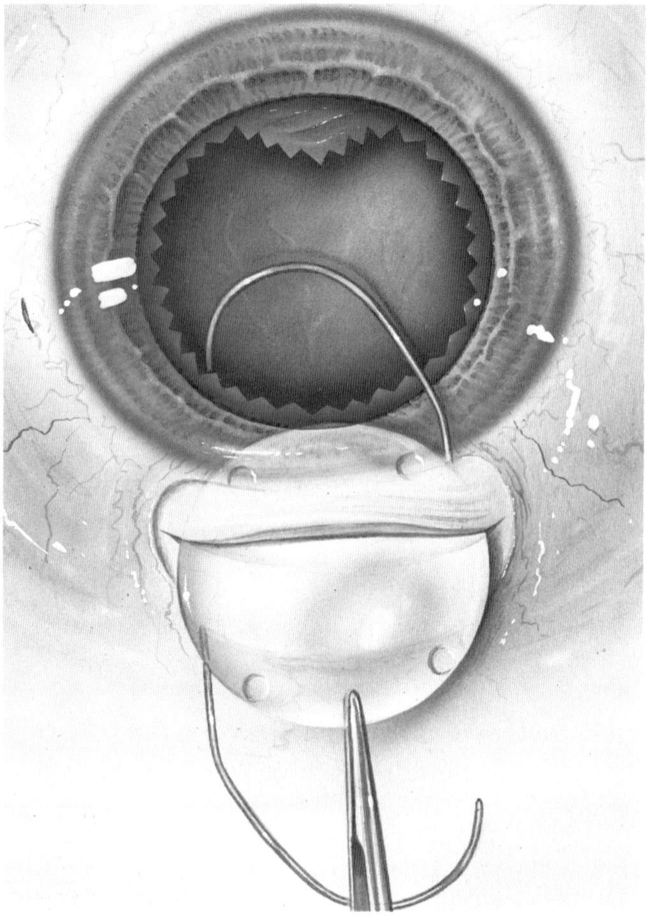

4.119 The optic is then grasped, and the 7 mm intraocular lens is introduced. If a 6.5 mm optic or a 6.0 mm optic intraocular lens is selected, then the initial incision should be similarly reduced.

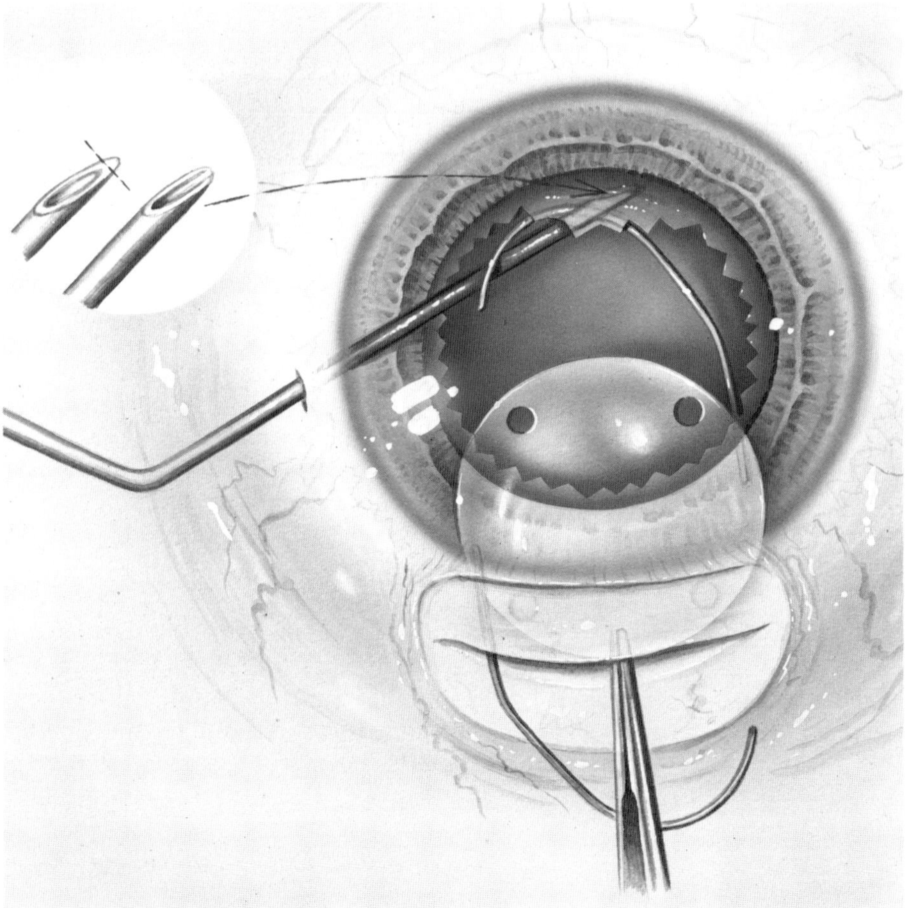

4.120 Usually, the inferior loop glides under the anterior capsule and into the bag without difficulty.

Sometimes it is helpful to use a cannula that has been prepared by cutting off and smoothing the tip of a 30-gauge needle. The cannula is placed on a 3 ml balanced salt solution syringe and is used as needed to manipulate the loop, iris, or anterior capsular flap. Since an inferior rim of capsule is allowed to remain, it is easy to visualize the loop entering the bag.

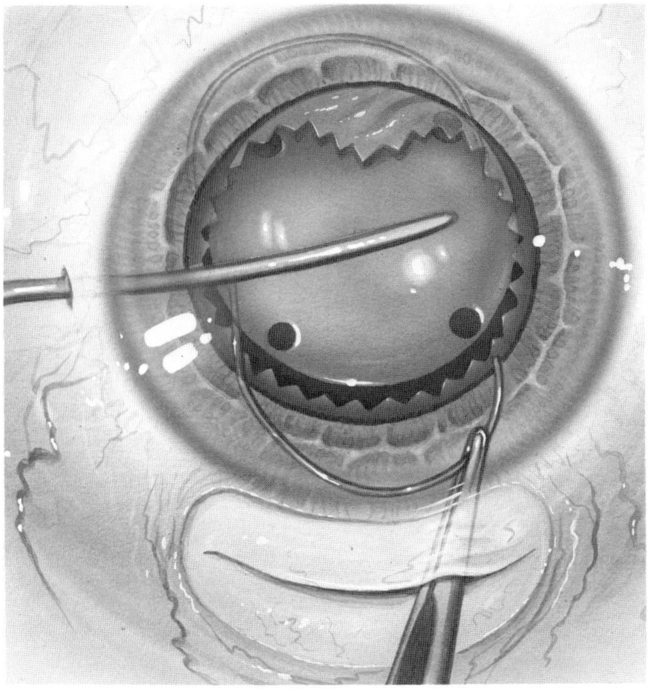

4.**121** The superior loop is grasped with the Kratz forceps and introduced into the anterior chamber. The right hand is partially pronated; this causes the left side of the optic and the loop to partially rotate posteriorly, permitting entry into the bag under direct visualization of the remaining capsular rim. Occasionally, it is helpful to use the 30-gauge irrigating cannula to push the optic posterior to facilitate entry of the superior loop into the bag.

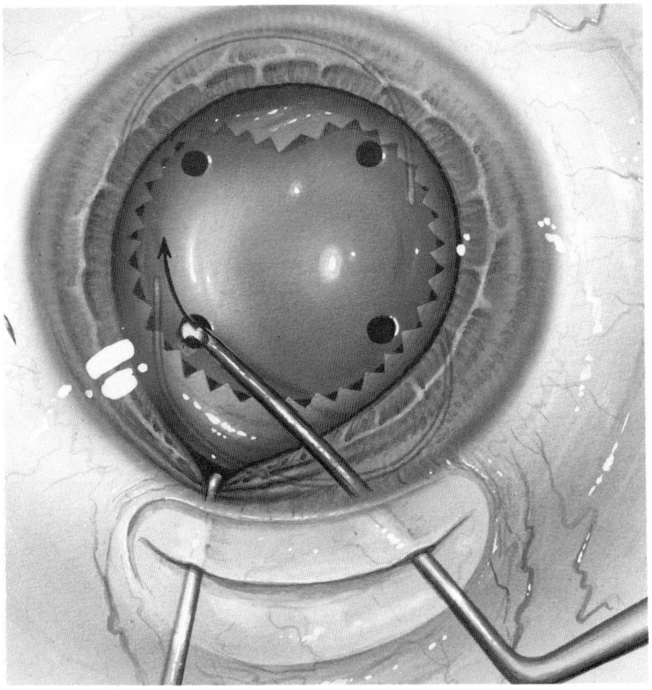

4.**122** An alternative technique is to dial the superior loop into place, and visualization may be facilitated by retracting the iris with a Bonn hook.

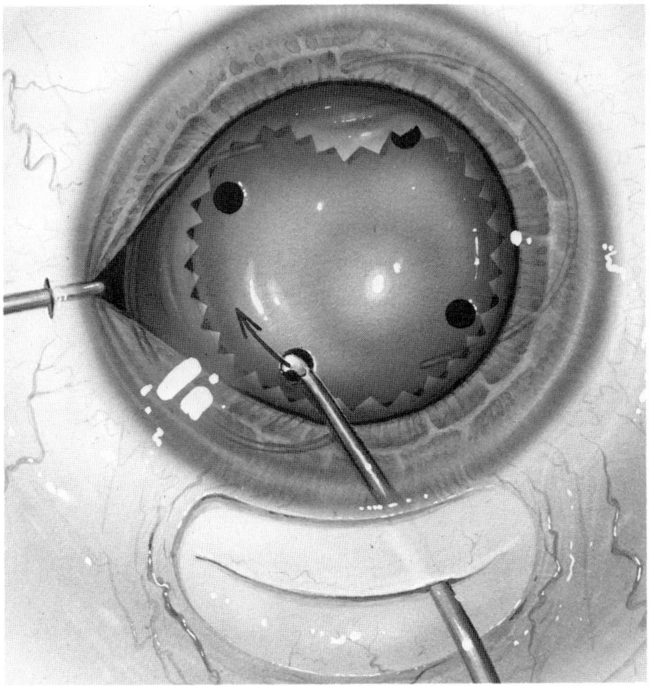

4.**123** Some ophthalmologists feel more secure if the intraocular lens is dialed into the horizontal position. I see no merit in this and only dial if the centering is not optimal.

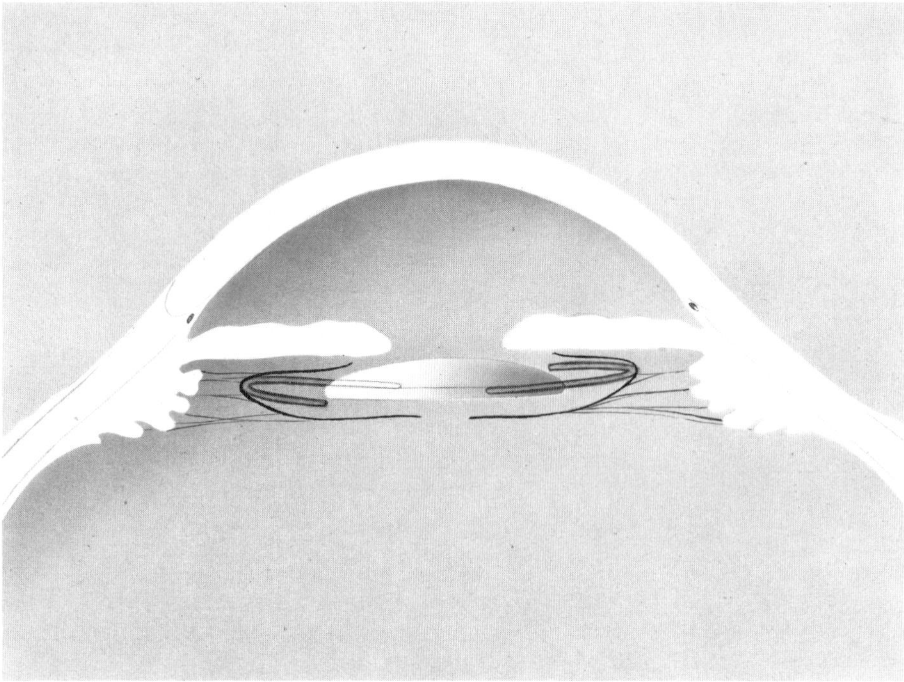

4.**124** The loops rest in the bag. If a low-compression-force intraocular lens is used, it is easy to compress the 14 mm overall length of the loops into the ± 10 mm diameter of the bag. It is wise to use the 14 mm intraocular lens, as it may still be inserted into the sulcus if a minor tear in the posterior capsule without vitreous loss has occurred. In that event, the full 14 mm will be needed.

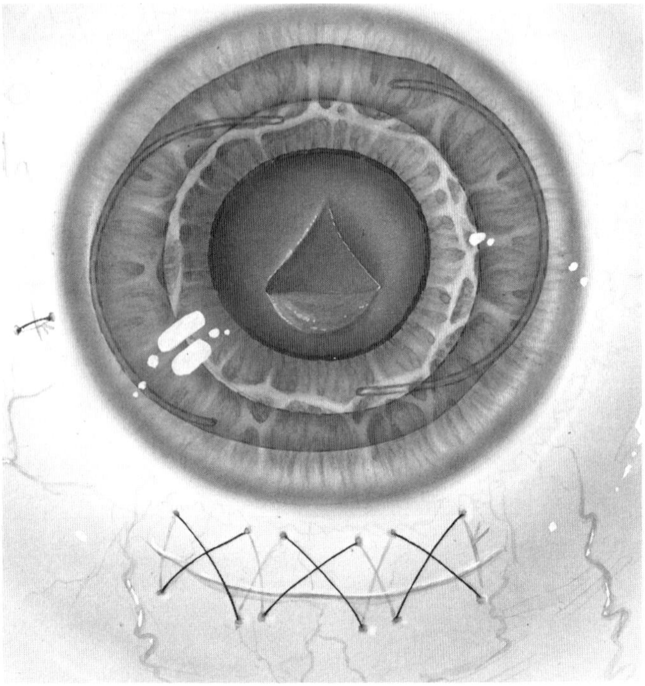

4.**125** Closure is with a 10-0 nylon suture. It is our experience that 10-0 nylon almost never requires removal if placed at or behind the Tenon's capsule insertion, whereas sutures placed in clear cornea or at the conjunctival insertion erode and require removal. We do not recommend 9-0 nylon, as it is much stiffer and erodes even if placed posterior to the Tenon's capsule insertion. The shoelace closure is started on the scleral side at the extreme right-hand corner of the incision. Three or more radial bites are added passing to the extreme left-hand side of the incision. Three or more radial bites are made passing to the right, and then the last half-bite is on the corneal side at the right-hand extreme of the incision. Healon is irrigated from the eye, and a temporary knot is tied. The eye is inflated to 21 mm Hg and checked with the Terry keratometer to properly adjust the tension on the sutures so that postoperative astigmatism may be minimized. Injections of gentamicin and dexamethasone are given subconjunctivally. The conjunctival flap is not sutured.

Complications

This technique requires familiarity with the use of a coaxial microscope. Practice is required to develop skill and comfort in the use of the machine. The greatest advantage of this technique is the control that the surgeon has in all parts of the procedure, which results in a low complication rate.

The scleral pocket incision should be carried into clear cornea for approximately 1 mm to avoid bleeding at the iris root and prolapse of the iris during emulsification. The emulsification incision should be carefully measured at slightly less than 3 mm to prevent iris prolapse when fluid is being infused into the anterior chamber.

If the posterior capsule is broken while a large part of the nucleus remains in the eye, the procedure should be converted into a standard planned extracapsular technique. If the posterior capsule is broken during irrigation and aspiration, and no vitreous enters the anterior chamber, it is possible to leave a small amount of cortex in the eye and proceed with the introduction of the intraocular lens with the help of Healon and a Sheets glide. If the posterior capsule is broken during cortical aspiration and vitreous enters the anterior chamber, it is wise to do an anterior vitrectomy before inserting an intraocular lens.

If the procedure has been traumatic to the eye, with or without an actual complication, then it is usually wise to delay the implantation of an intra-ocular lens until a later date.

Postoperative Management

The surgery is usually done on an outpatient basis. The eye is checked the next day for inflammation, intraocular lens centering and tension. It is then examined at one week, three weeks, and six weeks postoperatively. At the sixth week, final glasses are usually prescribed.

Bibliography

[1] Terry, C.: Advanced wound closure techniques utilizing the Terry keratometer so as to minimize postoperative corneal astigmatism, in *Cataract and Intraocular Lens Surgery*. Aesculapius, Birmingham (Ala.) 1984, pages 570–575.

[2] Kratz, R., Johnson, S.: Clinical results with the surgical keratometer. *Int. Ophthalmol. Clin.* 23 (4): 91–92, 1983.

[3] Kelman, C.: Phacoemulsification and aspiration. A new technique for cataract removal. A preliminary report. *Amer. J. Ophthalmol.* 64: 23, 1967.

[4] Thrasher, B., Keller, D.: Extracapsular cataract extraction, phacoemulsification and posterior chamber intraocular lens implantation, in *Cataract and Intraocular Lens Surgery*. Aesculapius, Birmingham (Ala.) 1984, pages 255–278.

[5] Colvard, D., Kratz, R. P., Mazzocco, T. R., Davidson, B.: Endothelial cell loss following phacoemulsification in the pupillary plane. *Amer. Intra-Ocular Implant Soc. J.* 7 (4): 334–336, 1981.

[6] Kraff, M. C., Sanders, D. R.: Planned extracapsular extraction versus phacoemulsification with IOL implantation: A comparison of concurrent studies. *Amer. Intra-Ocular Implant Soc. J.* 8 (1): 38–41, 1982.

[7] Johnson, S. M.: Emulsification of the nucleus: the bimanual technique in *Cataract Surgery*. McGraw-Hill, New York, 1986, pages 55–73.

Intracapsular Lens Implantation

Jörg Draeger

Surgical Principles

Intracapsular lens implantation by the method described in the following combines two fundamental factors: first, the implant is placed both safely and definitively at the physiological implantation site; second, the technique deliberately avoids using unnecessary apparatus.

Preparation for Surgery

The patient should be in possession of a certificate from his/her family physician stating that there are no contraindications to surgery. An ECG is done routinely on admission; a thorax roentgenogram is only necessary if general anesthesia is planned. A full ophthalmological examination is performed, including fundus, mydriasis, and contact lens examination. Ultrasound echometry is performed to calculate the required refraction of the implant.

Preoperative Medication and Anesthesia

The operation can be performed under either local or general anesthesia; in most cases the patient's wishes as regards the type of anesthesia can be accommodated. For good intraoperative mydriasis one drop of Cyclolat and one drop of 2.5 % Neo-Synephrine are instilled one hour, 30 minutes, 20 minutes, and 10 minutes before surgery. Additionally, when the procedure is performed under local anesthesia, 2 % and 5 % cocaine eye drops and one drop of naphazoline 1:1000 are given 10 minutes before surgery.

This results in a pronounced but reversible dilatation of the pupil. Epinephrine (0.5 %) is added to the intraocular collyrium. Preoperative intravenous administration of mannitol solution is advisable only in exceptional cases, in adipose patients with severe vis a tergo.

Instruments, Sutures, Needles

Aside from a powerful operating microscope, which must be equipped with a good coaxial illuminating system for pinpointing the red fundus reflex, the instrumentarium is confined to a few instruments packed together in a small set:

1. Lens implantation forceps with selective control of holding functions for lens optics and lens haptics
2. Angled Haab knife
3. Curved extrusion hook
4. Nucleus awl for harpooning the nucleus
5. Fine capsular spatula to detach the cortex from the anterior lens capsule
6. Microkeratotomy scissors
7. Ong capsule scissors
8. Flushing cannula set
9. Diamond knife or razor blade
10. Two pairs of suture-knotting forceps
11. Conjunctival forceps (may be needed for corneoscleral incision with a limbus-based conjunctival flap).
12. Atraumatic reinforced 10-0 nylon sutures.

To clarify the principle of the lens implantation forceps, their separate holding functions are explained here in brief:

The lens is held by thumb and middle finger via the branches of the forceps; a retractable "upper loop release" can be operated with the index finger, independently of the lens-holding function, via a lever fitted to the top of the forceps. During implantation the upper loop release is retracted: after placement of the intraocular lens the haptic which is pressed against the lens at 12 o'clock is released by removing the index finger from the lever. When the implant is positioned satisfactorily, the lens is then released by opening the forceps.

Surgical Technique

A holding suture (5-0 black silk) is placed in the tendon of the superior rectus muscle. A narrow, limbus-based conjunctival flap is then prepared with the conjunctival scissors and the corneoscleral border is traced with the hockey knife. The corneoscleral opening is now made in the form of an angled incision.

126

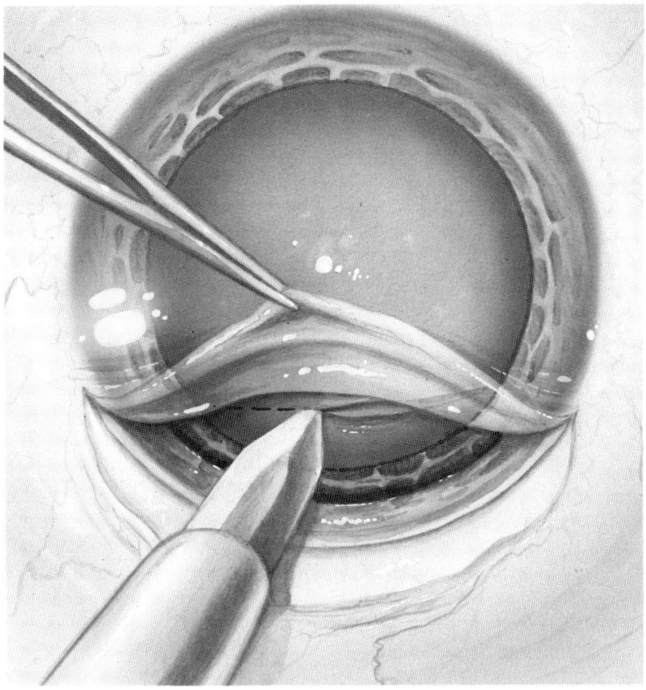

127

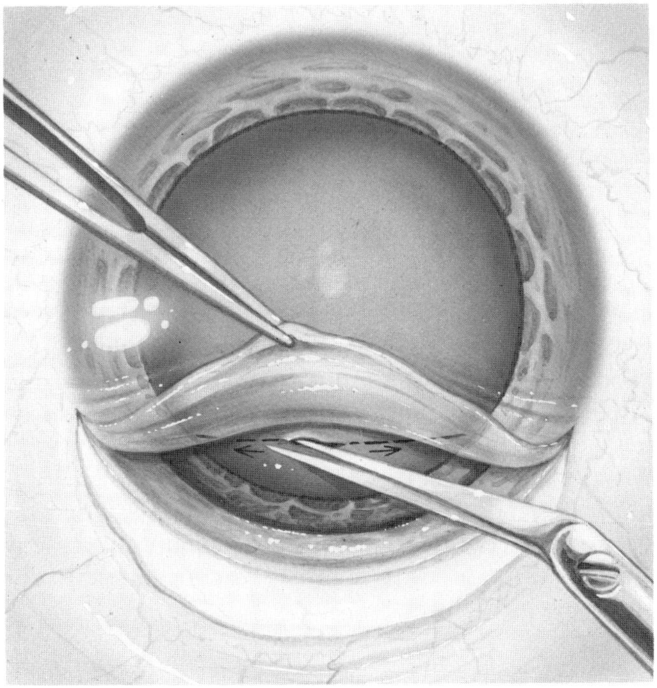

128

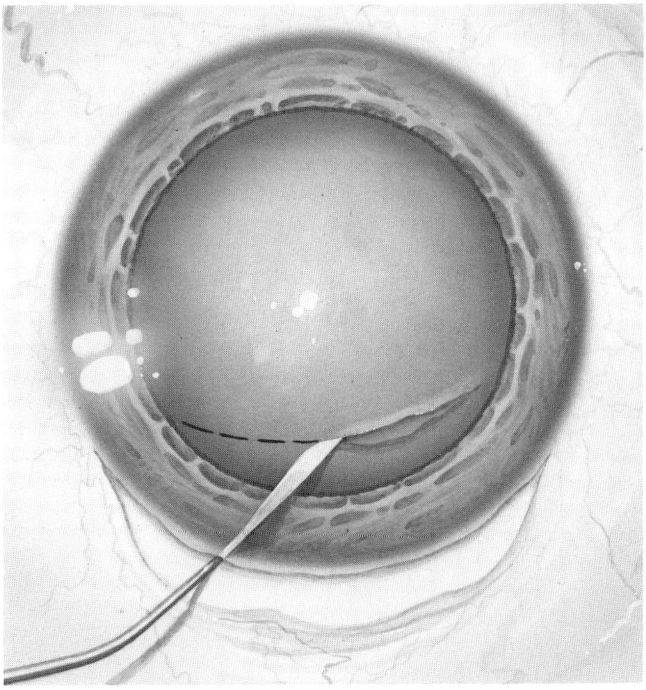

4.**126** and **127** When the open-sky method is used the cornea is next raised by applying gentle traction on the conjunctival flap with the conjunctival forceps. A horizontal capsulotomy is performed in the upper one-third of the lens, under direct vision, with a diamond, ruby, or Haab knife, unless YAG anterior discission was performed preoperatively.

4.128 In the closed-sky procedure a perforating incision with a capsulotomy is also possible.

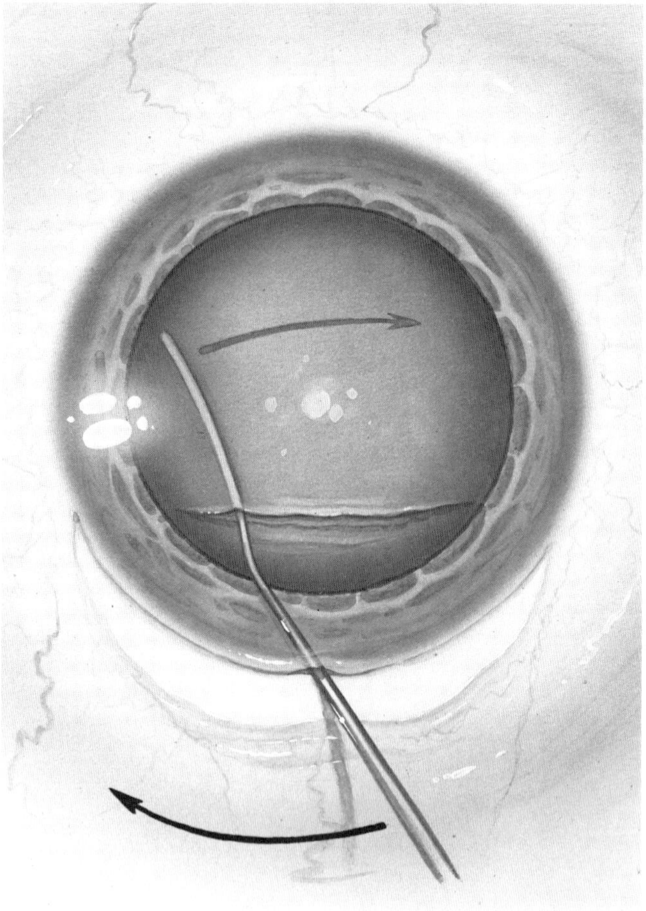

4.**129** Next, capsulolysis is performed, i.e., detachment of the anterior membrane of the capsule from the lens cortex. For this purpose a fine capsule spatula is introduced into the "mailing slit" and moved back and forth directly under the capsule. This greatly facilitates extrusion of the nucleus.

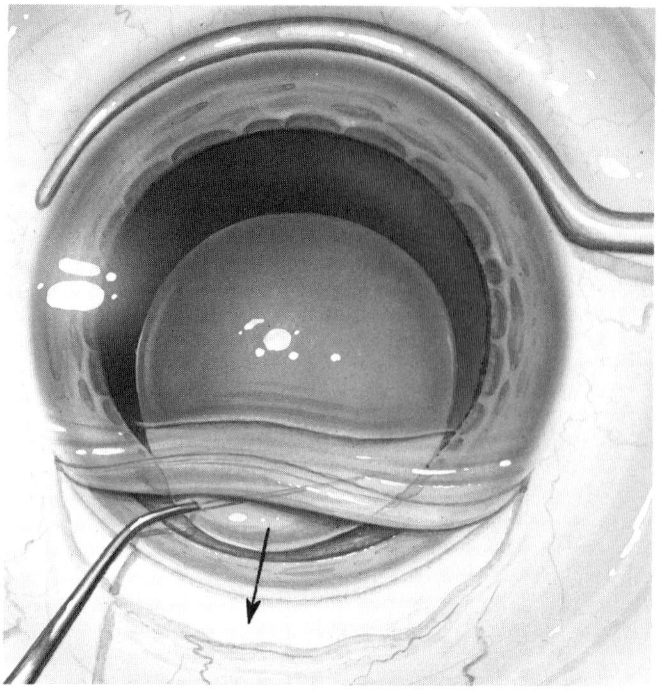

4.**130** In order to extrude the lens nucleus, counter-pressure is applied on the sclera at 6 o'clock with a curved extrusion hook; at the same time gentle pressure is applied at the scleral wound margin at 12 o'clock. As soon as the equator of the nucleus has come through the "mailing slit" a harpoon is inserted, with which detachment of the nucleus at 6 o'clock can be completed easily without any further pressure. Since, with the exception of the horizontal capsulotomy, the capsule is closed, an improved method of removing the remnants of the lens cortex can be used, in contrast to conventional capsulotomy procedures.

131

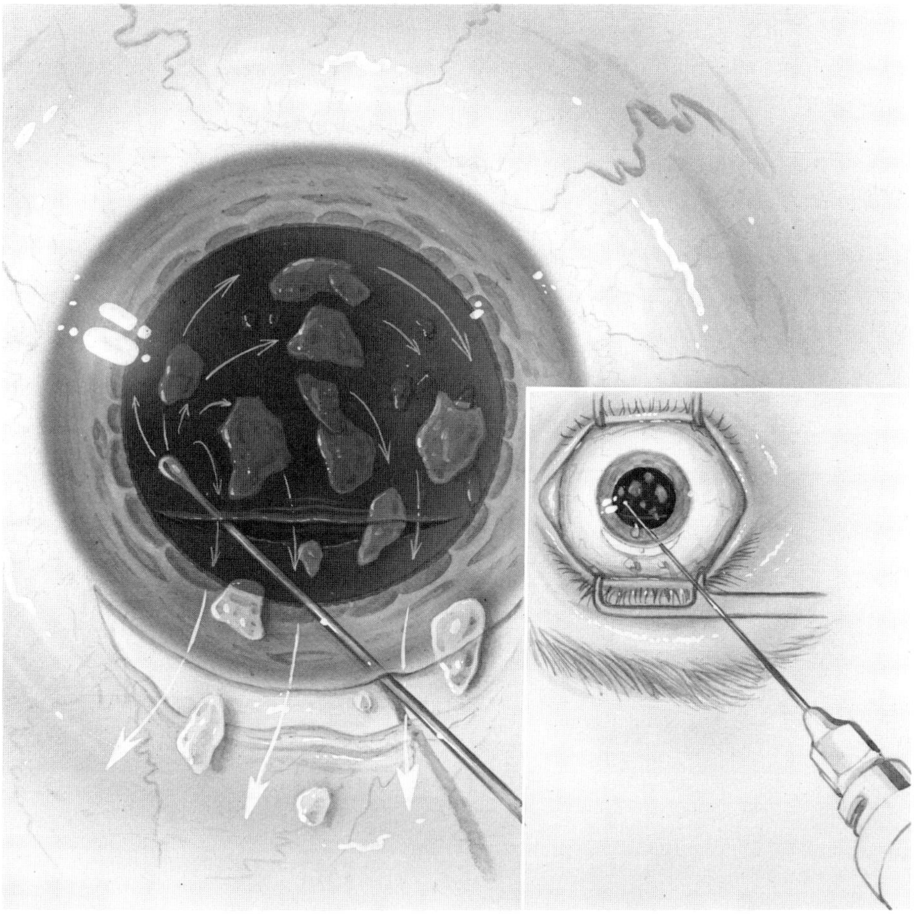

4.**131** and **132** Most of the cortex remnants can be removed by the powerful, turbulent flow of pressure flushing, practically without additional aspiration. Manual aspiration of the remnants is only necessary in exceptional cases. Flushing is performed first with a straight cannula and subsequently with one which is back-angled. The fact that the capsule is practically closed not only facilitates the removal of cortex remnants, but also gives the corneal endothelium additional mechanical protection against the turbulences during flushing.

132

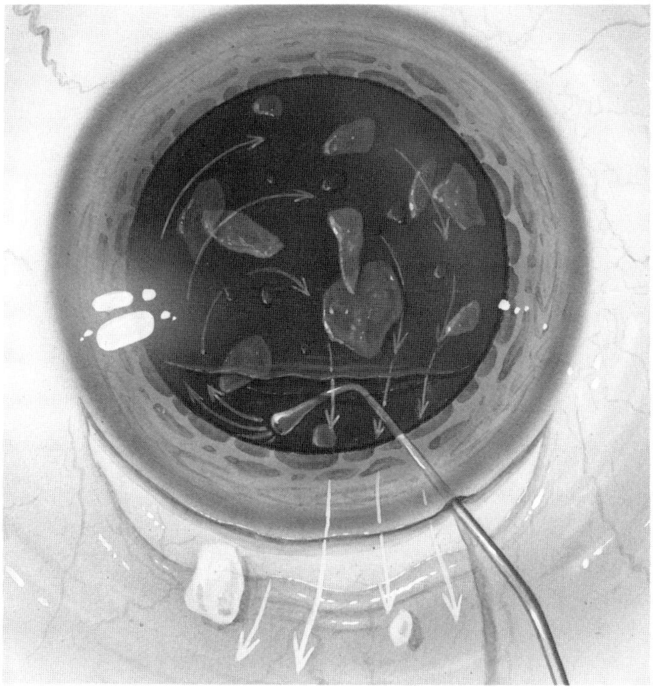

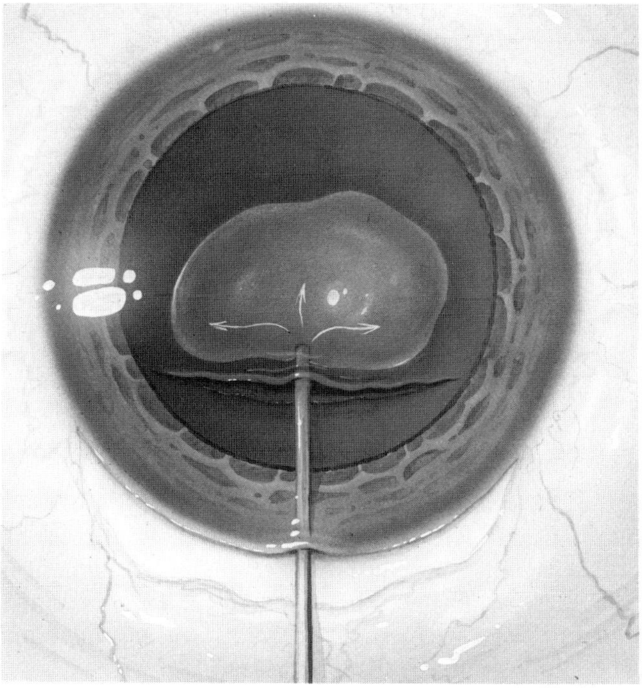

4.**133** In order to implant the intraocular lens in the capsule, the space between the anterior and posterior membranes of the capsule is enlarged by instilling 0.1–0.2 ml of highly viscous hyaluronic acid. With coaxial illumination of the microscope, good visual control of the membranes is possible.

134

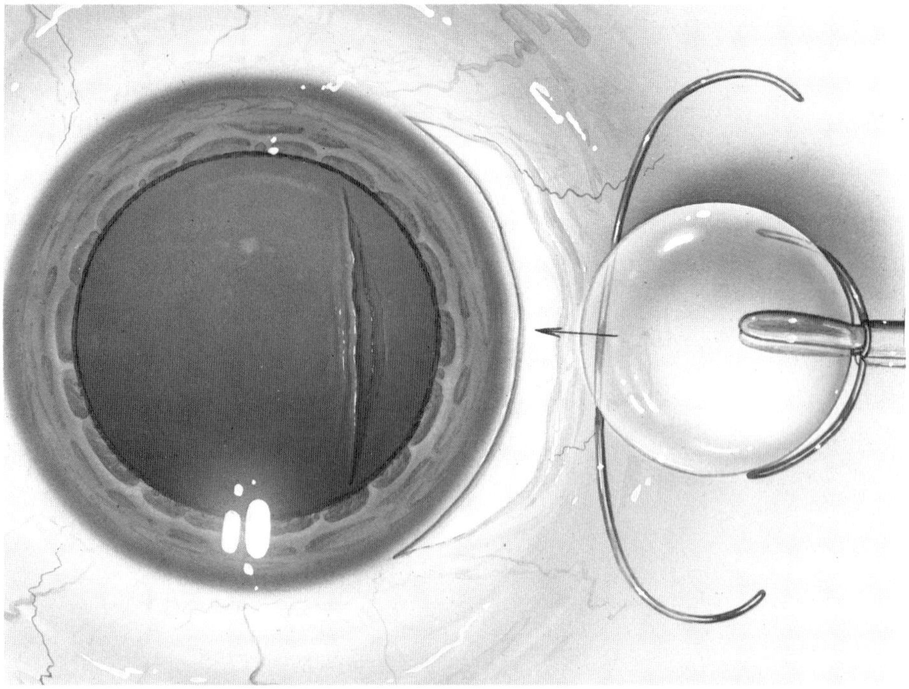

135 a

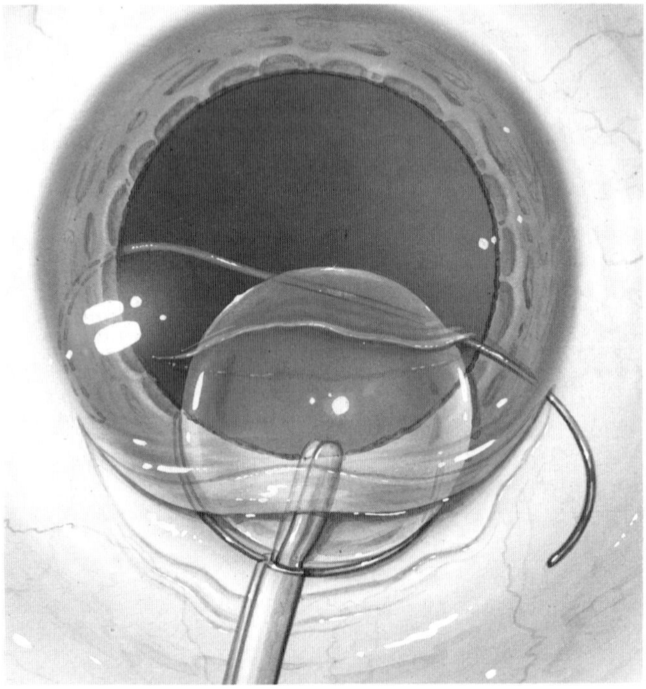

135 b

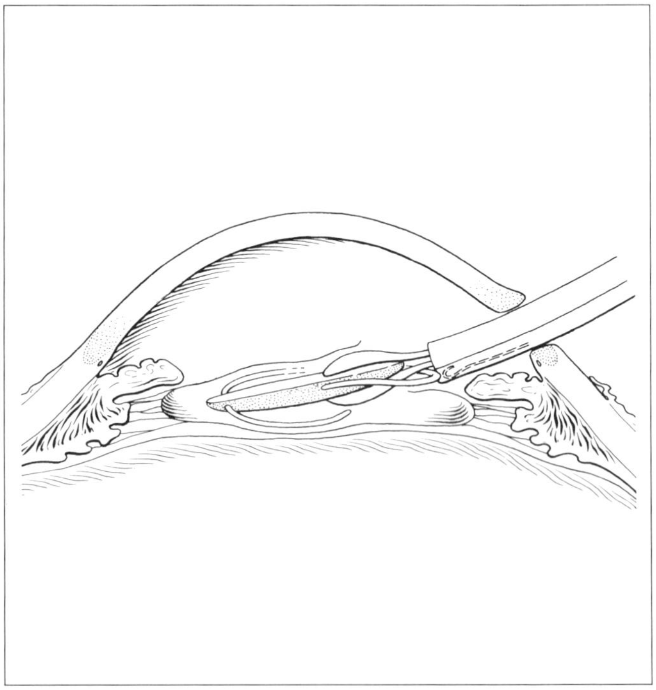

4.**134, 135 a** and **b** For implantation of the three-loop intracapsular lens, the haptic fixed at 12 o'clock is pressed against the lens itself with the special implantation forceps; the lens haptics, which are positioned uniformly upward, permit implantation in a straight line – rotation is completely unnecessary.

136 a

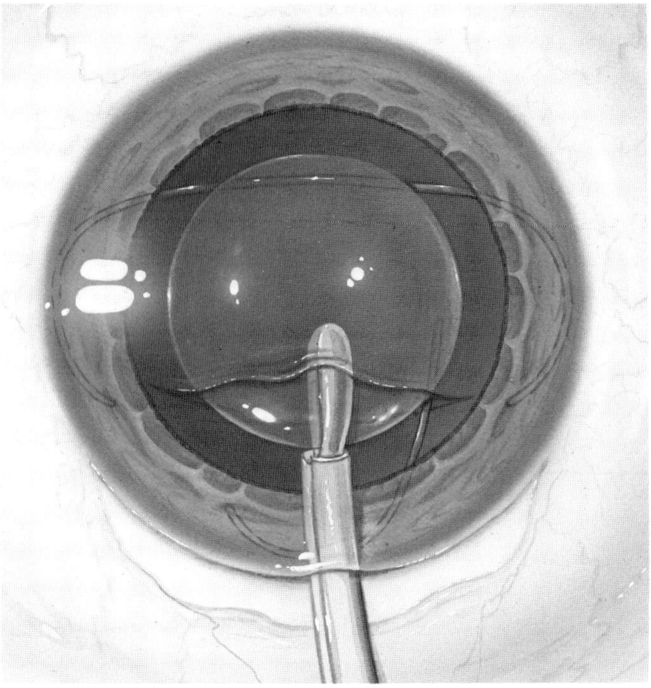

136 b

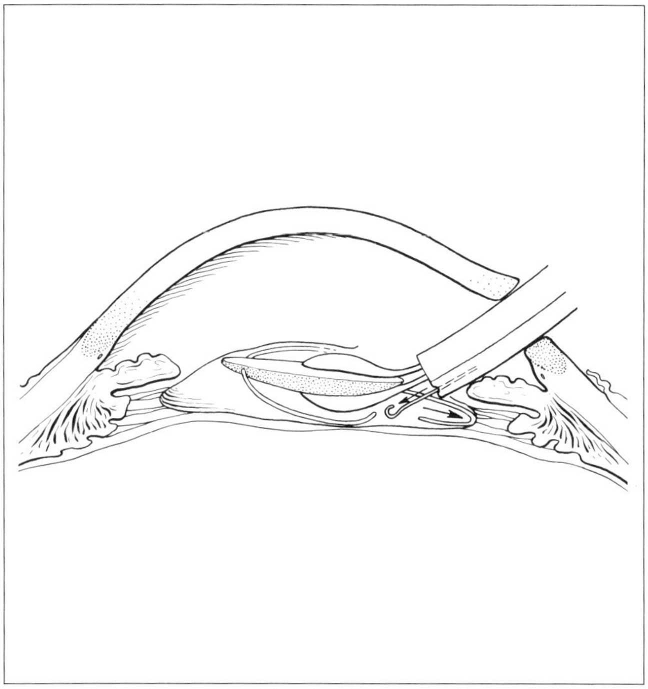

137

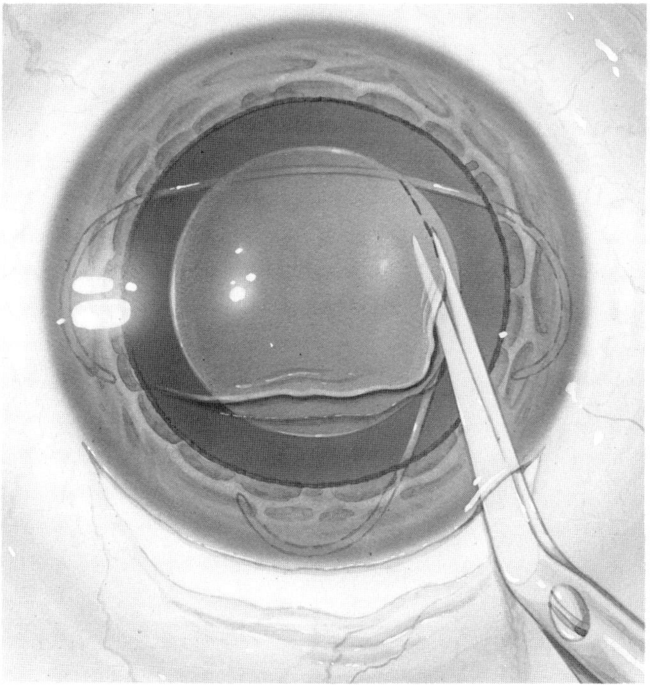

138

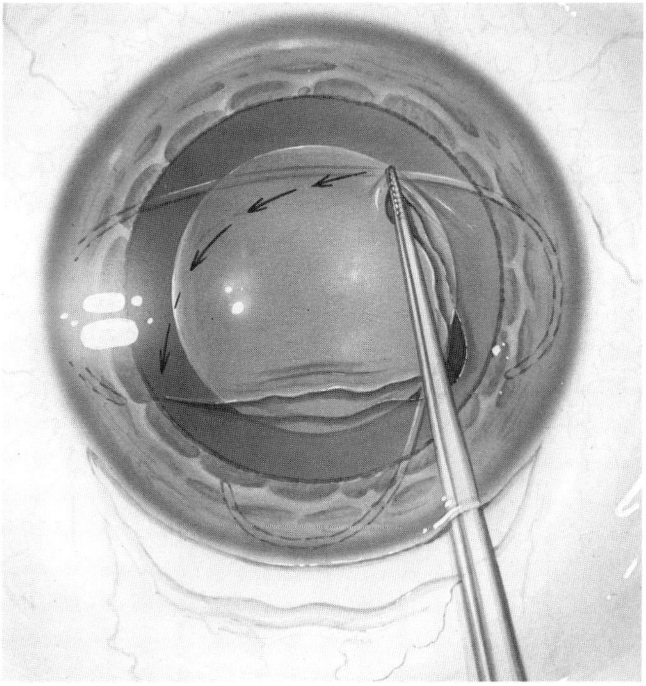

4.**136 a** and **b** As soon as the body of the lens and its upper equator have passed the "mailing slot," the upper loop release is activated so that the top haptic slides into the equator of the capsule at 12 o'clock by virtue of its spring force. The lens is then released and the forceps are withdrawn from the eye.

4.**137** Any manipulation of the uvea by retracting the iris with an iris hook is deliberately avoided throughout the procedure. Not until the implantation has been completed – the capsule and the anterior membrane of the capsule represent a physiological slipway – is the anterior capsule excised, by means of a slanting incision with scissors.

4.**138** and **139 a–d** The anterior capsule membrane is then grasped with fine-toothed forceps at the end of the scissors incision, and removed with an arcing movement in such a way that an opening of the desired size results in the anterior membrane of the capsule.

139 a **b** **c** **d**

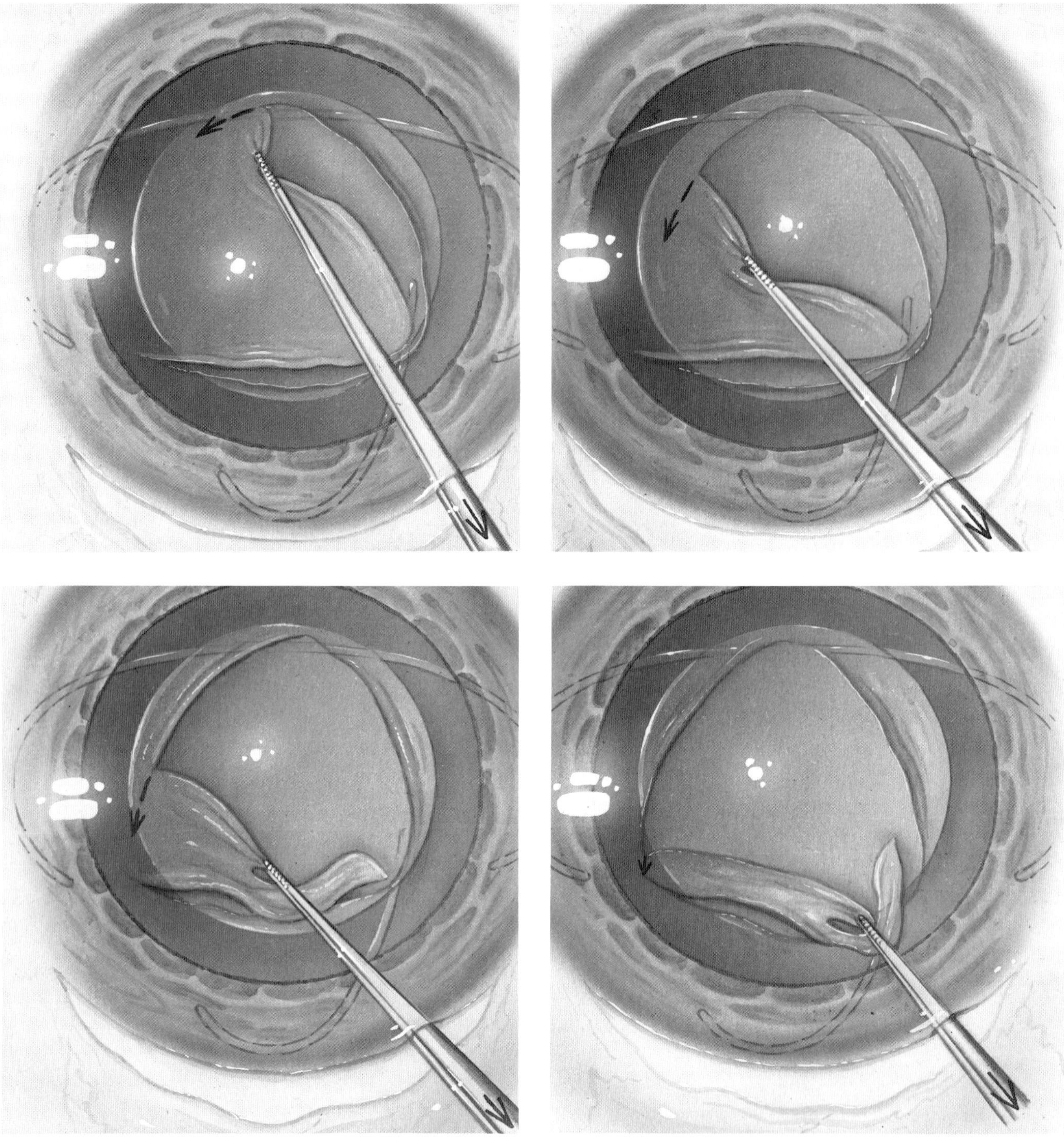

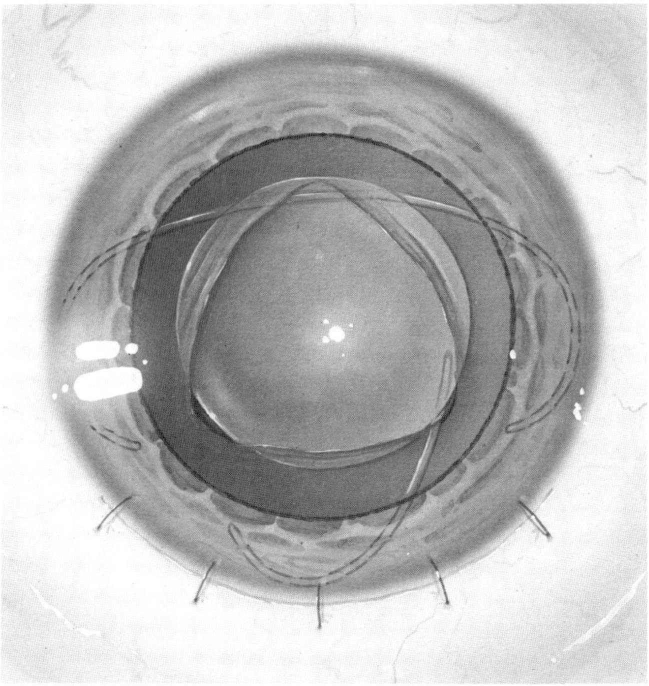

4.**140** Postoperative wound closure is effected with interrupted sutures of 10-0 nylon. If a limbus-based conjunctival flap was previously prepared, the conjunctiva is additionally closed with a continuous Dexon suture.

Modifications and Surgical Alternatives

As a primary incision a purely corneal incision is of course a perfectly acceptable alternative, as is a corneoscleral incision with a fornix-based conjunctival flap. Excision of the anterior membrane of the capsule can be effected by two scissors incisions instead of the arcuate movement with the toothed forceps; perforation of the anterior membrane from the interior of the capsule, followed by excision of the membrane with forceps, is also practicable.

Complications

Horizontal capsulotomy may be complicated by lateral tearing, especially if the instruments used are not sharp enough. These tears may become enlarged during extrusion of the nucleus, leading to a slanting anterior capsulotomy. However, even if this happens implantation between the anterior and posterior capsular membranes generally is possible; special consideration must then be given to the changed conditions when performing the capsule excision at the end of the procedure.

The same problems arise if the anterior capsulotomy is too short: when extruding the lens nucleus the side of the slit in the capsule may tear at the equator. In this eventuality the possibility of damage to the zonula must be considered: intracapsular lens implantation would then be out of the question.

No complications are experienced with extrusion and harpooning of the nucleus. Posterior capsular lesions usually are the result of unintentionally powerful aspiration. In such cases an initial attempt should be made to remove the cortex remnants by pressure flushing alone. If a central defect in the posterior membrane of the capsule occurs nevertheless, the decision whether or not to implant an intracapsular lens will depend on the size of the lesion. It is important to avoid instilling hyaluronic acid in front of the capsular membranes, to prevent the implant finding its way in front of the anterior membrane. One must, therefore, ensure that the anterior membrane moves forward during instillation of hyaluronic acid under regredient light.

After introducing the intraocular lens into the capsule, the lens itself must only be released when the upper haptic is safely in position. To accomplish this the lens is deliberately pressed down a little (at 12 o'clock). Otherwise sulcus fixation of the upper haptic would result. If, after excision of the anterior capsule, the desired arcuate configuration cannot be achieved with the toothed forceps after the first division with the scissors, and the line of the cut extends toward the equator, a second division with scissors from the opposite side is necessary.

Postoperative Management

The pupil is contracted intraoperatively, immediately after implantation of the lens, with acetylcholine; as a rule, no further pupillary medication is required. Gentamicin eye ointment and prednisolone 2.5 % eye ointment are applied to the conjunctival sac; after closing the lids with forceps, a gauze dressing is placed over the lids and a pad with capsule fixed with strips of plaster.

At the daily postoperative slit-lamp examination one should check for pupillary "play." If, as occasionally occurs, there is postoperative irritation, this author prescribes prednisolone 2.5 % eye drops, administered up to five times a day in the immediate postoperative period; generally, however, a single application of prednisolone 2.5 % and gentamicin eye drops is sufficient. Pupillary medication is only administered if there is a risk of development of synechiae.

Bibliography

[1] Baikoff, G.: Insertion of the Simcoe posterior chamber lens into the capsular bag. *AIOIS Journal* 7: 267–269, 1981.

[2] Binkhorst, C. D.: *Intracapsular Surgery and an Adapted new Lens Design*. Lecture read at the Second European Intraocular Implant Council Meeting, Giessen, 1983.

[3] Draeger, J.: Instrumentelle Erfordernisse für die Linsenimplantation in den Kapselsack. *Klin. Mbl. Augenheilk.* 1986 (in press).

[4] Draeger, J., Burk, R.: Überlegungen zum physiologischen Implantationsort von Kunstlinsen. *Klin. Mbl. Augenheilk.* 185: 200–203, 1984.

[5] Galand, A.: A simple method of implantation within the capsular bag. *AIOIS Journal* 9: 330–332, 1983.

Subluxated Lens: Intracapsular Aspiration

Douglas D. Koch and Jared M. Emery

Surgical Principles

Selection of the appropriate surgical technique for removal of a subluxated cataract depends upon several factors, including the age of the patient, the status of the vitreous, the degree of subluxation, and the extent of existing zonular support. The surgical technique for any particular case must be chosen on an individual basis. Listed below are our general guidelines for determining the surgical approach to a patient with a subluxated lens.

Vitreous in anterior chamber – over age 40. Vitreous loss usually occurs in these cases. If the lens is within reach and has adequate zonular support, the surgeon can first perform a vitrectomy with an automated vitrector or microsurgical sponges. Intracapsular extraction can then be completed. If the lens is excessively mobile or unstable, pars plana lentectomy and vitrectomy are preferred. This facilitates lens removal should posterior dislocation occur and also minimizes operative vitreous traction.

No vitreous in anterior chamber – over age 40. If zonular loss exceeds 90° or greater than one-third subluxation is present, intracapsular cataract extraction is preferred. If zonular loss or the degree of subluxation is minimal and the vitreous face is intact, an extracapsular extraction is attempted.

Vitreous in anterior chamber – under age 40. In most of these cases, pars plana lentectomy and vitrectomy are selected. Intracapsular extraction is not recommended because of vitreolenticular adhesions that predispose to excessive vitreous traction and vitreous loss.

No vitreous in anterior chamber – under age 40. If zonular loss exceeds 90° or greater than one-half subluxation is present, pars plana lentectomy and vitrectomy are selected.

In patients with lesser amounts of zonular loss and subluxation, we perform an intracapsular aspiration using an irrigation/aspiration instrument.[1, 2, 3] The surgical objective is to remove the cataract while preventing vitreous loss and minimizing anterior vitreous movement. The advantage of the technique is that irrigation and aspiration occur within the lens capsule; this minimizes fluid turbulence in the anterior chamber and thereby reduces potential zonular trauma. This technique is described below.

Preparation for Surgery

The preoperative routine is as for extracapsular cataract extraction.

Preoperative Medication and Anesthesia

Here again, the same procedure is followed as for extracapsular cataract extraction. It is essential to have a very soft eye to minimize vitreous pressure.

Instruments

Routine cataract instruments are required, together with an automated or manual irrigation aspiration system. Optional extras include: phacoemulsification instrument for soft but non-aspiratable nucleus; keratome; sodium hyaluronate (strongly preferred).

Surgical Technique

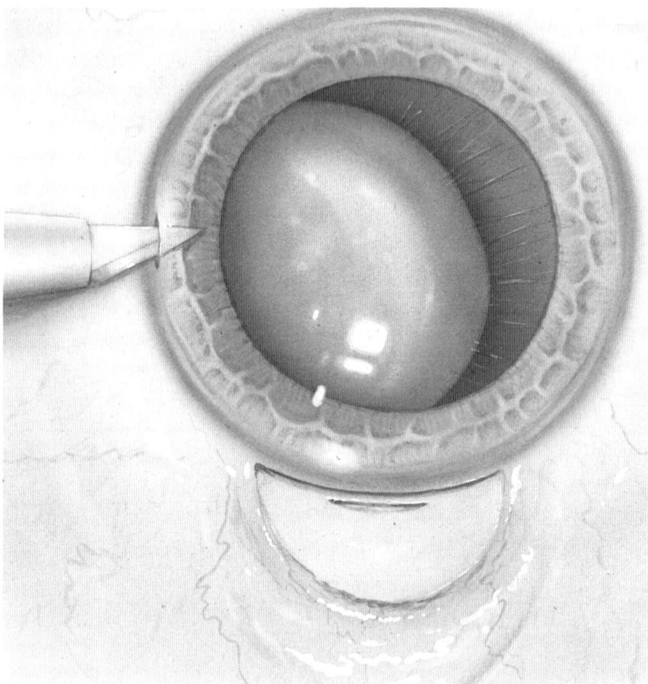

4.141 A small fornix-based conjunctival flap is prepared superiorly. The incision length should be determined by the size of the irrigation aspiration instrument to be utilized. A groove of appropriate length is made with a microsurgical steel knife, held vertically. This knife is used to make a 1 mm stab incision into the anterior chamber at the 3 o'clock position.

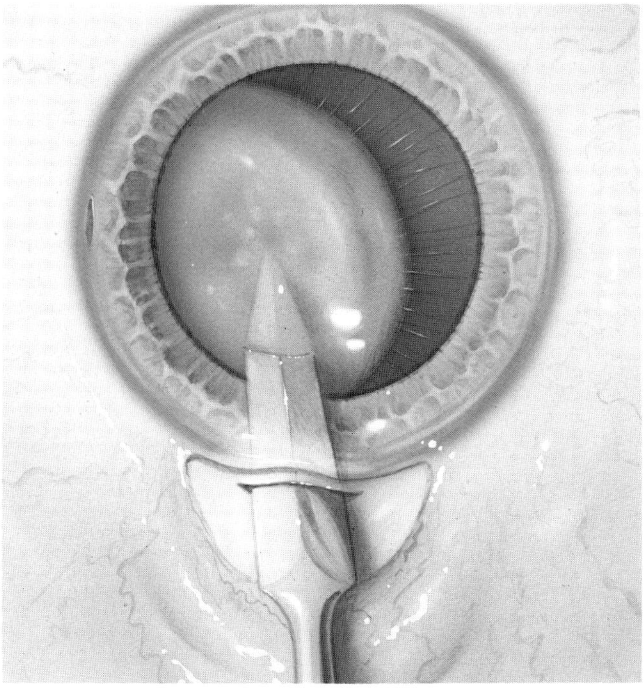

4.**142** The anterior chamber is filled with sodium hyaluronate (if available). It is especially important to cover the area that has stretched or missing zonules with the sodium hyaluronate. A sharp keratome is used to enter the anterior chamber and to incise the superior portion of the anterior lens capsule.

143

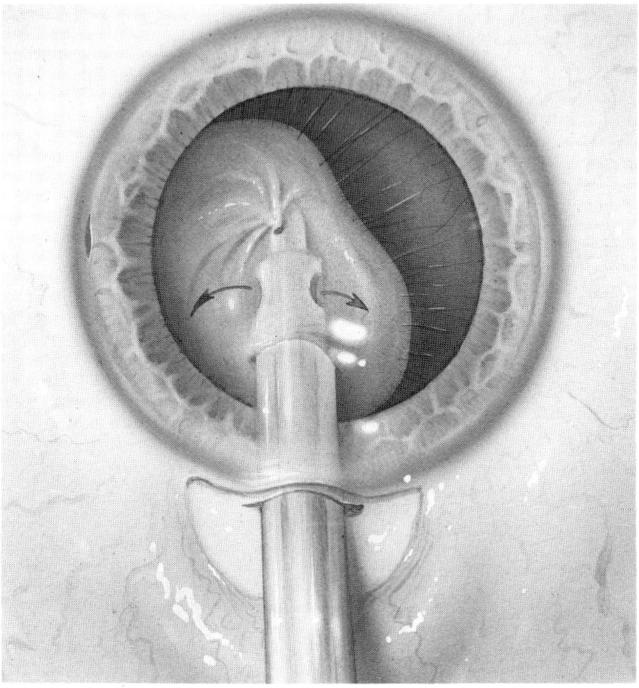

144

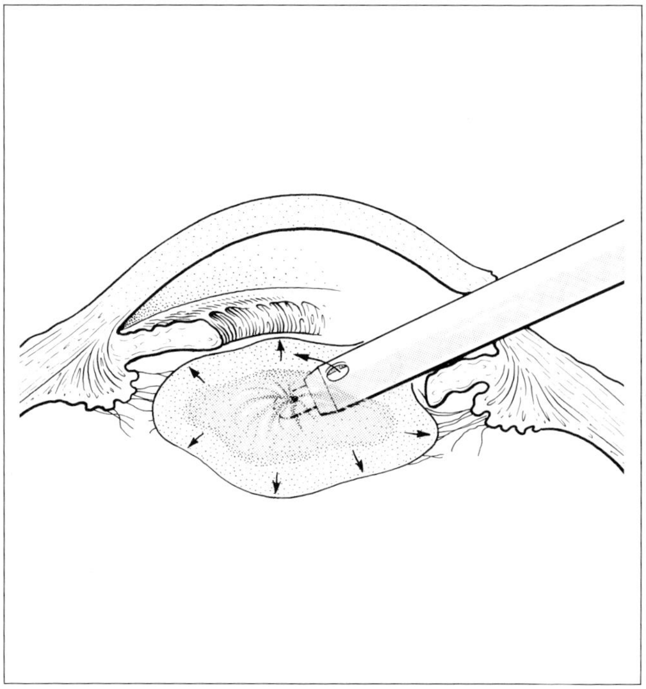

4.**143** and **144** The irrigation / aspiration instrument is inserted through the opening in the lens capsule. Using low-flow irrigation, the cortical material is aspirated.

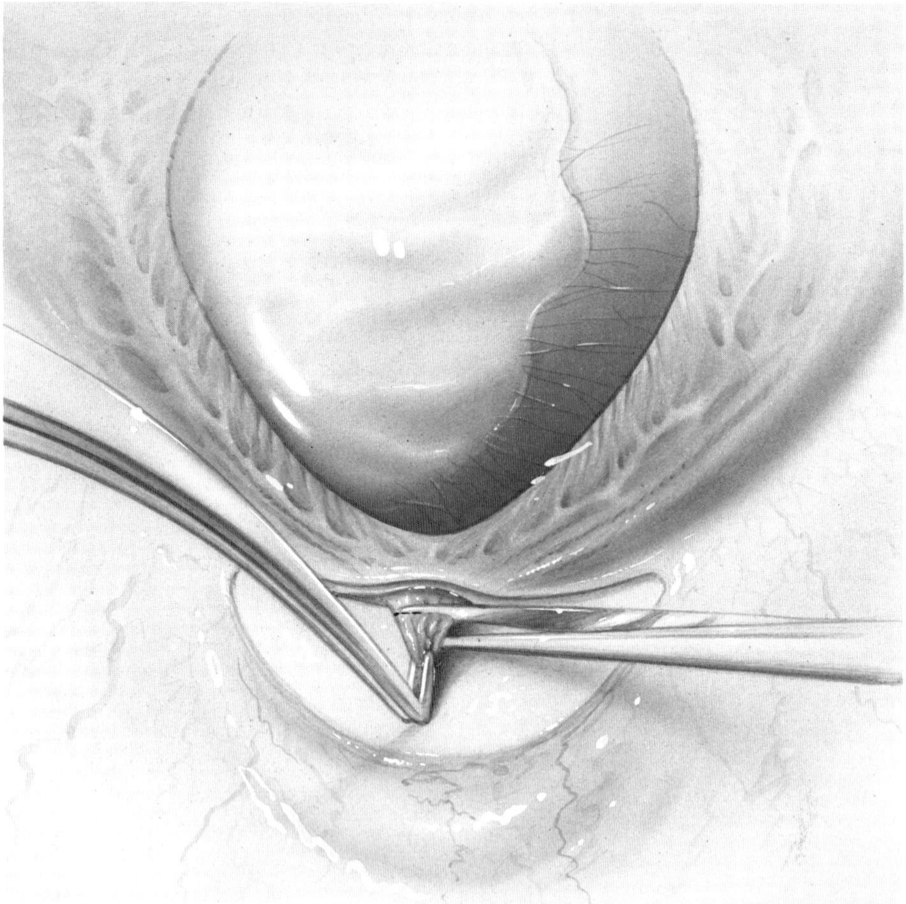

4.**145** A peripheral iridectomy is made superiorly.

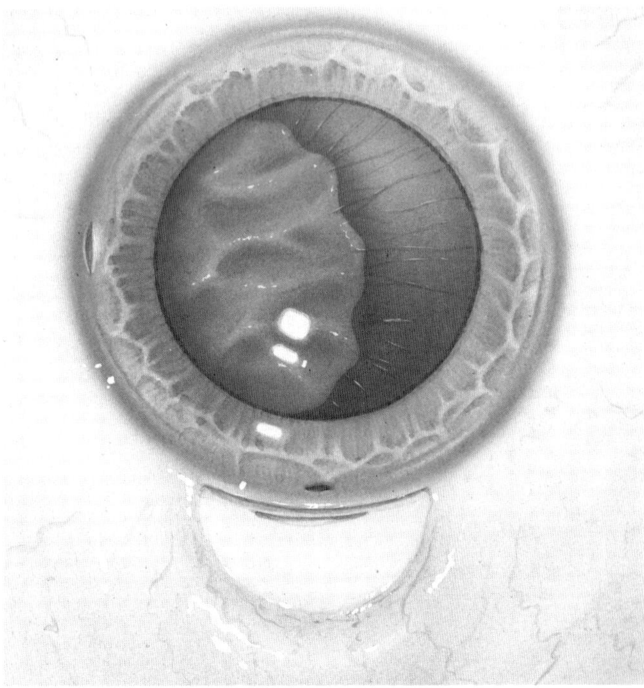

4.**146** The collapsed, wrinkled capsular bag still covers the visual axis. The sodium hyaluronate should be aspirated very gently using a 27-gauge cannula filled with balanced salt solution. It is not necessary to remove all of the sodium hyaluronate; overly aggressive hyaluronate aspiration can cause vitreous loss.

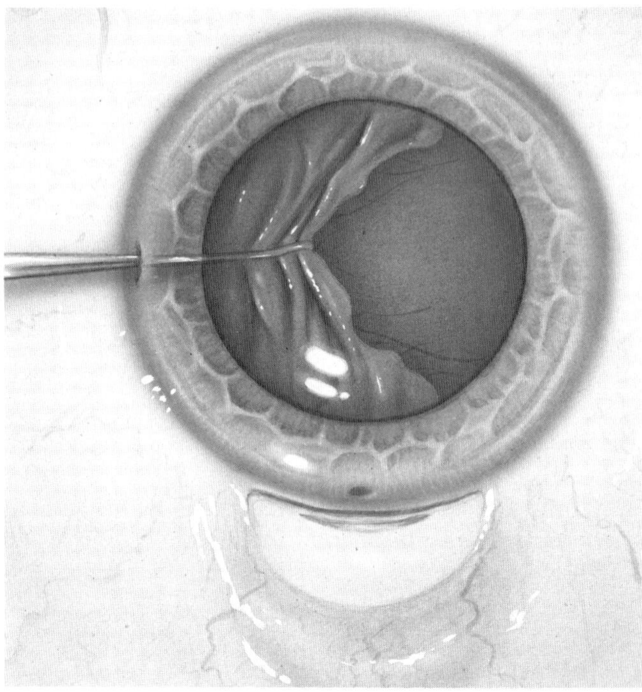

4.**147** A microsurgical iris hook is inserted through the 3 o'clock incision. The distal border of the capsular bag is grasped and retracted out of the visual axis.

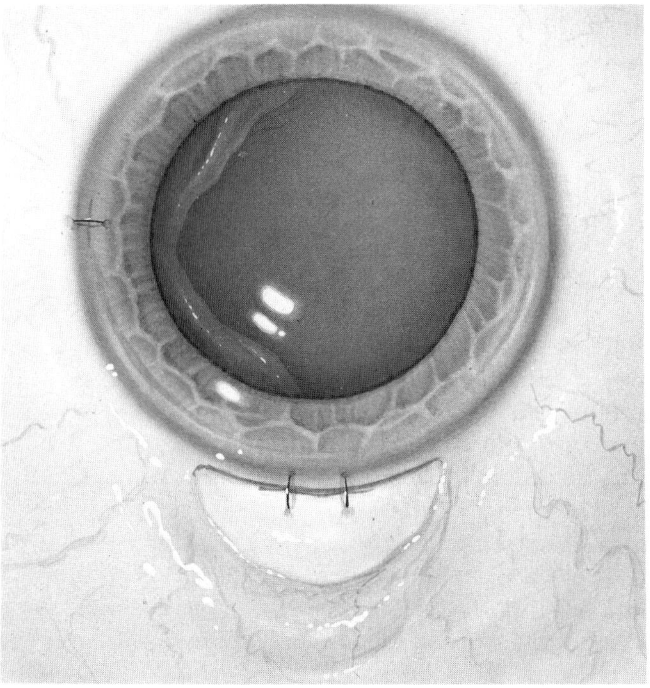

4.**148** The capsule has been retracted. Acetylcholine is injected to constrict the pupil. Vitreous adherence to either wound site will result in peaking of the pupil as miosis occurs. Before and after suturing both incisions, the surgeon should check each wound site to be certain that there is no vitreous to the wound. If a small amount of vitreous presents to the wound, this can be swept away using an iris sweep. If a greater amount of vitreous loss occurs, anterior vitrectomy should be performed with an automated vitrector or microsurgical sponges.

Modifications and Surgical Alternatives

The incision into the anterior capsule can also be made using a bent 25-gauge needle or a microsurgical steel knife, rather than a keratome. The critical factor is that the instrument should be extremely sharp in order to minimize traction on the zonules as the capsule is penetrated.

In rare instances, the nucleus cannot be aspirated with an automated or manual cortical aspiration instrument. If a phacoemulsification instrument is available, the phacoemulsification tip can be introduced through the opening in the anterior capsule, and the nucleus can be gently aspirated and emulsified. An alternative though less preferred option would be to enlarge the incision to 10 mm. The capsulectomy is then enlarged with a bent 25-gauge needle or Vannas scissors so that a routine capsulectomy is performed. An irrigating lens loop is gently inserted beneath the nucleus to extract it from the eye. There is a high risk of vitreous loss with this maneuver if the lens is not well fixated and if zonular disinsertion exceeds 60°. The surgeon must be alert to any suggestion of posterior lens movement so as to prevent loss of the nucleus into the vitreous.

If the extent of the zonular disinsertion is less than 60°, the vitreous face is solid, and there is little or no lens subluxation, a more typical anterior capsulectomy and extracapsular extraction can be attempted. A bent 25-gauge needle can be used to create a circular capsulectomy; the Nd: YAG laser may be preferred to minimize further zonular disruption while performing an anterior capsulectomy. The cortical material can be aspirated as in routine extracapsular extraction. If the patient is over age 30 or has a nucleus that is not aspiratable, then the nucleus can be expressed prior to cortical aspiration. The advantage of this approach is that a clear, intact posterior capsule can be preserved, thereby preventing anterior vitreous movement.

Complications

Possible complications include vitreous loss and dislocation of the lens into the vitreous, as well as other complications encountered during routine extracapsular extraction.

Vitreous loss can occur at any phase of the operation. If only a vitreous strand presents to the wound, this can be swept away as described. More extensive vitreous loss must be managed by anterior vitrectomy, preferably with an automated instrument. If vitreous loss occurs before the lens material has been aspirated; it is usually preferable to complete cortical aspiration following vitrectomy, to avoid mixing vitreous and cortical material in the aspiration tip.

If the lens begins to fall back into the vitreous cavity, the surgeon should immediately convert to a large-incision extraction. Sodium hyaluronate is injected underneath the lens to provide an additional cushion against its posterior movement. The wound is then enlarged to at least 10 mm. A lens loop is inserted into the eye underneath the lens, and the entire lens is extracted. A partial anterior vitrectomy is performed to remove the greater part of the vitreous from the wound. The wound is then partially sutured, and the vitrectomy is completed using a closed chamber technique. Because of the vitreous traction these maneuvers generate, these patients must be closely followed postoperatively for the development of any retinal breaks.

If the lens falls into the vitreous cavity, it is usually advisable to terminate the operation and suture the wound. If the lens capsule is still intact, the dislocated lens might be well tolerated and not require removal. The patient is at risk for developing pupillary block, however, should the lens prolapse anteriorly and occlude the pupil. If the lens capsule has been opened prior to lens dislocation into the vitreous cavity, then the lens material will often cause chronic inflammation and glaucoma. Pars plana lentectomy is advisable in these instances, either at the time of the initial surgery or as a secondary operation.

Postoperative Management

Routines after extracapsular cataract extraction also apply here. The intraocular pressure should be measured on the morning following surgery. Marked elevation in intraocular pressure can be induced by residual sodium hyaluronate in the anterior chamber, and this elevation can persist for several days. It should be controlled with topical timolol, oral acetazolamide and, if necessary, oral osmotic agents.

If indicated, contact lens fitting can be initiated three weeks postoperatively. Astigmatism induced by tight sutures can be modified by selective suture removal beginning as early as three weeks following surgery.

Results

The visual prognosis in general is similar to that for eyes that have undergone intracapsular cataract extraction. However, these patients often have other factors that can complicate visual recovery. Patients with Marfan's syndrome and homocystinuria are at risk for developing retinal detachment and must be followed closely for the development of postoperative retinal breaks. Traumatized eyes are also at risk for retinal problems and can have pre-existing ocular pathology that will limit postoperative acuity.

References

[1] Maumenee, A. E., Ryan, S. J.: Aspiration technique in the management of the dislocated lens. *Am. J. Ophth.* 68: 808–811, 1969.

[2] Boniuk, M.: A new technique for removal of subluxated lenses. *Tr. Am. Acad. Ophth. & Otol.* 78: 60–64, 1974.

[3] Emery, J. M., Little, J. H.: Operative technique for subluxated lenses. In: *Phacoemulsification and aspiration of cataracts.* Mosby, St. Louis 22: 214–215, 1979.

Posterior Capsulotomy

Stephen H. Johnson and Douglas D. Koch

Surgical Principles

Postoperative opacification of the posterior capsule is one of the most common complications of extracapsular surgery, and it is certainly the most frequent indication for surgical reintervention. Its incidence has been reported to be as high as 50 % by five years following cataract surgery. There are two mechanisms of capsular opacification: Elschnig pearl formation, and capsular fibrosis or wrinkling. Elschnig pearls can be managed by aspiration or by posterior capsulotomy; a fibrotic capsule can be treated only by the latter approach.

The standard discission technique has been to use a needle-knife or hollow-bore needle to make the capsular opening. More recently, the neodymium: YAG laser has supplanted knife discission as the preferred approach for many surgeons for us, too. The main advantages of laser capsulotomy are the elimination of the risk of endophthalmitis, the greater precision with which the capsular opening can be made, the lack of patient discomfort, and the rapidity of visual rehabilitation. Disadvantages of laser capsulotomy include higher incidences of acute intraocular pressure rise and marking of intraocular lenses.

Knife Discission

Preparation for Surgery

The patient is examined with the slit lamp biomicroscope prior to dilatation in order to determine the position of the pupil and intraocular lens (if present), the location and extent of posterior capsule opacification, and the center of the visual axis. These may not be readily identifiable following pupillary dilatation, especially if iris trauma and synechia formation have caused pupillary distortion. A drawing or photograph can be taken to the operating room if necessary to assist the surgeon in localizing the region to be incised.

Preoperative Medication and Anesthesia

The surgery is performed under topical or retrobulbar anesthesia. The latter is often preferable because it eliminates unexpected eye movements. Tropicamide drops (1 %) are instilled to dilate the pupil.

Instruments

Discission knife, such as Haab needle-knife (Storz E 0182) or Girard-Swan needle-knife (Storz E 0162); 0.12 mm forceps; 30- or 27-gauge cannula for intraocular injection.

Surgical Technique

The technique is illustrated for a patient with a posterior chamber intraocular lens. Technically, this is the most difficult situation the surgeon encounters, because of the proximity of the lens and posterior capsule. The same technique is used for aphakic patients and patients with more anteriorly positioned intraocular lenses.

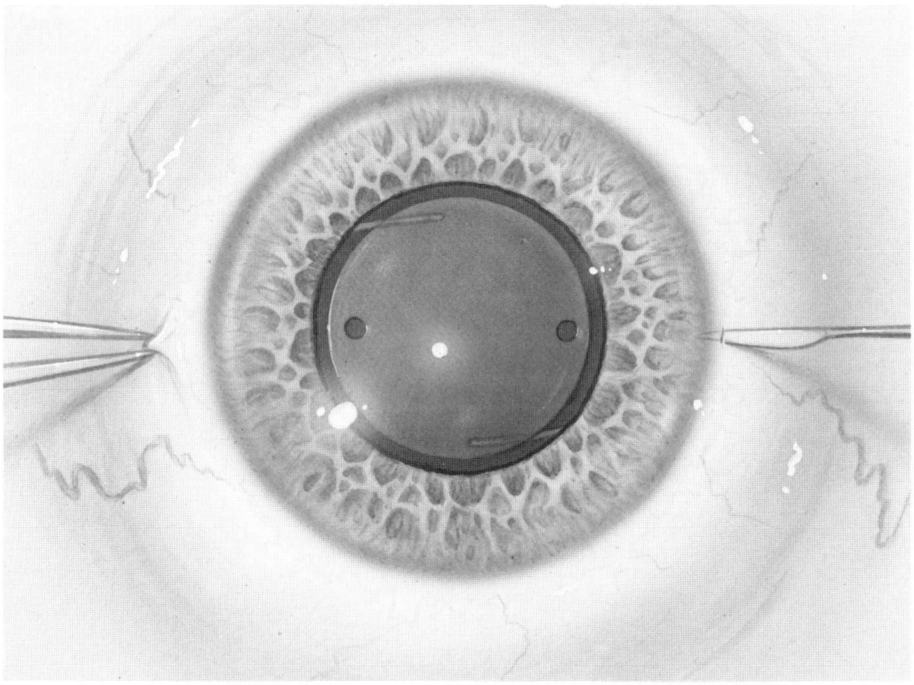

4.**149** The limbus is grasped with a 0.12 mm forceps directly opposite the planned anterior chamber entry site. The needle-knife is held with the blade directed inferiorly, and a stab incision is made at the limbus or just into the clear cornea. The blade is directed slightly posteriorly during this procedure to facilitate penetration of Descemet's membrane.

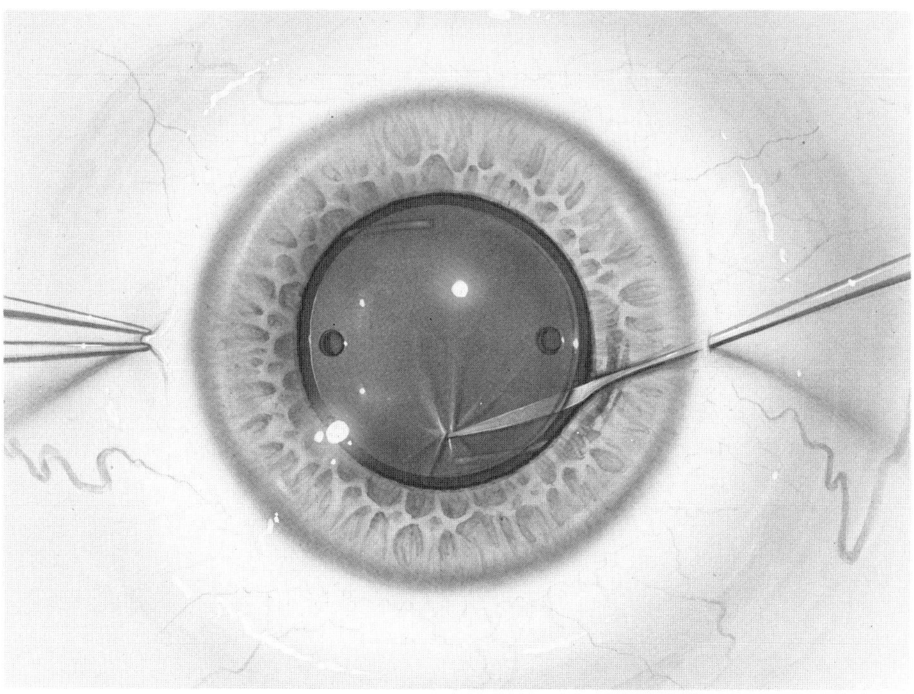

4.**150** The tip of the knife is eased under the edge of the implant at the 9 or 10 o'clock position. The knife is then rotated superiorly, using the limbus as the center of rotation. The blunt face of the knife remains directed superiorly and forms the leading edge as the knife is rotated upwards.

The knife is positioned with its tip 1–1.5 mm below the upper edge of the implant. The tip of the knife is vertically aligned superior to the center of the visual axis.

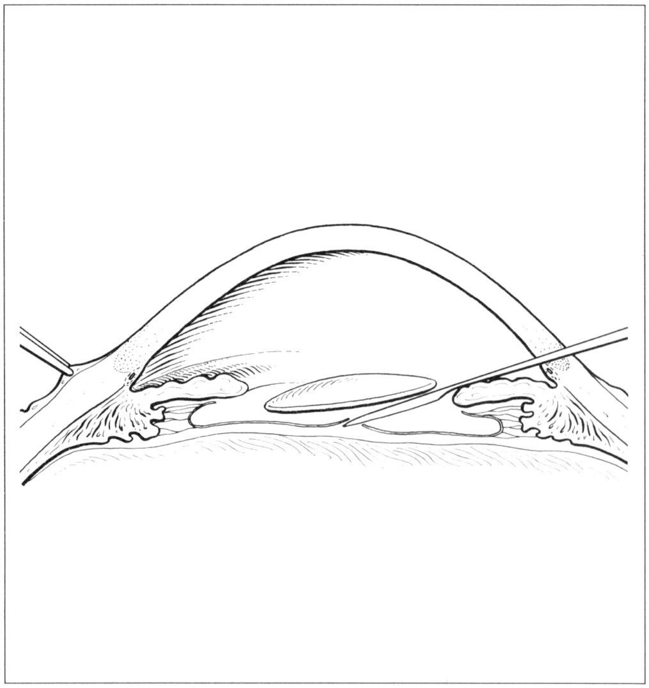

4.**151** A stab incision is made through the posterior capsule. After the tip of the knife has penetrated the capsule, the knife is elevated slightly, thereby lifting the posterior capsule away from the vitreous face. This minimizes the chances of rupturing the vitreous face.

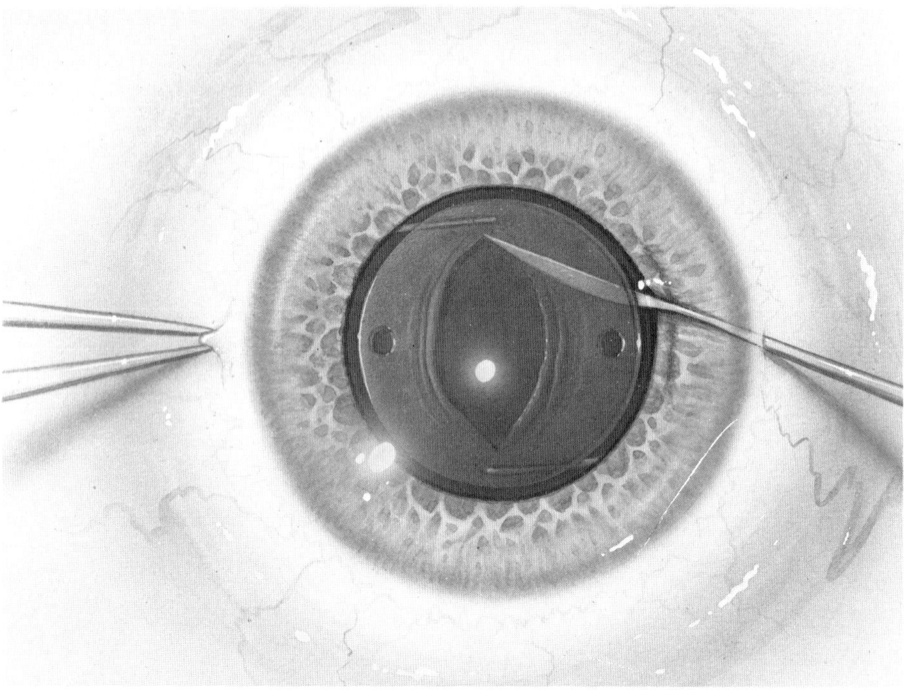

4.**152** The knife is passed inferiorly while maintaining the slight elevation of the capsule. The capsulotomy is terminated 1–1.5 mm above the inferior edge of the intraocular lens. The knife is then brought out from beneath the implant without passing over the area of open capsule. If a vitreous strand is engaged on the knife tip, it can be released by moving the knife tip centrally or superiorly. The knife is then quickly removed from the eye.

Balanced salt solution may be injected to deepen the chamber or to dislodge a vitreous strand that has followed the knife tip to the incision site. Acetylcholine may be injected to constrict the pupil; this can also pull a vitreous strand away from the wound. The wound is checked to determine if it is sufficiently watertight. Suturing of the incision is rarely required.

Complications

In rare instances, the anterior chamber shallows during the discission. If excessive chamber collapse occurs, the knife must be withdrawn immediately. The chamber should then be reformed with balanced salt solution. It may be necessary to maintain the anterior chamber depth with intermittent injection or gravity infusion of balanced salt solution through a separate stab incision site. Alternatively, sodium hyaluronate can be injected, although this is less desirable because removal of the hyaluronate following the discission can predispose to anterior vitreous movement and migration of vitreous strands to the wound.

A certain amount of elevation or rocking of the posterior chamber intraocular lens commonly occurs when the knife is behind it, but it is rare for significant displacement of the implant to occur. The stab incision site should be planned carefully so that the knife movement is not restricted by an intraocular lens loop.

The major vision-threatening complications are persistent cystoid macular edema (incidence 1.9 %)[1] and retinal detachment (incidence 0–3.6 %).[1,2]

Admonitions and Suggestions

It is important to use a knife that has a sharp tip and blade. A blunt knife will not penetrate Descemet's membrane and can cause its detachment. Also, a blunt knife will not penetrate the posterior capsule without excessive force. If a sharp needle-knife is not available, a 25- or 27-gauge needle can be used. The needle tip should be bent to a 45° or 90° angle. On advantage of a needle is that balanced salt solution can be infused through it if necessary.

It is sometimes difficult to determine when the posterior capsule has been penetrated, particularly in patients with heavy Elschnig pearl formation. In these instances, it may appear that the capsule has been penetrated when in fact the knife tip is positioned between the Elschnig pearls and posterior capsule. Inferior rotation of the knife in this instance will remove the Elschnig pearls from the central capsule, reinforcing the impression that a capsulotomy has been achieved. Examination under high magnification, however, should reveal that there are no distinct edges to this central area, confirming that the capsule is still intact.

A single, accurately positioned 3–4 mm slit in the capsule usually provides an adequate capsulotomy, since the edges of the slit will retract to widen the opening over the next few days. However, if the opening is not in the visual axis or is eccentric to the pupil, postoperatively the patient may have suboptimal visual acuity or problems with glare. Unfortunately, additional incisions in the capsule are more likely to result in a broken vitreous face and anterior vitreous movement; hence they should be attempted only when necessary.

The capsulotomy can be enlarged in two ways. If the discission is too short, the knife can be inserted at either end of the capsulotomy and the incision extended. Alternatively, small oblique or horizontal cuts may be made in the capsule, creating small flaps of capsule that will retract in the first few days postoperatively. To perform this, the knife is reintroduced beneath the implant, and a gentle stab incision is made in the capsule 1–2 mm away from the capsulotomy; this should be done ipsilateral to the limbal entry site to avoid passing the knife tip over the exposed vitreous face. The knife is then swept toward the capsulotomy, thereby creating a horizontal or oblique tear.

Postoperative Management

Topical corticosteroids are administered for one to four weeks postoperatively; the latter period of administration may provide greater prophylaxis against development of cystoid macular edema.

Laser Capsulotomy

S. H. Johnson and Douglas D. Koch

Preparation for Surgery

The patient is examined under the slit lamp with the pupil in an undilated state. The presence of factors that would alter the size, shape or method of the intended capsulotomy, and their relationship to the visual axis, are noted. These factors may include abnormalities of pupil shape or size, intraocular lens type and position, retained corticonuclear material, and ocular movements. Not all patients are good candidates for neodymium: YAG laser capsulotomy. A patient who is unable to control his eye movements satisfactorily, or who has a lens implant of glass or other vulnerable material, may do better with the needle-knife approach.

Preoperative Medication and Anesthesia

Pupillary dilatation is unnecessary and may make it more difficult for the surgeon to accurately determine the location and appropriate size of the capsulotomy. A contact lens and anesthetic drops may be used at the discretion of the surgeron, but neither are routinely necessary. The contact lens is useful in cases where further concentration of the energy of the laser beam or tamponading of ocular movements are needed.

Instruments

Q-switched (our preference) or mode-locked neodymium:YAG ophthalmic laser; contact lens (optional).

Surgical Technique

The technique is illustrated with a pseudophakic patient whose posterior capsule has been clouded by pearls. A slight alteration in technique is necessary in patients with capsular fibrosis. Pupillary dilation is not desirable and is only shown for clarity of illustration.

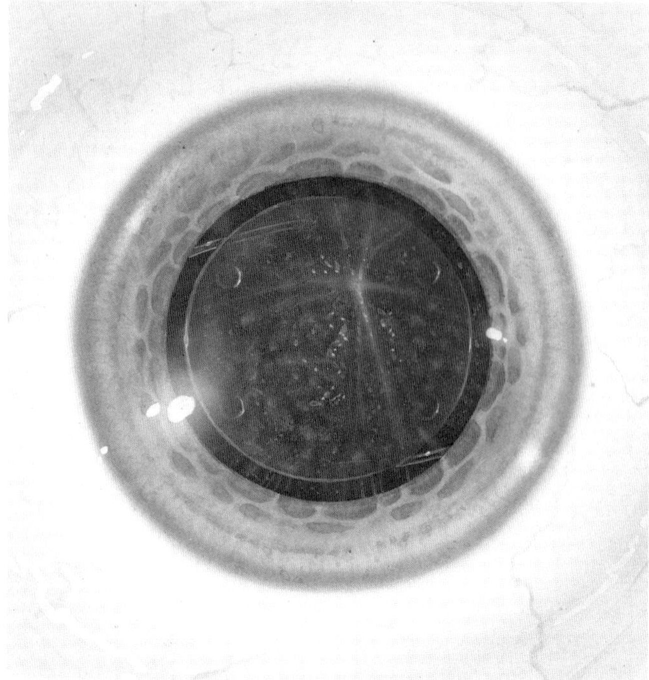

153

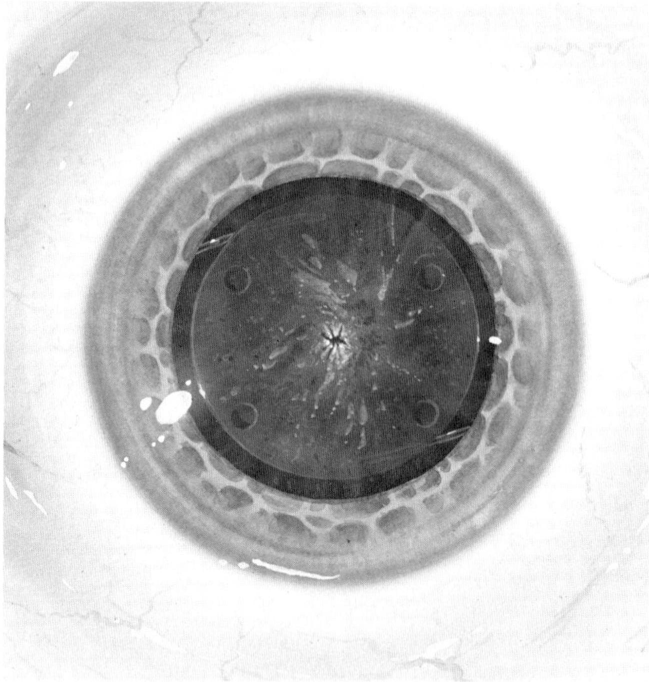

154

4.**153** The posterior capsule is examined for stress lines which may cross the visual axis and for topographic features marking the center of the visual axis.

4.**154** The patient is asked to direct gaze slightly to one side of the laser beam axis, and a single laser burst is used to open the posterior capsule at the center of the visual axis. The non-alignment of visual axis and laser beam axis may also be accomplished by altering the angle of the laser beam delivery system while the patient looks straight ahead.

The initial opening created in the posterior capsule is a small hole surrounded by a series of short tears produced by tissue tension; it is similar to the hole created in a piece of paper under stretch when it is stabbed with a sharp pencil.

The energy level of the bursts applied should be adjusted to create the desired intraocular effect. There are no statistically significant differences in visual outcome or complications whether a smaller number of larger energy bursts are used. e.g., 12 spots at 3 mJ, or a large number of shots are given at a lower energy level, e.g., 36 spots at 1 mJ.

However, to minimize vitreous face disruption and intraocular lens damage, the energy setting of the laser should be adjusted to the lowest level that creates an effective burst.

155

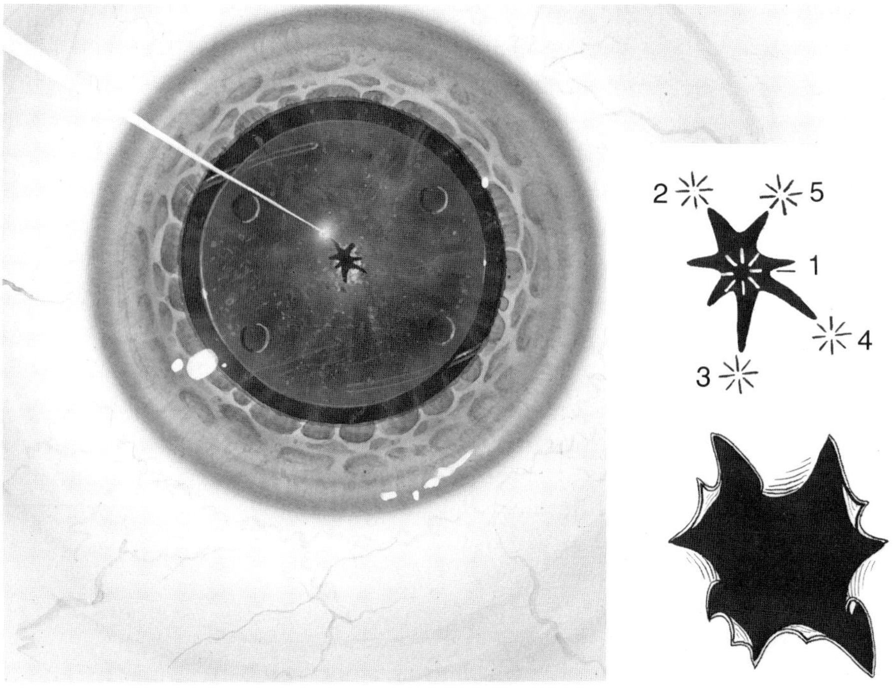

156

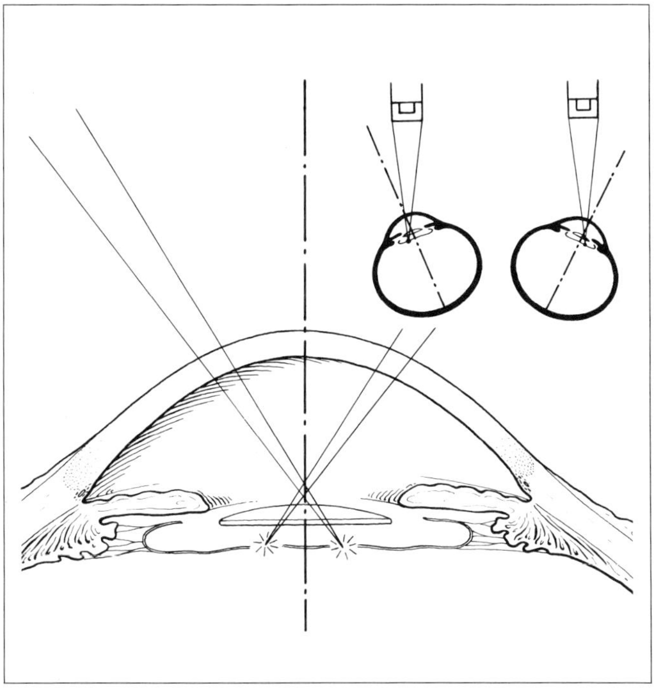

157

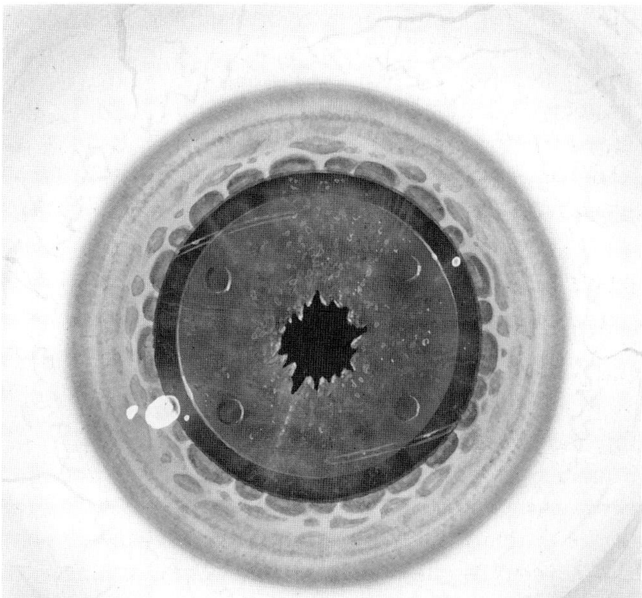

4.**155** The opening is extended to the size and shape desired. Capsular stress lines enhance the effect of initial laser bursts. The creation of a large capsular flap is avoided by utilizing existing tissue tension and by placing additional single laser bursts at the peripheral ends of the existing small capsular tears. The small flaps created scroll up upon themselves, providing an unobstructed opening. Close attention should be paid to laser burst location to ensure that any extension of the opening created includes the visual axis, rather than obstructing it by leaving a large, central capsular flap whose tissue tension has been released.

The size of the capsulotomy should approach the size of the pupil under photopic conditions; for the great majority of patients, a capsular opening of 3–3.5 mm is sufficient.

4.**156** In rare instances the surgeon may wish to make the capsular opening larger than the photopic pupil size. Placement of the additional laser bursts behind the pupillary margin is facilitated by having the patient slightly direct his gaze first to one side and then to the other while the surgeon completes extension of the capsular opening in each direction.

4.**157** The resultant central opening is surrounded by small flaps peripheral to the visual axis.

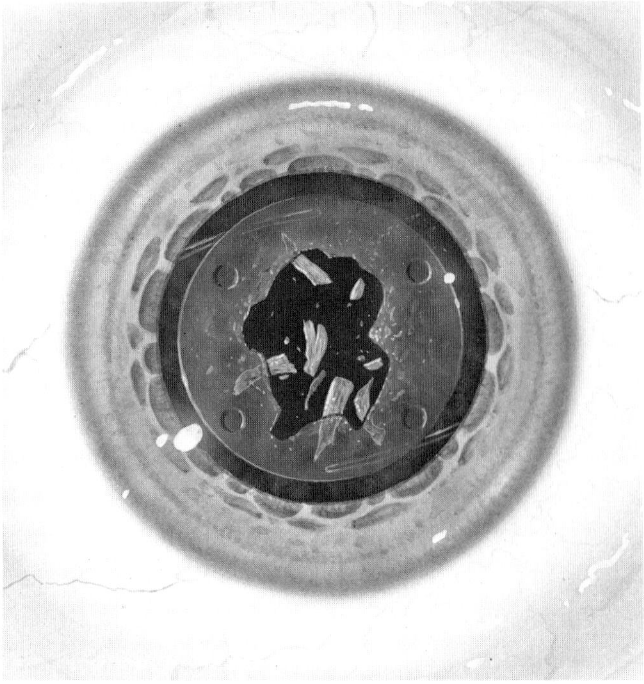

4.**158** Fibrotic capsules have no useful tissue tension and resist the extension of the central opening described above. The surgeon will need to use more bursts with closer spacing to chip away pieces of the capsule, much as an ice pick chips away pieces of ice. The resultant loose capsular debris remains in the visual axis only transiently.

Complications

The most frequent complications of neodymium:YAG laser capsulotomy are acute intraocular pressure elevation and intraocular lens damage. In a recent study, one of us has shown that the induced intraocular pressure increase (incidence 61 %; highest net rise + 39 mmHg) can be dramatically reduced in both incidence (28 %) and severity (maximal increase of 10 mmHg) by perioperative treatment with hypotonic agents such as timolol maleate[3]. Occasional patients will develop persistent intraocular pressure elevation with associated glaucomatous visual field loss.[4]

Intraocular lens damage is minimized if the surgeon carefully focuses each ocular of the laser so that his plane of focus coincides with the plane of focus of the neodymium:YAG beam. Some lasers are constructed with the helium neon aiming beam and the neodymium:YAG beam focused at disparate points; the surgeon must be familiar with the focusing system of his particular unit.

If the central posterior capsule is in contact with the posterior surface of the lens implant, lens damage can be minimized by discharging the laser bursts slightly posterior to the posterior capsule, using the anterior extension of the shock wave created to fashion the initial capsular opening.

Other serious, but much less frequent, complications include cystoid macular edema (incidence 0.4 % –1.2 %), and retinal detachment (incidence 0.4 % – 0.8 %)[1, 5, 6].

Postoperative Management

The intraocular pressure should be checked two to six hours after the procedure, since the majority of patients who develop elevated intraocular pressure will have done so within this time.[7]

Results

With either technique, over 80 % of patients attain improved vision, and the incidence of vision-threatening complications is less than 5 %.[1, 5, 6] The major causes of persistent visual loss are cystoid macular edema and retinal detachment. Both techniques provide effective means of restoring good vision following opacification of the posterior capsule.

References

1 Keates, R. H., Steinert, R. F., Puliafito, C. A. et al.: Long term follow-up of Nd:YAG laser posterior capsulotomy. *Amer. Intra-Ocular Implant Soc. J.* 10: 164–168, 1984.

2 Coonan, P., Fung, W. E., Webster, R. G. et al.: The incidence of retinal detachment following extracapsular cataract extraction. *Ophthalmology* 92: 1096–1101, 1985.

3 Johnson, S. H.: Perioperative treatment of ND:YAG laser induced IOL elevation. Presented at the American International IOL Congress, Boston Mass., April 10–13, 1985.

4 Demer, J. L., Koch, D. D., Smith, J. A. et al.: Persistent elevation in intraocular pressure after Nd:YAG laser treatment. *Ophthalmic Surg.* (in press).

5 Johnson, S. H., Kratz, R. P., Olson, P. F.: Clinical experience with the neodymium:YAG laser. *Amer. Intra-Ocular Implant Soc. J.* 10: 452–460, 1984.

6 Stark, W. J., Worthen, D., Holladay, J. T. et al.: Neodymium:YAG lasers. An FDA report. *Ophthalmology* 92: 209–212, 1985.

7 Terry, A. C., Stark, W. J., Maumanee, A. E., Fagadau, W.: Neodymium-YAG laser for posterior capsulotomy. *Amer. J. Ophthalmol.* 96: 716–720, 1983.

5

Corneoscleral Lacerations and Anterior Segment Reconstruction

C. Stephen Foster and David B. Mark

Surgical Principles

The primary goal in the surgical treatment of anterior segment trauma is to maintain the integrity of the globe so as to preserve vision and prevent the serious sequelae which may occur. One must obtain a careful history and perform a thorough examination prior to surgery. It is equally important to document in detail all of the information obtained prior to surgical intervention.

Loss of Corneal Stroma

In the case of a significant loss of corneal stroma after injury, the use of tissue adhesive can be a very useful therapeutic modality.

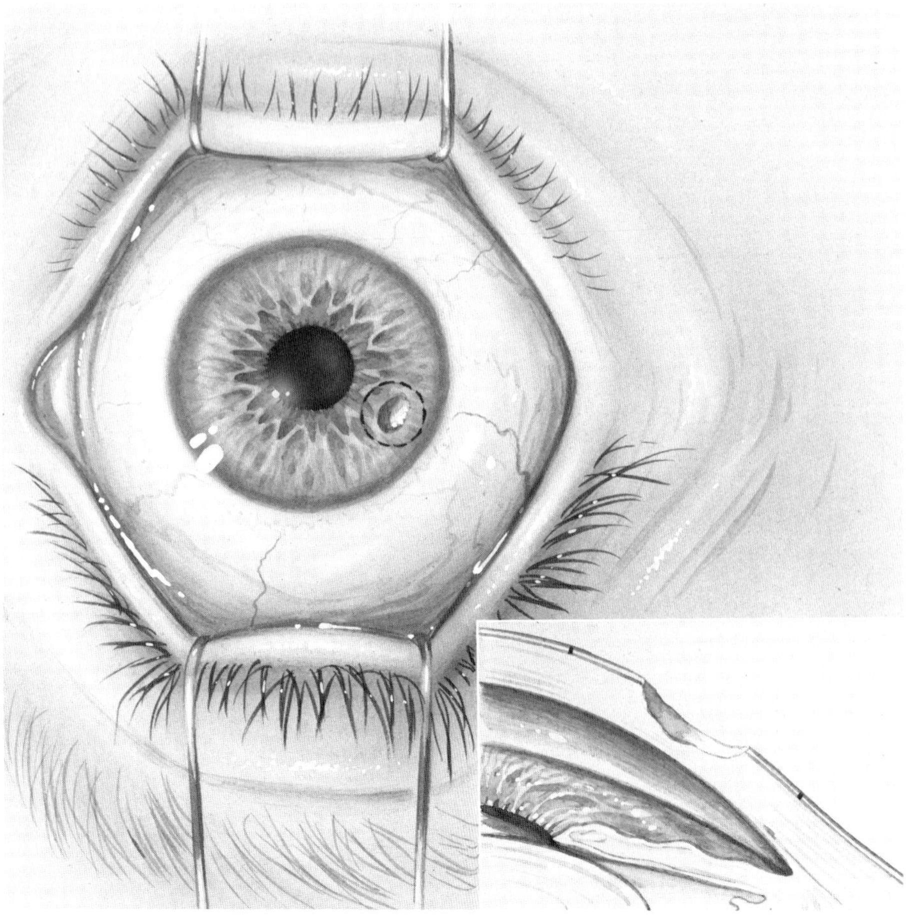

5.1 The situation depicted is similar to deep corneal ulceration caused by infection or autoimmune melting. A Bard-Parker knife is used to outline the affected area 1–2 mm from the wound edge. Only the epithelium is incised (inset).

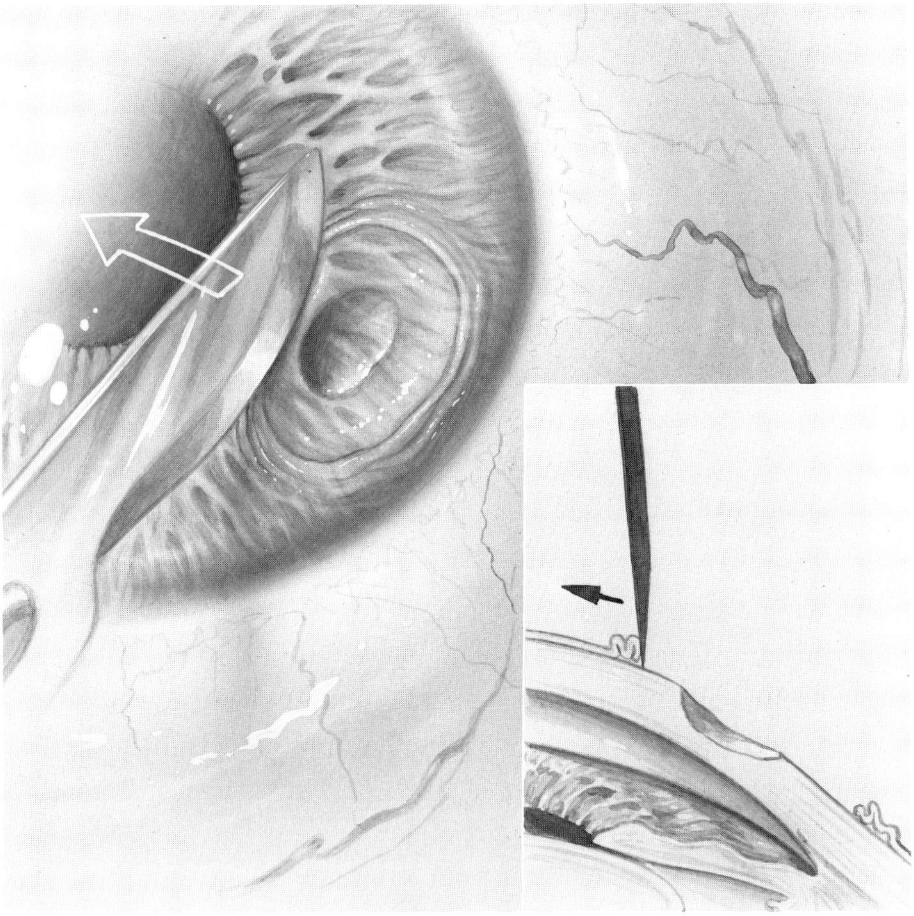

5.**2** The epithelium is then debrided from the wound margin outward. The blade is angled so as to avoid damage to the basement membrane of the epithelium.

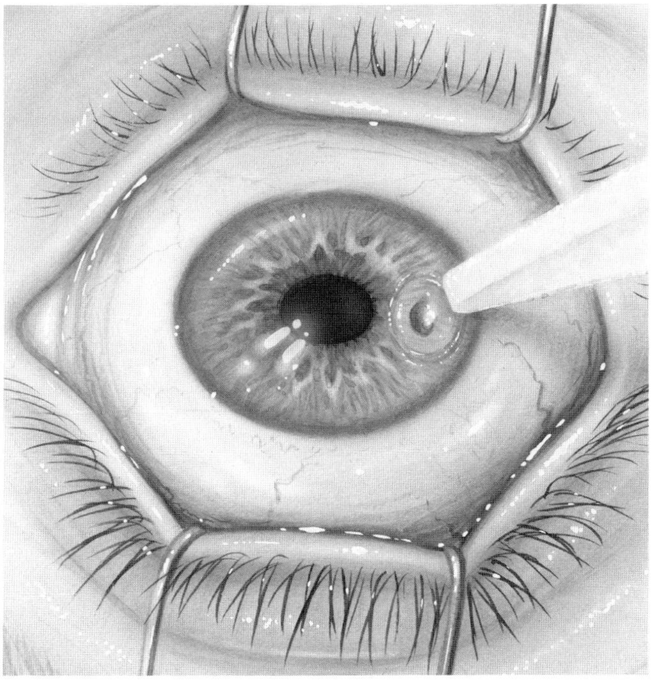

5.**3** The surface must then be thoroughly dried to allow firm adhesion of the adhesive (usually cyanoacrylate).

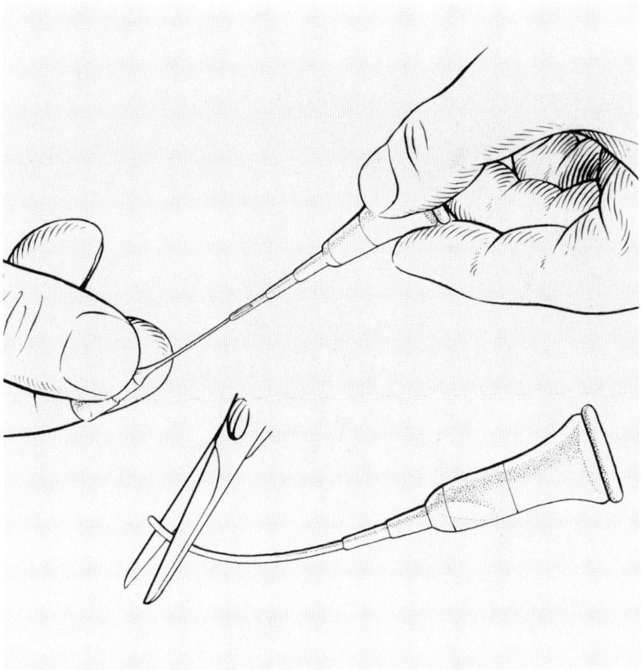

5.**4** The tip of the tissue adhesive container is then cut, and the adhesive is placed into the hollow applicator by the method of capillary action.

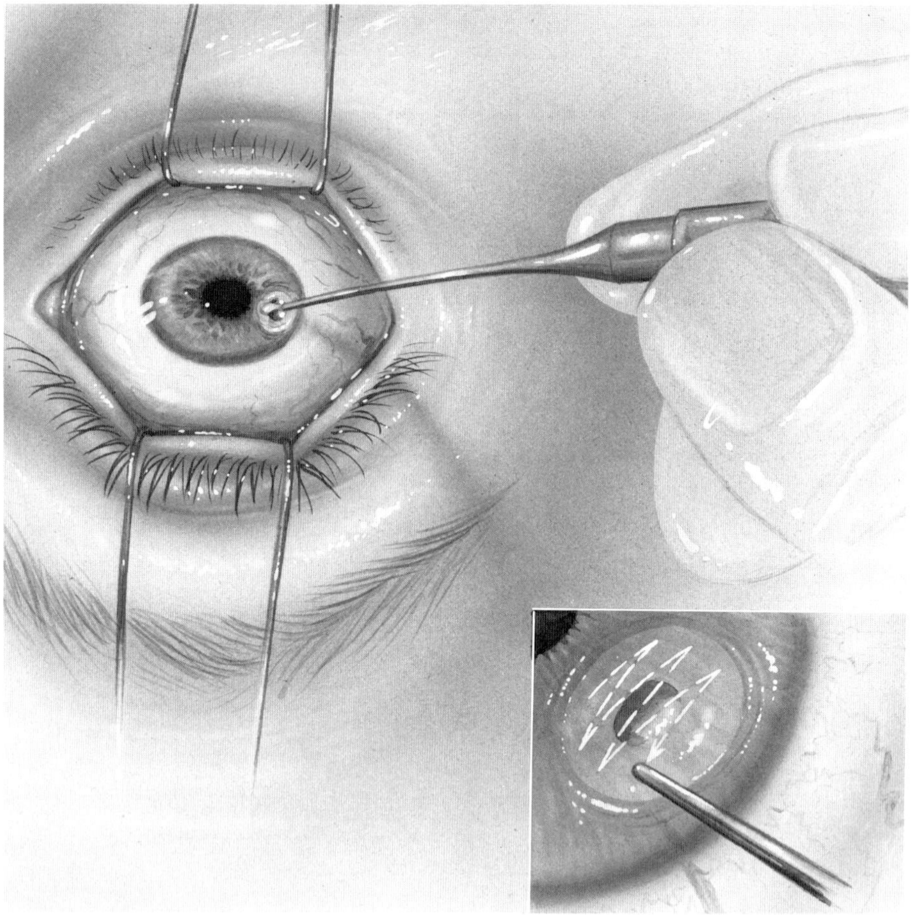

5.5 The adhesive is then applied to the surface with small sweeping motions. A thin layer is all that is necessary to promote good healing.

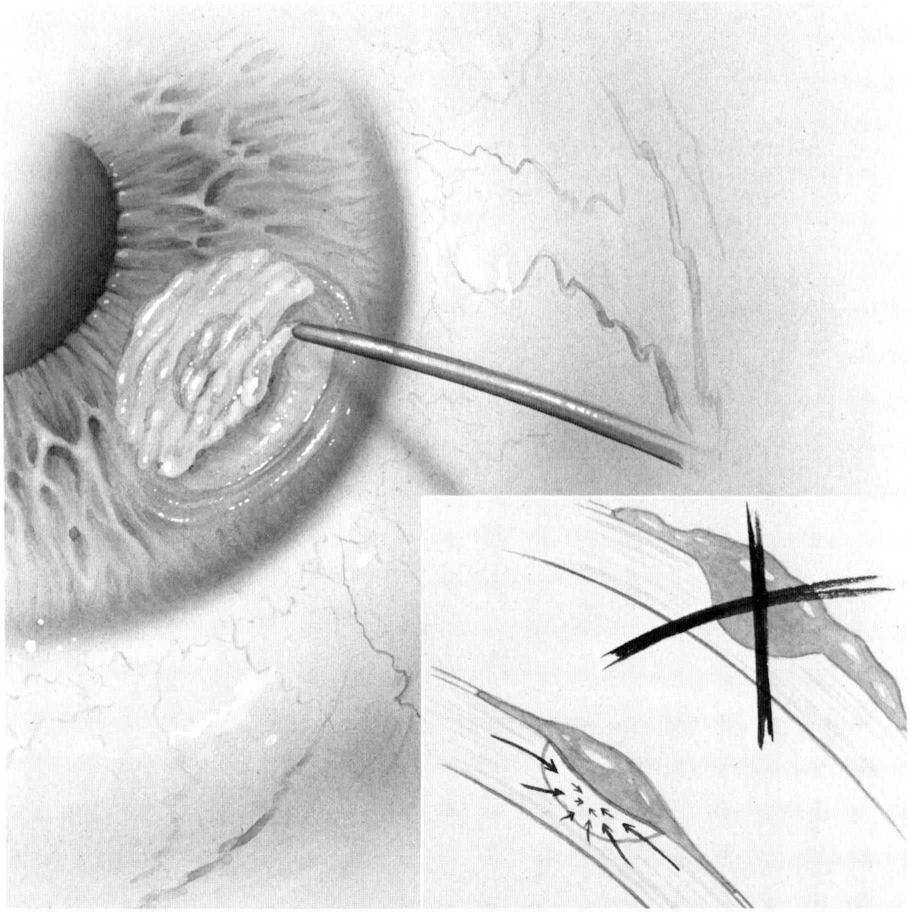

5.6 A thick, elevated mound of adhesive should be avoided. The corneal stroma heals from below the adhesive over a period of weeks to months.

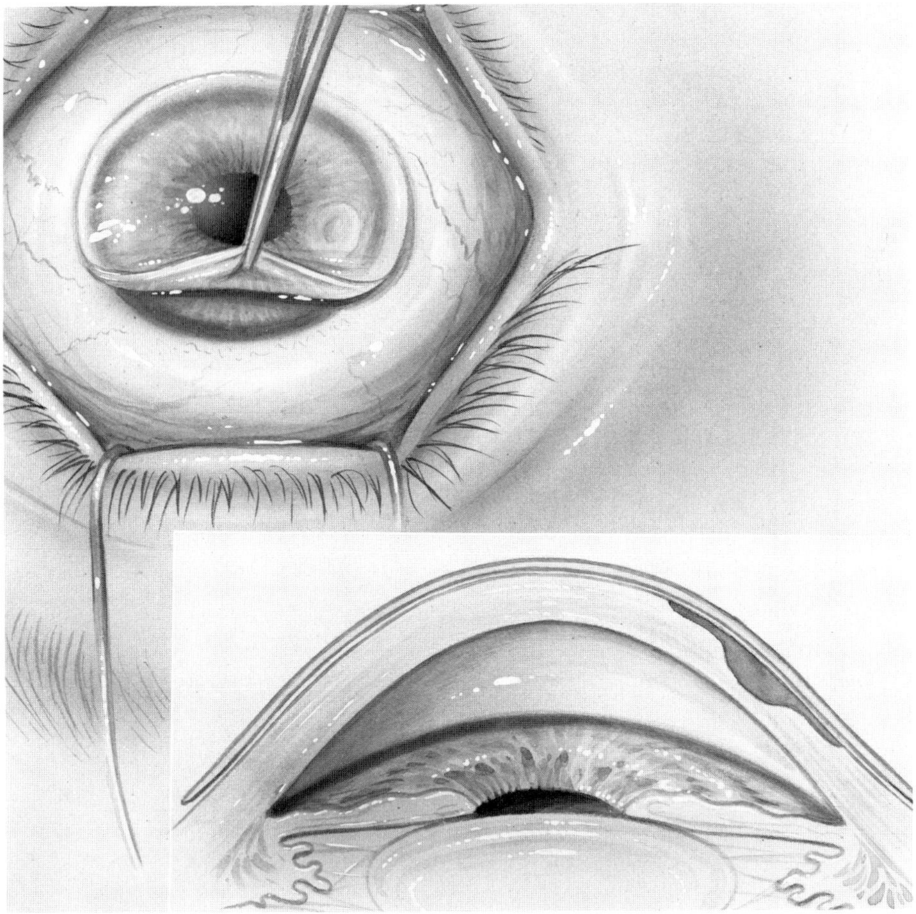

5.**7** A bandage soft contact lens is placed on the eye to protect the adhesive and prevent irritation caused by its irregular surface.

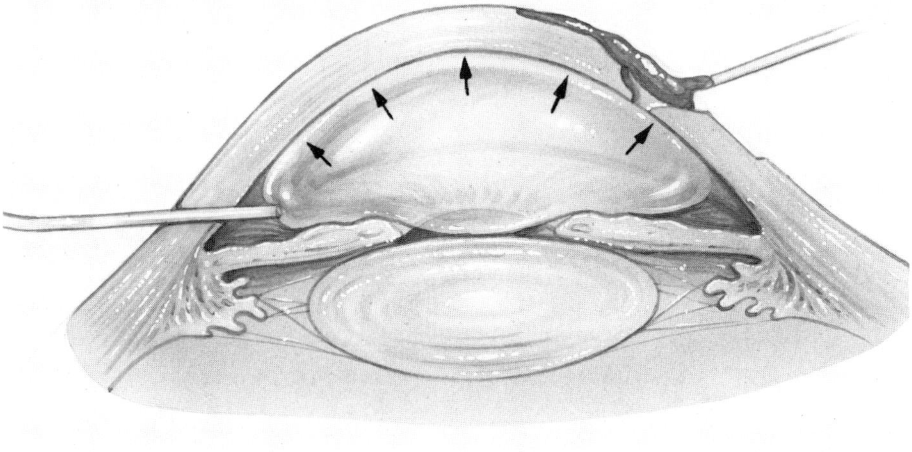

5.**8** If the cornea is perforated at the time of injury, tissue adhesive can still be used if air is injected into the anterior chamber when the adhesive is applied.

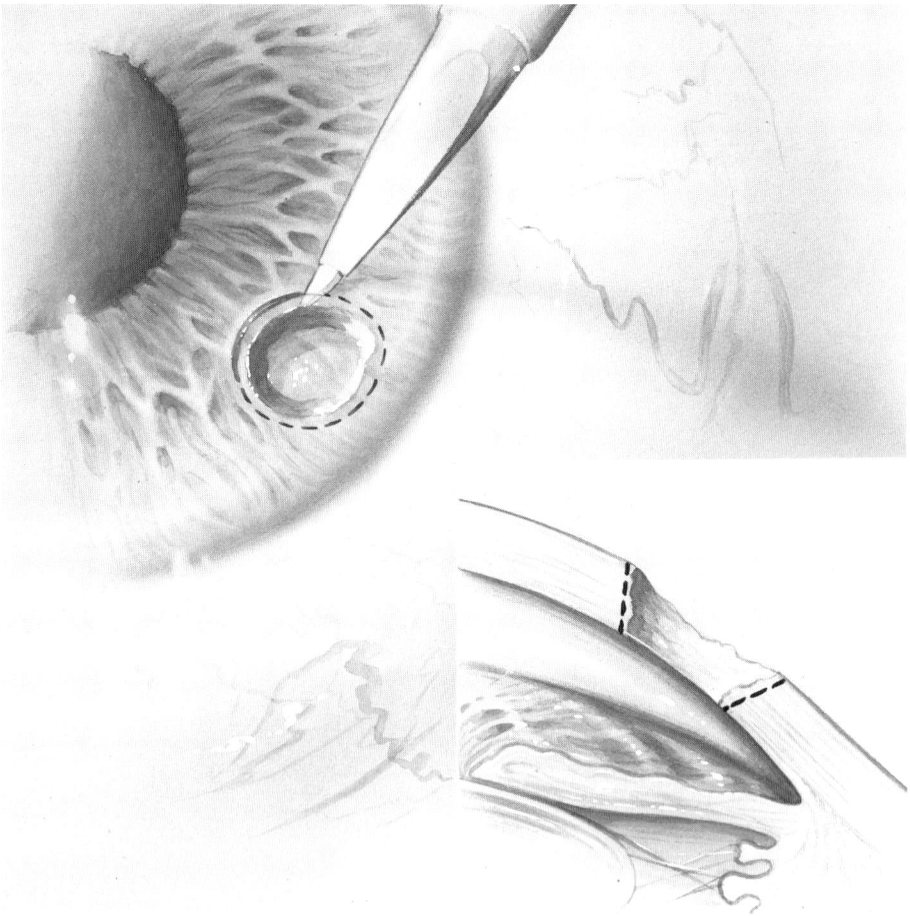

5.**9** A lamellar corneal graft can also be used to treat very deep and large corneal defects. Here, the defect extends to Descemet's membrane. A thin, sharp blade is used to create a regular wound margin.

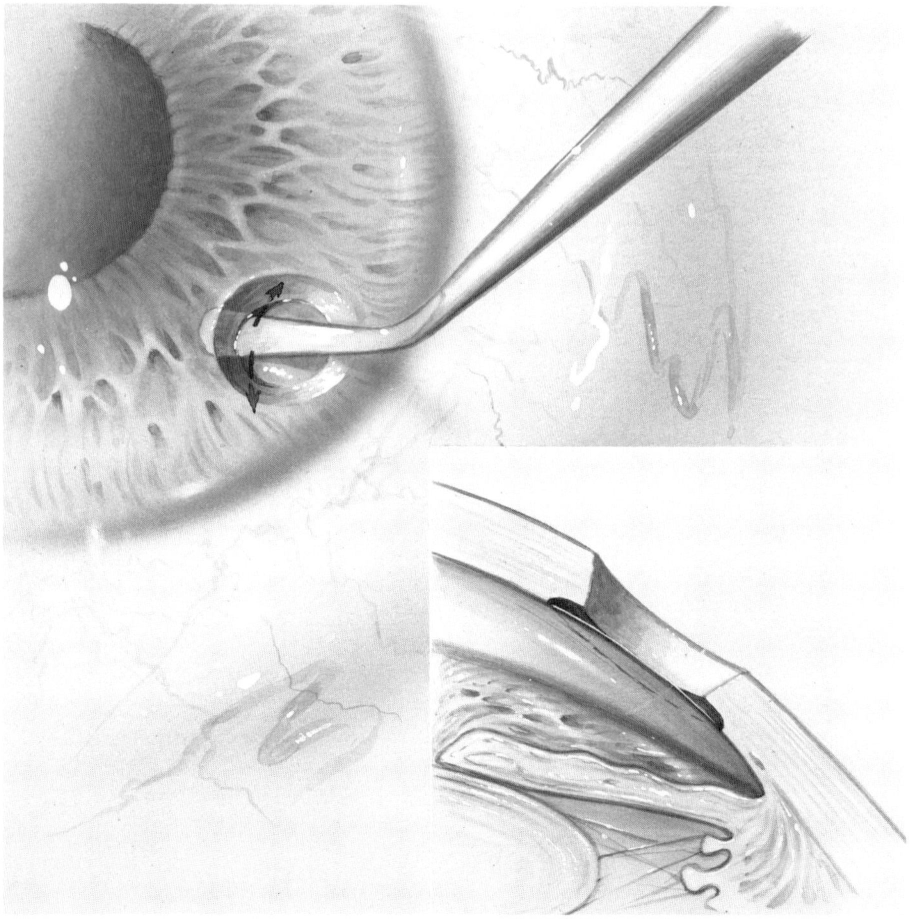

5.**10** A thin, angled spatula is then used to separate the posterior stromal layers at the deep margin of the wound.

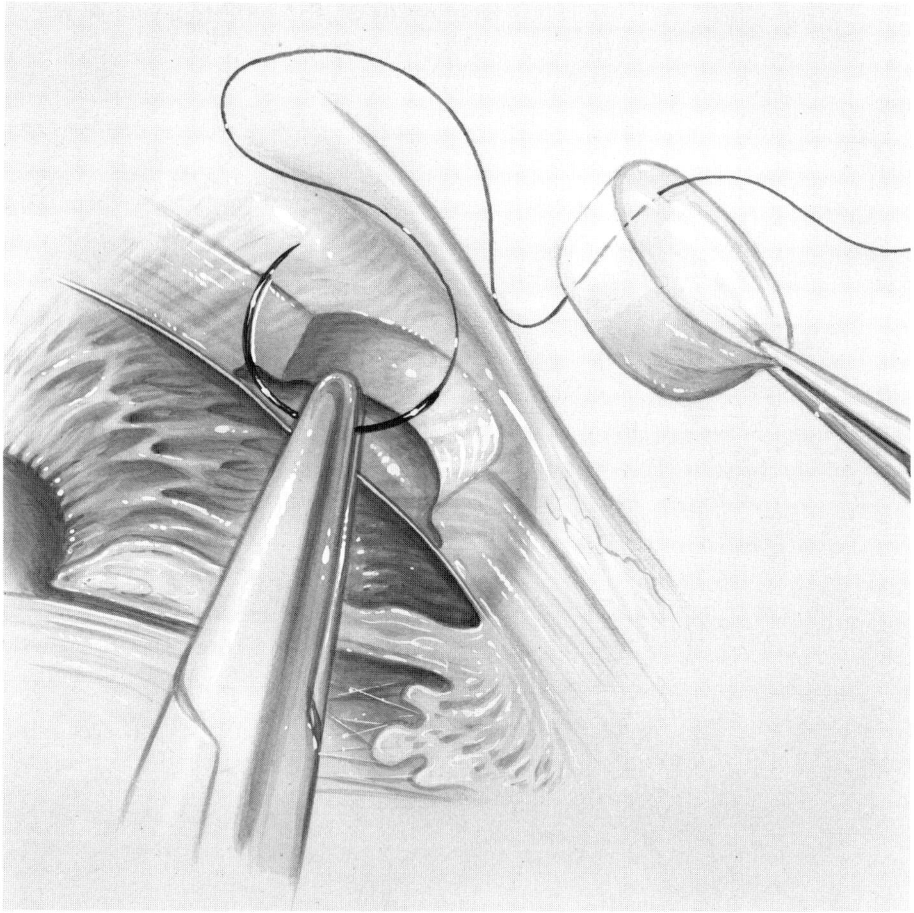

5.**11** Nylon suture (10-0) is then passed through the full thickness of the donor tissue and brought upwards through the host bed.

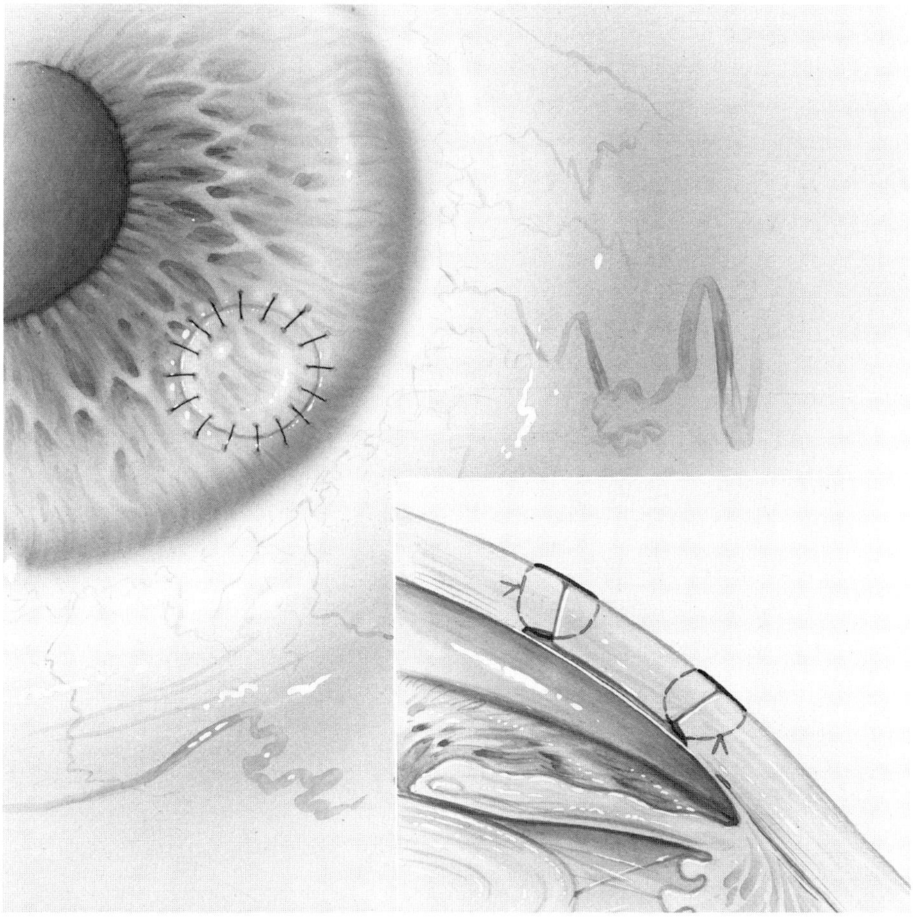

5.**12** This technique allows excellent appositional wound healing.

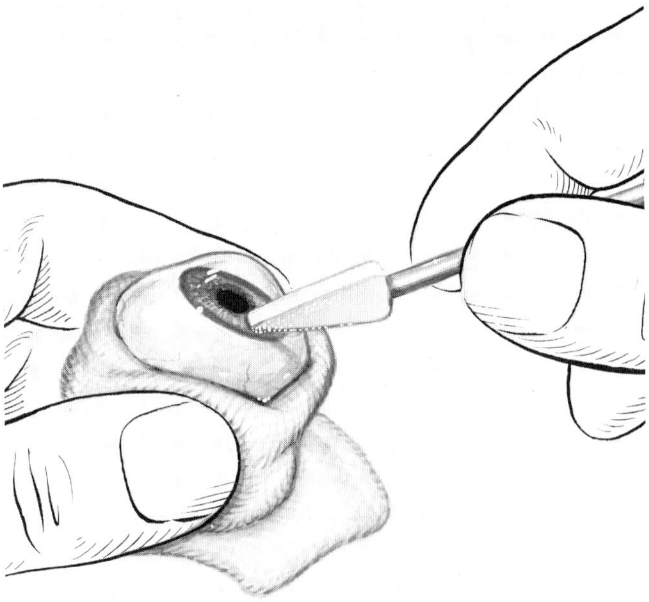

5.**13** The technique of preparation of lamellar corneal tissue for grafting is as follows. The donor surface is thoroughly dried before an incision is made.

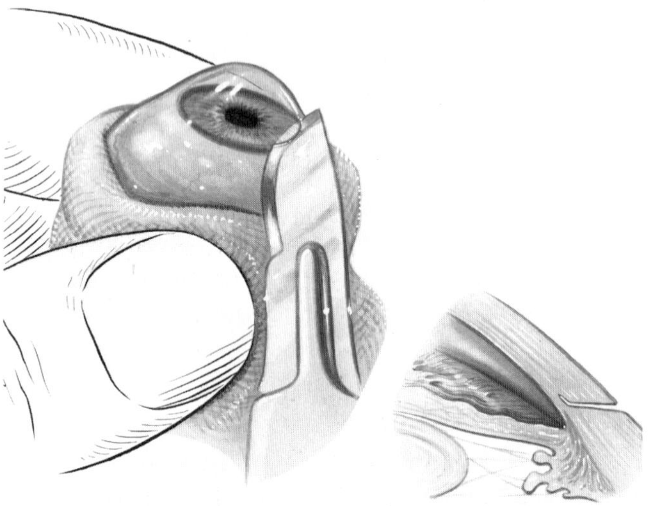

5.**14** A Bard-Parker blade is then used to create an angled groove in the deep stroma over 90 degrees of the circumference.

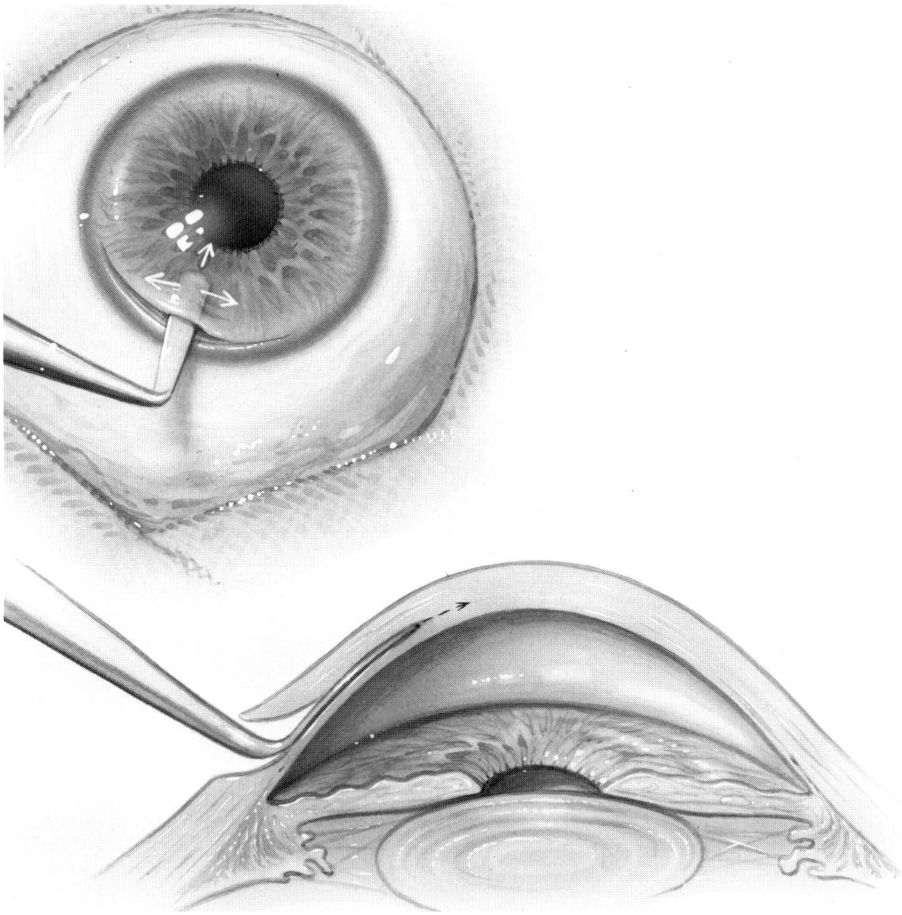

5.**15** An angled corneal spatula is then used to separate the posterior stromal lamellae following the curve of the cornea.

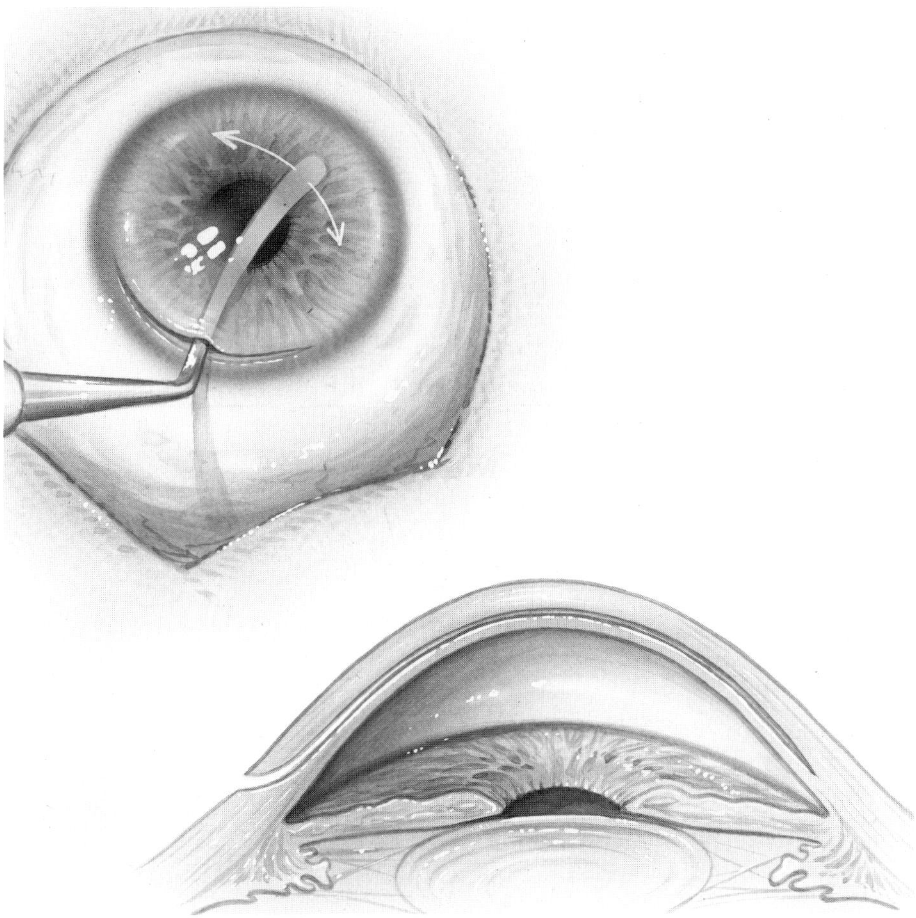

5.**16** Broad sweeping motions are used to split the lamellae by blunt dissection.

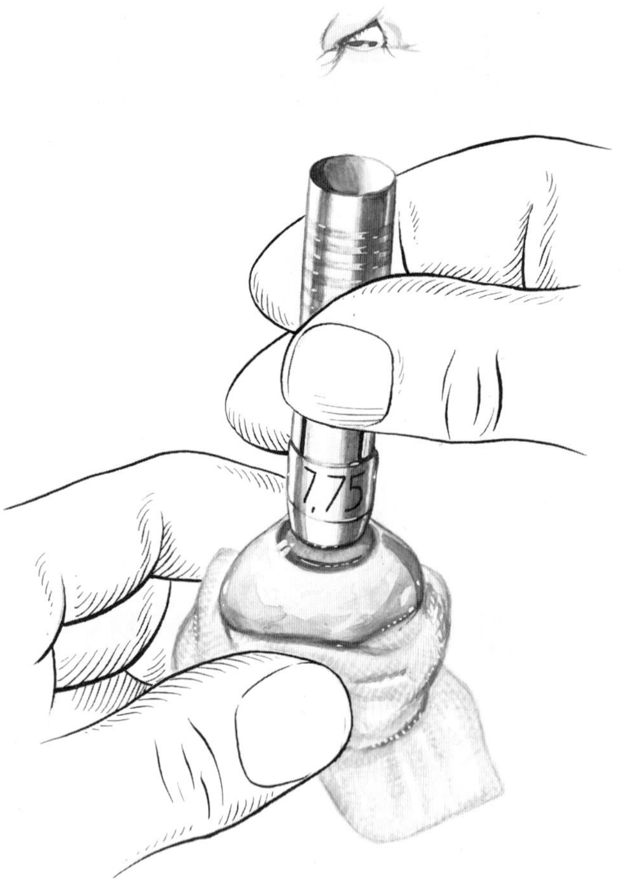

5.**17** A corneal trephine is then used to obtain the desired donor button; the trephination is centered by direct observation.

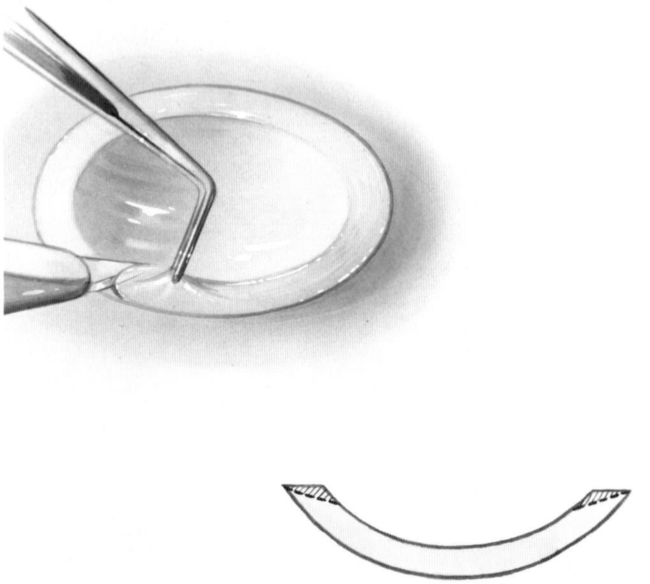

5.**18** A thin, sharp blade is used to create a groove for the placement of curved corneal scissors.

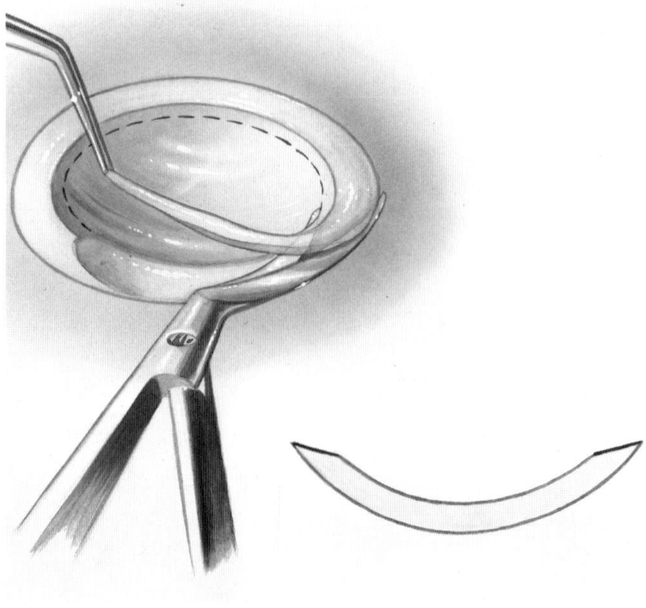

5.**19** These are then used to fashion a posterior bevel of the donor tissue.

Conjunctival Flap

Occasionally it is necessary to cover the cornea with a conjunctival flap. It is important when creating a flap to provide maximal amount of tissue in order to limit tension on the conjunctiva and to avoid buttonholing the flap. The corneal epithelium should be removed.

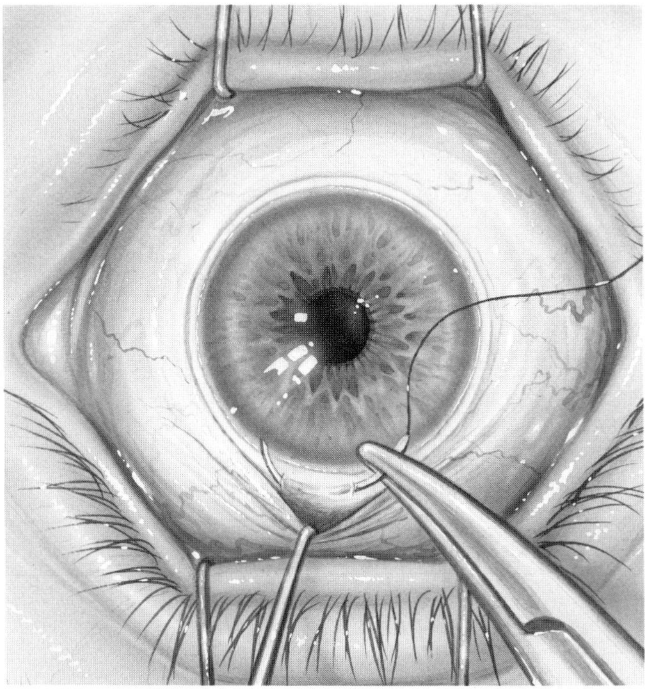

5.**20** A 360 degree peritomy is then made at the limbus and a traction suture (6-0 silk or vicryl) is placed at the 12 o'clock limbus to pull the globe downward and facilitate dissection of the conjunctiva.

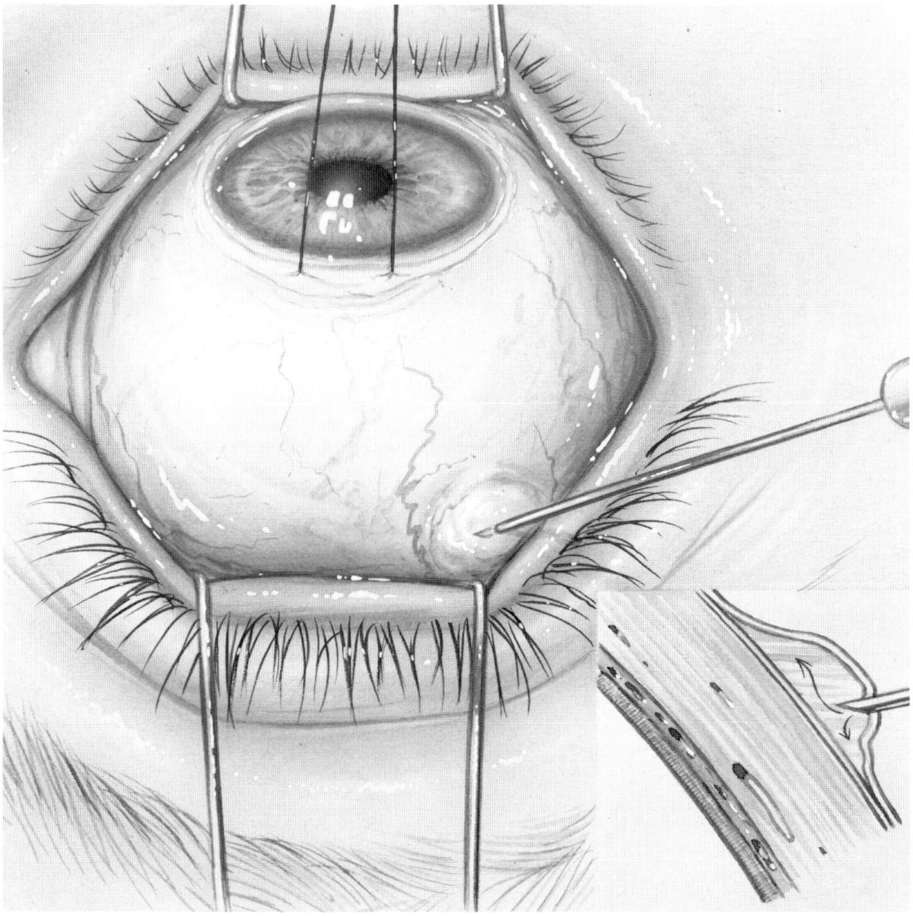

5.**21** Balanced salt solution is then used on a 30-gauge needle to separate the conjunctiva from Tenon's capsule. The injection site should be near the fornix so as not to perforate the eventual flap.

22

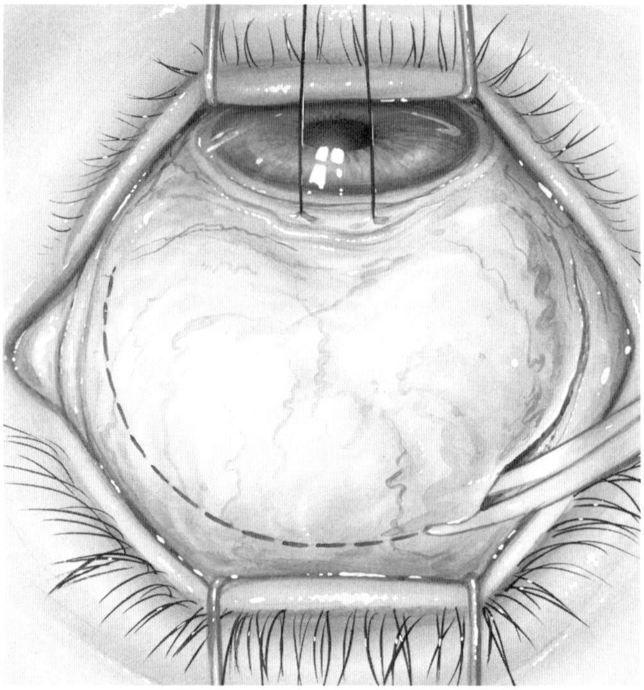

23

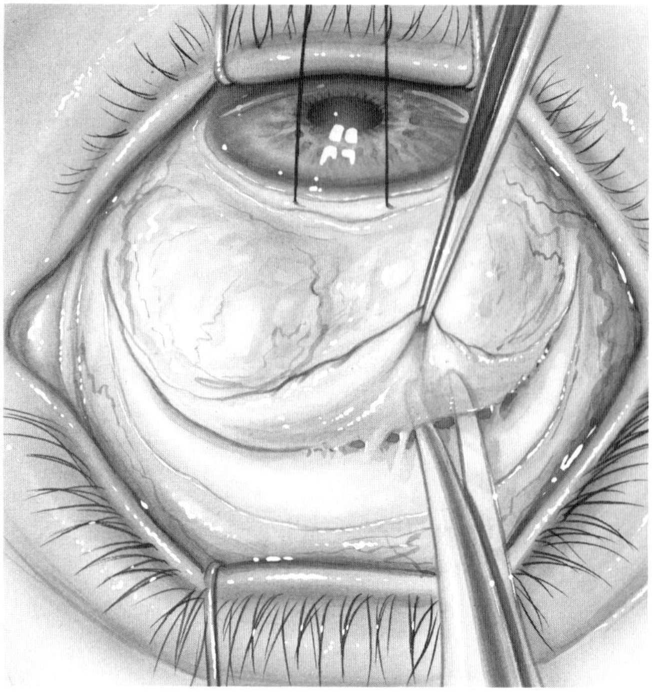

24

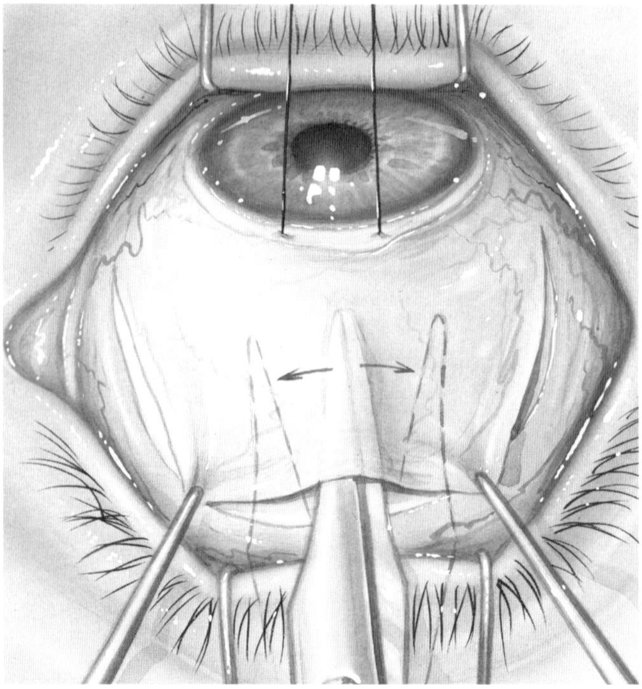

25

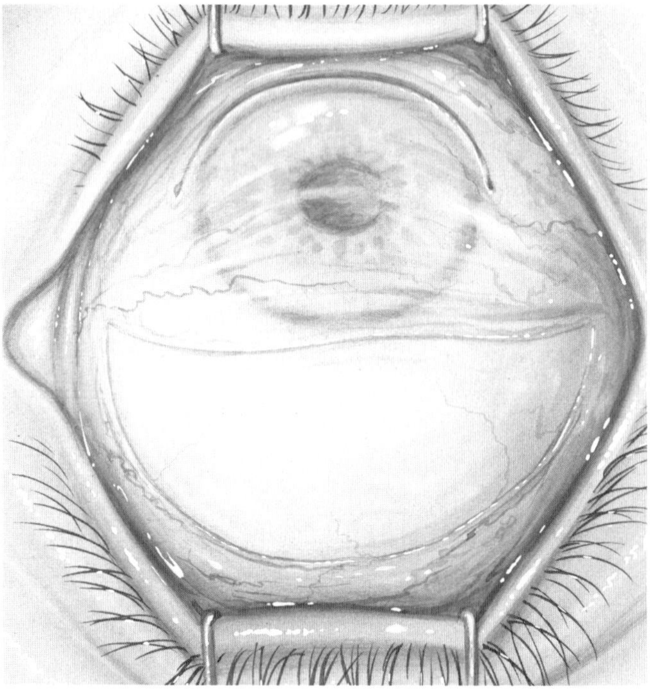

5.**22** Scissors are then used to create a large conjunctival flap superiorly, obtaining the maximal amount of tissue for the flap. One should be careful not to injure Müller's muscle.

5.**23** The flap is then undermined beginning superiorly and mobilizing only conjunctiva and not Tenon's capsule.

5.**24** Countertraction using smooth forceps facilitates the dissection. Blunt dissection is used, employing a closed-open technique under the conjunctiva.

5.**25** The flap is then brought down across the cornea.

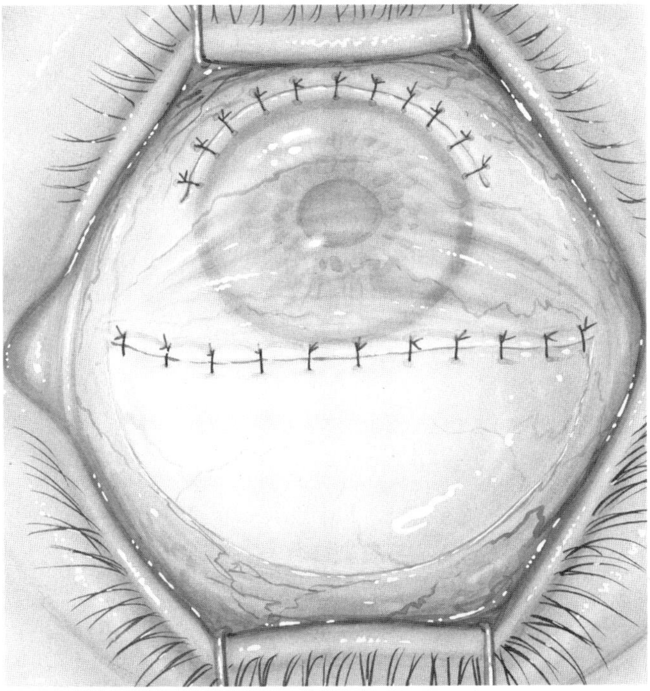

5.**26** It is sutured with interrupted 10-0 nylon sutures.

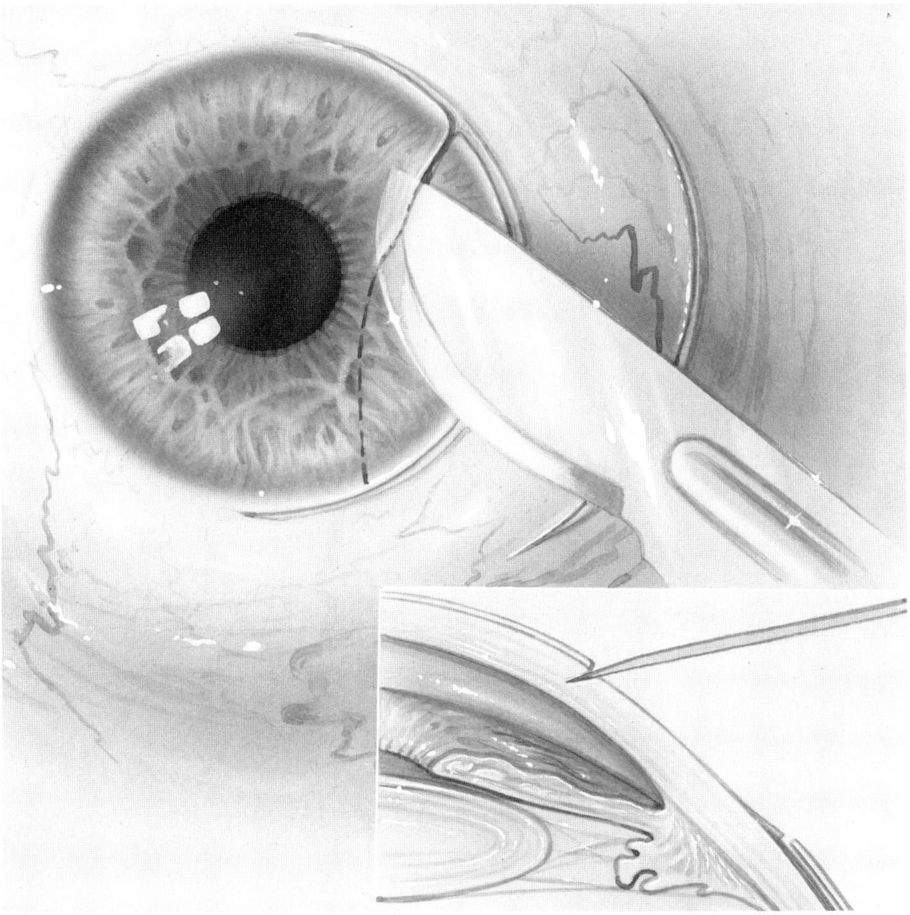

5.**27** When only a partial vertical flap is necessary, the peritomy is made 180 degrees with a circumferential incision away from the limbus. Again, the corneal epithelium is removed and a partial-thickness lamellar incision is made at the future margin of the flap.

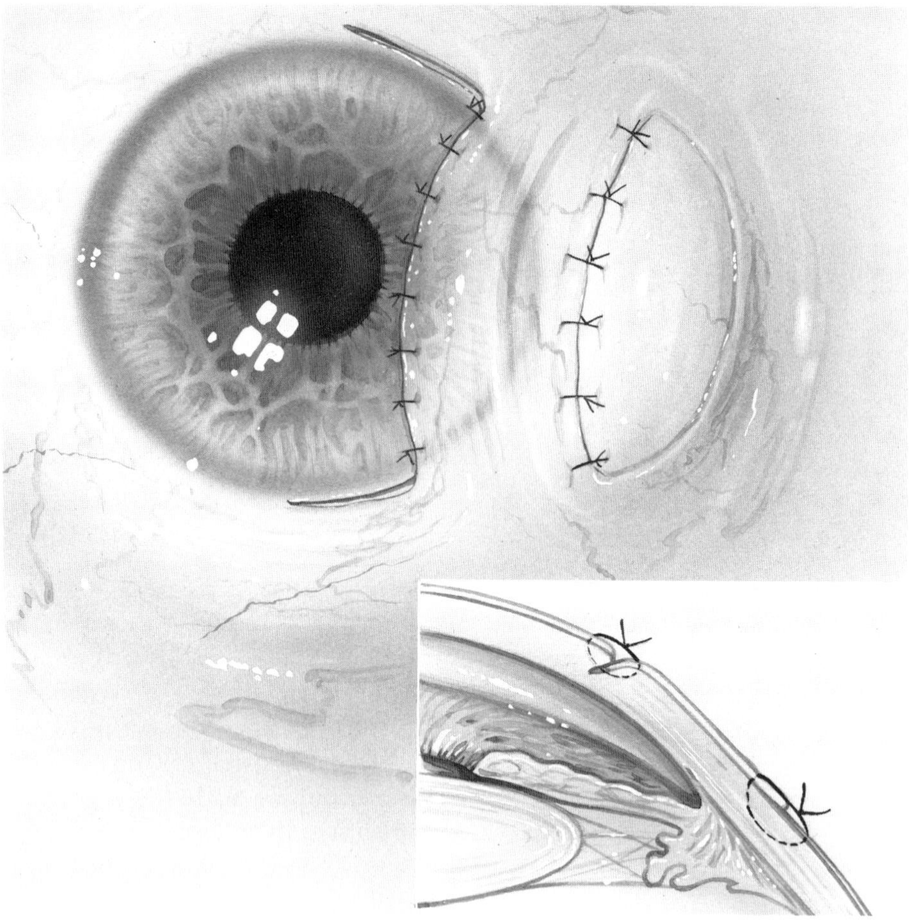

5.28 When the flap is brought across the cornea, the sutures should include the corneal stroma to facilitate healing.

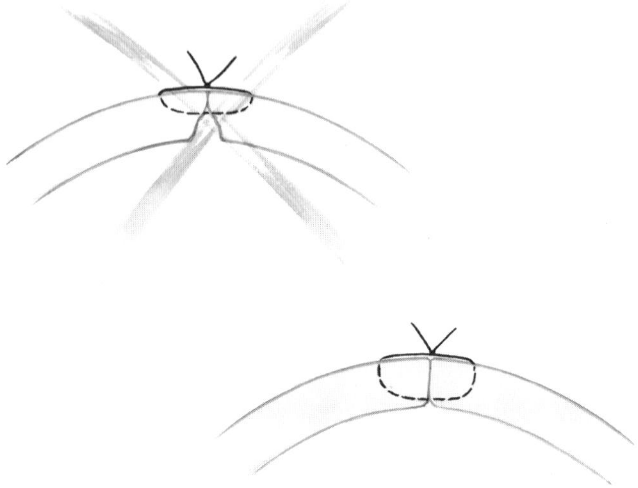

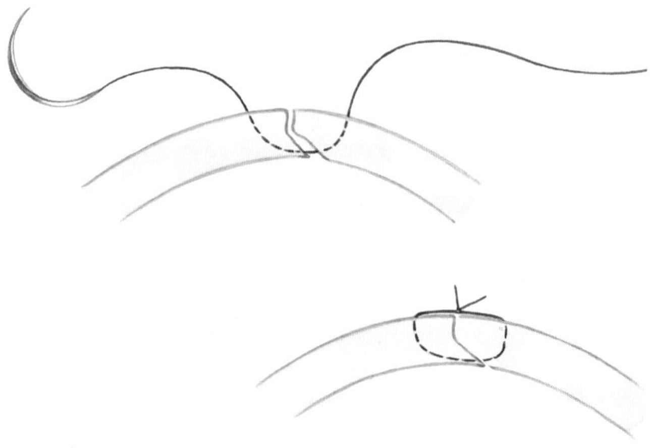

5.29 It is important when repairing even simple lacerations of the cornea to avoid placing superficial sutures; these can cause posterior gaping. Proper, deep suture placement prevents this from occurring.

5.30 When an irregular wound is present, adequate closure can be obtained by apposing the deeper edges of the wound as illustrated.

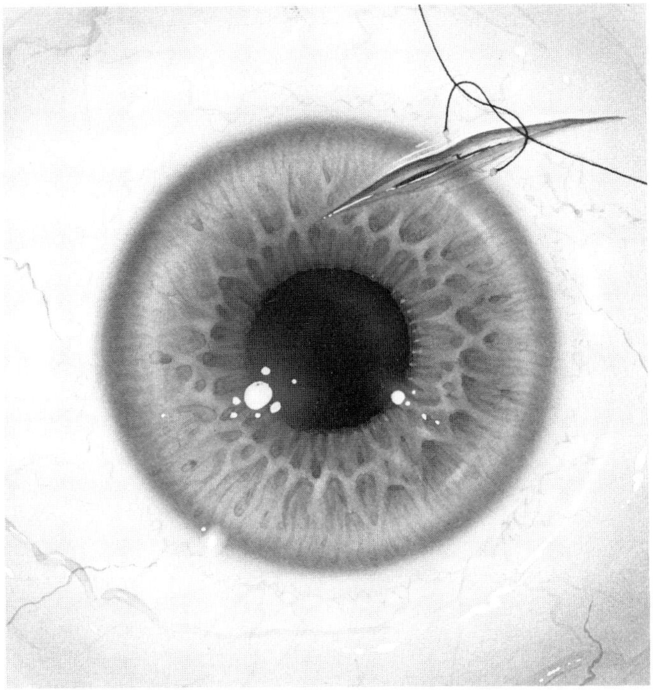

5.**31** In the case of a simple laceration without iris incarceration, interrupted nylon sutures are used initially.

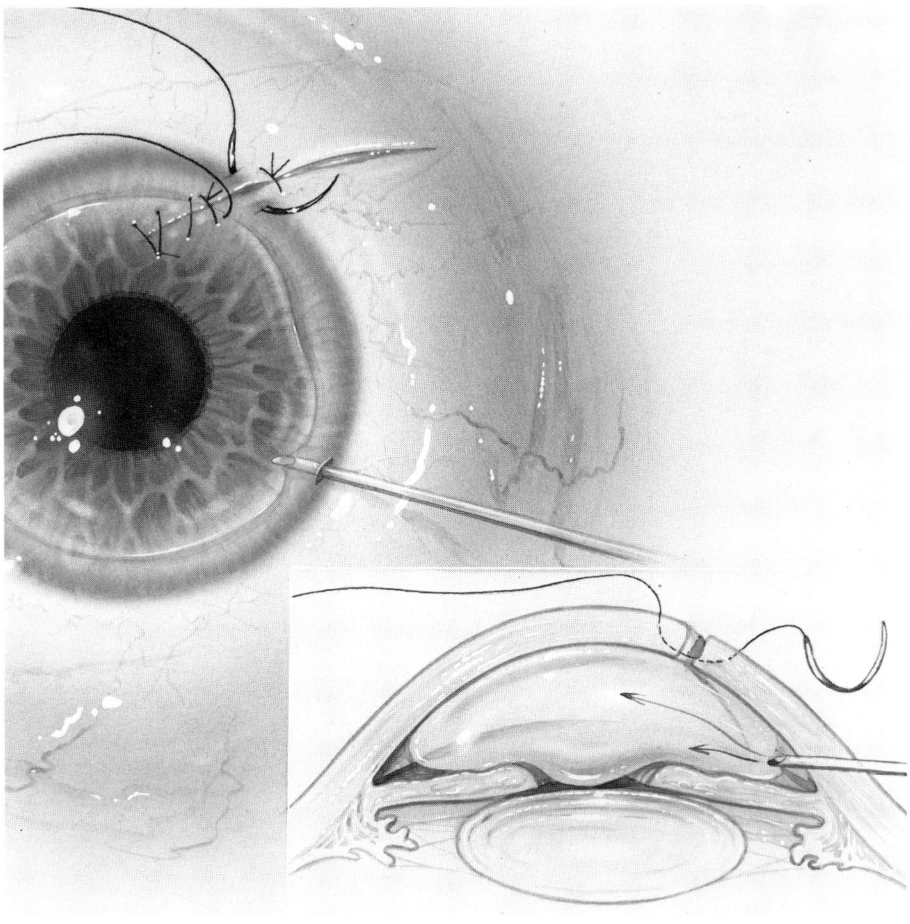

5.**32** A 30-gauge needle on an air-filled syringe can then be used to form the anterior chamber. Running sutures can then be employed. Viscoelastic gel (e. g., sodium hyaluronate) can also be used when the chamber does not remain formed with air.

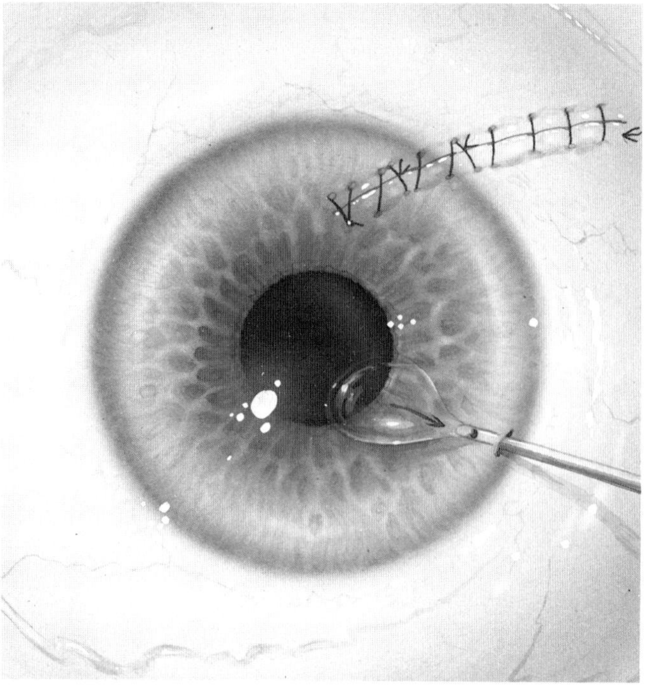

5.**33** The advantage of air is that it can more easily be removed and replaced with saline at the end of the procedure, but one must approach each case individually.

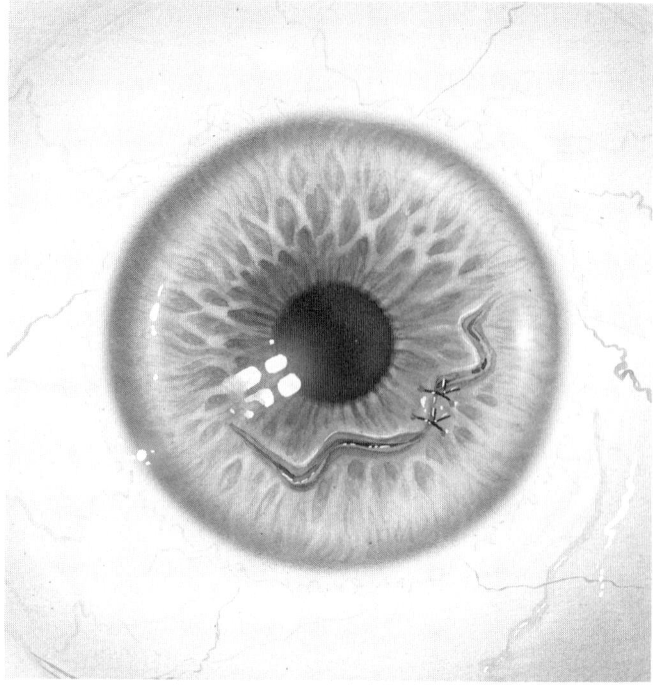

5.**34** When an irregular laceration is present, interrupted sutures should be placed centrally to align the wound before the more peripheral aspect of the wound is closed.

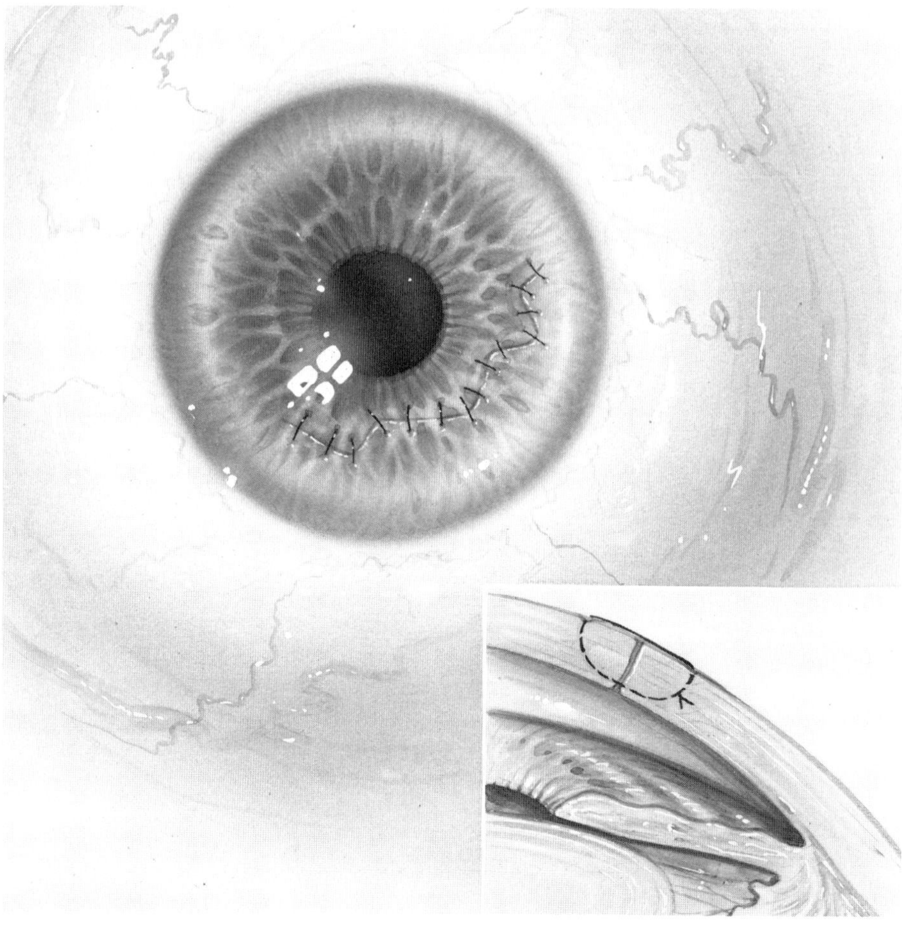

5.**35** Once again, all of the sutures should be placed deep for best healing.

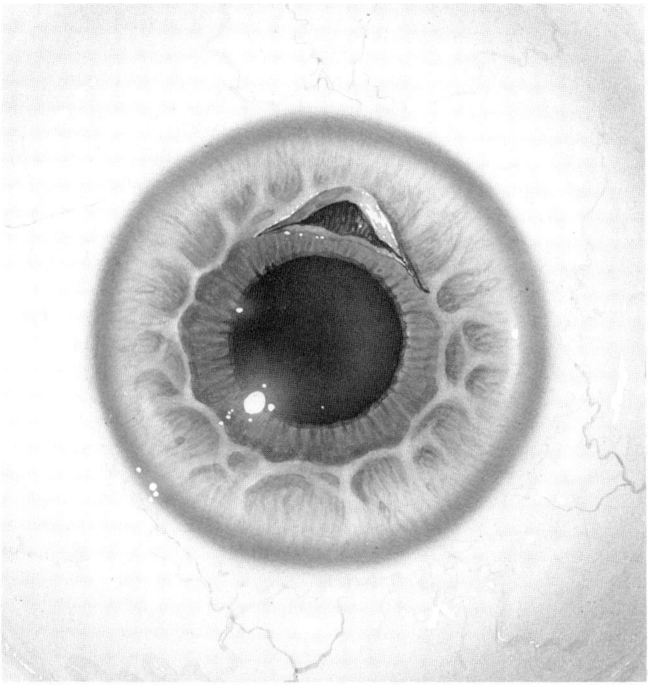

5.**36** Here, a large amount of tissue has been lost.

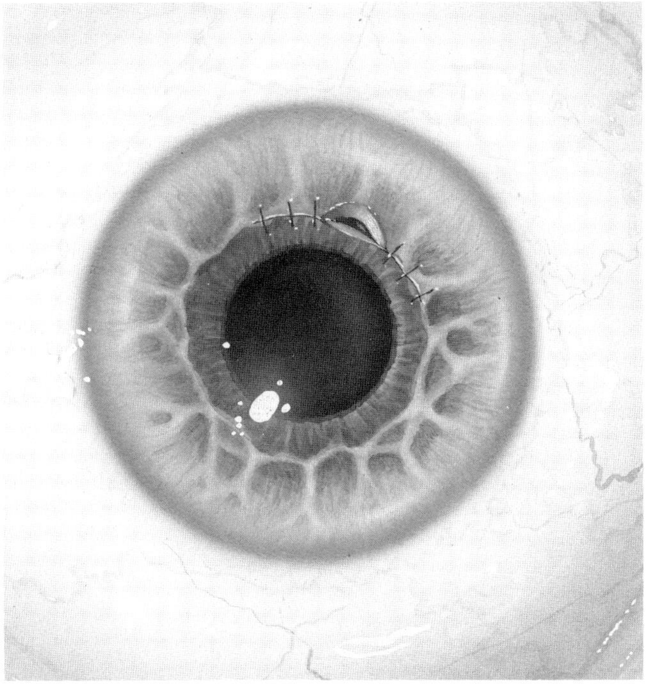

5.**37** Interrupted sutures should be used to close as much of the wound as possible.

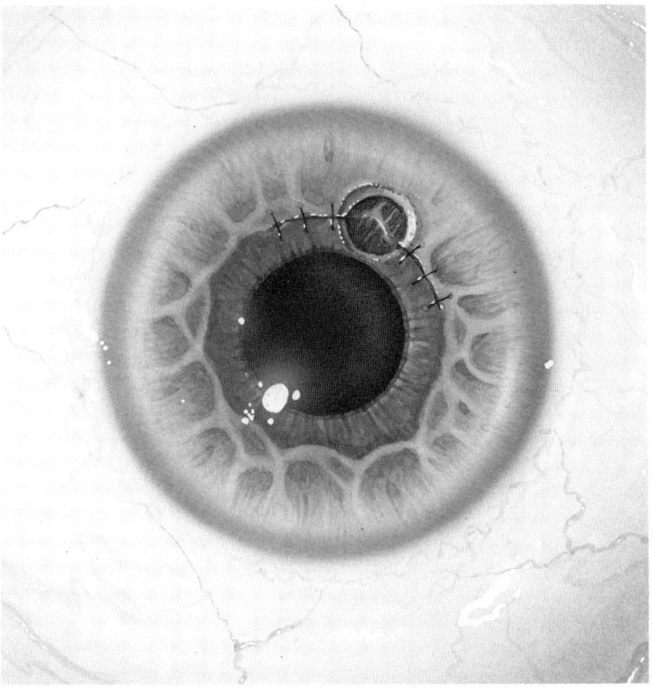

5.**38** A small tissue graft can then be used to complete the procedure.

39

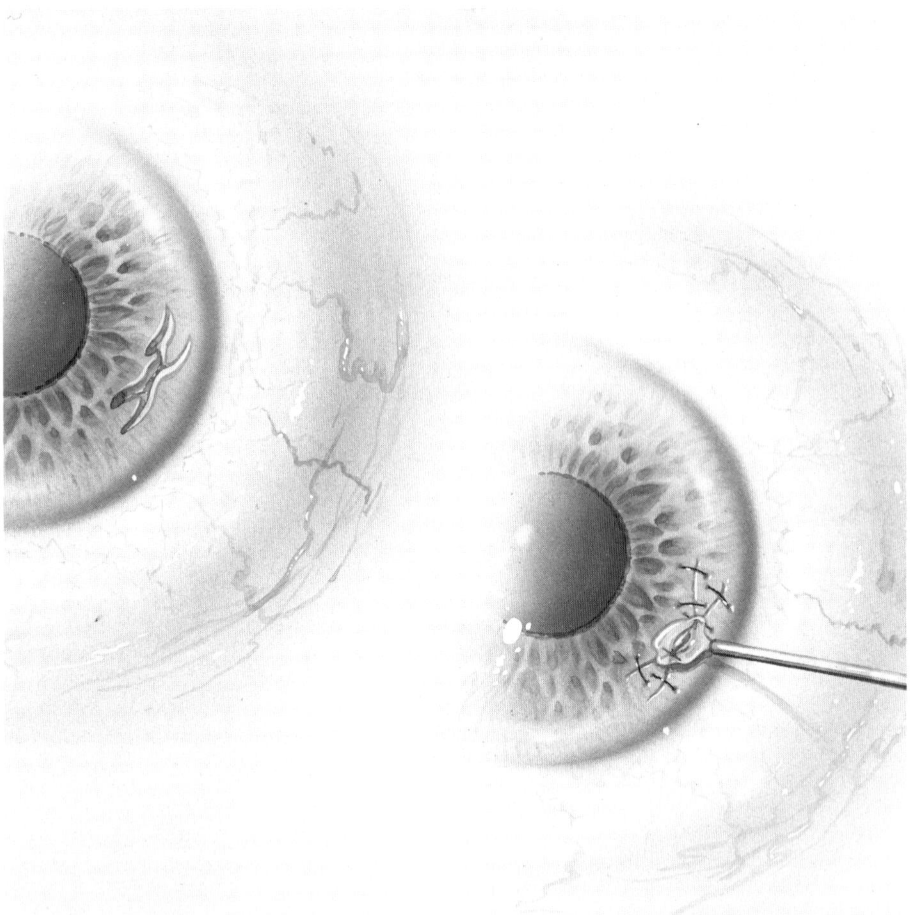

5.39 If only a tiny defect remains tissue adhesive can be used in the manner described above. Again, one should denude the corneal epithelium before application of the adhesive.

5.40 When iris incarceration is present, a decision must be made whether or not to excise the extruded tissue. In general, it is best to reposit the iris tissue unless there is clear evidence of substantial necrosis or there is evidence of infection.

5.41 The iris can often be reposited through a small wound with the use of a fine, smooth spatula.

40

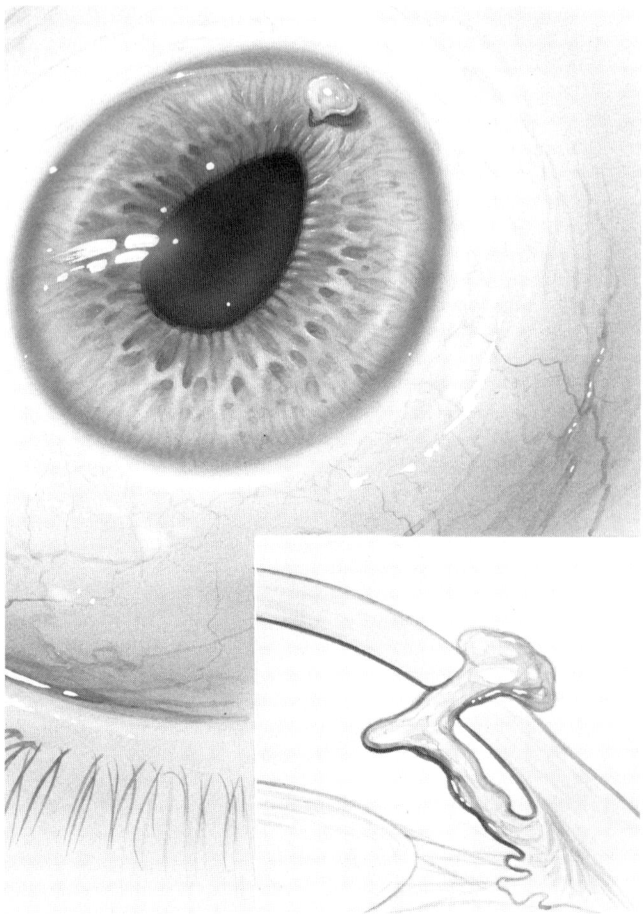

41

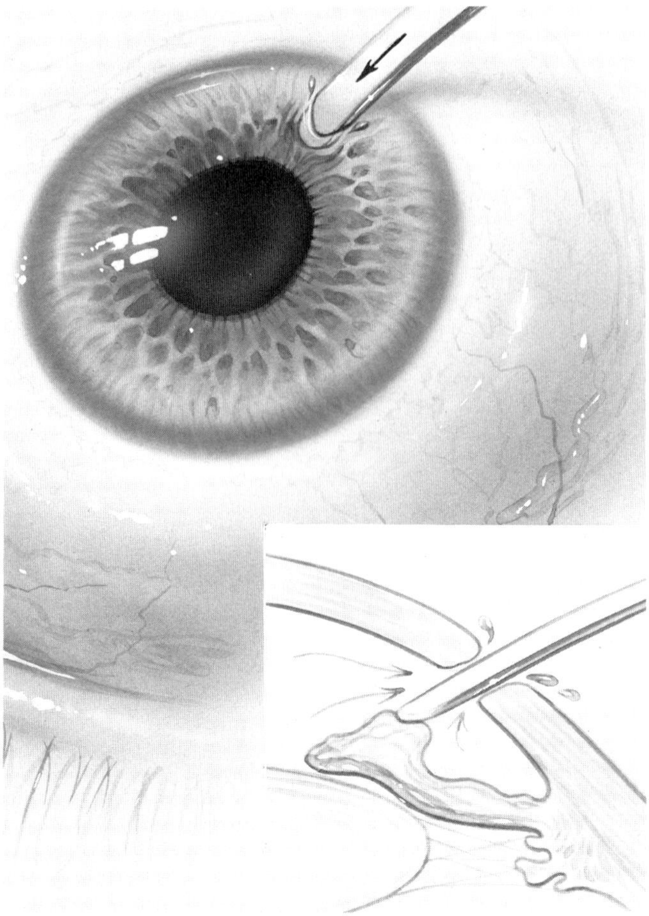

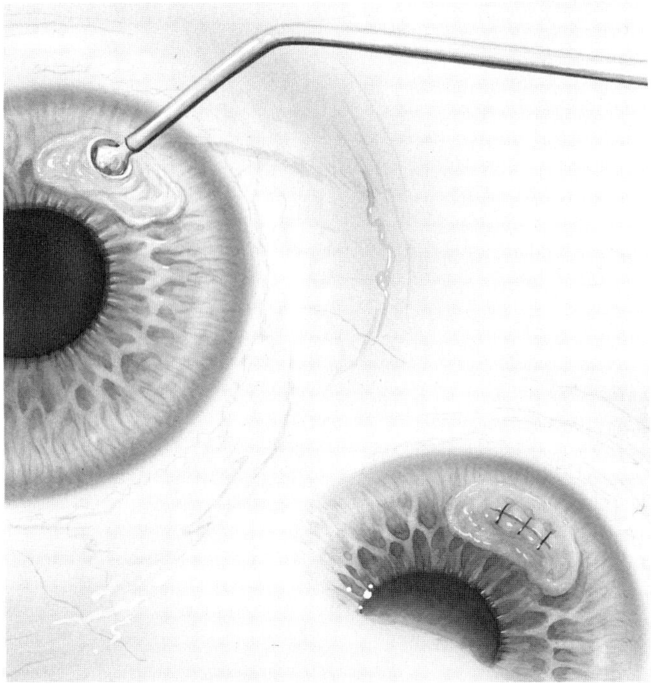

5.**42** Often a small amount of viscoelastic gel will allow wound closure without iris adherence.

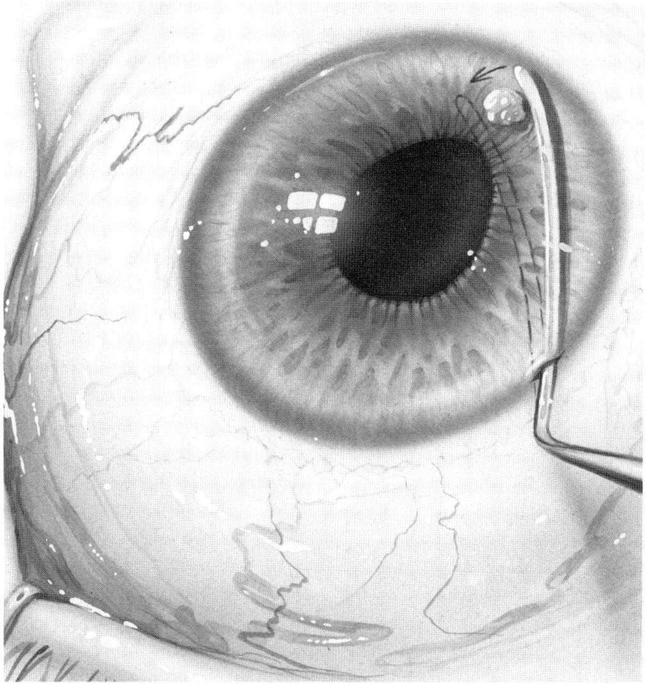

5.**43** When it is not possible to reposit the iris directly through the wound, a separate entry site can be used to introduce a thin, smooth spatula to sweep the iris away from the cornea. Care is taken to avoid the corneal endothelium and, in particular, the central cornea.

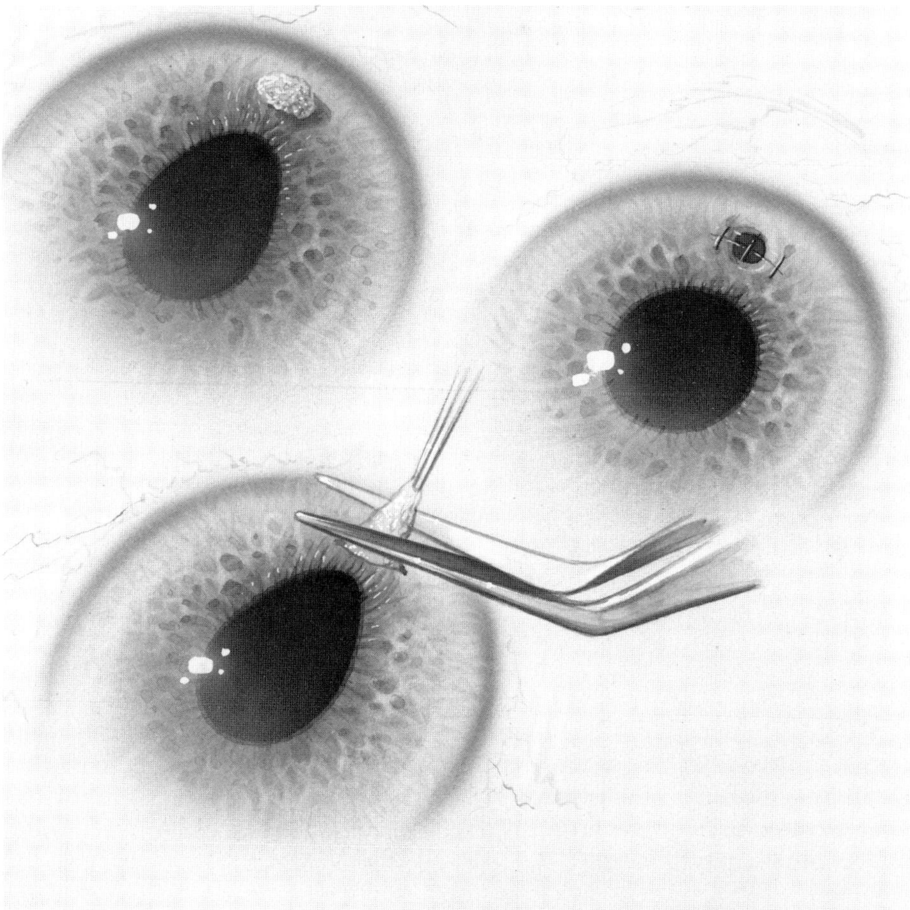

5.**44** When it is necessary to excise the incarcerated iris, smooth forceps are used to pull the iris slightly upward so that all of the necrotic or infected tissue can be excised.

Traumatic Cataract

When a capsule rupture is present in an older patient, it is often advantageous to perform an intracapsular cataract extraction.

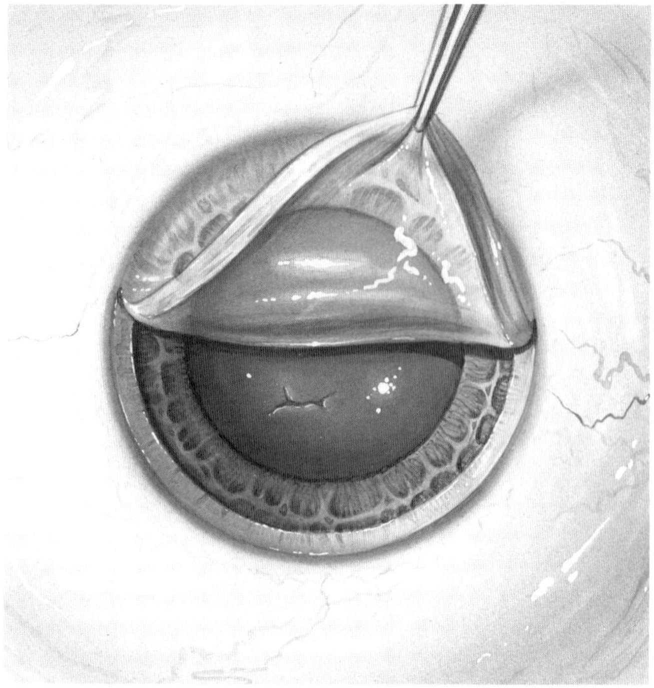

5.**45** A limbal wound is created to allow good exposure and access for the cryoprobe.

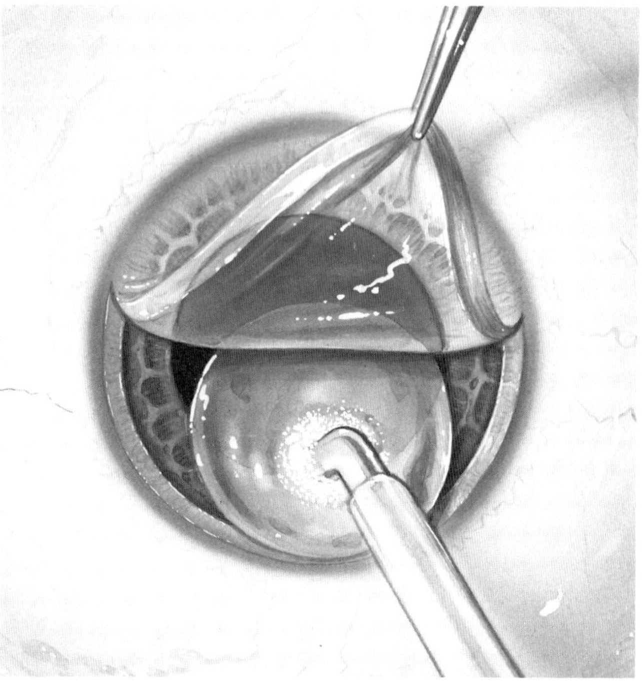

5.**46** The anterior capsule is dried using a sponge, and the cryoprobe tip is placed directly over the capsule rupture. The entire lens can then be removed.

In many instances, an extracapsular extraction is the treatment of choice. While surgical techniques may vary, the basic principles remain the same.

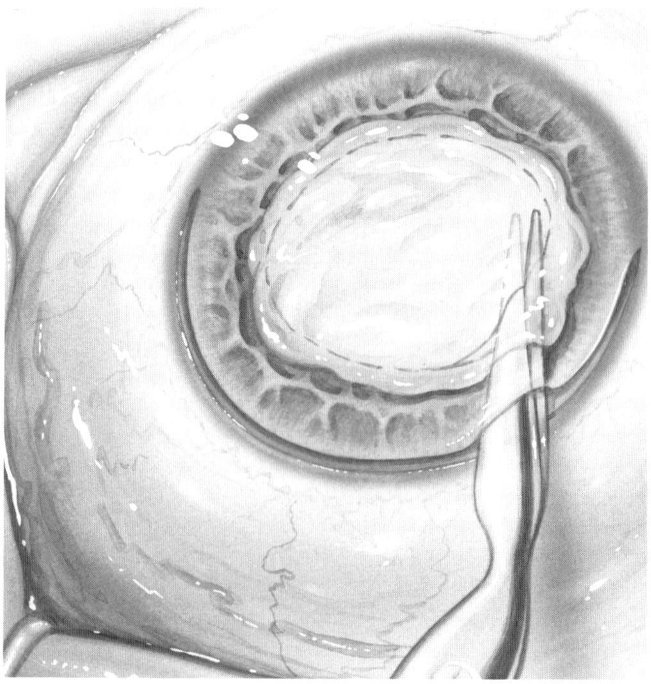

5.**47** An anterior capsulotomy is made using fine scissors after introduction of viscoelastic gel to protect the corneal endothelium. The lens nucleus can then be partially dislodged using saline or gel on a smooth needle.

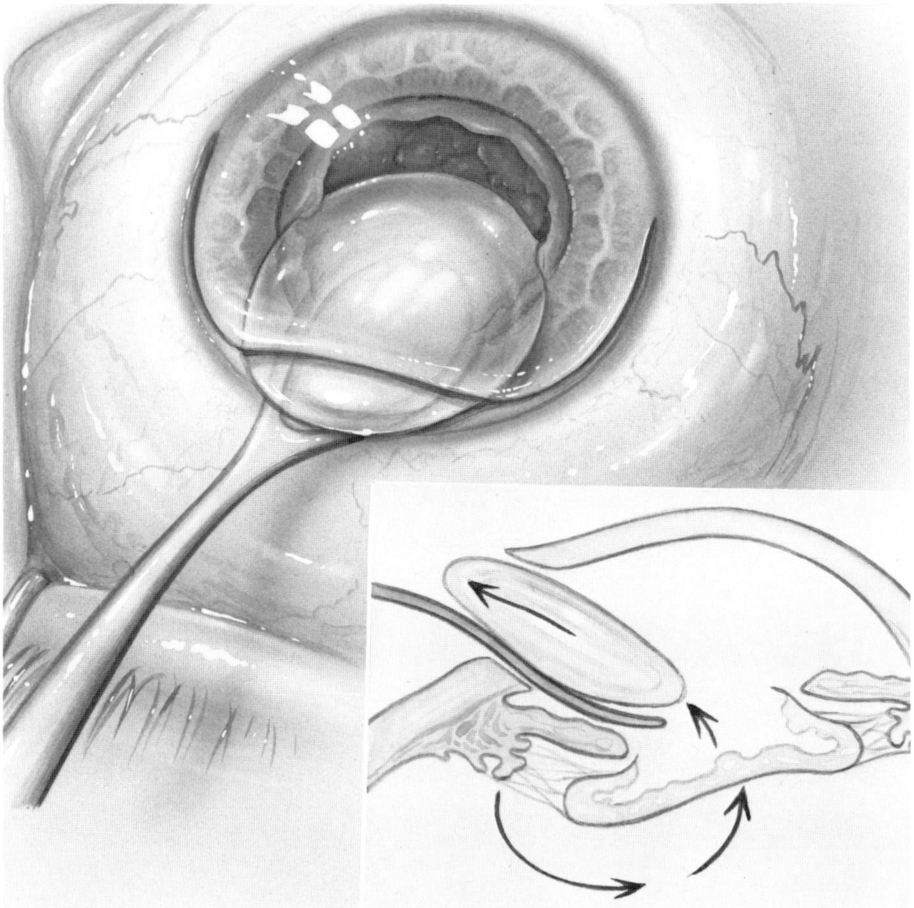

5.**48** An irrigating vectis spatula can be used to remove the lens nucleus. It may be necessary to apply pressure on the posterior wound margin and occasionally counterpressure at the inferior limbus.

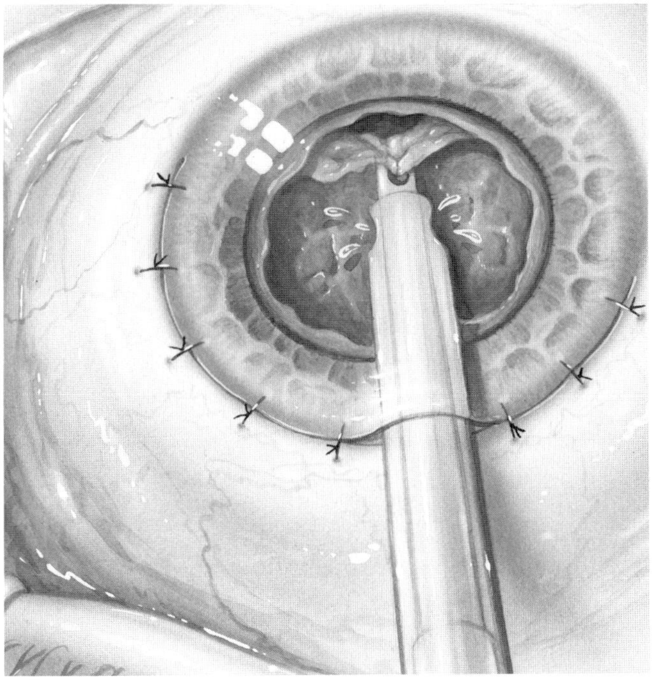

5.**49** The remaining lens cortex is removed using an irrigating-aspirating device in a "closed-system", with the wound partially sutured to create a deep anterior chamber during the procedure.

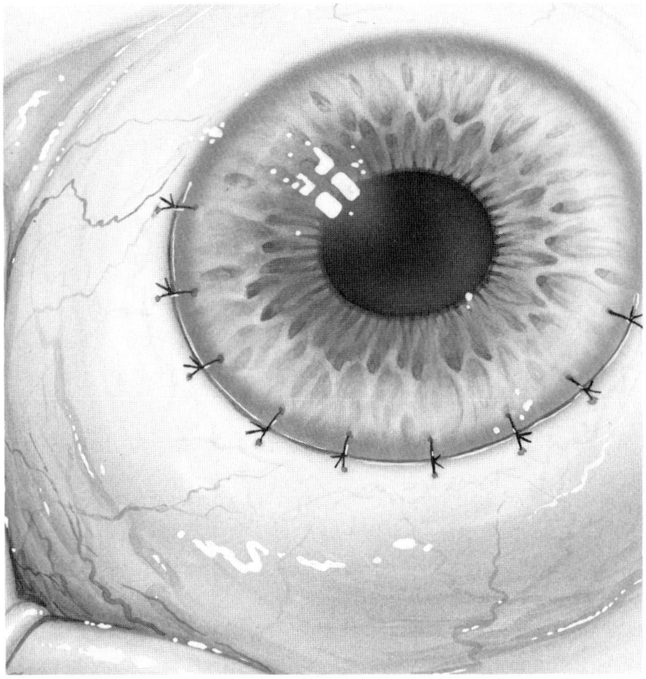

5.**50** An intact posterior capsule is desired in most cases of traumatic cataract. The aspiration port should thus face anteriorly during cortical clean-up.

51

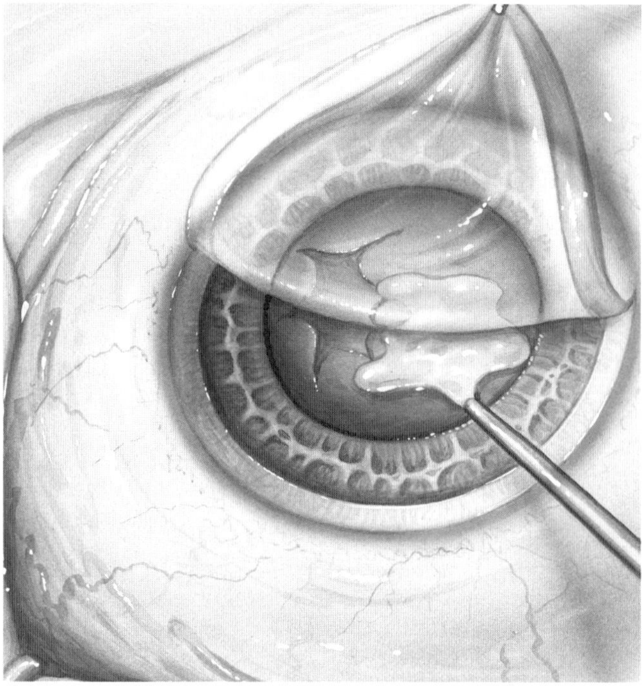

52

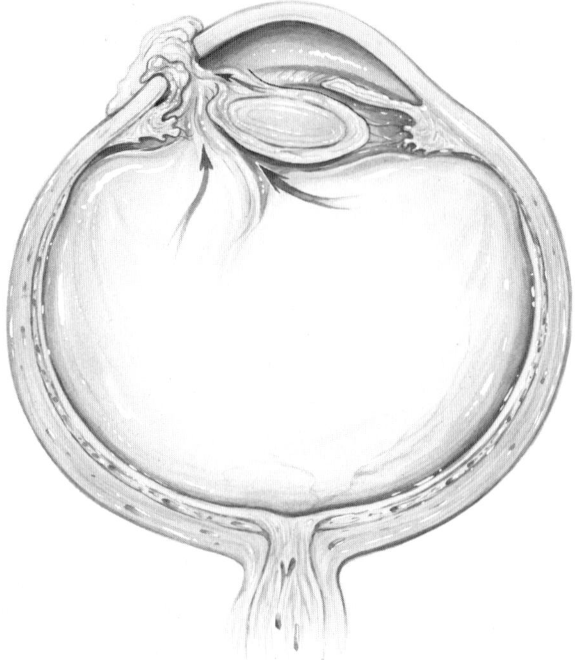

53

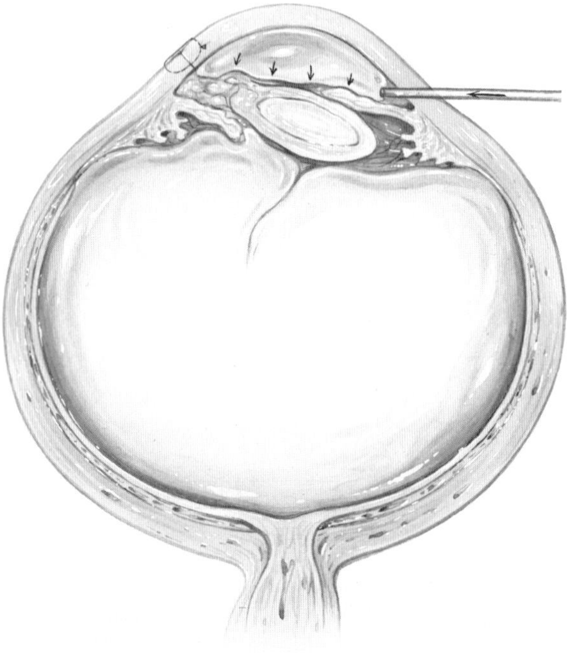

54

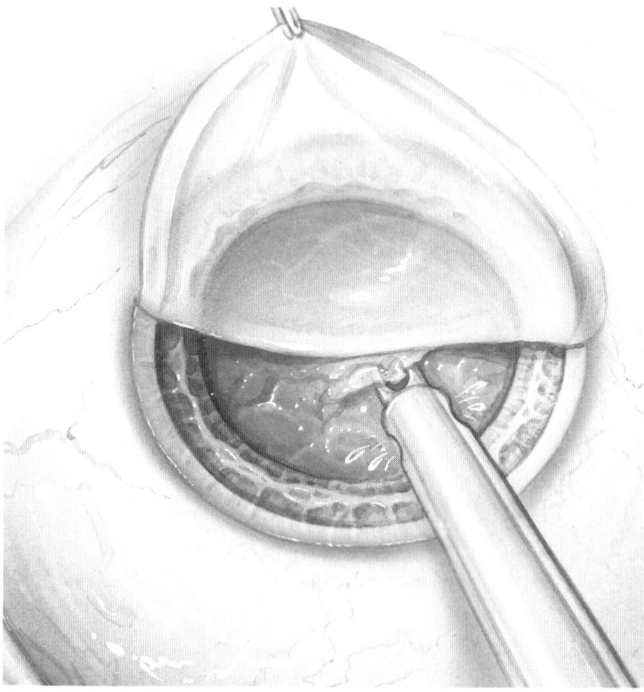

5.**51** If a relatively small rent is present in the posterior capsule, it is not always necessary to perform an anterior vitrectomy. By placing viscoelastic gel in the capsular bag at the end of the procedure and checking the wound after closure, it is usually possible to leave a capsular rent and avoid the complications of vitreous protrusion.

5.**52** When a laceration is present with extruded vitreous and traumatic cataract as well, however, it is necessary to perform a vitrectomy. It is preferable to remove the vitreous and lens material via a closed system.

5.**53** The laceration is sutured and the anterior chamber formed using air or gel. One can then enter the anterior chamber through the wound or a separate limbal incision for clean-up of lens material and vitreous.

5.**54** However, direct visualization is not always possible as the cornea may be opacified. In this circumstance it is necessary to retract the cornea and perform the procedure via an "open sky" technique. If there are not significant amounts of vitreous in the central anterior chamber, much of the lens material can be removed using an irrigation-aspiration unit.

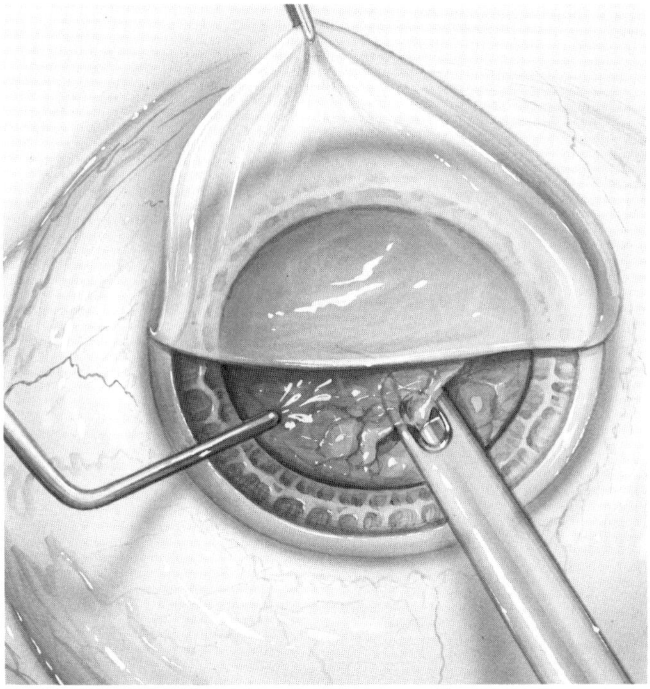

5.**55** However, often it is necessary to perform the entire procedure using a vitrectomy device. It may be necessary to have additional irrigation to maintain some chamber depth during the procedure. Care is taken not to excise iris when using the vitrectomy instrument. Again, the aspiration port should face anteriorly. One must also be careful in cases of trauma with associated severe inflammation, as dense fibrin may be adherent to the cornea. Gentle irrigation or aspiration should be used with care to avoid increased trauma to the endothelium. All of the anterior vitreous should be removed at the time of traumatic wound repair.

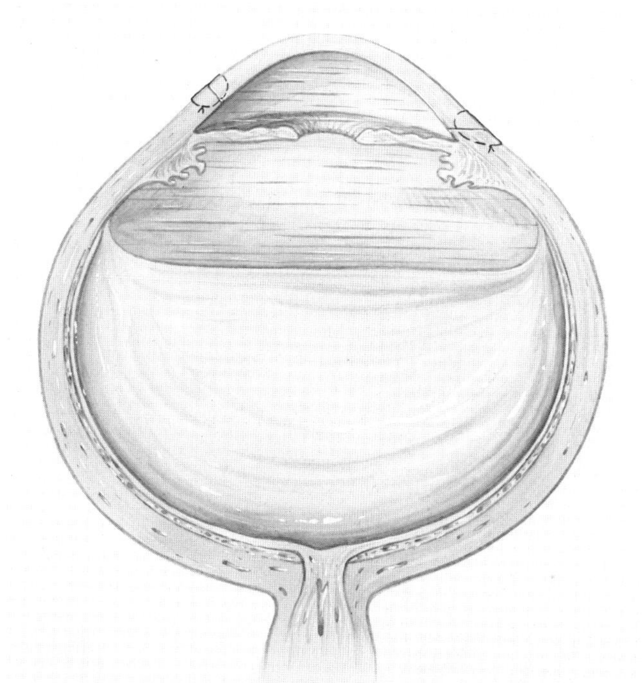

5.**56** With the vitrectomy device placed in the center of the pupil and very high suction settings avoided, the anterior vitreous can be removed while avoiding trauma to the posterior segment, especially the vitreous base where retinal tears are likely to occur with vitreous traction.

Uveal Prolapse

When presented with a corneoscleral wound with uveal prolapse, one must approach the question of uveal excision cautiously. In a severe wound it is occasionally necessary to remove not only the iris, but also portions of the ciliary body and ciliary processes. Blood and debris should be carefully irrigated from the wound, the possibility of retinal incarceration in the wound being borne in mind.

57

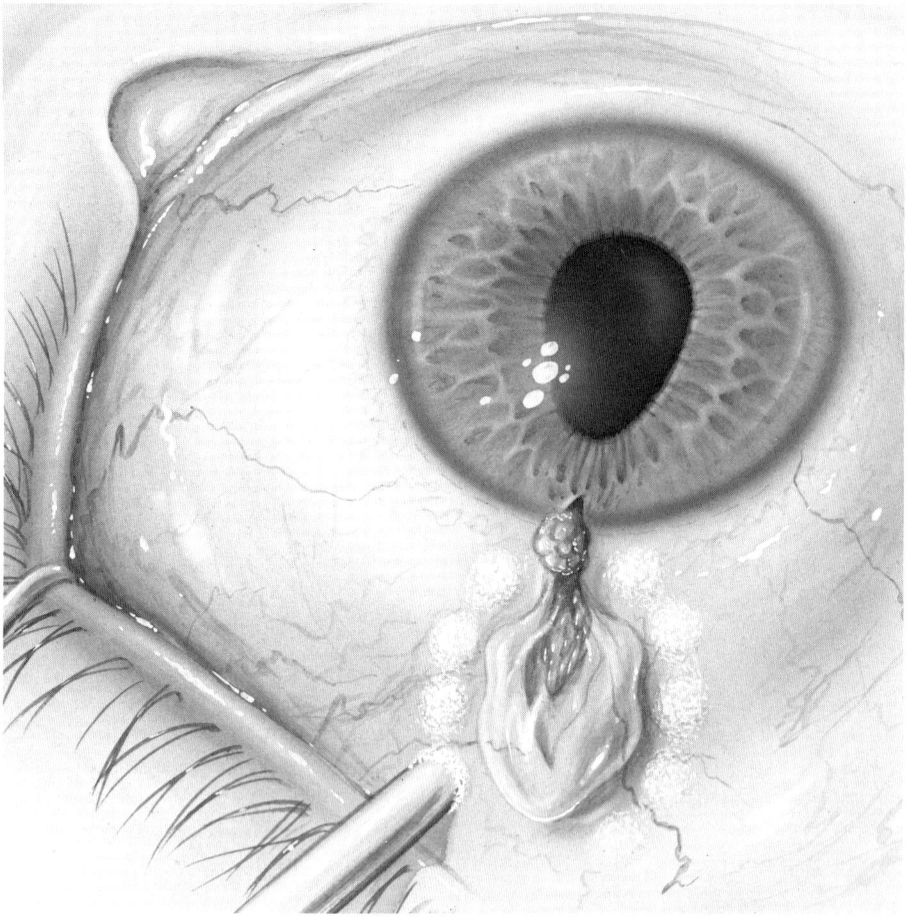

5.57 External vitreous should be removed and preparation made to create better exposure for surgical repair.

5.58 A limbal wound should be made and conjunctiva undermined and pulled from the wound site for better exposure and proper healing.

5.59 The prolapsed iris should be excised initially.

58

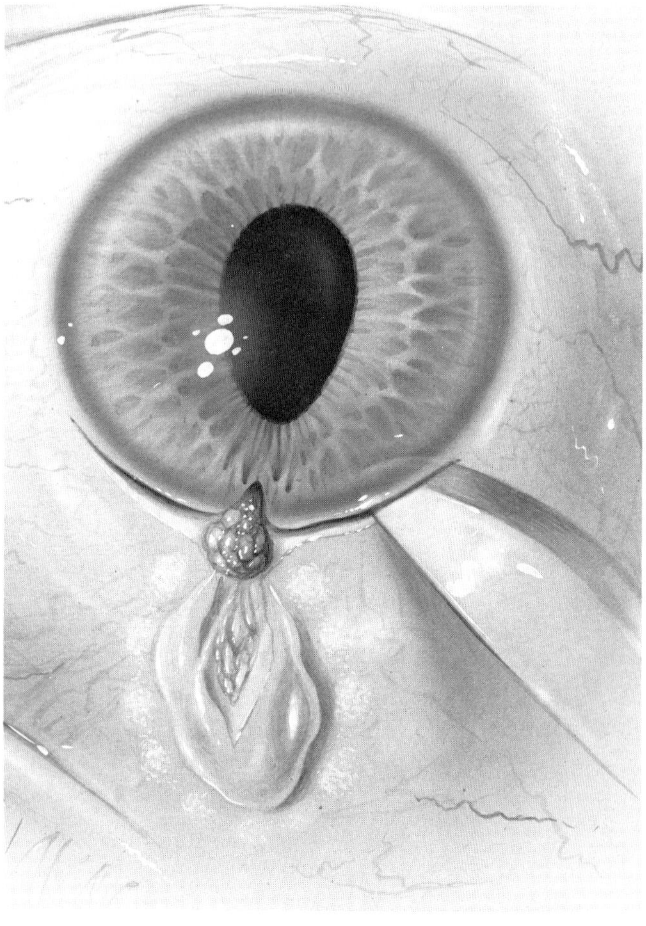

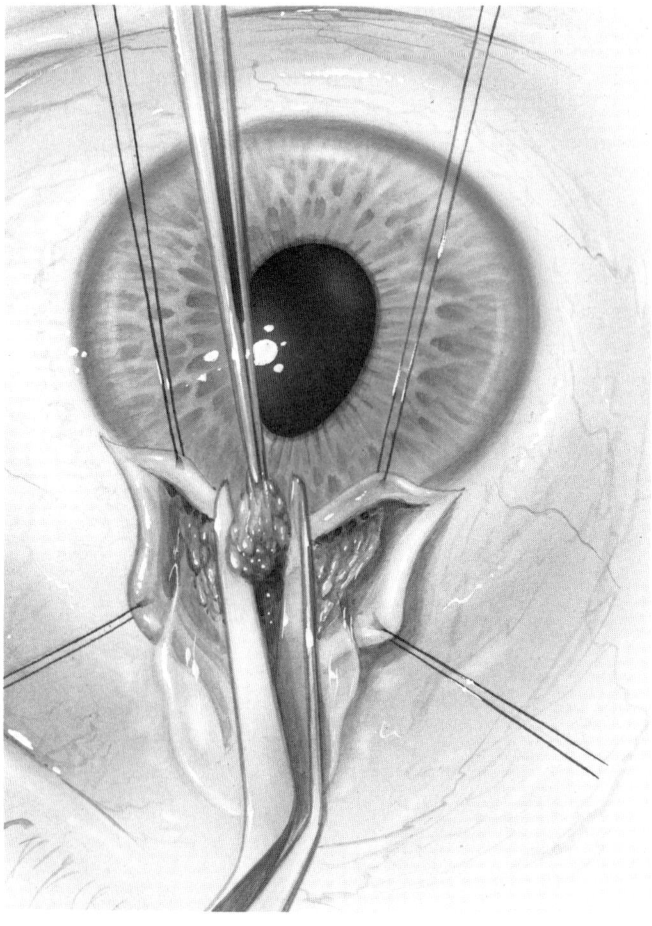

59

60

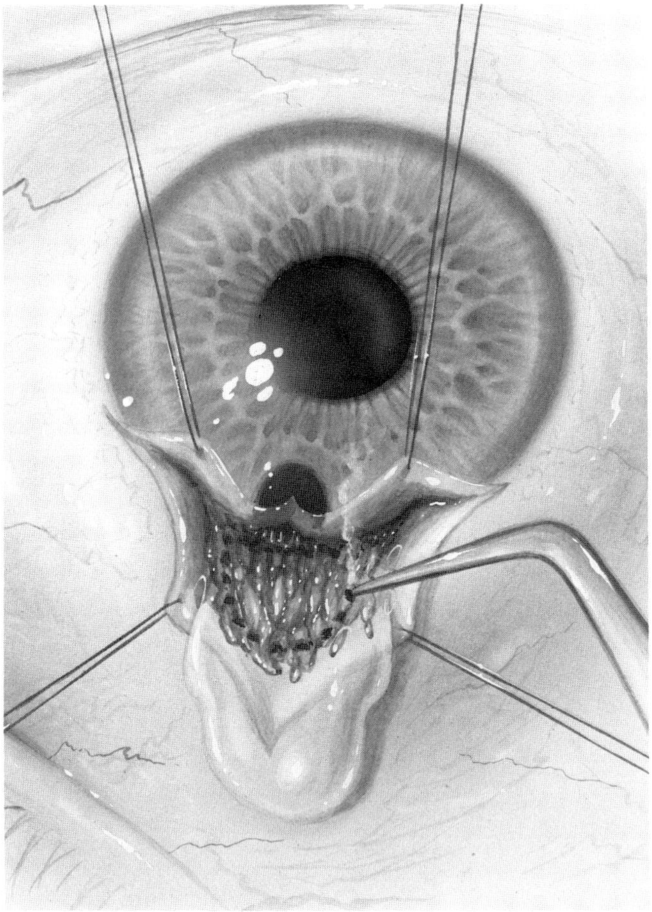

61

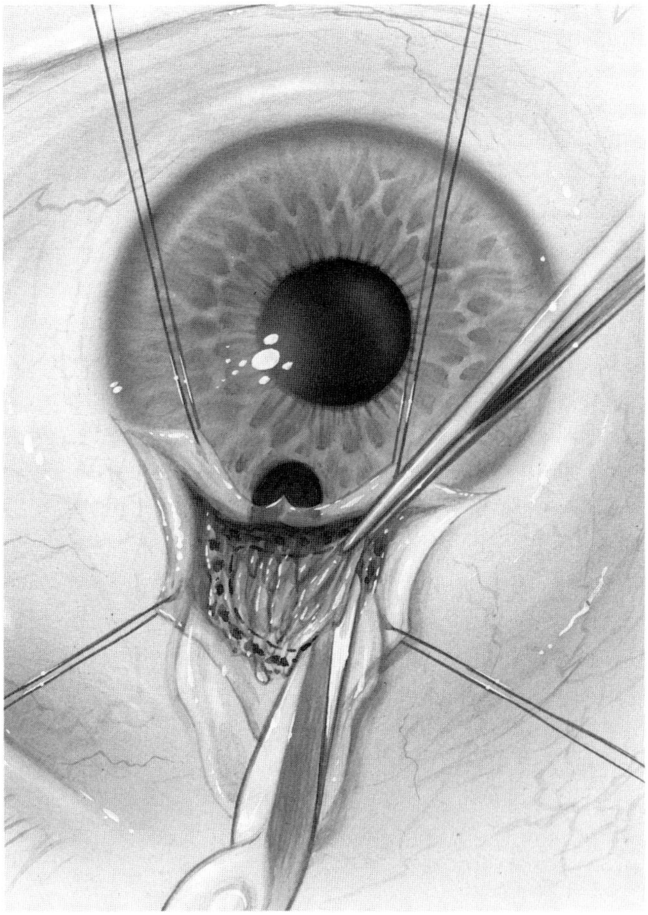

62

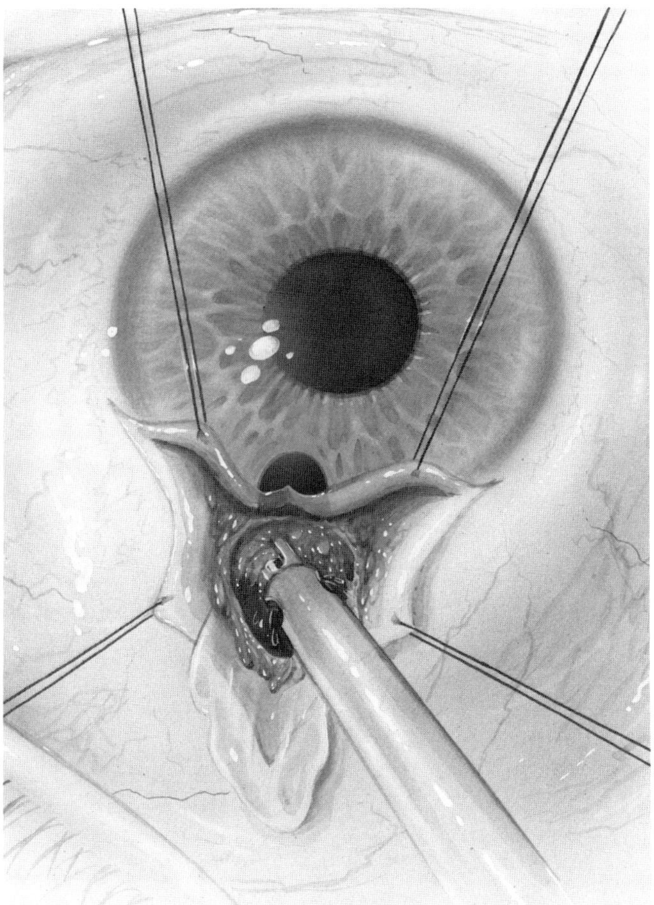

5.60 The ciliary processes and ciliary body should then be cauterized before incising to minimize the bleeding which can ensue.

5.61 The cyclectomy is then completed using delicate forceps and scissors inside the cautery areas.

5.62 A vitrectomy can then be performed through the cyclectomy site and, if necessary, lens material can also be removed. The deeper layers of the wound are closed first, beginning at the limbus. After wound closure, the adjacent peripheral retina should be treated with cryotherapy or diathermy.

Corneal Transplantation

5.**63** After initial repair of severe lacerations, it is sometimes advisable to perform corneal transplantation after acute injury. The corneal wound should be closed to allow formation of the anterior chamber and restore intraocular pressure.

5.**64** The eye is often soft, however, and standard trephination of the cornea may produce an irregular corneal host bed. In this situation, a suction trephine can be very useful. After placement of the trephine over the cornea, the plunger is depressed and pulled back to create a vacuum on the corneal surface. This maintains the shape of the host bed during trephination.

63

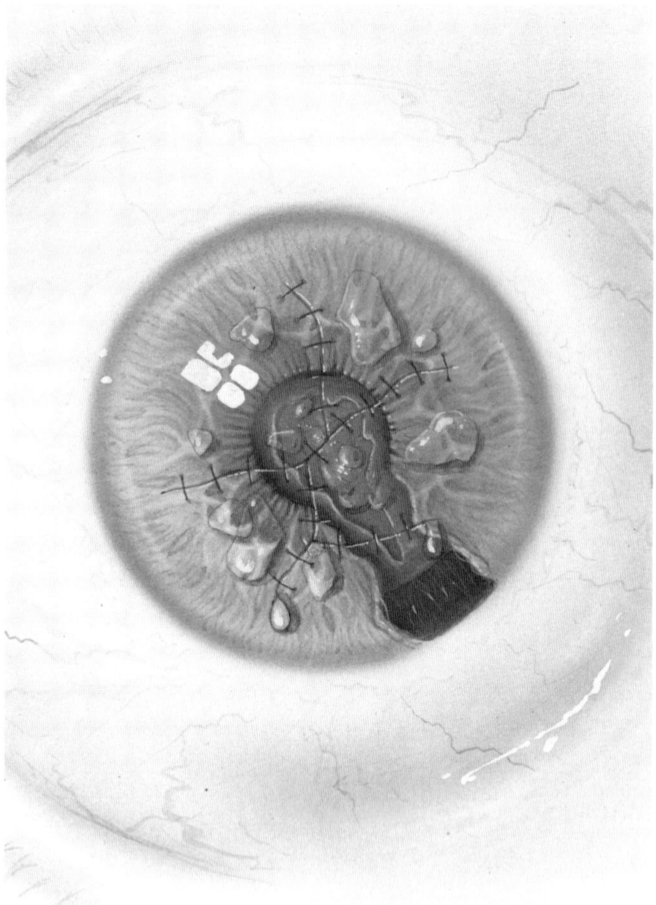

64

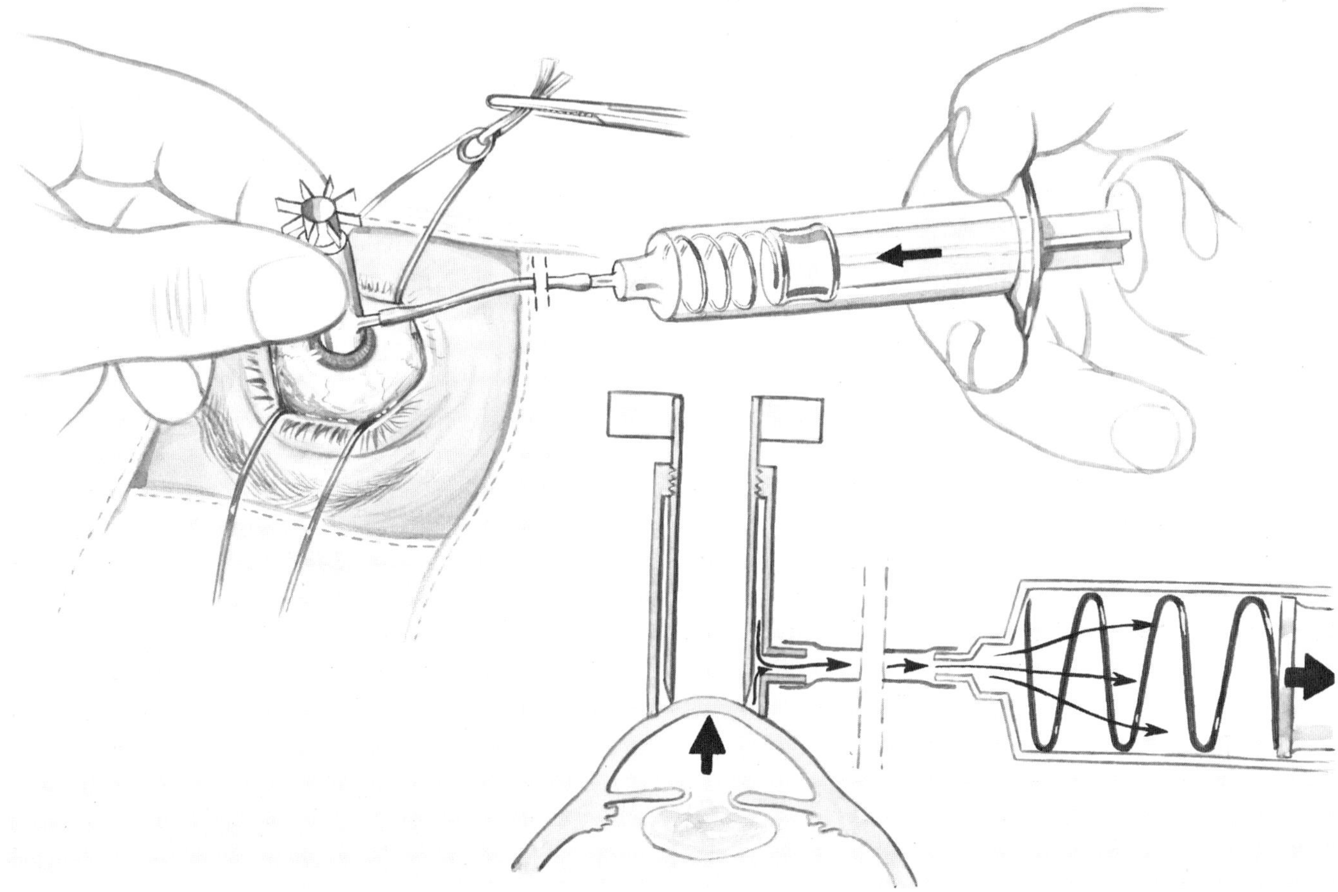

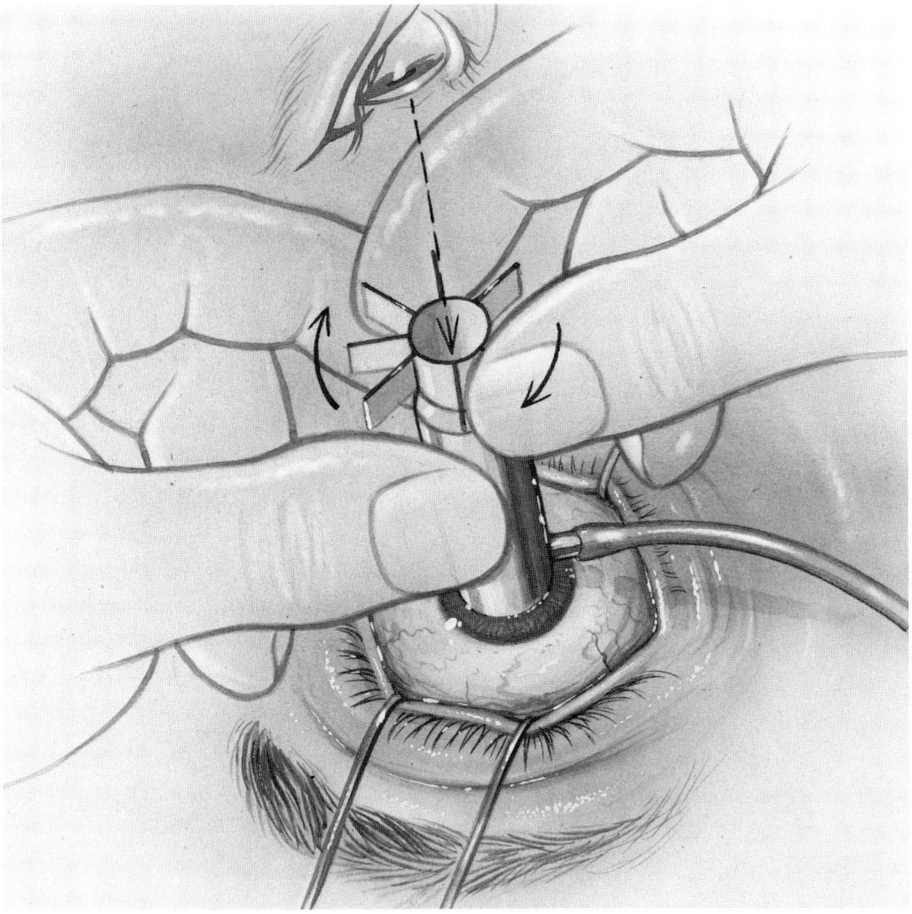

5.**65** The actual trephining can be observed directly through the hollow viewing port as the blade is lowered and rotated at the top of the trephine.

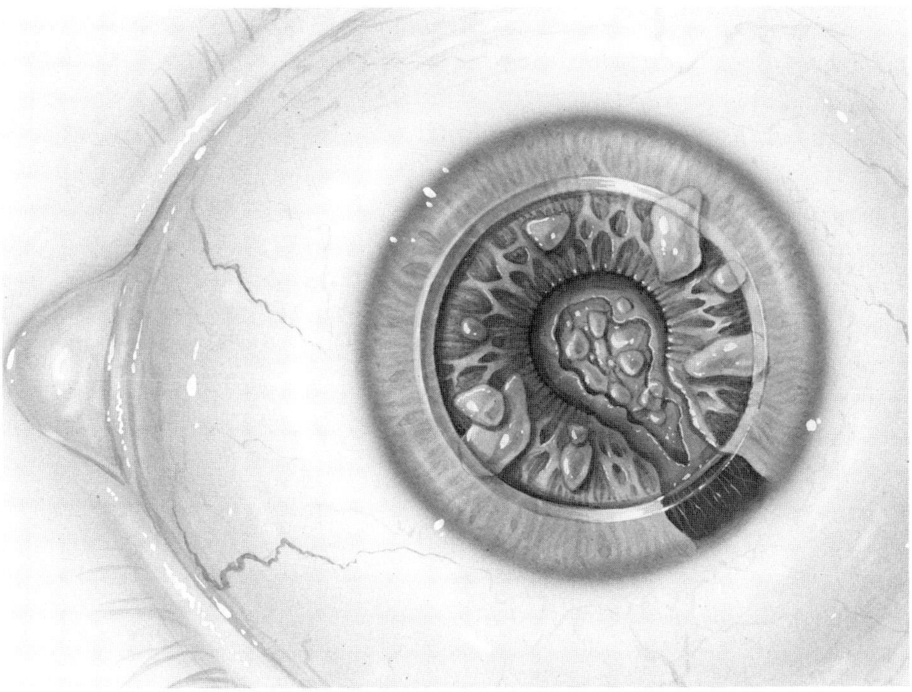

5.**66** Once the wound has been created, the chamber is entered with either the trephine or a fine blade, and the wound completed with curved corneal scissors. The trephine itself should not be used to complete the wound, to prevent damage to the iris.

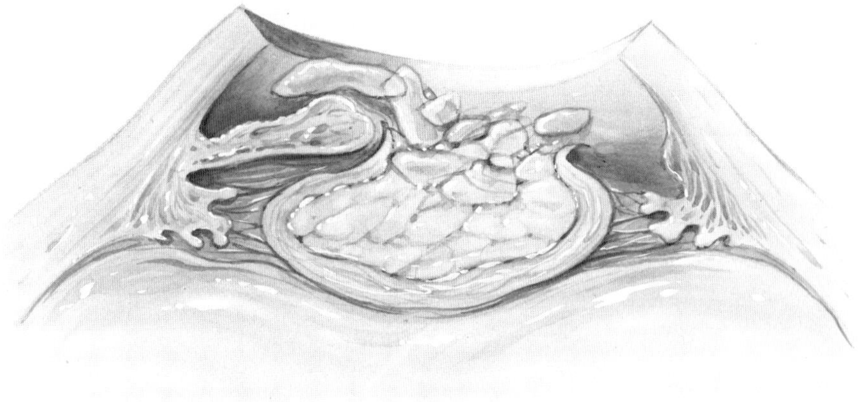

5.**67** Traumatic cataract may be found.

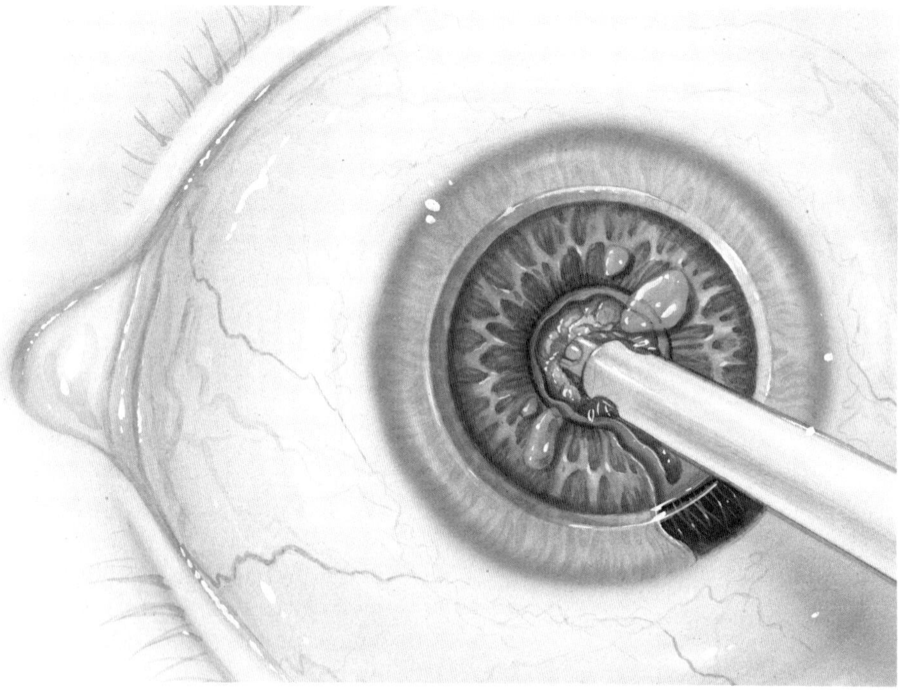

5.**68** The lens material can be removed via an "open sky" technique. As previously described, an anterior capsulotomy can most conveniently be done with scissors. In the open sky technique the lens nucleus is easily delivered after separation from the cortex, usually by means of an olive-tip cannula.

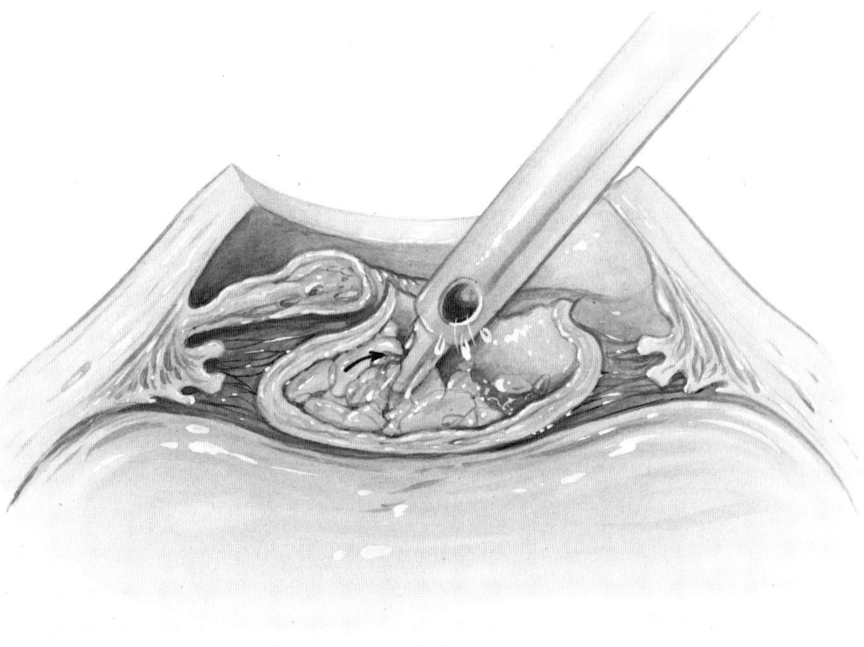

5.**69** Small portions of lens nucleus can be removed using the irrigation-aspiration device.

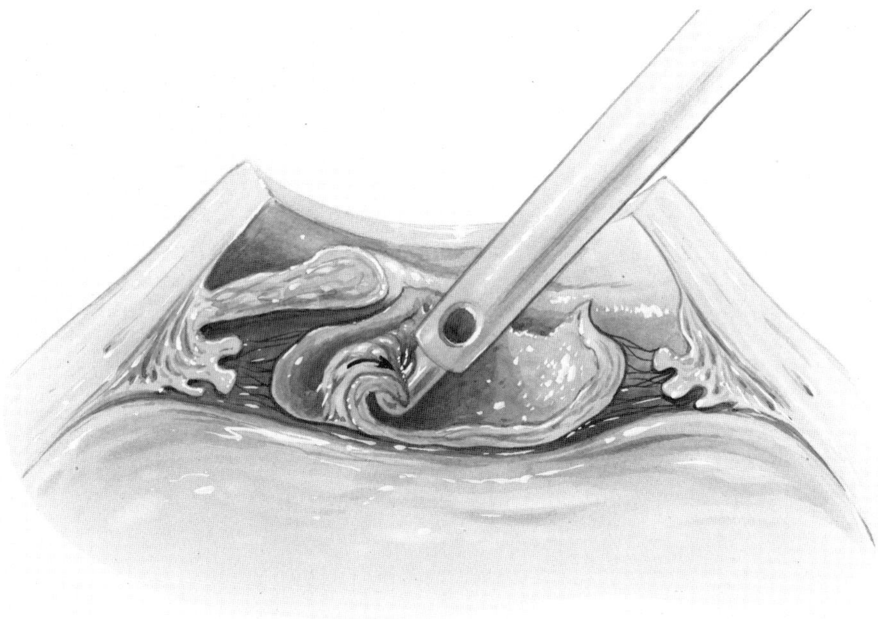

5.70 The cortex is then cleaned up. As in a standard operation, the lens cortex should be peeled from the capsule sulcus and brought into the central pupil when aspirated. The lens capsule can be polished using a polishing device or can be vacuumed using mild suction with the irrigation-aspiration instrument. It is important to have profuse irrigation when using this device so as not to aspirate the posterior lens capsule.

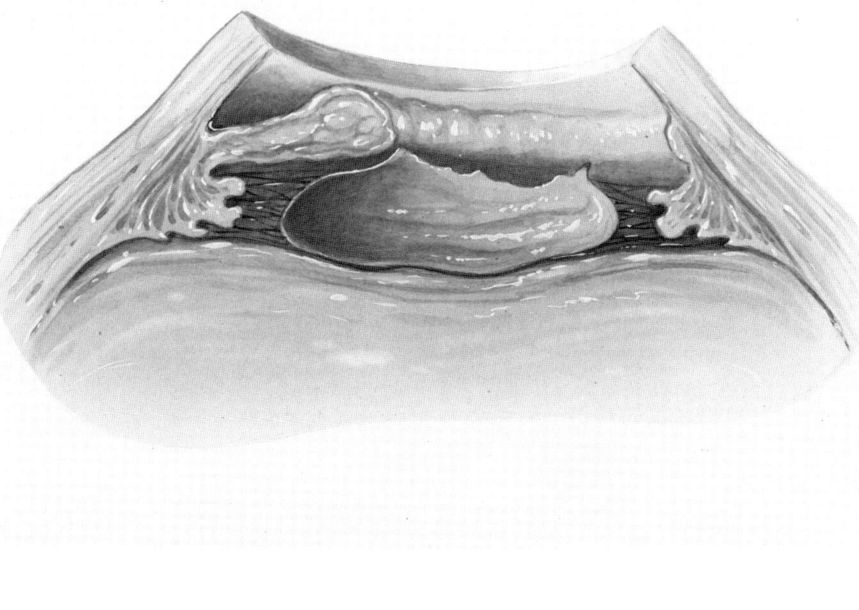

5.71 Preservation of an intact posterior lens capsule may prevent posterior segment disease in the long run. If one can avoid disrupting the vitreous, there is a lower incidence of these complications.

72

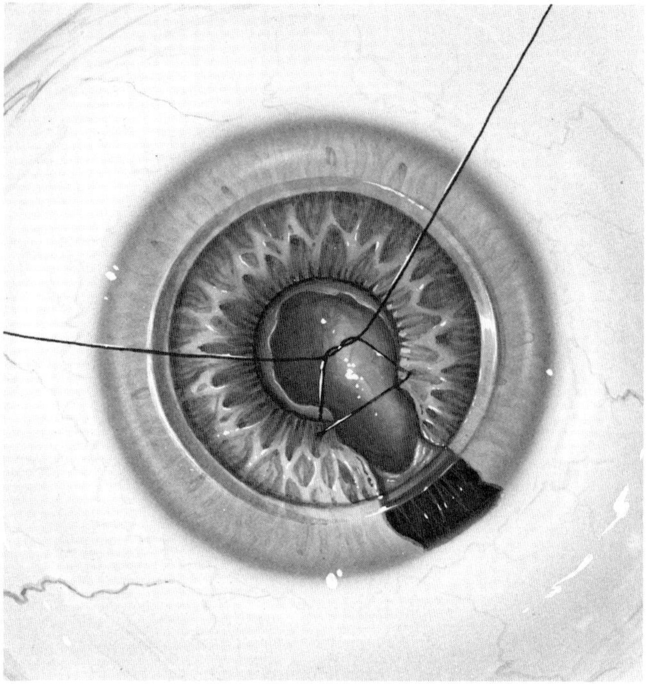

73

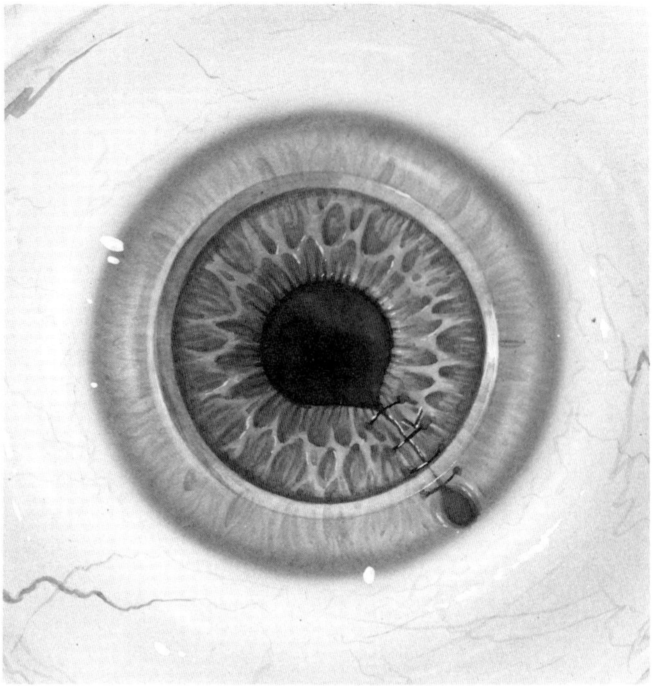

74

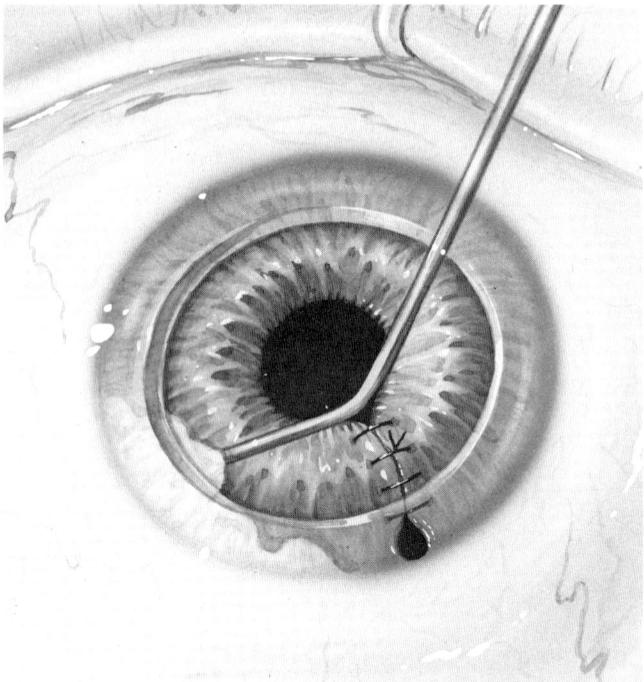

5.**72** In the case of a traumatic sector iridectomy, it may be useful to suture the iris. Nylon suture (10-0) may be used to form the pupil margin with the first suture.

5.**73** After suturing, the iris remains on a level plane, lowering the risk of subsequent peripheral anterior synechiae.

5.**74** and **75** Viscoelastic gel can then be used to form the peripheral anterior chamber.

75

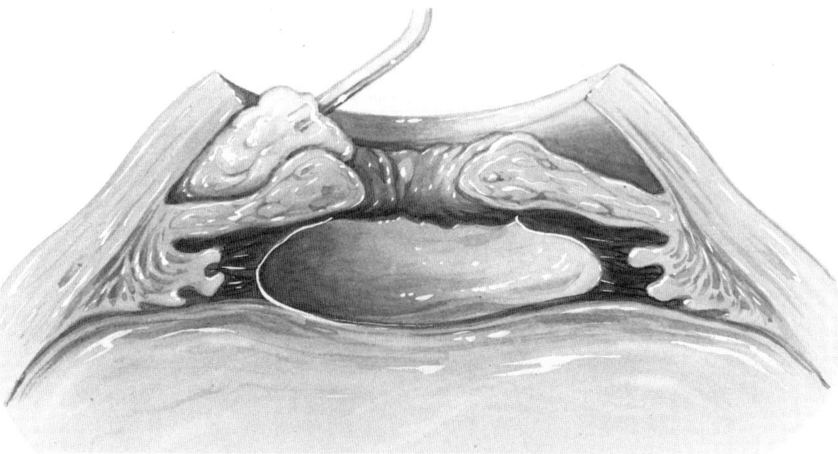

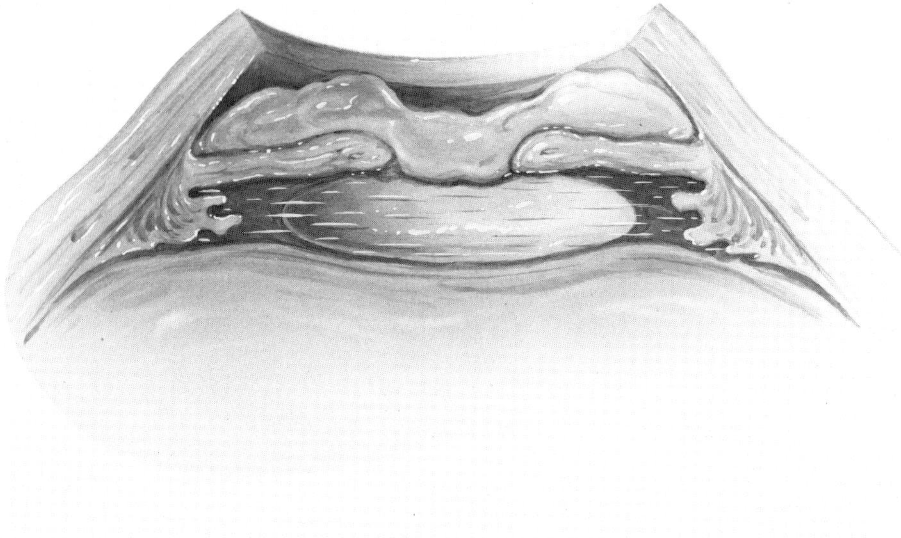

5.**76** A layer of gel will protect the corneal endothelium and keep the chamber formed during suturing.

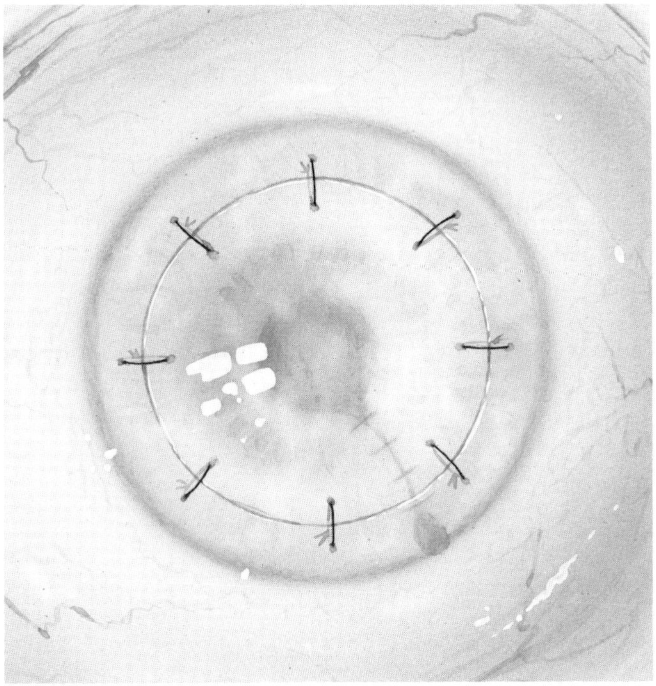

5.**77** Interrupted sutures can then be placed with buried knots.

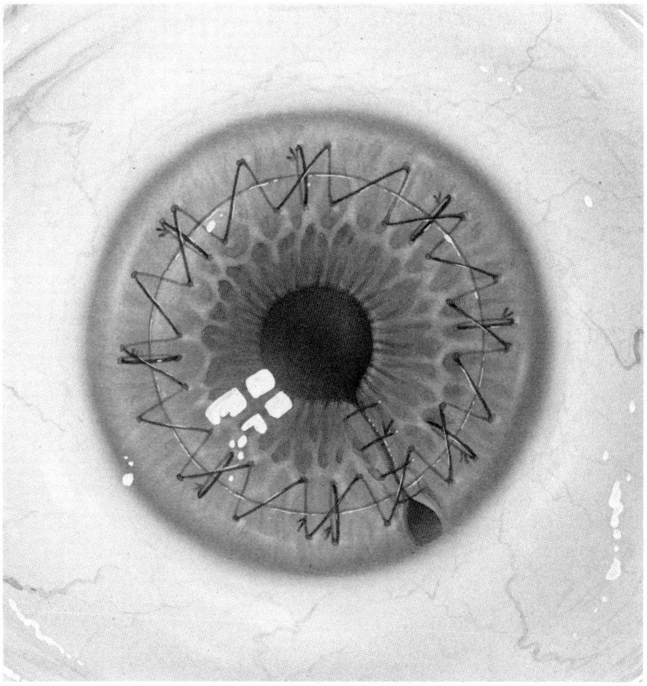

5.**78** A running suture is placed in addition to the interrupted sutures.

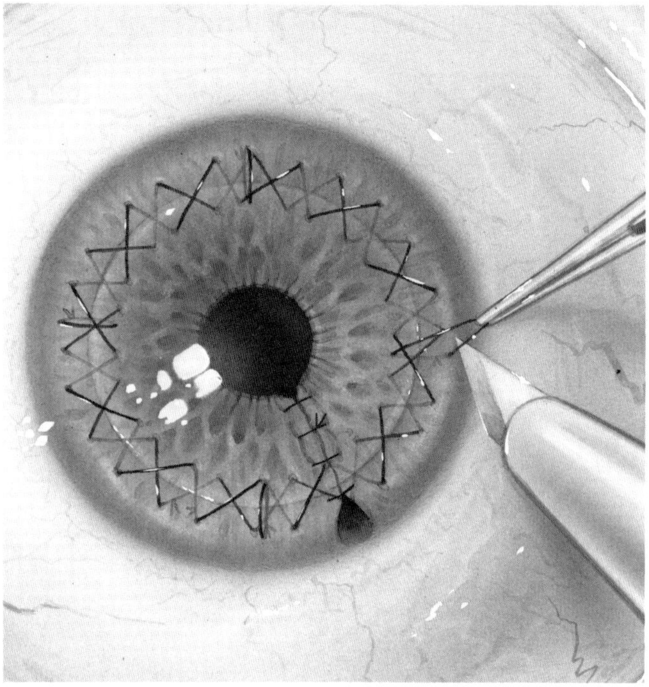

5.**79** A double running suture can then be accurately positioned and the interrupted sutures removed.

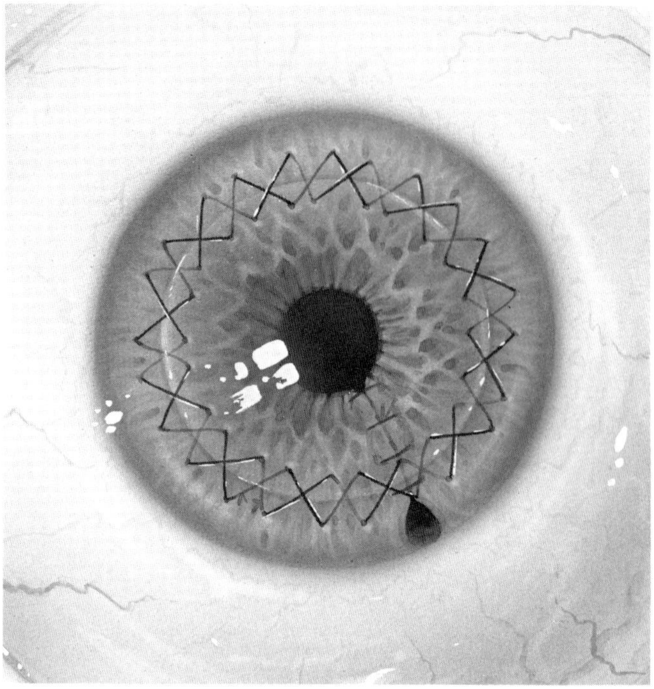

5.**80** The final suture pattern is shown.

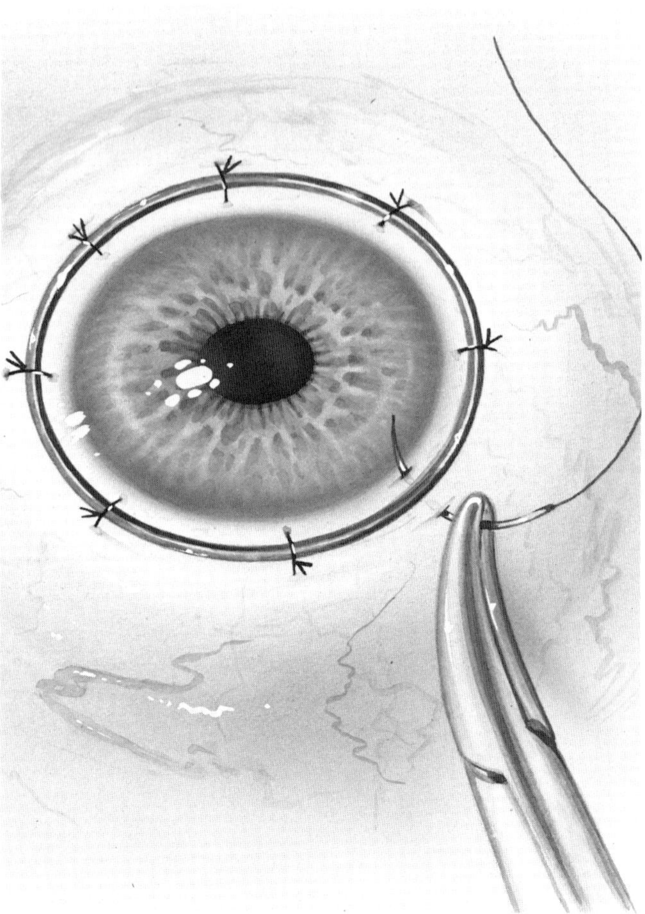

5.**81** Although it is not mandatory, a metal support ring can be used during penetrating keratoplasty for trauma. Interrupted sutures on a cutting needle (e.g., 7-0 vicryl) are used to secure the ring, which should be 3-4 mm greater in diameter than the cornea. The sutures are placed through episclera and superficial sclera for secure fixation.

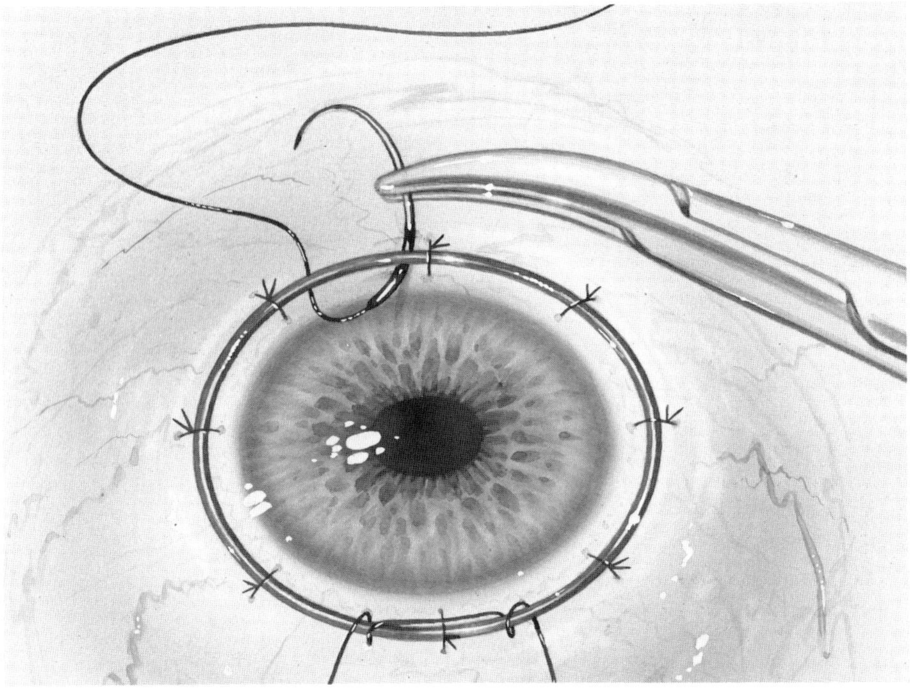

5.**82** A 4-0 silk suture is passed beneath the ring at the 6 and 12 o'clock positions. The needle is passed under the ring in a reverse direction on either side of the interrupted suture to provide support and exposure. A scleral support ring can be useful in many cases of anterior segment trauma and should be seriously considered when performing penetrating keratoplasty on an aphakic patient. It is most useful in cases where vitreous loss is present as in the following circumstances.

If the vitreous is present with lens material, it is advisable to use a vitreous cutting and aspiration device through the "open sky" wound. The lens material should be removed first so as to prevent lens remnants from sinking posteriorly.

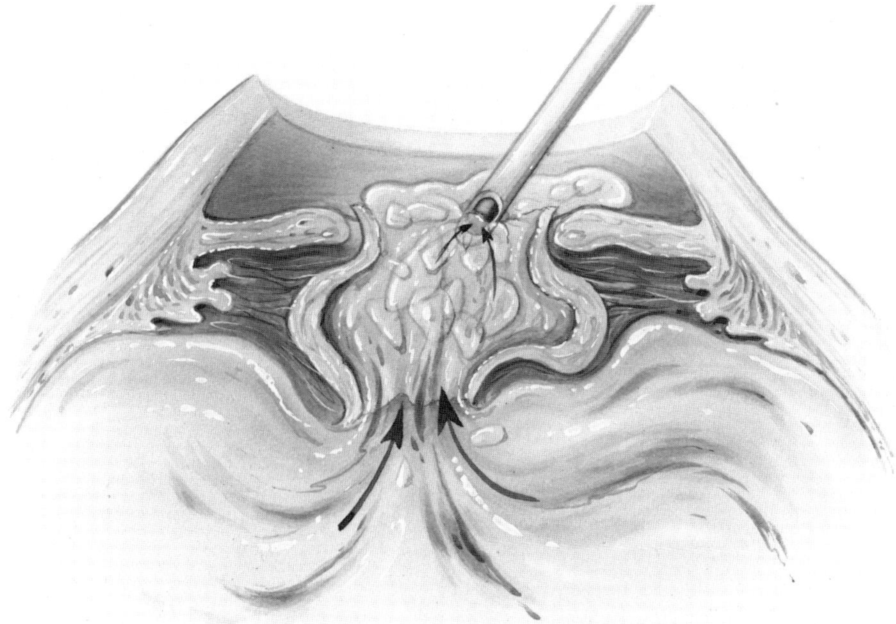

5.**83** The tip of the device should be kept in the center of the pupil as much as possible to avoid excessive peripheral vitreous traction. If a large amount of lens material is present posteriorly, a pars plana vitrectomy is the best approach.

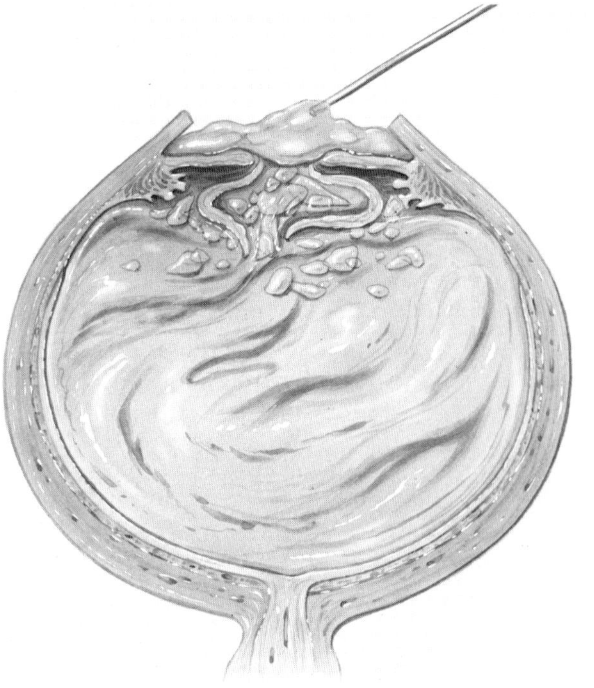

5.**84** The anterior chamber is filled with viscoelastic gel before placement of the donor button.

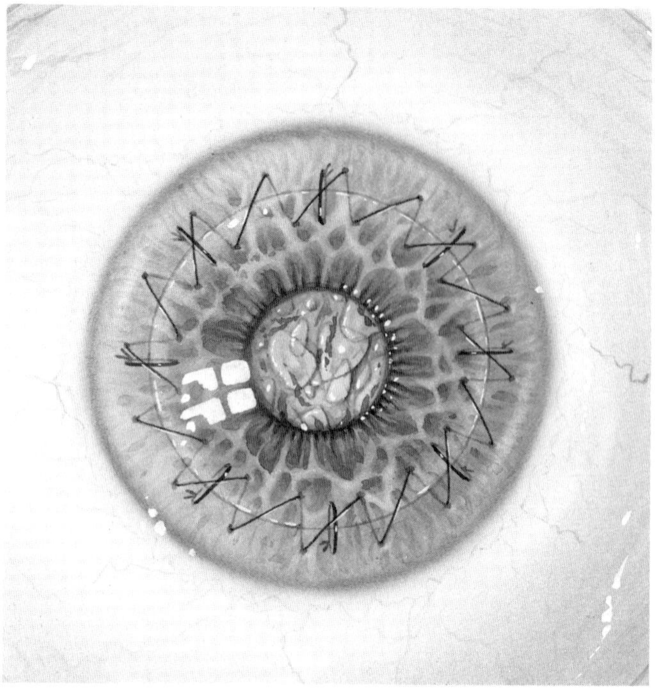

5.**85** The corneal graft is sutured in place as described previously.

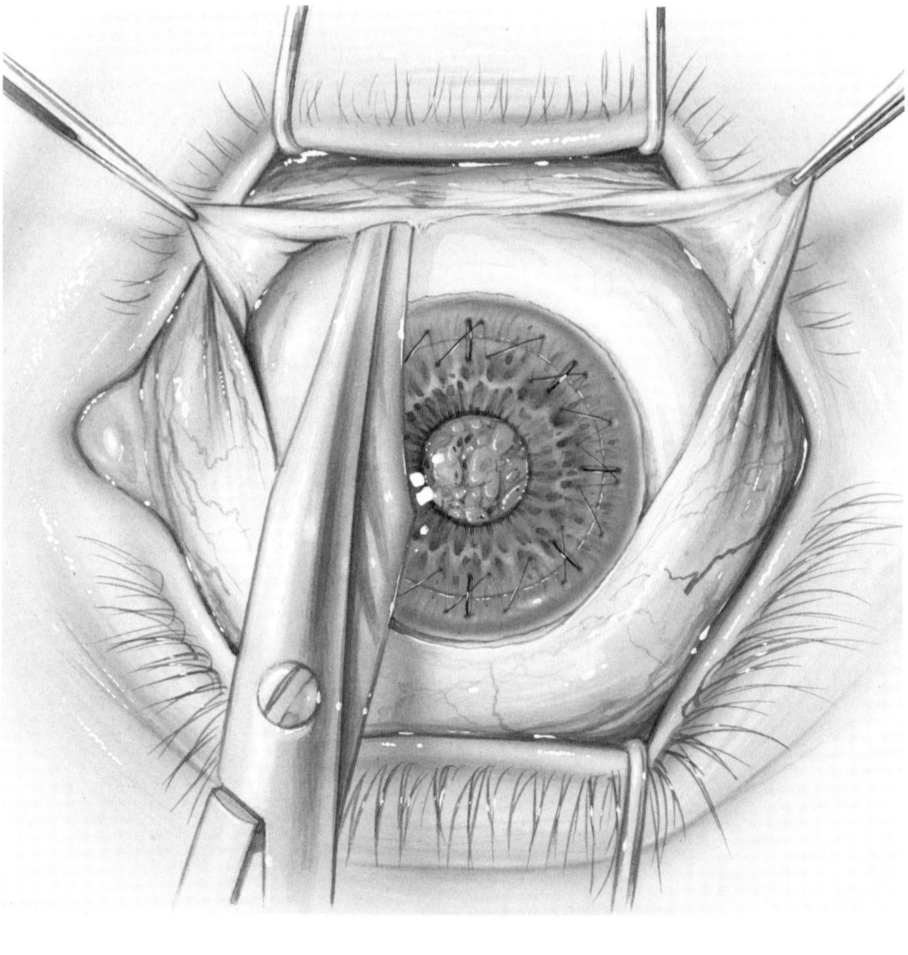

5.**86** The conjunctiva is retracted after a 360 degree peritomy.

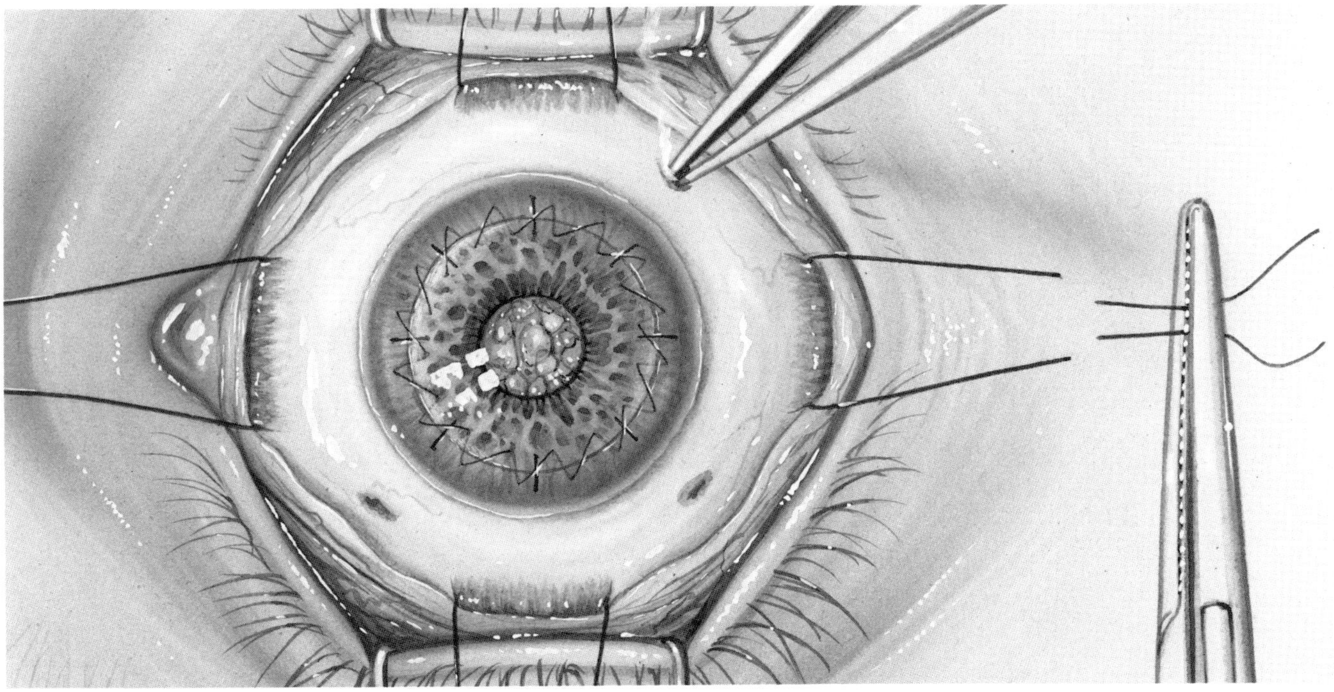

5.**87** Silk sutures are placed beneath the rectus muscles for traction and support. The pars plana is then marked using cautery 3.5 mm posterior to the limbus in three quadrants.

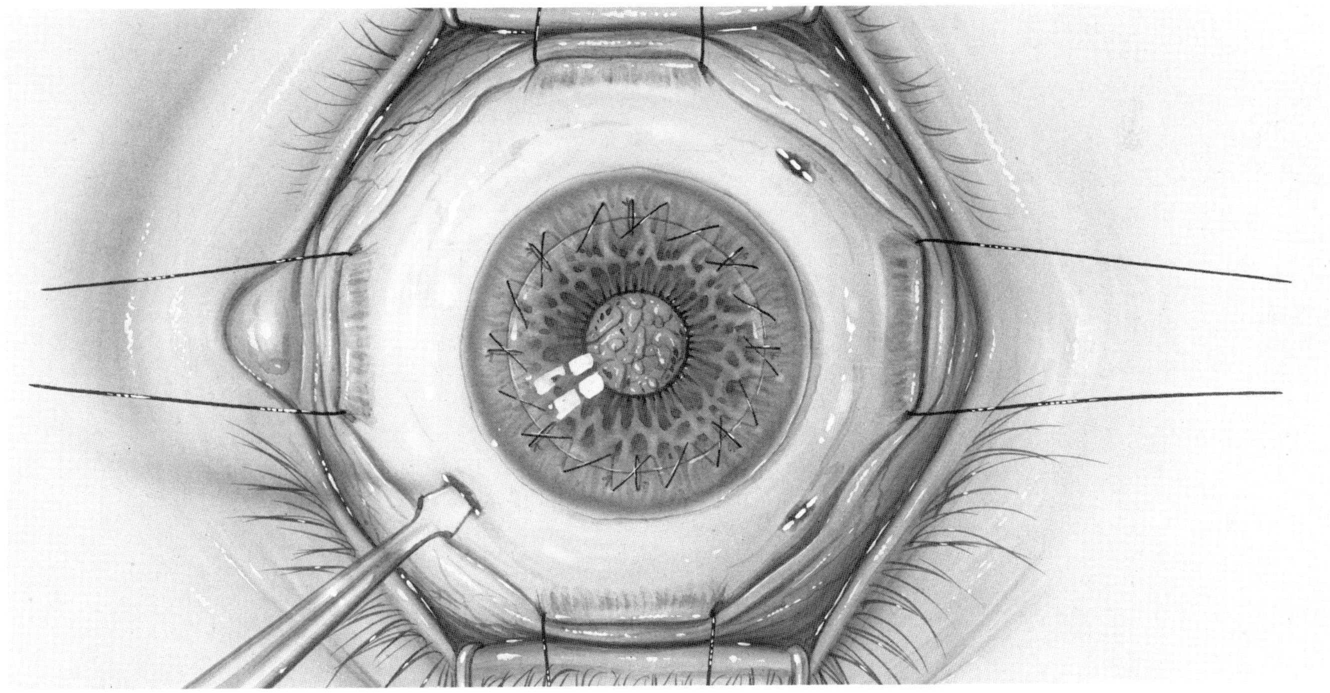

5.**88** A myringotomy blade is used to enter the sclera.

89

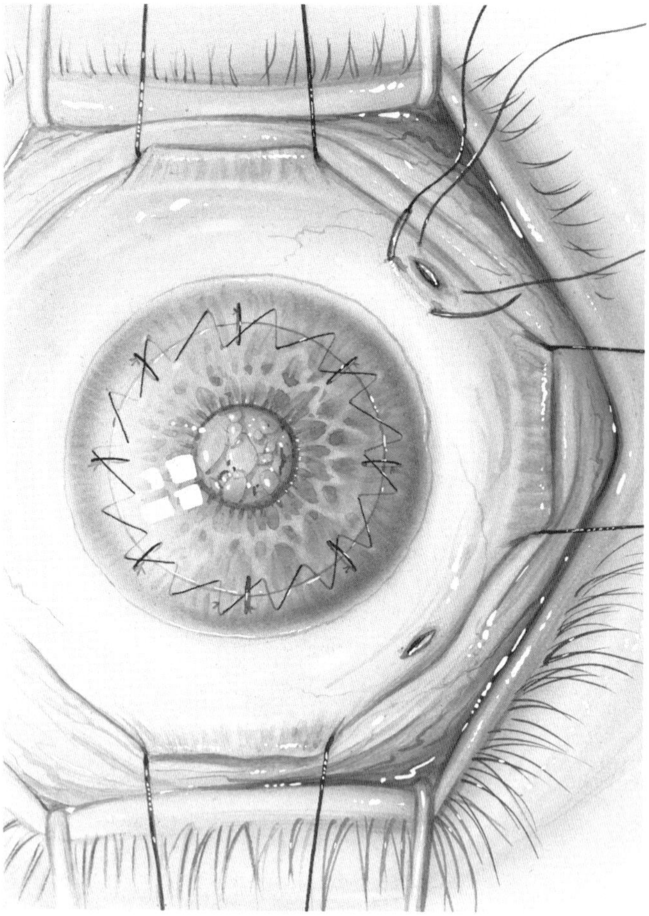

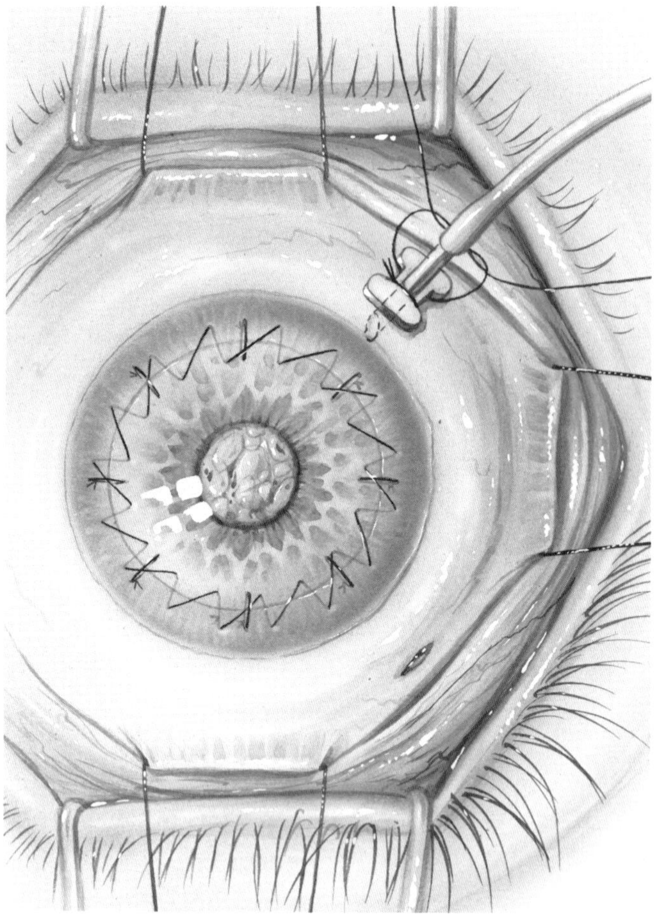

90

91

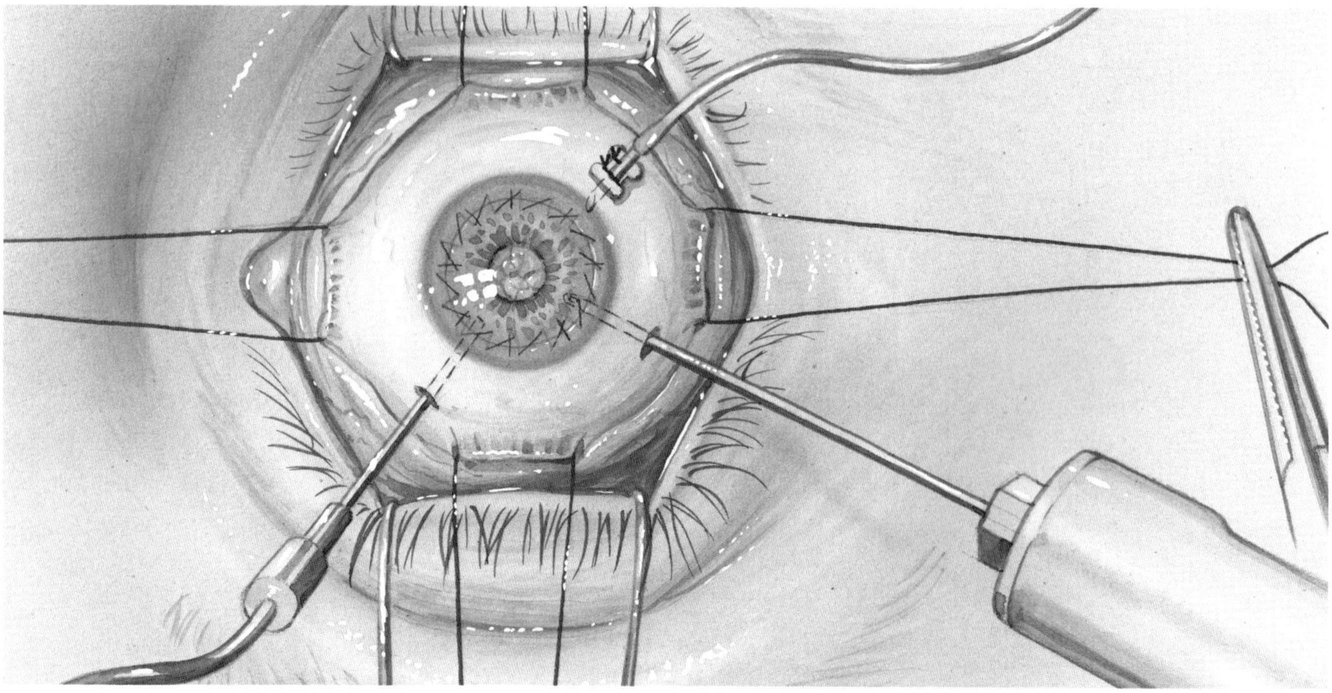

5.**89** A 5-0 mersilene suture is then placed in a mattress fashion over the inferior entry site for placement of the infusion cannula.

5.**90** The cannula infusion is not turned on until this suture, which will be temporary, is secured.

5.**91** The two superior wound sites are used for the fiberoptic illuminating instrument and the vitreous aspiration unit.

92

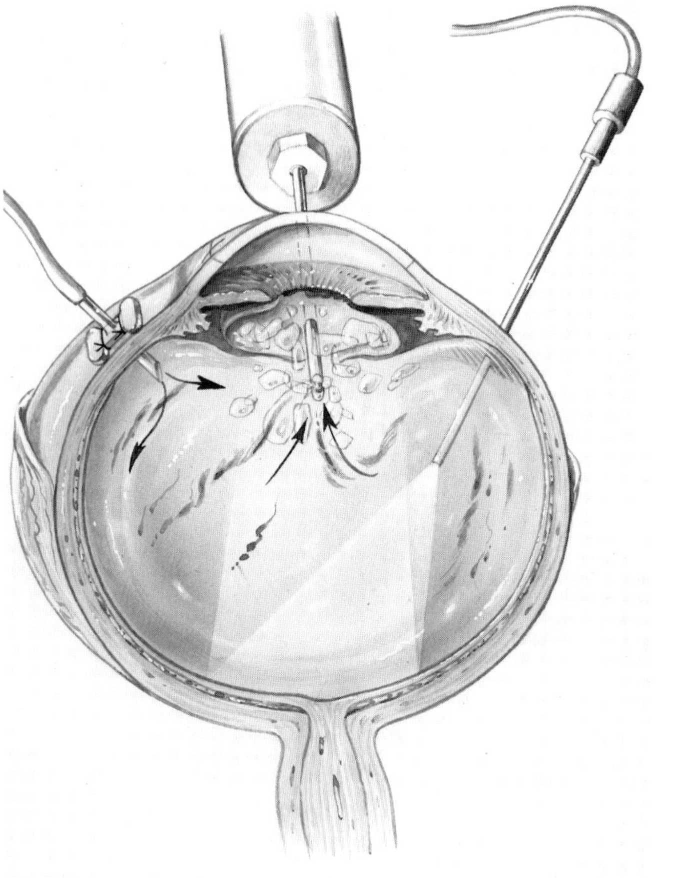

93

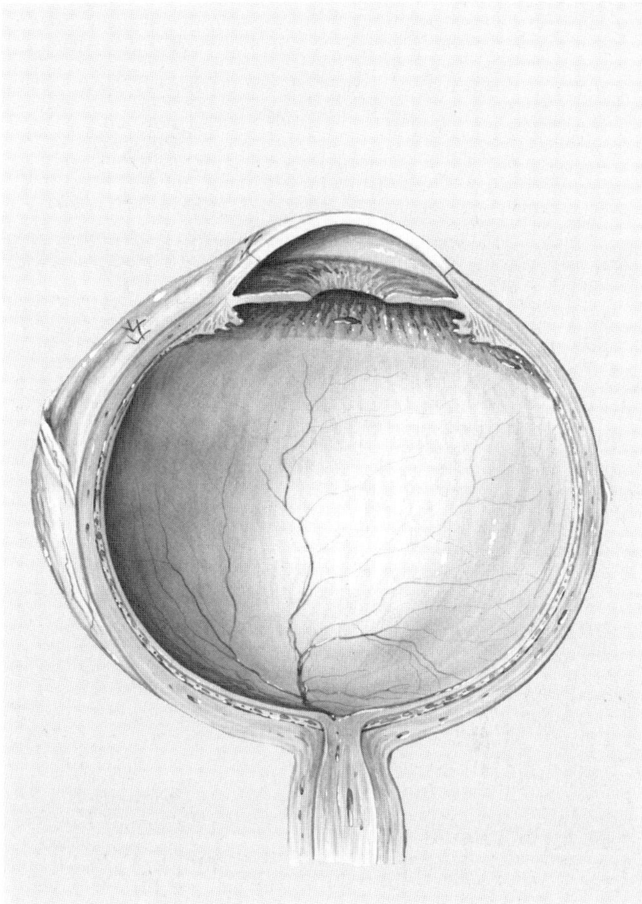

94

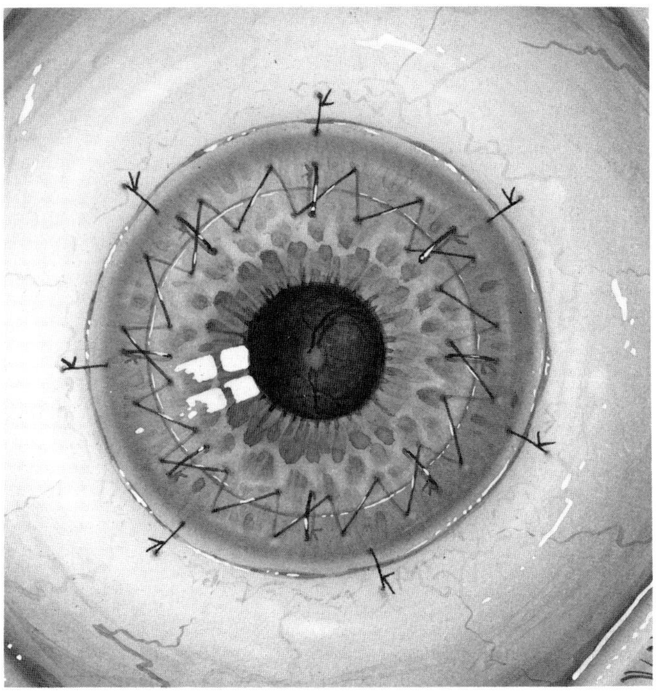

5.**92** In cases of trauma, the initial portion of the procedure may be poorly visualized and the aspiration unit should be kept anterior and towards the center of the pupil. The suction setting should not be too high so as to avoid traction on the vitreous base.

5.**93** It is not necessary to spare the posterior lens capsule, and the majority of the vitreous may be removed at this time. A contact lens with irrigation may be used during surgery to remove posterior vitreous and lens fragments. One should refer to the chapter on vitreous surgery regarding the use of gas-fluid exchange. The instrument entry sites are closed with nylon suture, with the infusion cannula the last to be removed; the infusion is shut off prior to removing the cannula.

5.**94** The conjunctiva is then closed in an interrupted fashion.

Lamellar Corneoscleral Graft

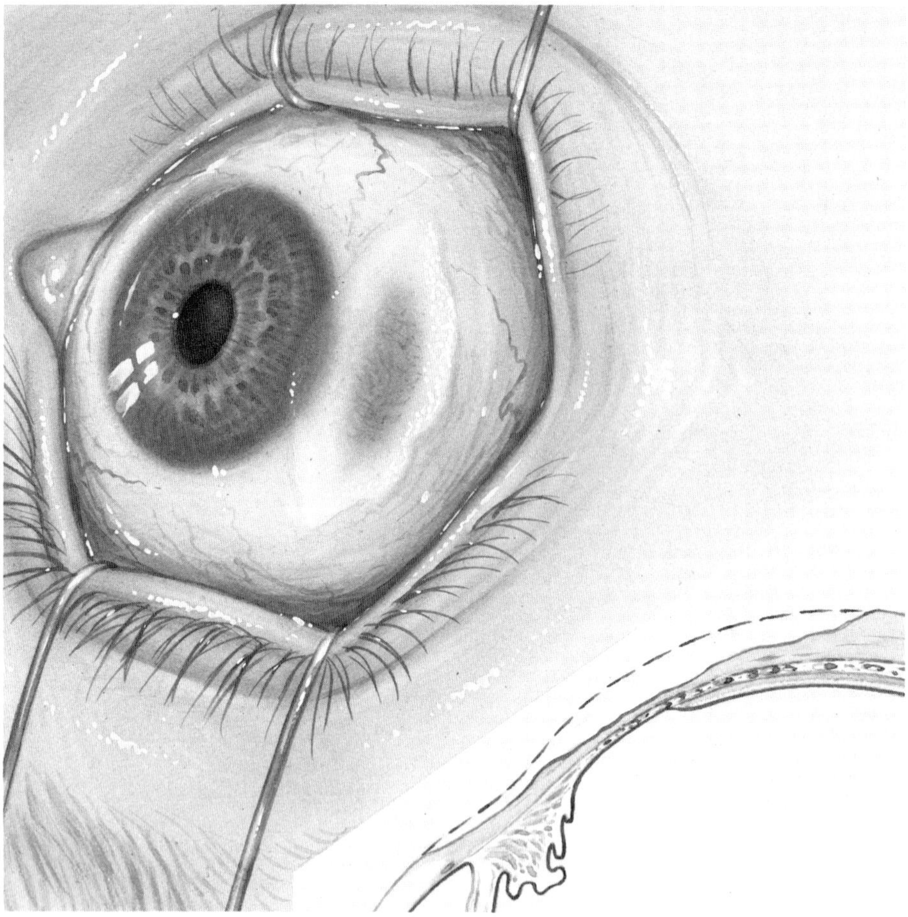

5.**95** Extensive loss of scleral tissue can also occur after trauma. A thin sclera with uveal bulge and ectasia may lead to severe consequences, the least of which is marked astigmatism. The entire area must be reinforced and stabilized.

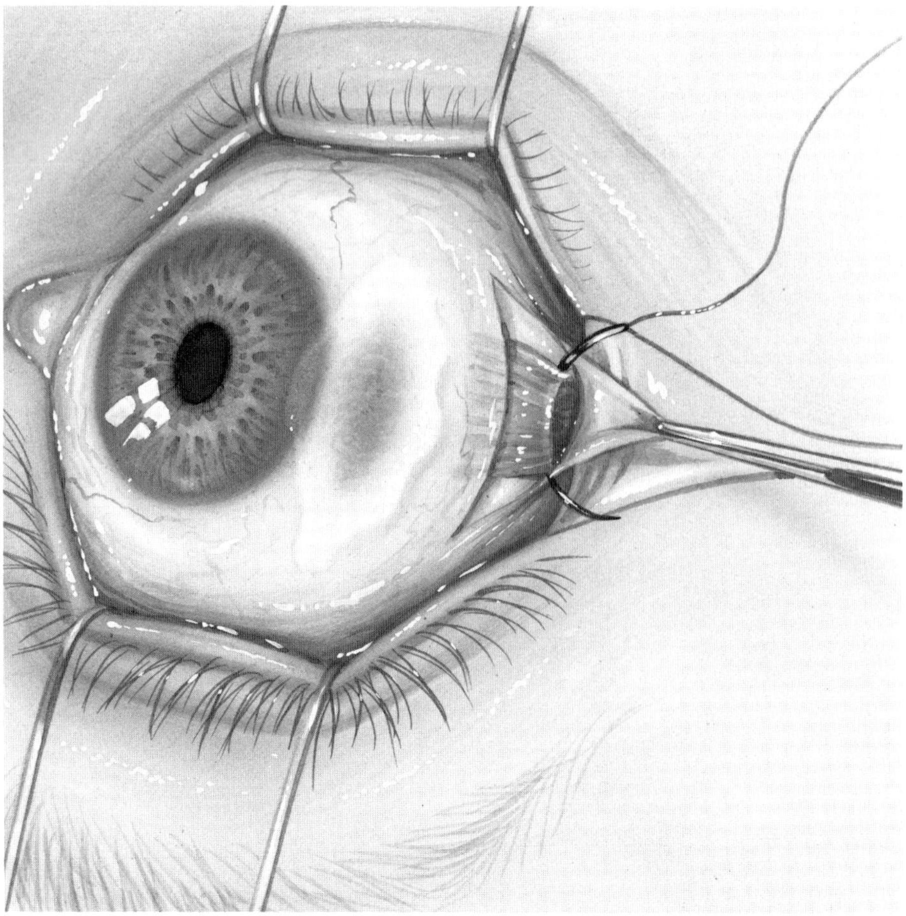

5.**96** Good exposure is achieved by the use of a traction suture.

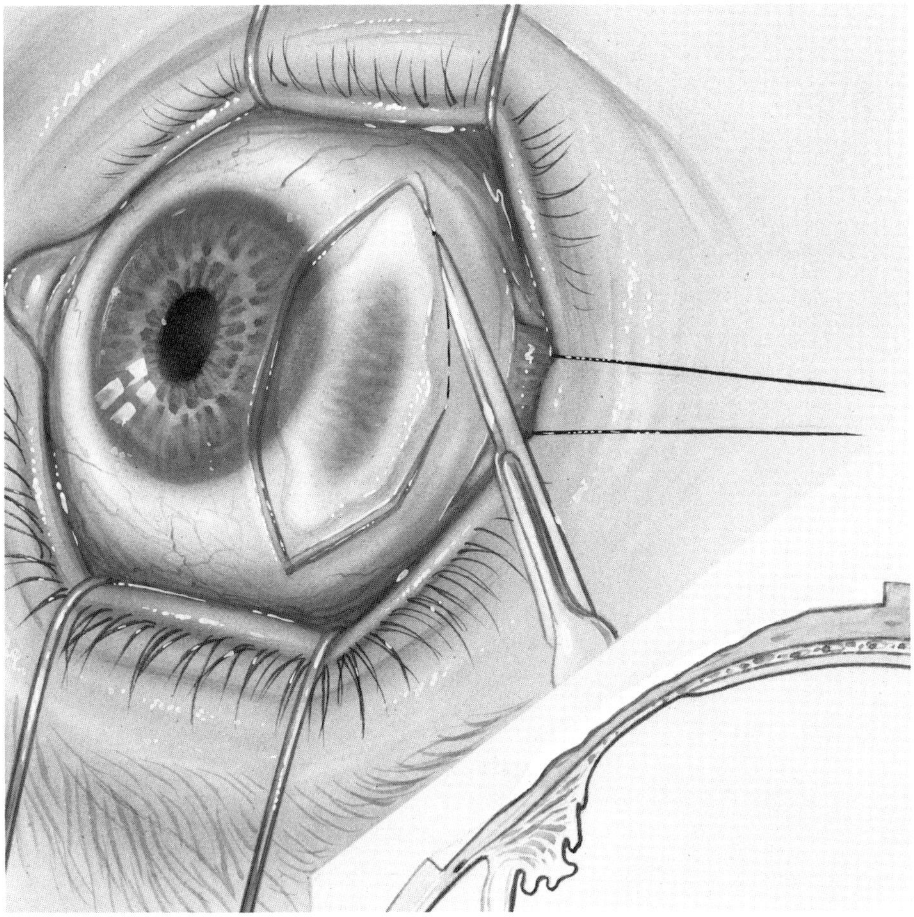

5.97 A broad area is undermined by means of sharp dissection half the thickness of the sclera.

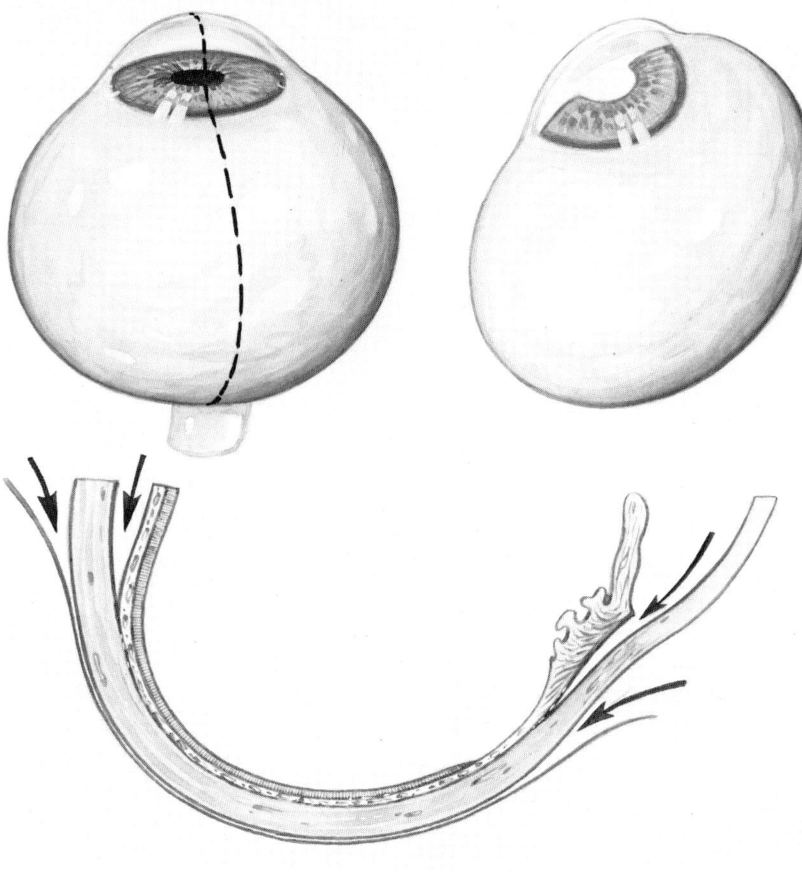

5.98 The donor tissue is prepared by bisecting a donor eye. Uvea and epithelium are removed prior to grafting.

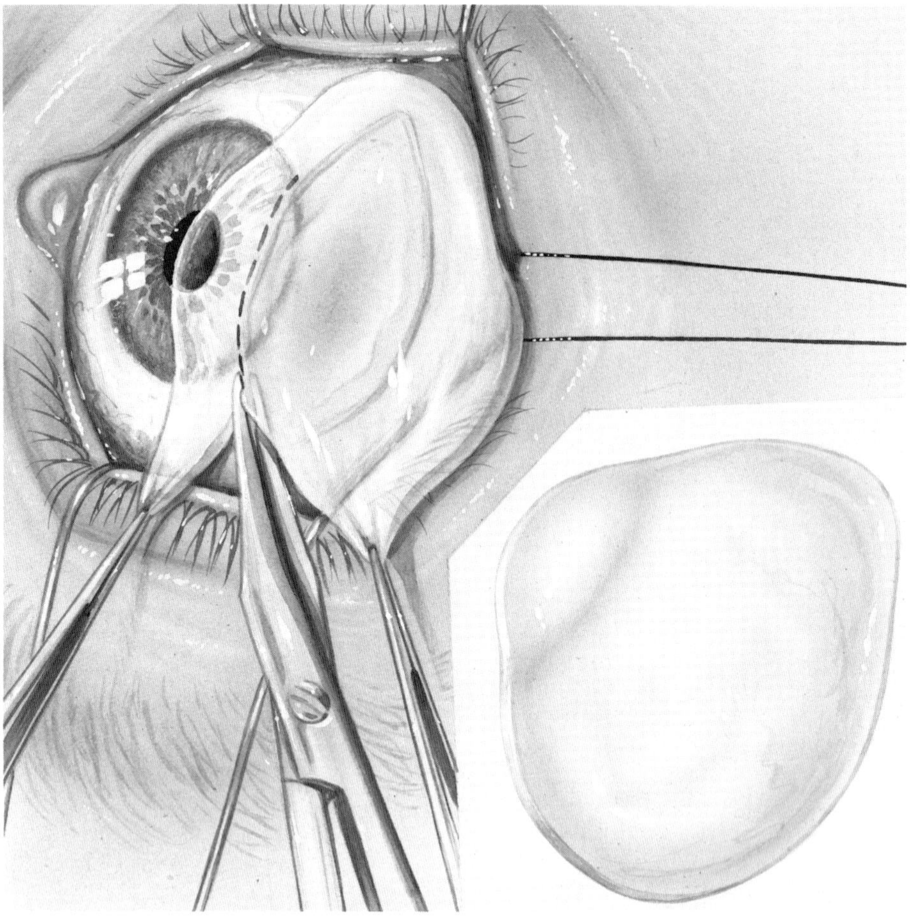

5.**99** The larger donor tissue is then placed over the recipient eye and shaped using a freehand technique. The corneal side is fashioned first and sutured into place. A very beveled edge is created using scissors as illustrated; interrupted sutures are used to secure the corneal side of the graft.

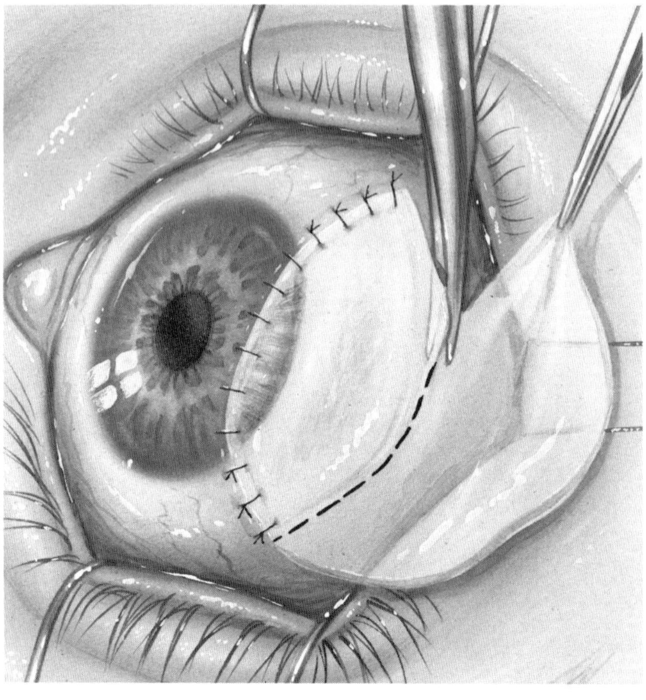

5.**100** The remainder of the graft is then fashioned similarly.

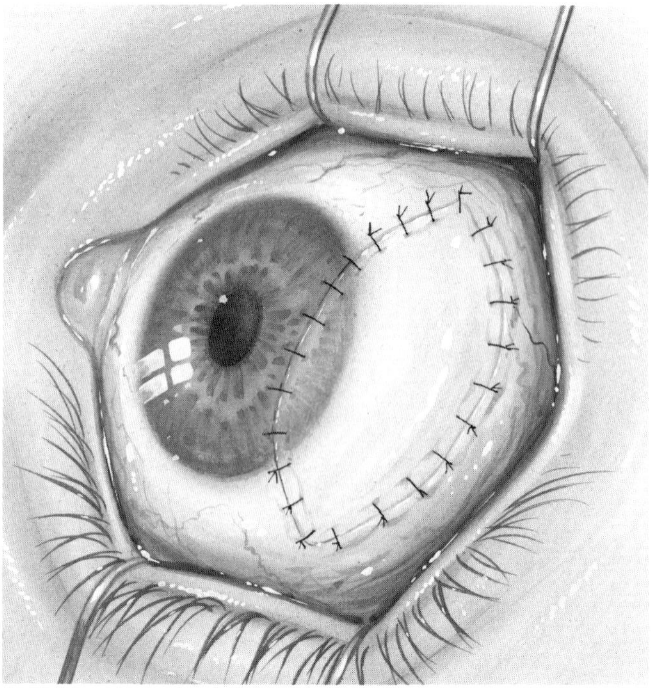

5.**101** The broad lamellar graft provides support for the weakened tissue.

Conjunctival Transplantation for Previous Trauma

After severe trauma, such as chemical burn, there is often poor epithelial healing. Often, after prolonged healing, a scar is formed, which may consist of a superficial pannus; or a conjunctival flap may be used to cover the surface of the cornea to prevent ulceration and infection. After healing in these circumstances it is often possible to restore vision by providing a healthy epithelium for the cornea from another site.

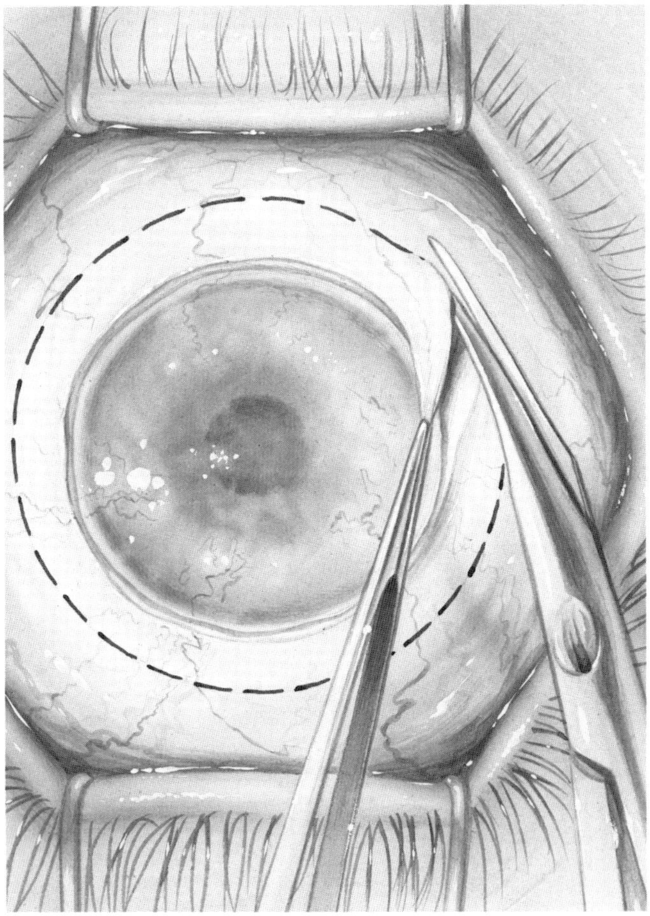

5.**102** The host bed is prepared by removing the conjunctival epithelium 2 mm from the limbus circumferentially.

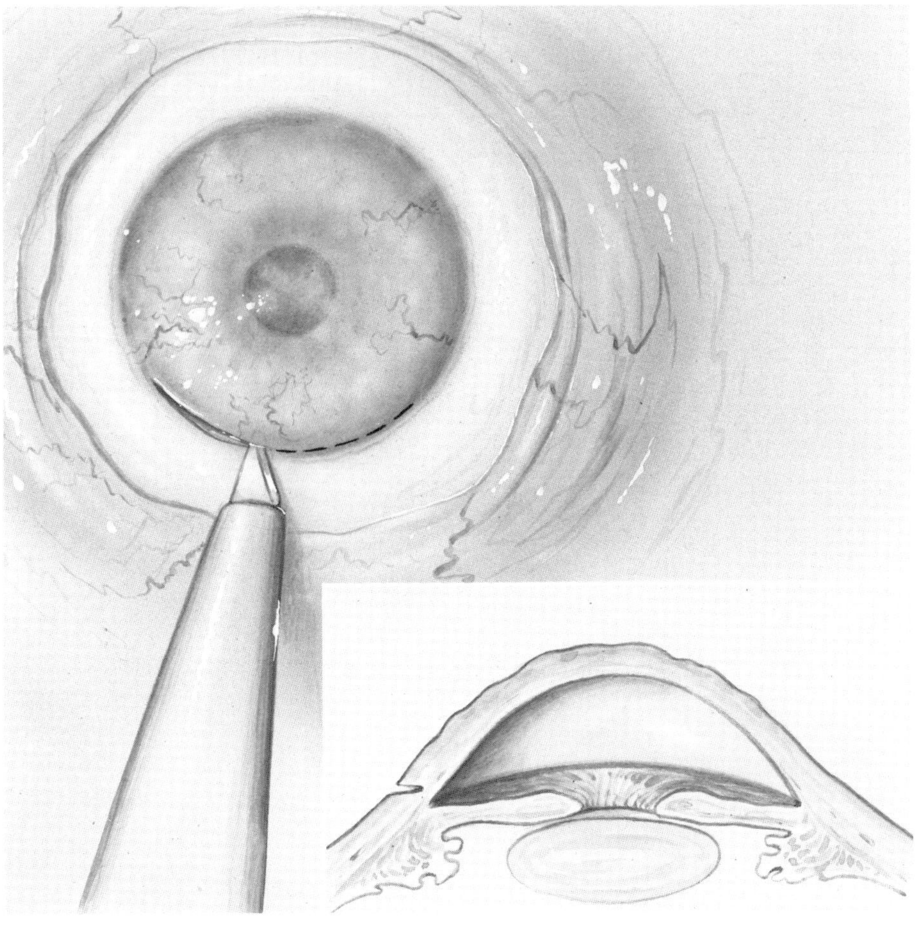

5.**103** An incision is carried into the corneal stroma at the limbus.

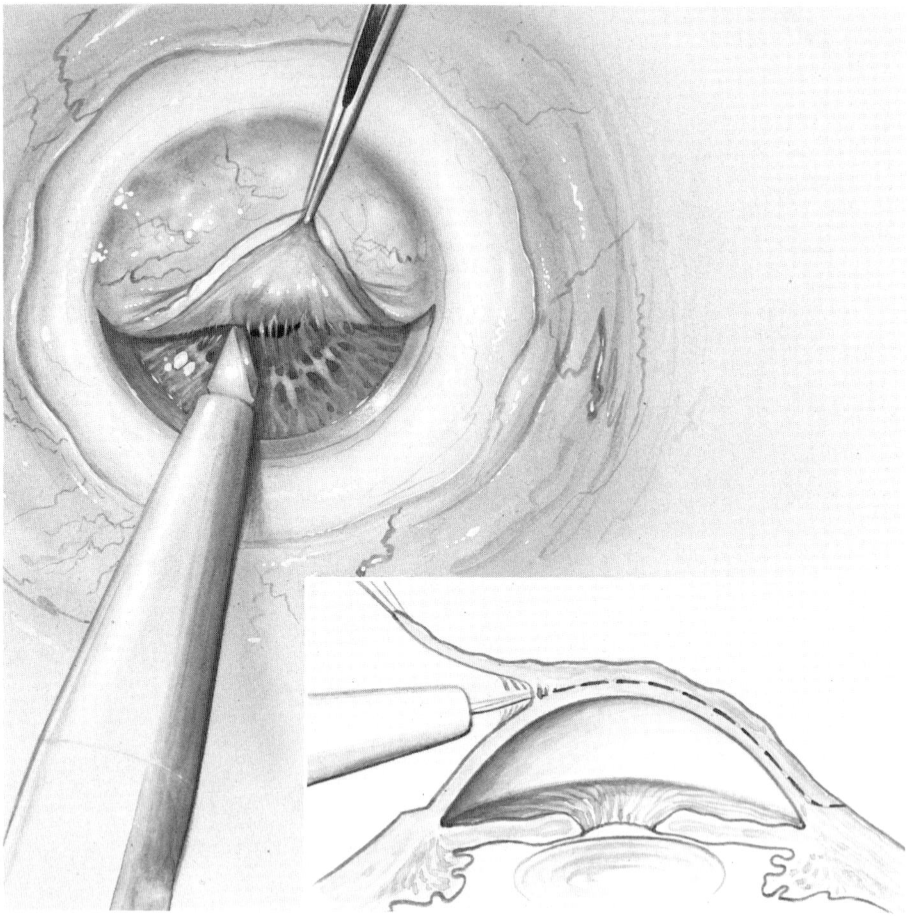

5.**104** The pannus is excised meticulously with a sharp blade.

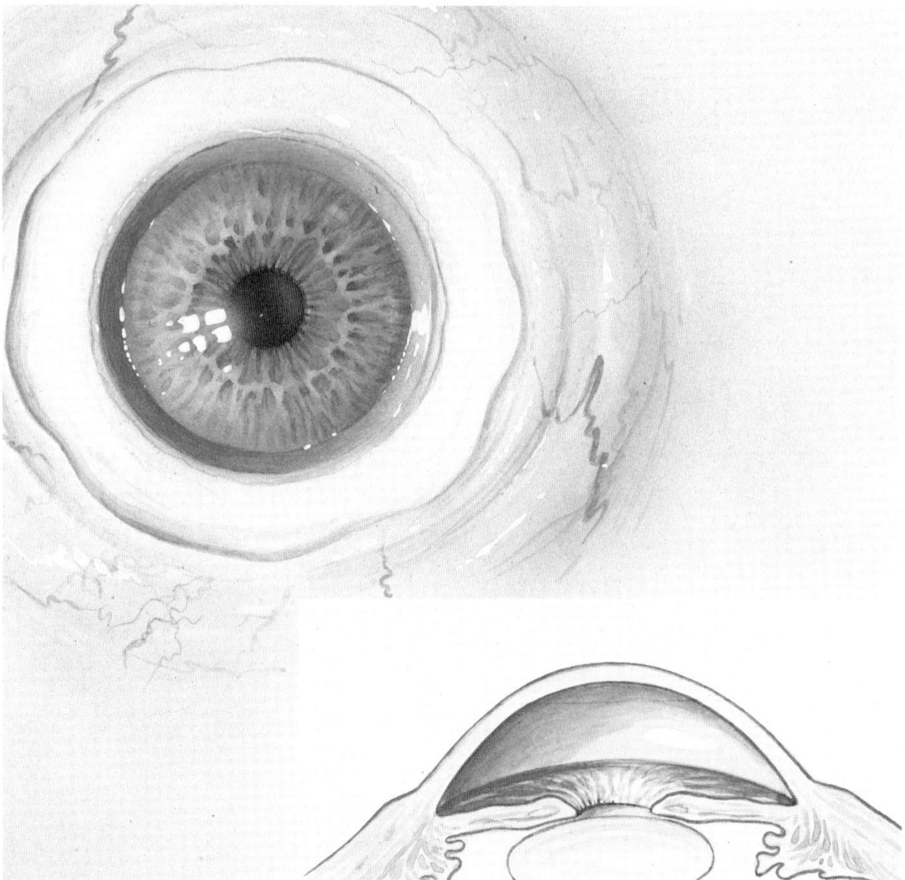

5.**105** The scar should be so removed that only clear cornea remains, expecially in the central area.

106

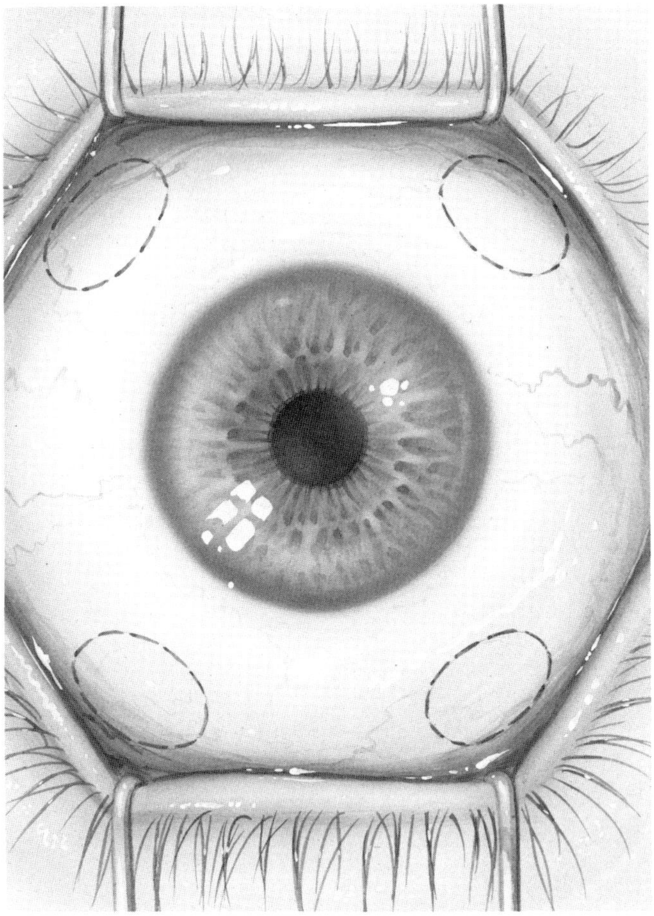

5.**106** The other, healthy eye is then approached. Four donor sites will be obtained from the healthy eye, and these areas can be outlined using cautery for future reference, as will be seen.

5.**107** The areas of conjunctiva are separated from Tenon's capsule by injection with either air or saline. The injection site should be away from the proposed donor tissue to avoid buttonholing.

5.**108** The conjunctiva is then excised.

107

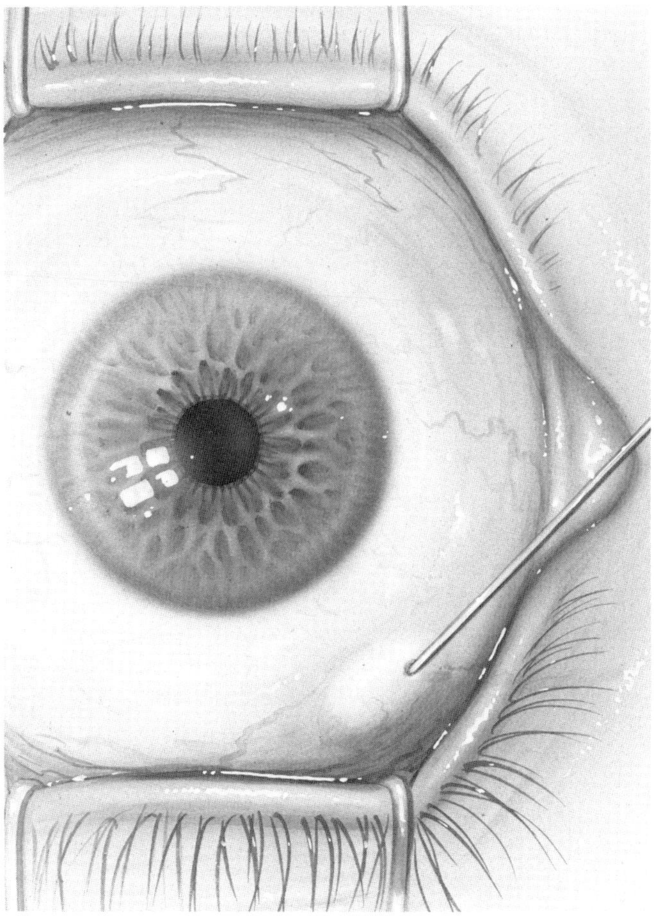

108

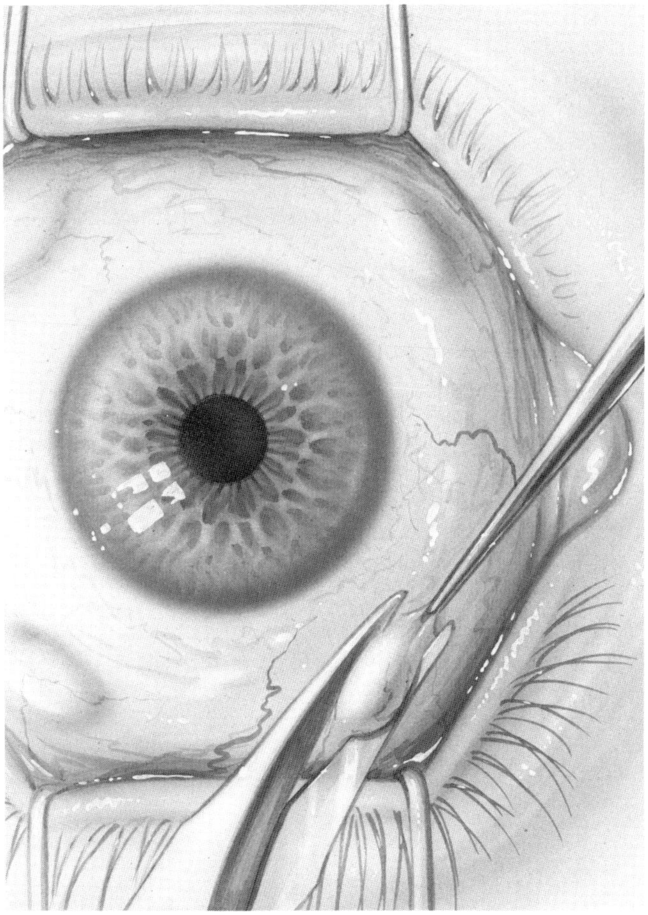

109

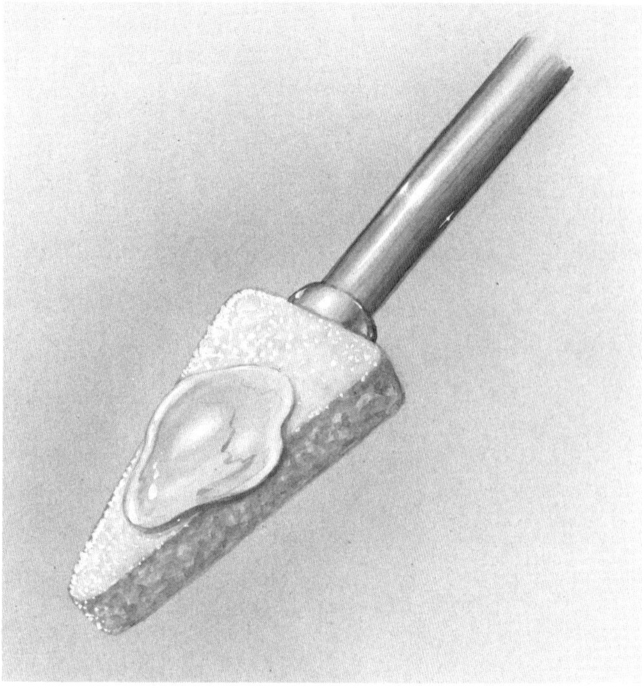

110

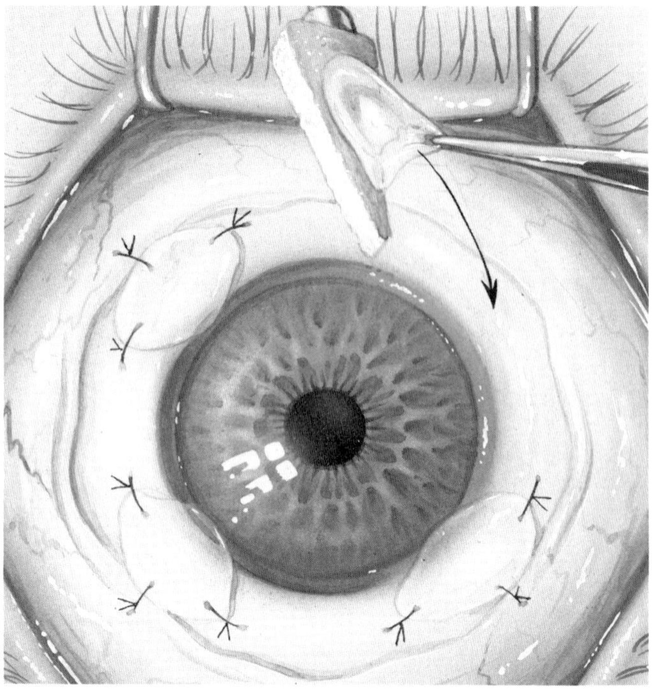

111

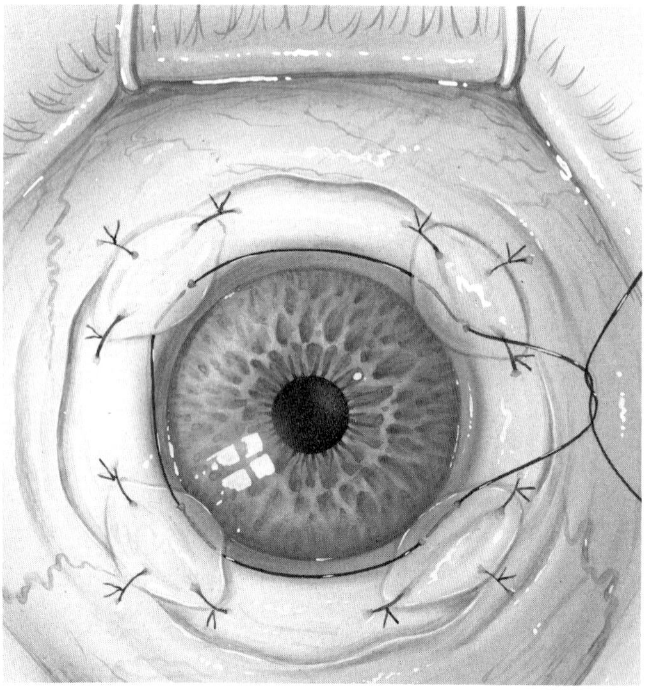

112

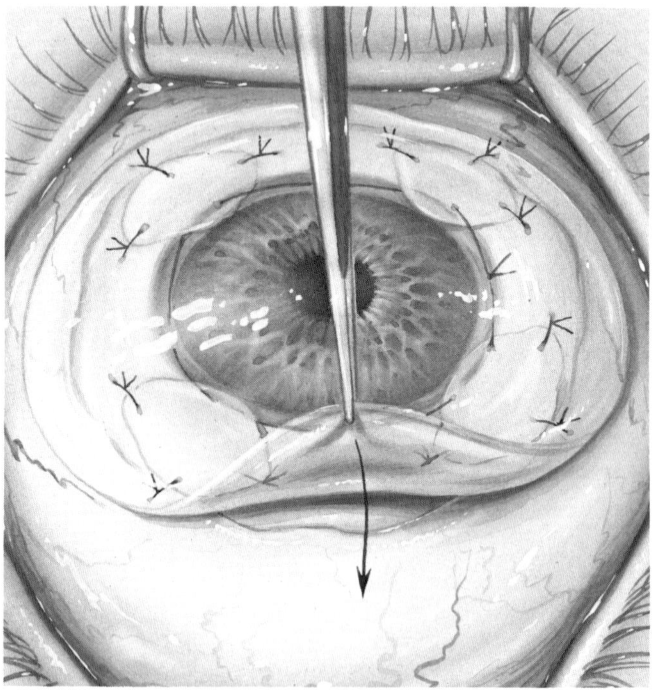

5.**109** If cautery is done on the anterior surface, this more readily identifies the anterior surface when transporting the donor tissue to the recipient bed.

5.**110** The donor conjunctiva is then sutured into the previously prepared site by means of interrupted 10-0 nylon sutures.

5.**111** The corneal edges of the grafts are sutured to the limbal episclera using a circumferential suture.

5.**112** A large-diameter, bandage extended-wear soft contact lens is placed over the cornea and donor conjunctiva. This lens can be left in place for several months while the host bed is re-epithelialized.

113

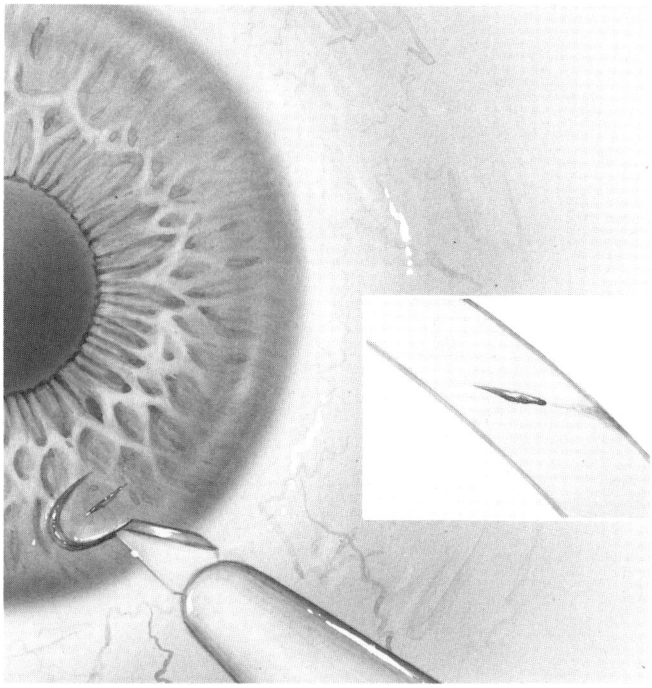

114

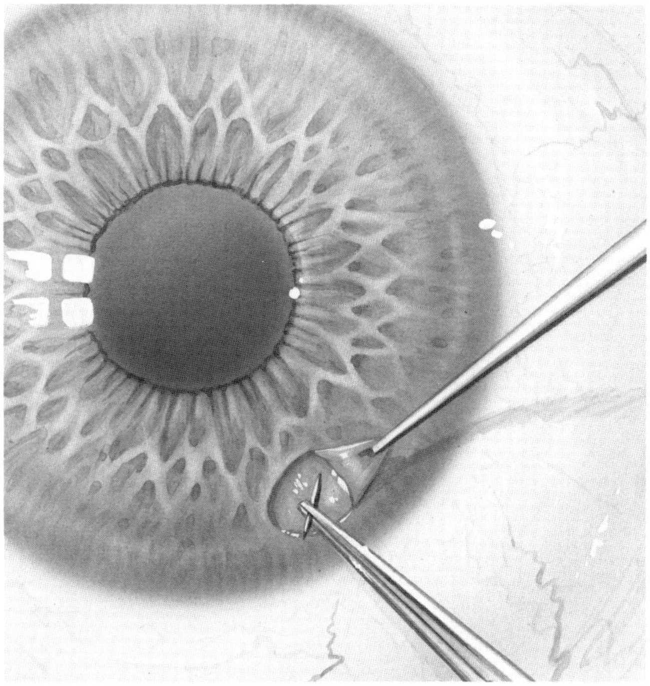

115

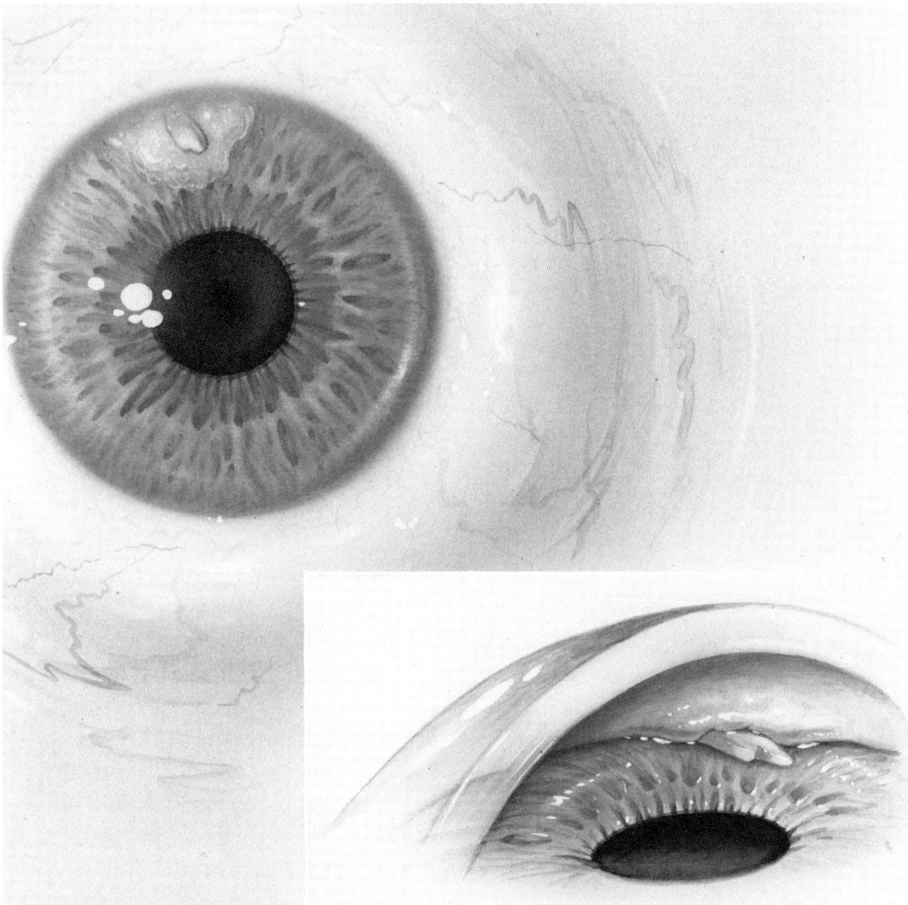

Intracorneal Foreign Body

5.**113** When a foreign body is embedded in the corneal stroma, it is often not possible to retrieve it via a direct approach. In this situation, a small corneal flap is made which will prevent excessive manipulation of the cornea and possible loss of the object into the anterior chamber. A semicircular flap of stroma is created using a sharp blade.

5.**114** When this flap is retracted, one can easily remove the foreign body without damaging the endothelium.

5.**115** When a foreign body is present in the inferior angle, a patient may present only with inferior corneal edema. In such a situation, gonioscopy may reveal the inciting agent.

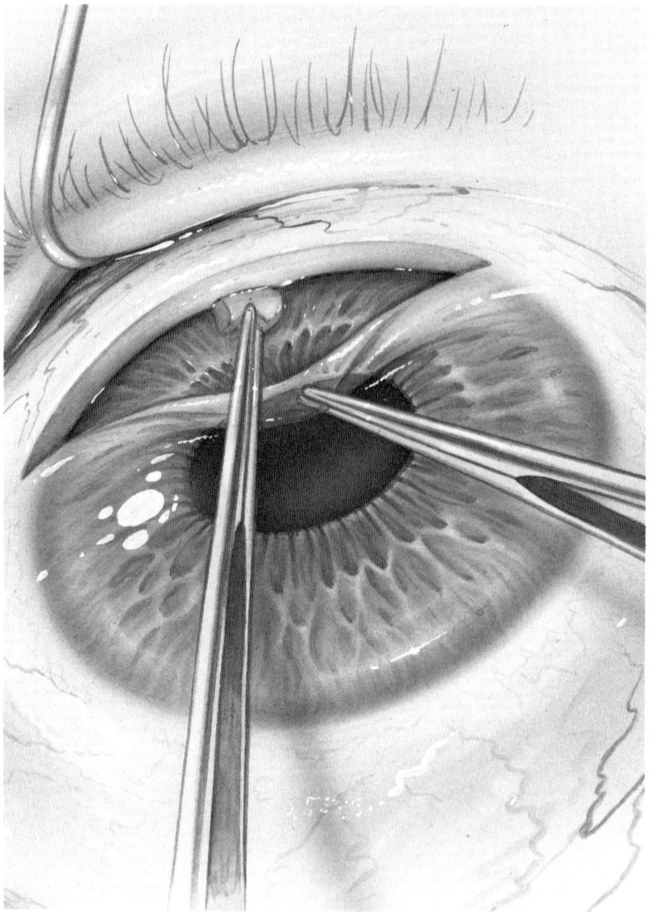

5.**116** A limbal wound should be made directly over the object for retrieval. The use of viscoelastic gel during this technique may prevent slippage of the object during the procedure and protect the corneal endothelium.

Detached Descemet's Membrane

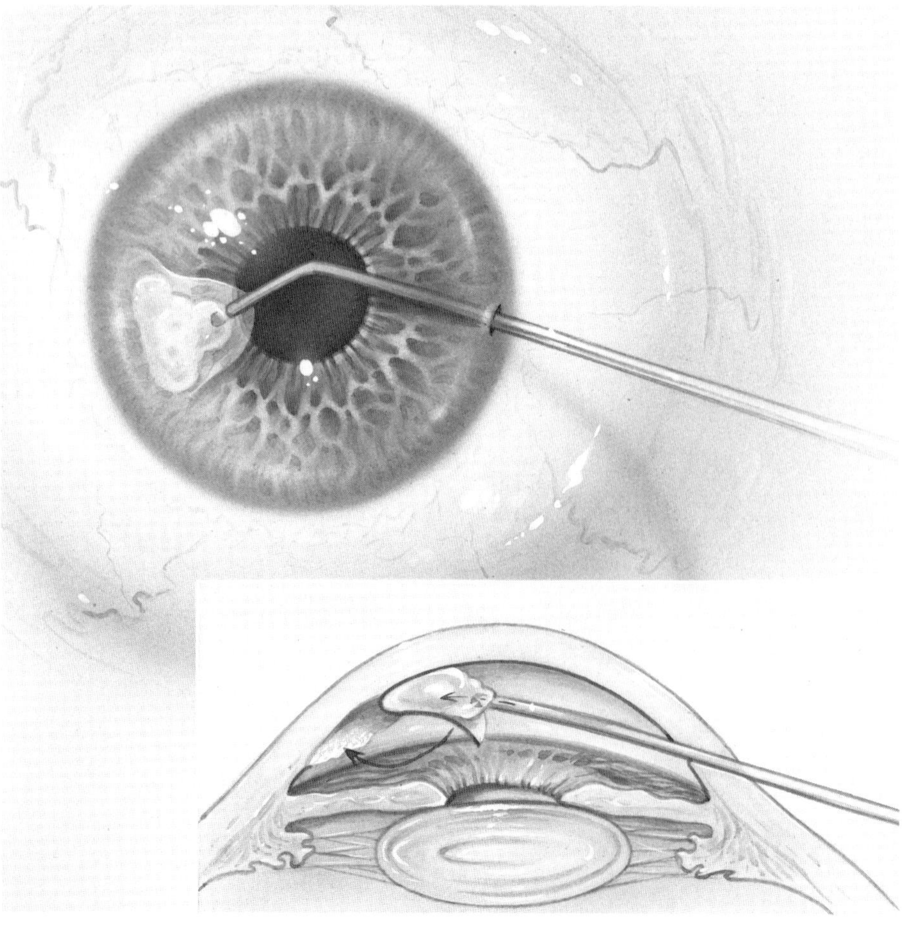

5.**117** Occasionally after trauma a large portion of Descemet's membrane will be detached, as a result of either the initial trauma or excessive surgical manipulation. Local corneal edema is present which, even though persisting for a long period of time, can be reversed. One can enter the anterior chamber from the opposite limbus and, using viscoelastic gel, reposition Descemet's membrane as illustrated. The patient should be positioned after the procedure to allow reattachment on the early postoperative phase. It is also possible to use air for repositioning. One must be careful not to place air behind the flap during this procedure.

Tarsorrhaphy after Trauma

Two types of tarsorrhaphy are illustrated.

118

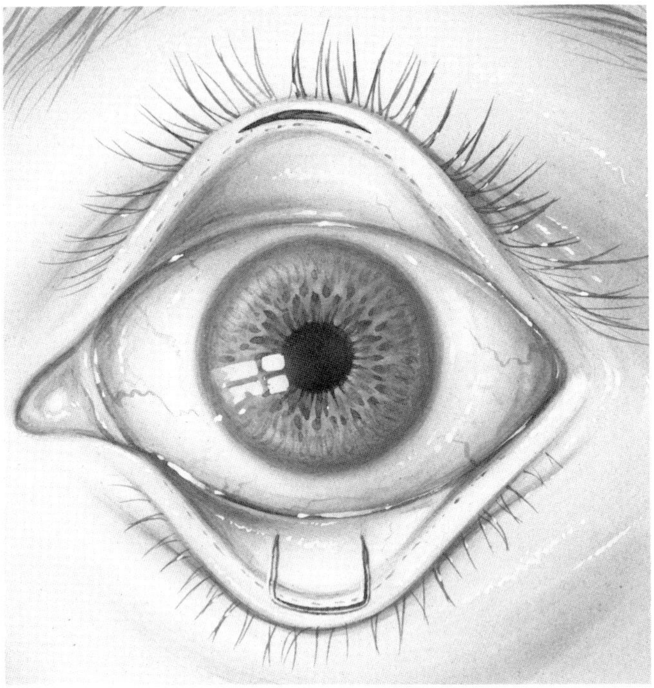

119

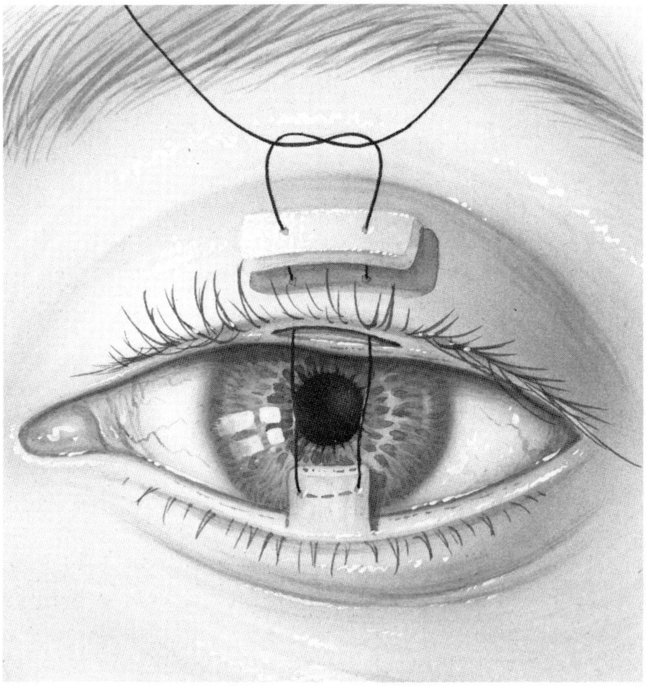

120

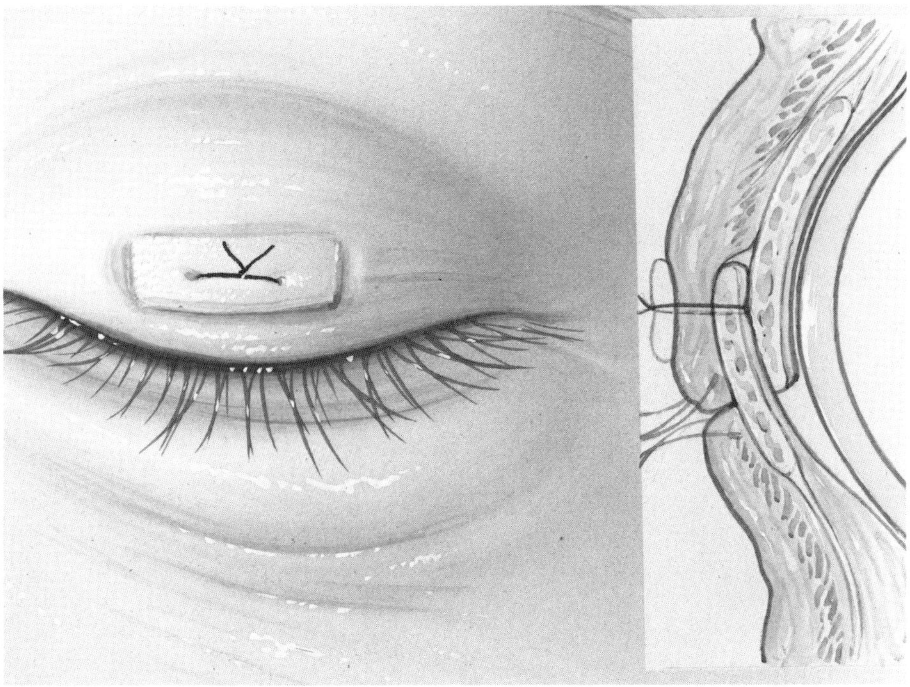

5.**118** In the first instance, a more permanent procedure is performed by creating a flap of tarsus and conjunctiva in the inferior lid. The superior lid is bisected so that a pocket is created for the inferior lid flap. The upper lid is divided into skin and orbicularis anteriorly and tarsus and conjunctiva posteriorly.

5.**119** The sutures are brought through the upper lid and sutured above a bolster to prevent damage to the upper lid skin.

5.**120** This method of tarsorrhaphy is very secure and is indicated when prolonged lid closure is necessary. The suture, either silk or nylon, is removed after two weeks.

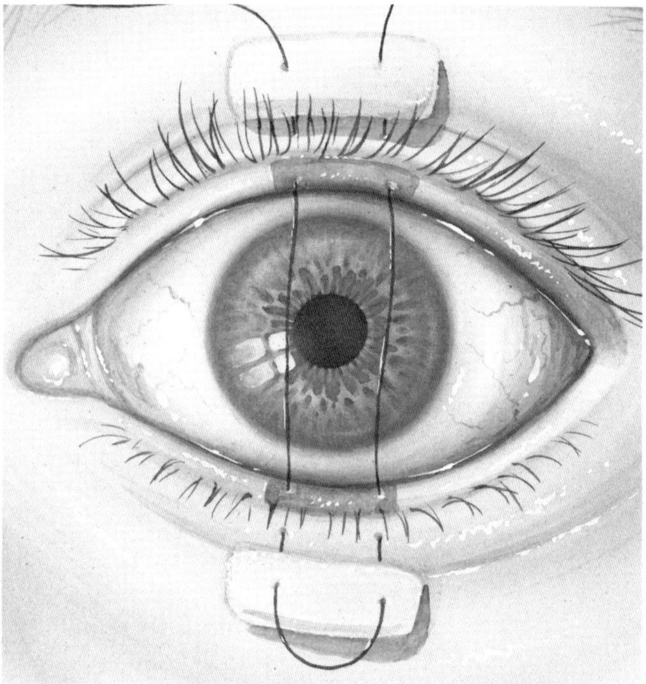

5.**121** A more temporary marginal tarsorrhaphy is performed by excising 1 mm of lid margin of both upper and lower lids. Care should be taken to avoid the lash follicles. The gray line can be split to provide greater surface area for healing purposes. The double-armed suture is brought through a bolster and then the lid skin 3 mm below the lash line, through the gray line, and then through the opposite lid in reverse order. The needles are brought through a bolster, and the suture is tied and left in place for 2 weeks.

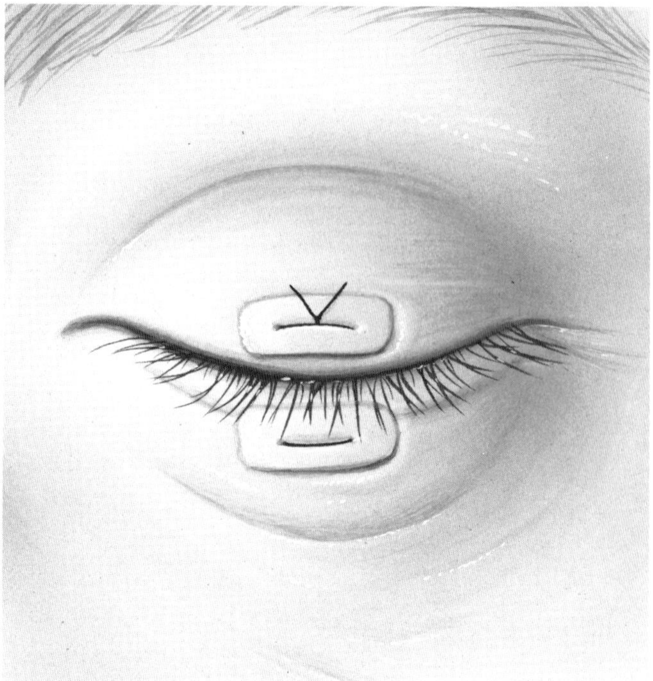

5.**122** This marginal tarsorrhaphy can be left intact for many months or can be easily reversed in the office.

Index

Total number of pages: XVI, 268